# Personal Health

## PERSPECTIVES AND LIFESTYLES

**Patricia A. Floyd**
*Alabama State University*

**Sandra E. Mimms**
*Alabama State University*

**Caroline Yelding**
*Alabama State University*

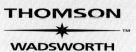

THOMSON
™
WADSWORTH

Australia • Brazil • Canada • Mexico • Singapore • Spain
United Kingdom • United States

## THOMSON

### WADSWORTH

Acquisitions Editor: *Peter Adams*

Development Editor: *Nedah Rose*

Assistant Editor: *Kate Franco*

Editorial Assistant: *Elizabeth Downs/Jean Blomo*

Technology Project Manager: *Ericka Yeoman-Saler*

Marketing Manager: *Jennifer Somerville*

Marketing Assistant: *Jessica Capizano*

Marketing Communications Manager: *Shemika Britt*

Content Project Manager: *Teresa L. Trego*

Creative Director: *Rob Hugel*

Art Director: *John Walker*

Print Buyer: *Doreen Suruki*

Permissions Editor: *Roberta Broyer*

Production Service: *Pre-PressPMG*

Text Designer: *Ellen Pettengill*

Photo Researcher: *Terri Miller*

Copy Editor: *Pre-PressPMG*

Illustrator: *Pre-PressPMG*

Cover Designer: *Ellen Pettengill*

Cover Image: © *Getty images, The Image Bank Collection, Photographer: Superstudio.*

Cover Printer: *Courier*

Compositor: *Pre-PressPMG*

Printer: *Courier*

Printed in the United States of America

1  2  3  4  5  6  7  11  10  09  08  07

For more information about our products, contact us at:
Thomson Learning Academic Resource Center
1-800-423-0563
For permission to use material from this text or product, submit a request online at
http://www.thomsonrights.com.
Any additional questions about permissions can be submitted by e-mail to thomsonrights@thomson.com.

ExamView® and ExamView Pro® are registered trademarks of FSCreations, Inc. Windows is a registered trademark of the Microsoft Corporation used herein under license. Macintosh and Power Macintosh are registered trademarks of Apple Computer, Inc. Used herein under license.

Library of Congress Control Number: 2007926466

Student Edition:
ISBN-13: 978-0-495-11157-3
ISBN-10: 0-495-11157-0

**Thomson Higher Education**
10 Davis Drive
Belmont, CA 94002-3098
USA

**Asia**
Thomson Learning
5 Shenton Way
#01–01 UIC Building
Singapore 068808

**Australia/New Zealand**
Thomson Learning Australia
102 Dodds Street
Southbank, Victoria 3006
Australia

**Canada**
Thomson Nelson
1120 Birchmount Road
Toronto, Ontario M1K 5G4
Canada

**UK/Europe/Middle East/Africa**
Thomson Learning
High Holborn House
50/51 Bedford Row
London WC1R 4LR
United Kingdom

**Latin America**
Thomson Learning
Seneca, 53
Colonia Polanco
11560 Mexico D.F.
Mexico

**Spain/Portugal**
Thomson Paraninfo
Calle Magallanes, 25
28015 Madrid, Spain

# Brief Contents

# Contents

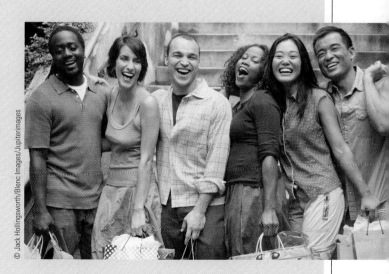

© Jack Hollingsworth/Blenc Images/Jupiterimages

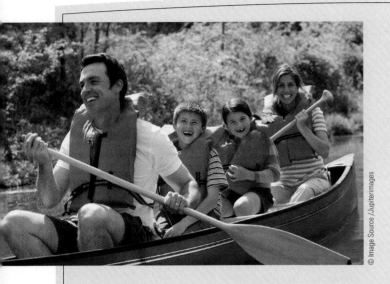

© Image Source /Jupiterimages

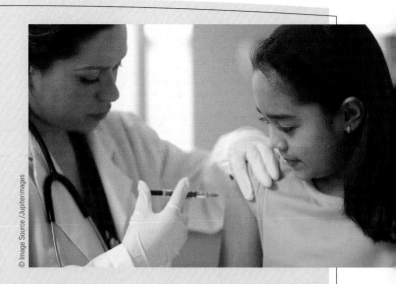

© Image Source /Jupiterimages

# 6  Communicable Diseases 147

## 7 Noncommunicable Diseases  197

## 8 Cardiovascular Disease  243

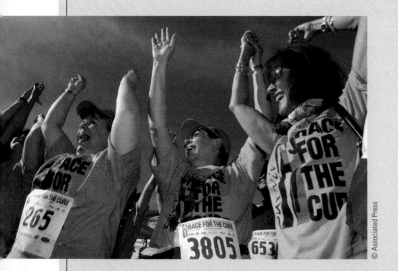

© Associated Press

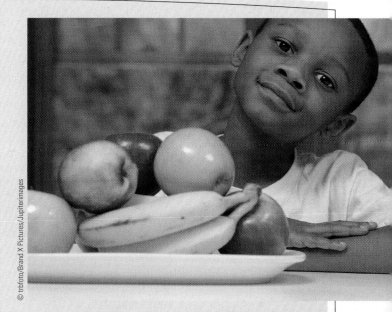

© trbfoto/Brand X Pictures/Jupiterimages

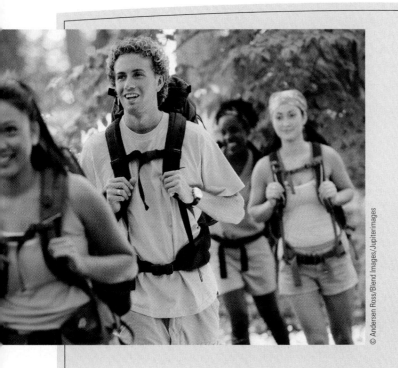

© Andersen Ross/Blend Images/Jupiterimages

## 11 Physical Activity and Health 355

## 12 Psychoactive Drugs and Medications   399

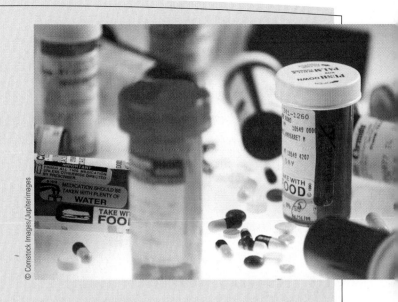

© Comstock Images/Jupiterimages

## 13 Alcohol and Tobacco   433

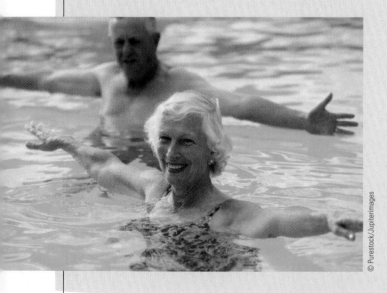

© Purestock/Jupiterimages

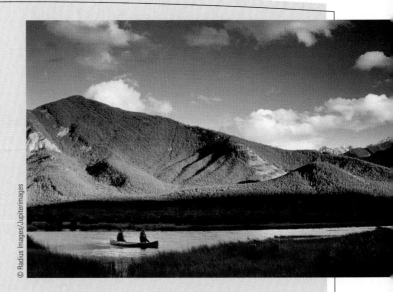

# Preface

Health in today's world is much different than it was a century ago. The infectious diseases that killed people in large epidemics and from which few families escaped have been all but eradicated. In their place are noncommunicable diseases, led by cardiovascular conditions and cancer. The bad news is that these diseases take great numbers of people each year and reduce the quality of life for many others. The good news is that these diseases are largely preventable. Therefore, the contemporary focus is on prevention. The role of the fourth edition of *Personal Health: Perspectives and Lifestyles* is to set forth the most current information readers can use to take control of their lives. "Tips for Action," "Self Assessments," and "FYI" features appear in each chapter to provide students with practical advice, empowering readers to assess themselves and make good decisions. A distinctive feature of this text in past editions was the emphasis on health as it relates to various cultural differences. The fourth edition continues to promote diversity as it relates to health and wellness. This text covers macro issues such as worldwide tobacco use and micro issues such as the shaving differences between African-Americans and Caucasians. In researching the text, we have come to appreciate the concept of diversity more fully; therefore we have added "Focus on Diversity" features in each chapter. These boxes provide information on topics including stress as it relates to age, gender differences in communication, heart attack trends around the world, and HIV/AIDS in the African-American community. Regardless of culture, gender, race or age, each person must take control of his or her own life in order to live a long and healthy life.

Features in each chapter include:

**Objectives**—At the beginning of each chapter, these provide a guide to the content within each chapter.

**Key Terms**—In boldface type and defined in boxes close to their use in the text, these terms also are combined in a complete glossary at the end of the book.

**Focus on Diversity**—This feature provides relevant research about diversity and health issues. Topics include stress as it relates to age, gender differences in communication, heart attack-prone areas of the world, HIV/AIDS in the African-American community, and many more.

**Tips for Action**—Integrated throughout every chapter of the text, this feature gives readers practical advice and encourages students to take action and apply what they have learned.

**Figures, tables, and photos**—These are located throughout the text to enhance the content and make it clearer.

**ViewPoint**—This critical thinking feature contains hot topics in health to stimulate discussion. Topics include pro- and anti-gun proponents, circumcision, needle exchange, embryonic stem cell research, and many more.

**FYI**—This boxed feature presents facts and statistics about health to pique the readers' interest.

**Personal Health Resources**—Included at the end of every chapter are relevant Web URLs and brief descriptions of the resources located at that site.

**Self-Assessments**—At the end of each chapter, these give students the opportunity to assess themselves and apply the knowledge gained from reading the chapter, to their own life.

**Chapter Summary**—Located at the end of each chapter, it consists of a bullet point synopsis of the chapter's main ideas.

**It's Your Turn—Study and Review Questions**—This feature contains questions relevant to chapter objectives.

All these features are designed to be reader-friendly. The focus is on practicality and relevance to today's reader. In our contemporary perspective we reflect the changing student population, which now includes more nontraditional students. They may be simultaneously in the workplace, or at home rearing families, or retired and looking to expand their mental horizons.

This text is flexible enough to accommodate courses that carry from one to three hours of credit. It highlights the major health issues—emotional health and personal relations; stress management; sexuality and contraception; communicable and noncommunicable diseases; physical activity; nutrition and weight management; use and abuse of psychoactive drugs, including tobacco and alcohol; aging, dying and death; and consumer and environmental issues—that impact everyone. Because health science is rapidly changing and keeping up with the latest information is imperative, this fourth edition incorporates the most recent research you will find in a college health textbook. Notice the selected bibliography at the end of each chapter, which includes 1999–2001 citations from federal agencies, not-for-profit organizations, current serial publications, professional journals, and other sources.

## ANCILLARY PACKAGE

**HealthNow ™ (NEW!).** Class-tested and student praised, HealthNow offers a variety of features that support course objectives and interactive learning. This online tutorial for students, available with new texts, offers a Personalized Change Plan, pre- and post- tests, a wellness journal and a variety of activities, all designed to get students involved in their learning progress and to be better prepared for class participation and class quizzes and tests. Students log on to HealthNow by using the access code available with the text.

**Instructor's CD-ROM.** This CD-ROM includes Instructor Manual and Test Bank resources, PowerPoint® presentation, and ABC videos for Health and Wellness.

- **Instructor's Manual with Test Bank.** This contains objectives, key terms, chapter outlines, instructor activities, Web-based student activities and Web resources. The Test Bank consists of over 600 multiple-choice, true-false, and essay questions.

- **PowerPoint® Presentation.** This tool contains lecture slides to correspond with every chapter of the text; also included are figures and art from the text. New to this supplement are the Chapter Objectives featured at the beginning of each chapter.

- **ABC Videos for Health and Wellness (NEW!).** These videos allow you to integrate the newsgathering and programming power of the ABC News networks into the classroom, showing students the relevance of course topics to their everyday lives. The video clips included correlate with the text and can help you launch a lecure, spark a discussion, or demonstrate an application, Students can see first-hand how the principles they learn in the course apply to the stories they hear in the news.

**ExamView®—Computerized Testing.** Create, deliver, and customize tests and study guides (both print and online) in minutes with this easy-to-use assessment and tutorial system. ExamView offers both a Quick Test Wizard and an Online Test Wizard that guide you step-by-step through the process of creating tests, while its unique "WYSIWYG" capability allows you to see the test you are creating on the screen exactly as it will print or display online.

**Walk4life Elite Model Pedometer (NEW!)** This pedometer tracks steps, elapsed time, distance, and includes a calorie counter. The pedometer includes an extra large digital display with a hinged protective cover, and comes with instructions on how to use the tool most effectively. Whether to be used as an activity in class or as a tool to encourage students to simply track their steps and walk toward better fitness awareness, this is a valuable resource for everyone *and* at $10.50 when bundled with the text, this pedometer a deal!

**Diet Analysis Plus 8.0 CD-ROM (NEW!).** The market – leading diet assessment program used by colleges and universities allows students to create personal profiles based on height, weight, age, sex, and activity level. Its new dynamic interface makes it easy for students to track the types and serving sizes of foods they consume, from one day to 365 days! Now including even more exciting features, the updated 8.0 version includes a 10,000 food database, nine reports for analysis, a new food recipe feature, the latest Dietary References, and goals and actually percentages of essential nutrients, vitamins, and minerals. Students can use this information to adjust their diet and gain a better understanding of how nutrition relates to their personal health goals. Thoroughly revised and updated, the software is available online or on a new Windows/Mac® CD-ROM.

**Careers in Health, Physical Education, and Sport.** Co-authored by *Personal Health: Perspectives and Lifestyles* author Patricia Floyd, this book is the essential manual for majors who are interested in pursuing a position in their chosen health-related field. It guides them through the complicated process of picking the right type of career, includes suggestions on how to prepare to the transition to the working world, and offers information about career paths, education requirements, and reasonable salary expectation. This supplement also describes differences in credentials in the field, and testing requirements for certain professions.

**http://www.thomsonedu.com/health.** When you adopt *Personal Health: Perspectives and Lifestyles*, you and your students will have access to teaching and learning resources you will not find anywhere else. This site features student and instructor resources for this text, including self-quizzes, Web links, suggested online readings, and discussion forums—as well as downloadable supplementary resources, PowerPoint® presentations, and more for instructors. You will also find an online catalog of Wadsworth's health, fitness, wellness, and physical education books and supplements.

**InfoTrac® College Edition.** This extensive online library gives professors and students access to the latest news and research articles online—updated daily and spanning four years. Conveniently accessible from students' own computers or the campus library, InfoTrac College Edition opens the door to the full text of articles from hundreds of scholarly and popular journals and publications.

**Infotrac College Edition Student Guide for Health/Wellness.** This handy booklet assists students using Infotrac College Edition for research. It includes 24 pages of detailed guidance for students on how to use the InfoTrac College Edition database. Includes log-in help, a complete search tips "cheat sheet," and a topic list of key word search terms for health, fitness and wellness. This supplement also features activities for each chapter that challenge the student to critically read articles and studies relating to key topics in the chapters. These activities help guide students through the vast database and answer questions relating to specific articles.

**Health and Fitness Wellness Internet Explorer.** This handy trifold contains relevant Web sites related to health and fitness and wellness. Topics include stress, nutrition, alternative medicine, and much more.

**Trigger View Series (Fitness or Stress).** Exclusive to Wadsworth/Thomson Learning, this video is designed to promote classroom discussion on a variety of important topics related to physical fitness or stress. Each 60-minute video contains five clips of eight to 10 minutes, followed by questions for answer or discussion and material appropriate to the chapter in this text.

**Relaxation: A Guide to Personal Stress Management.** This 30-minute video shows students how to manage their stress and recognize what a healthy stress is in their lives. Experts explain relaxation techniques and guide the student through progressive relaxation, guided imagery, breathing, and physical activity.

**Wadsworth Video Library for Fitness, Wellness, and Personal Health.** A comprehensive library of videos is available to adopters of this textbook. Topics include weight control and fitness, AIDS, sexual communication, peer pressure, compulsive and addictive behaviors, and the relationship between alcohol and violence. Contact your local Wadsworth/Thomson Learning representative for a detailed list of video options.

**Personal Daily Log.** This contains an exercise pyramid, food pyramid, study and exercise tips, time-management strategies, and goal setting worksheets, as well as **Get Connected,** a list of interactive health and wellness-related Web sites. The **Personal Daily Log** also includes record forms so students can gauge their successes in cardiorespiratory exercise, strength training, and daily nutrition.

**Testwell.** This online assessment tool allows you to complete a 100-question wellness inventory related to

the dimensions of wellness. Complete the personal assessments in order to evaluate your personal health status related to nutrition, emotional health, spirituality, sexuality, physical health, self-care, safety, environmental health, occupational health, and intellectual health.

**Health and Wellness Resource Center at http:// www.gale.com/health.** Gale's Health and Wellness Resource Center is a new comprehensive website that provides easy-to-find answers to health questions.

**Behavior Change Workbook.** This engaging supplement includes a brief discussion of the current theories behind making positive lifestyle changes, along with exercises to help students effect those changes in their everyday lives.

## Acknowledgments

We are grateful to those who participated in the preparation of this new edition. We especially want to express our appreciation to our colleagues across the country who took time to review each edition. Their comments have greatly enhanced this fourth edition. **Fourth Edition Reviewers:** Denise Colaianni, Western Connecticut State University; William Kelley, Green Mountain College; Amy Rowland, John Jay College of Criminal Justice; Tammy J. Wyatt, University of Texas at San Antonio. **Third Edition Reviewers:** Angela Burroughs, North Carolina Central University; Dianne Davis, Bowie State University; Bernard Griego, University of California at Berkley; and Marilyn Wells, Hampton University. **Second Edition Reviewers:** Sharon Dittman, Cornell University; Brent Hafen, Brigham Young University; Werner Hoeger, Boise State University; and Virginia Utermohlen, Cornell University. **First Edition Reviewers:** Troy Adams, Oklahoma State University; Judy Baker, East Carolina University; G. Robert Bowers, Tallahassee Community College; Jerry Braza, Western Oregon State College; Susan Burge, Cuyahoga Community College; Carol Johnson, University of Richmond; Vince Minor, Utah Valley Community College; Susan Mitchell, University of Central Florida; Kathy M. Wood, Butler County Community College; and Karen M. Camarata, Eastern Kentucky University.

We also wish to thank Ravi and Jai Howard; Courtney Zinke; Sie Gearl Cho; Ronnie Floyd; Evelyn Nettles; Linda Hockett McClellan, Service Learning Coordinator, HBCU Wellness Program Meharry Medical College; Patricia Wingfield McCarroll, Biology department, Fisk University; Loretta Fairley; Cora Coley; Mary Smith and Heidi Hataway, Alabama Department of Public Health; and John A Jernigan, M.D.

Further, we wish to thank the members of the Department of Health, Physical Education, and Recreation, especially Barbara Williams, Charlie Gibbons, Ritchie Beene, Cyrenthia Crawford, instructors of Personal Health and Wellness at Alabama State University, for their comments and assistance and Doris P. Screws and Kathy J. Neely. We are grateful to the following for their technical assistance:

Kristen Webster, Lynn Smith, Monique Chatfield, Jacqueline Hill, Amanda Thompson, Taylor Thompson and Harrietta Colvin.

We especially want to thank Stephanie Kling and Kate Franco for continuing to promote a health textbook with strong emphasis on diversity as it relates to national health issues. We appreciate the staff, technical and editorial, for completion of such a mammoth task.

Thank you all.

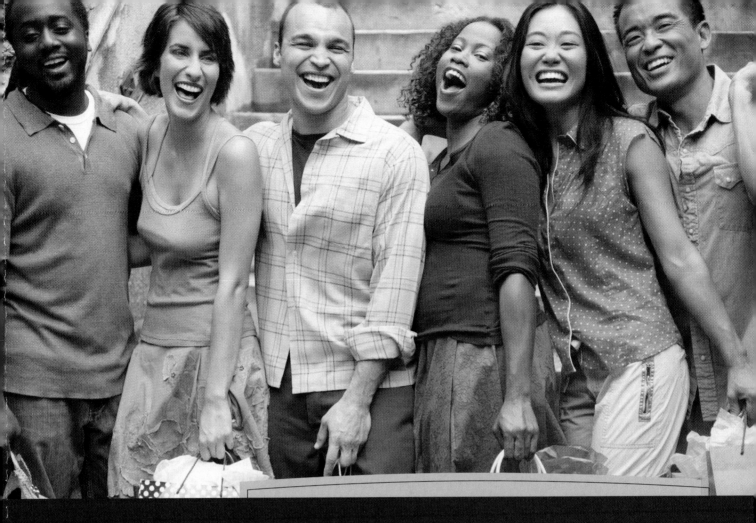

©Jack Hollingsworth/Blend Images/Jupiterimages

# Chapter One Introduction to Personal Health

**OBJECTIVES** ■ Write two definitions or descriptions of health. ■ Define wellness and list its components. ■ Differentiate the three phases of prevention. ■ Name the 10 leading causes of death for adults in the United States. ■ Identify two reasons why knowing your family's health history is important to your health. ■ List the top 10 underlying causes of death identified in the *Journal of the American Medical Association*. ■ Indicate one National Health Observance (include the month and days, if applicable) that you are willing to promote to family members or to friends.

ThomsonNOW  Log on to ThomsonNOW at http://thomsonedu.com/thomsonnow to access and explore self-assessments, interactive tutorials, and practice quizzes.

Health is a personal quality. It is unique to each person. At the same time, health is a universal quality. It applies to everyone. In *Webster's Dictionary*, health is defined as "the condition of being sound in body, mind, and spirit . . . freedom from physical disease or pain." The World Health Organization (WHO) defines health as "a state of complete physical, mental, and social well-being, not merely the absence of disease or infirmity."

Definitions of health have evolved over the years. The earliest definitions were synonymous with hygiene and sanitation, in keeping with the prevailing concerns at the time—the devastating toll taken by highly infectious diseases carried throughout community water supplies and in sewage.

Now that many of the deadliest infectious diseases are under control, the meaning of health has changed. **Health** no longer means simply the absence of illness. Contemporary Americans are more likely to define health as "the energy to do the things I care about."

**Wellness** is a relatively new term reflecting the positive emphasis on health. A definition of wellness that has been widely used is "the adoption of healthy lifestyle habits that will enhance well-being while decreasing the risk of disease." Wellness encompasses more than physical health. It is a state of being with several interrelated dimensions.

## Components of Wellness

Wellness has physical, mental/intellectual, emotional, social, environmental, and spiritual components, as depicted in Figure 1.1. Balancing these components is necessary to achieve a high level of wellness.

1. **Physical.** Physical health is the component most often associated with health. It includes disease prevention and management of health conditions (topic of Chapters 5, 6, 7, and 8). Also, it encompasses cardiovascular endurance, muscular flexibility, muscular strength and endurance, and body composition (topic of Chapters 10 and 11).

2. **Mental/intellectual.** More than 5,000 years ago philosophers including Homer, Plato, and Aristotle speculated that the mind exerts a powerful influence over the body. Among the attributes of mental wellness are alertness, creativity, logic, curiosity, open-mindedness, and keen memory.

3. **Emotional.** Emotions, the topic of Chapter 2, bridge the gap between the mind and the body. Emotions are interrelated with complex physical changes that affect the immune system. Negative emotions such as chronic stress (topic of Chapter 3) can lead to serious illness and death. Emotional wellness means the

**FIGURE 1.1 ▶** The Components of Wellness

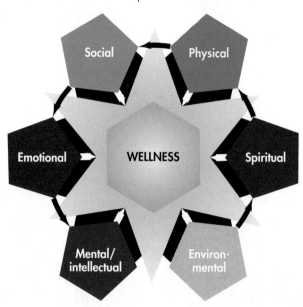

ability to adjust to change, face challenges and problems, and enjoy life.

4. **Social.** Social wellness is characterized by a concern for and affinity with others and the world in general. Social wellness requires the ability to relate to other people, communicate effectively with them, show respect, and give of self. Socially healthy people have friends and are members of groups—families, neighborhoods, churches. The old axiom applies here: Before you can love others, you must be able to love yourself.

5. **Environmental.** Environmental health concerns those aspects of health that are external to our bodies and over which we have very limited control. This would include the immediate physical surroundings, climate and geography, the community, and other factors such as the economic environment.

6. **Spiritual.** Spiritual wellness combines a person's ethics, values, and morals. This component is what gives life meaning and purpose. It is based on faith, hope, love, optimism, and forgiveness.

Wellness, then, encompasses the entire lifestyle: sound nutrition, fitness, stress management, not using tobacco or other psychoactive drugs, moderate (if any) use of alcohol, weight management, sexuality, and spirituality. How people manage these lifestyle factors determines in large part how well they will be.

Health and wellness range along a continuum, illustrated in Figure 1.2. At one end is the condition of total illness or disease, ending in death. At the opposite extreme is the condition of total well-being or wellness. Each person moves back and forth along this continuum from day to day as his or her health status fluctuates.

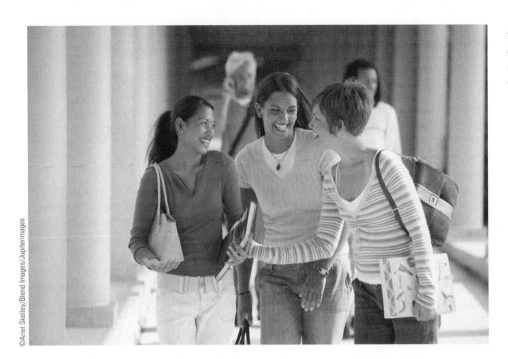

◄ *Wellness has physical, mental, emotional, social, intellectual, and spiritual components.*

©Ariel Skelley/Blend Images/Jupiterimages

## FACTORS THAT INFLUENCE HEALTH

Personal health is a dynamic state of being. Thus it is influenced by multiple factors. However, the four major factors influencing personal health are heredity, environment, personal behavior, and access to professional health care practitioners and other health services.

*The Family Tree—"Your Antecedents":* A person may be tempted to dismiss heredity as a health factor that cannot be altered and say, "You can choose your friends, but you can't choose your relatives." To the contrary, knowing one's family health history is a key to assessing and improving personal health. To focus attention on the importance of knowing one's family health history, U.S. Surgeon General Richard Carmona, M.D., M.P.H., in cooperation with other U.S. Department of Health and Human Services (HHS) agencies, launched a national public health campaign entitled "U.S. Surgeon General's Family History Initiative," and declared Thanksgiving 2005 the second annual National Family History Day. According to a survey cited in the initiative document, 96% of Americans believe that knowing one's family health history is important, but only 33% of those surveyed reported that they have "tried to gather and write down their family's health history."

Since a family health history is vital information needed by a person's health care providers, the surgeon general created a new Web-enabled program that organizes and saves the user's family history. The tool is called "My Family Health Portrait" and can be accessed at www.familyhistory.hhs.gov/. This revised version of the tool has several advantages: 1) it is accessible on any computer connected to the Web that uses an up-to-date version of a major Internet browser; 2) the family health history can be saved to the user's computer; 3) it can be printed to share with family members and health care providers; and 4) it can create and print a graphical representation of your family's generations and health conditions that may affect other generations. The online version of "My Family Health Portrait" is available without cost (in English and Spanish); no user information is

### KEY TERMS

**Health** the condition of being fit in body, mind, and spirit, free from pain or disease, with the ability to adapt to the environment

**Wellness** adoption of healthy lifestyle habits that enhance well-being and reduce the risk of disease

**FIGURE 1.2** ► Wellness Continuum

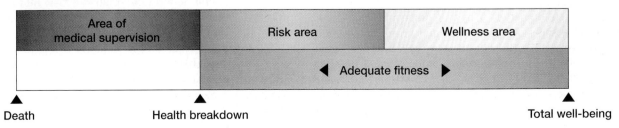

One of the overarching goals of *Healthy People 2010: Understanding and Improving Health* is to eliminate health disparities. The sections titled "Race and Ethnicity" and "Income and Education" in the introduction to the U.S. Department of Health and Human Services document say: "Current information about biological and genetic characteristics of African Americans, Hispanics, American Indians, Alaska Natives, Asians, Native Hawaiians, and Pacific Islanders does not explain the health disparities experienced by these groups compared with the white, non-Hispanic population in the United States. These disparities are believed to be the result of the complex interaction among genetic variations, environmental factors, and specific health behaviors. . . . Inequalities in income and education underlie many health disparities in the United States. . . . Higher incomes permit increased access to medical care, enable people to afford better housing and

live in safer neighborhoods, and increase the opportunity to engage in health-promoting behaviors."

The following is a selection of the disparities.

- African-American women have a higher death rate from breast cancer despite having a mammography screening rate that is nearly the same as the rate for white women.
- Hispanics living in the United States are almost twice as likely to die from diabetes as are non-Hispanic whites.
- American Indians and Alaska natives have disproportionately high death rates from unintentional injuries and suicide.
- Asians and Pacific Islanders, on average, have indicators of being one of the healthiest population groups in the United States. However, women of Vietnamese origin suffer from cervical cancer at nearly five times the rate of white women.

---

saved on any computer of the U.S. federal government (see Privacy and Security Policy on the tool).

Many of the health conditions discussed in this text link the generations, or run in families (Chapters 5, 6, 7, and 8). Awareness of any predisposition to a specific health problem and the familial link allows the person to cultivate healthy behaviors and make lifestyle changes that will reduce the risk for developing that health problem. For example, a 22-year-old African-American male may know that prostate cancer runs in his family, and he plans to begin prostate-specific antigen (PSA) testing at age 50. However, the American Cancer Society recommends that screening for prostate cancer in asymptomatic persons begin at age 45 if one **first degree relative** has prostate cancer. In this situation, if the relative is the young man's brother, then he should begin his screening before age 50.

*Personal Behavior—"Pay Now or Pay Later":* Lifestyle choices (food intake, physical activity, drug use) have a direct impact on a person's health status. In many instances, the choices result in the development of diseases or conditions that might have been avoided. To paraphrase the poet Maya Angelou, people who know better do better. Reliable health, fitness, and nutritional information is readily accessible. Many people read it, discuss it, and enroll in classes about it; they "know better" and intend to "do better." Why then do people armed with knowledge and skills to protect and promote personal health and reduce the risk of many chronic conditions and premature death adopt behaviors that put them at risk? Since behavior is influenced by the interrelation of multiple factors, one explanation used by health educators is the **health belief model (HBM),** an intrapersonal behavior theory.

Developed in the 1950s by a group of psychologists, the HBM's focus is that of the influence of intrapersonal factors (knowledge, skills, attitudes, beliefs/values, past experiences, motivation) on a person's health behaviors or actions. According to the HBM, a person's decision to act (or not act) to conserve and improve personal health is influenced by that person's assessment of the benefit of the act weighed against the person's perception of risk. The concepts or constructs of the HBM are **cue,** perceived susceptibility, perceived seriousness/severity, perceived benefits, perceived barriers, and **likelihood of taking recommended action.** The following is an example of the application of the health belief model: Eric is a 21-year-old African-American man and a sports fan. During a televised broadcast of the playoffs, Eric views a commercial about the benefit of early detection of cancer. The commercial is the prompt (cue to action) that initiates Eric's thinking about his family members who have been diagnosed with prostate cancer. Eric even remembers the "cancer survivor" who spoke about the importance of the cancer screening test in his health issues class. Eric has an "A-ha" moment and realizes that the possibility that he might develop prostate cancer in his fifties is "real" (perceived susceptibility). Because Eric has one first degree relative with the disease he recognizes that he has more than one **risk factor** for prostate cancer, and if it were to develop, the cancer could be life threatening (perceived seriousness/severity). Eric has read that he should reduce his intake of saturated fat, use his "MyPyramid" guidelines for meals, increase his intake of water, and have an annual PSA screening test beginning at age 45 to reduce his risk (perceived benefits). Although Eric exercises regularly, he hates to drink water, it's "too hard to eat all those servings" of fruit and veggies,

**Tips for Action** How to Live a Healthy, Longer Life

■ **Exercise regularly.** Engage in 30 to 60 minutes of aerobic exercise four to five days per week to enhance cardiovascular health, relieve stress, and increase blood flow to your brain.

■ **Lift weights and stretch.** The benefits include increased strength and bone density, more lean muscle mass (which you begin losing around age 35), and more efficient burning of calories. Stretching improves flexibility and is a tension buster.

■ **Eat healthy.** A great place to begin is by following the nutrient and serving suggestions on MyPyramid.gov for daily meal planning. Keep your weight within the normal range (obesity is a risk factor for medical problems that shorten life expectancy); significantly limit saturated fat in your diet; and watch your portions—stop "Super Sizing."

■ **Exercise your brain.** Keep your mental functioning sharp by reading, playing games, or learning a new skill.

■ **Exercise moderation.** Use alcohol in moderation. (If you have an addiction, do not use it at all.) Do not use tobacco products. The surgeon general says that the single biggest preventable risk factor that contributes to premature death is cigarette smoking. There is no health benefit to using tobacco products.

■ **Exercise your libido.** Healthy sexual activity is important and need not stop as you get older. Healthy sex is consensual and responsible. Communication is vital, and the use of prophylactics is necessary to reduce the risk of sexually transmitted diseases (STDs).

■ **Cultivate spirituality.** Faith or spirituality is important to longevity. Connect with your spiritual sovereign daily through prayer, meditation, or your customary ritual. Keep a gratitude journal. Many people who live past 75 list faith practice as an important part of their lives.

■ **Take action.** Engage in activities that improve your life. Pursue your dreams by engaging in activities or hobbies that you enjoy. Remember to help others. Sharing your gifts and giving back are always rewarding.

and turning 45 is a long way off (perceived barriers). At this point, Eric will analyze the difference between the benefits (diet, exercise, future PSAs) and barriers. Eric's actions (likelihood of taking the recommended action) will be determined by weighing the perceived threat against the reduction of the threat. Will Eric "do better"?

Fortunately, people can do much to prevent illness and promote health and wellness by taking responsibility for their health through wise lifestyle choices, behavior patterns, and behavior modification. Nutritional intake and weight management are particularly important. These areas are covered in Chapters 9 and 10. Also, the importance of physical activity is the topic of Chapter 11.

## Prevention

The emphasis on prevention in promoting wellness is clear and is reflected in the 2000 *A Report of the Surgeon General: Physical Activity and Health* (see Appendix) and in *Healthy People 2010: Understanding and Improving Health*, both of which are cited throughout this book. Crucial to prevention is a change in attitude by health care providers and patients alike. Patients have to stop demanding medication as well as hospitalization and surgery for every ache and pain. Health care providers have to be less eager to dispense medication and advise hospitalization and surgery for conditions that can be treated in less extreme ways.

Joseph Califano, former secretary of Health and Human Services, stated that American doctors should be "more skeptical in resorting to surgery and less promiscuous in dispensing pills." Of the people who die each year in the United States, only 10% die because of inadequate health care and only 20% die because of biological and environmental factors combined; the remaining 70% die from a combination of lifestyle behaviors.

Preventive measures take place on three levels.

1. **Primary prevention**—taking measures to stop a health problem before it begins. Preventive measures include getting recommended immunizations,

### KEY TERMS

**First degee relative** a family member that is a person's biological parent, sibling, or offspring

**Health belief model (HBM)** an intrapersonal theory that analyzes the relationship between a person's perception of a threat to health and the willingness of the person to reduce the perceived threat by changing behavior

**Cue** (to action) a construct of the health belief model that addresses a circumstance or event that motivates a person to act

**Likelihood of taking action** a construct of the health belief model that addresses the chances a person will behave or take certain actions

**Risk factor** a familial or environmental situation or a behavior that increases the likelihood that a person will develop a health problem

**Primary prevention** taking steps to prevent health problems from developing

never starting to smoke, getting the right kind and amount of exercise, eating nutritionally healthy foods, using prophylactics wisely to prevent sexually transmitted diseases, and following recommended safety procedures.

2. **Secondary prevention**—detecting a health problem early so intervention may deter or lessen the negative consequences of an undesirable condition. For example, a long-term smoker who develops a chronic cough, attends a clinic, and subsequently quits smoking has reduced the risks for acquiring cancer, heart disease, and other diseases attributable to smoking.

3. **Tertiary prevention**—taking care of people after they get ill. This, unfortunately, is the established pattern of medical delivery. The monetary cost of health care, along with the physical cost, could be reduced dramatically if the focus were to change to primary and secondary prevention.

## LEADING CAUSES OF DEATH

The significance of the three levels of prevention is illustrated clearly in the leading causes of death in the United States as percentages of overall deaths, depicted in Figure 1.3. Factors over which a person has absolutely

**FIGURE 1.3 ▶** Leading Causes of Death in 1900 and 2004.

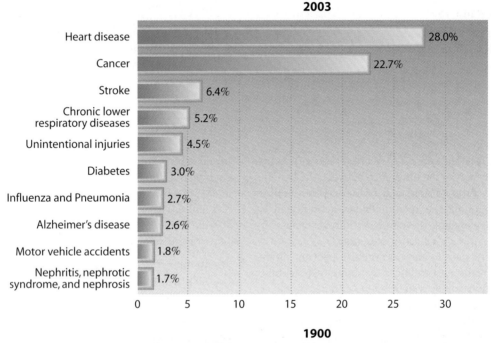

**2003**

- Heart disease — 28.0%
- Cancer — 22.7%
- Stroke — 6.4%
- Chronic lower respiratory diseases — 5.2%
- Unintentional injuries — 4.5%
- Diabetes — 3.0%
- Influenza and Pneumonia — 2.7%
- Alzheimer's disease — 2.6%
- Motor vehicle accidents — 1.8%
- Nephritis, nephrotic syndrome, and nephrosis — 1.7%

(0, 5, 10, 15, 20, 25, 30)

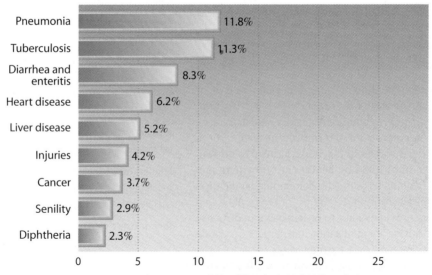

**1900**

- Pneumonia — 11.8%
- Tuberculosis — 11.3%
- Diarrhea and enteritis — 8.3%
- Heart disease — 6.2%
- Liver disease — 5.2%
- Injuries — 4.2%
- Cancer — 3.7%
- Senility — 2.9%
- Diphtheria — 2.3%

(0, 5, 10, 15, 20, 25)

Percentage of Total Deaths/100,000 Population

no control account for only a fraction of the total deaths, whereas more than half of all disease can be entirely self-controlled.

At the beginning of the 20th century, almost a third of all deaths in the United States resulted from tuberculosis, influenza, and pneumonia. Less than 5% of deaths were the result of cancer, and only about 10% were from cardiovascular diseases. In the 1990s, according to the U.S. Department of Health and Human Services, approximately 70% of all deaths in the United States were attributable to diseases of the heart and circulatory system and cancer. Up to 80% of those deaths might have been prevented by lifestyle changes as basic as eating a diet lower in fat, getting regular exercise, not abusing alcohol, and not smoking. The data in Figure 1.3 compare leading causes of death in 1900 and 2004.

From another perspective, the *Journal of the American Medical Association* has translated the numbers of deaths into underlying causes of death. These are shown in Figure 1.4. The three lifestyle-related factors of tobacco, poor diet coupled with inactivity, and alcohol all overshadow infectious diseases, the fourth leading cause of death.

**Trends in Longevity.** On the upside, the Centers for Disease Control and Prevention (CDC) data indicate that people in the United States are living longer than ever before and that the infant death rate has reached an all-time low. The average person in 2004 could expect to live 77.9 years, up from 77.3 in 2002. Women still live

### KEY TERMS

**Secondary prevention** early detection and intervention to reduce the consequences of a health problem

**Tertiary prevention** taking care of a health problem that has already caused illness

**FIGURE 1.4** ▶ Underlying Causes of Death

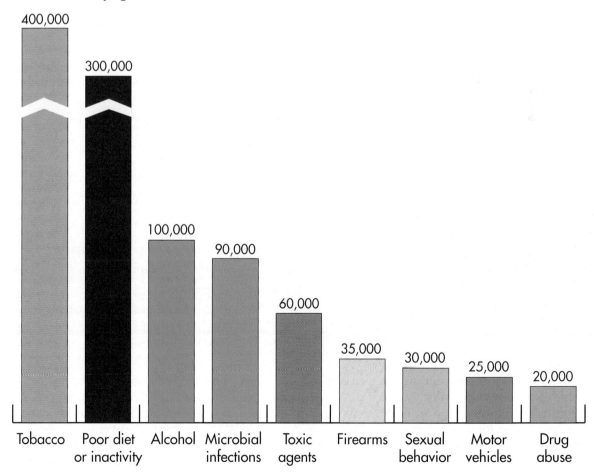

*Source:* Modified from the *Journal of the American Medical Association,* 1993, 270: 2207–2212. © 1993 American Medical Association. Used with permission.

## HEALTHY PEOPLE 2010 Selected Health Objectives

### Mental Health and Mental Illness

- Reduce the suicide rate.
- Reduce the proportion of homeless adults who have serious mental illness.
- Increase the number of states, including the District of Columbia, and territories with an operational plan that addresses mental health crisis interventions, ongoing screening, and treatment services for elderly persons.

### Maternal and Child Health

- Reduce fetal and infant deaths.
- Reduce maternal illness and complications due to pregnancy.
- Increase the proportion of pregnant women who receive early and adequate prenatal care.
- Increase the proportion of mothers who breastfeed their babies.

### Family Planning

- Increase the proportion of pregnancies that are intended.
- Increase the proportion of females at risk of unintended pregnancy (and their partners) who use contraception.
- Increase the proportion of adolescents who have never engaged in sexual intercourse.
- Reduce the proportion of married couples whose ability to conceive or maintain a pregnancy is impaired.

### Injury and Violence Prevention

- Reduce maltreatment and maltreatment fatalities of children.
- Reduce the rate of physical assault by current or former intimate partners.
- Reduce the annual rate of rape or attempted rape.
- Reduce deaths caused by motor vehicle crashes.
- Increase use of safety belts.
- Increase functioning residential smoke alarms.

### HIV

- Reduce the incidence of acquired immune deficiency syndrome (AIDS) among adolescents and adults.
- Increase the proportion of sexually active people who use condoms.
- Increase the number of people testing positive for the human immunodeficiency virus (HIV) who know their serostatus.
- Reduce deaths from HIV infection.
- Reduce new cases of perinatally acquired HIV infection.

### Sexually Transmitted Diseases

- Reduce the proportion of adolescents and young adults with *Chlamydia trachomatis* infections.
- Reduce gonorrhea.
- Eliminate sustained domestic transmission of primary and secondary syphilis.
- Reduce the proportion of persons with human papillomavirus infection.
- Reduce the proportion of females who have ever required treatment for pelvic inflammatory disease.

### Immunizations and Infectious Diseases

- Reduce or eliminate indigenous cases of vaccine-preventable diseases.
- Reduce hepatitis A; reduce hepatitis C.
- Reduce Lyme disease.
- Reduce tuberculosis.
- Reduce the number of antibiotics prescribed for the sole diagnosis of the common cold.

### Cancer

- Reduce the overall cancer death rate.
- Reduce the lung cancer death rate.
- Reduce the breast cancer death rate.
- Reduce the prostate cancer death rate.

---

longer—80.4 years—the **life expectancy** for men is up to 75.2 years, which closes the gap slightly.

Although the life expectancy for whites is six years longer on average than for blacks, the gap is narrowing, as shown in Figure 1.5. In 1998 blacks could expect to live an average of 71 years, up from 69.5 years in 1995. For 2004 (latest available), blacks could expect to live an average of 73.1 years.

Despite overall reductions in homicide and suicide rates, these causes of death remain the second and third leading causes of death, respectively, among young people ages 15–24. The leading cause of death for this age group continues to be motor vehicle traffic crashes. For the first time, deaths from acquired immune deficiency syndrome (AIDS) showed a decline, and now AIDS is the fifth leading cause of death (after suicide) of adults between ages

## HEALTHY PEOPLE 2010 Selected Health Objectives (*continued*)

### Diabetes

- Prevent diabetes.
- Increase the proportion of persons with diabetes who receive formal diabetic instruction.
- Reduce deaths from cardiovascular disease in persons with diabetes.
- Increase the proportion of adults with diabetes who self-monitor their blood glucose at least once daily.

### Arthritis, Osteoarthritis, and Chronic Back Conditions

- Reduce the proportion of adults with chronic joint symptoms who experience a limitation in activity due to arthritis.
- Reduce activity limitations due to chronic back conditions.

### Heart Disease and Stroke

- Reduce coronary heart disease deaths.
- Reduce stroke deaths.
- Reduce the proportion of adults with high blood pressure.

### Nutrition and Overweight

- Increase the proportion of adults who are at a healthy weight.
- Reduce the proportion of children and adolescents who are overweight or obese.
- Increase the proportion of persons aged two years and older who consume at least two daily servings of fruit.

### Physical Fitness and Activity

- Increase the proportion of adults who engage regularly, preferably daily, in moderate physical activity for at least 30 minutes.

- Increase the proportion of the nation's public and private schools that require daily physical education for all students.

### Substance Abuse

- Reduce deaths and injuries caused by alcohol- and drug-related motor vehicle crashes.
- Reduce cirrhosis deaths.
- Reduce the proportion of persons engaging in binge drinking of alcoholic beverages.
- Reduce past month use of illicit substances.

### Tobacco Use

- Reduce tobacco use by adults and adolescents.
- Increase smoking cessation during pregnancy.
- Reduce the proportion of children who are regularly exposed to tobacco smoke at home.
- Reduce the illegal sales rate to minors through enforcement of laws prohibiting the sale of tobacco products to minors.

### Environmental Health

- Reduce the proportion of persons exposed to air that does not meet the U.S. Environmental Protection Agency's health-based standards for harmful air pollutants.
- Eliminate elevated blood lead levels in children.
- Reduce waterborne disease outbreaks arising from water intended for drinking among persons served by community water systems.

*Source:* Adapted from U.S. Department of Health and Human Services, *Healthy People 2010: Understanding and Improving Health* (Washington, DC: U.S. Government Printing Office, January 2000).

---

25 and 44. As with 15- to 24-year-olds, accidents rank as the leading cause of death for persons 25 to 44.

**Risks by Age Group.** Statistically, people outgrow the risks for some conditions. The things people do during their younger years are no longer as life threatening in middle age and older. Table 1.1 summarizes the ten leading causes of death by age group (infants under 1 year to seniors 65+ years).

**Age Group 19–39.** Between ages 19 and 39 disease is not the leading cause of death, and the most common

medical conditions typically are not serious. The risks of death can be reduced primarily by living safely. The single most important thing to do is to practice safety on the roads. That means wearing seat belts and bicycle helmets,

### KEY TERMS

**Life expectancy** the average number of years of life remaining to a person at a particular age; the average number of years at a given year of birth that a person is expected to live

**FIGURE 1.5 ▶** Trends in Life Expectancy for Whites and Blacks

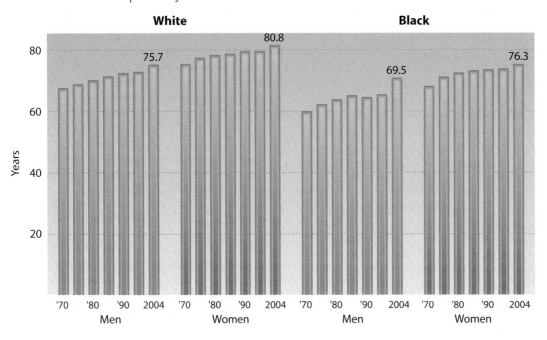

**TABLE 1.1 ▶** Top 10 Leading Causes of Death in the United States for 2003, by Age Group

### nhtsa
National Highway Traffic Safety Administration's
National Center for Statistics and Analysis

## Top 10 Leading Causes of Death in the United States for 2003, by Age Group[1]

| RANK | Infants under 1 | Toddlers 1–3 | Young Children 4–7 | Children 8–15 | Youth 16–20 | Young Adults 21–24 | Other Adults 25–34 | Other Adults 35–44 | Other Adults 45–64 | Elderly 65+ | All Ages | Years of Life Lost[2] |
|---|---|---|---|---|---|---|---|---|---|---|---|---|
| 1 | Perinatal Period 14,254 | Congenital Anomalies 480 | MV Traffic Crashes 479 | MV Traffic Crashes 1,582 | MV Traffic Crashes 5,988 | MV Traffic Crashes 4,312 | MV Traffic Crashes 6,675 | Malignant Neoplasms 15,509 | Malignant Neoplasms 145,535 | Heart Disease 563,390 | Heart Disease 685,089 | Malignant Neoplasms 23% (8,672,799) |
| 2 | Congenital Anomalies 5,621 | Accidental Drowning 401 | Malignant Neoplasms 444 | Malignant Neoplasms 859 | Homicide 2,489 | Homicide 2,744 | Suicide 5,065 | Heart Disease 13,600 | Heart Disease 102,792 | Malignant Neoplasms 388,911 | Malignant Neoplasms 556,902 | Heart Disease 21% (8,027,887) |
| 3 | Heart Disease 439 | MV Traffic Crashes 385 | Congenital Anomalies 168 | Suicide 412 | Suicide 1,813 | Suicide 2,012 | Homicide 4,516 | MV Traffic Crashes 6,780 | Diabetes 16,389 | Stroke 138,134 | Stroke 157,689 | MV Traffic Crashes 5% (1,725,870) |
| 4 | Homicide 341 | Homicide 333 | Accidental Drowning 149 | Homicide 389 | Accidental Poisoning 752 | Accidental Poisoning 1,221 | Malignant Neoplasms 3,741 | Suicide 6,602 | Stroke 16,073 | Chronic Lwr. Resp. Dis. 109,139 | Chronic Lwr. Resp. Dis. 126,382 | Stroke 5% (1,641,883) |
| 5 | Influenza/ Pneumonia 322 | Malignant Neoplasms 272 | Exposure to Smoke/Fire 145 | Congenital Anomalies 320 | Malignant Neoplasms 749 | Malignant Neoplasms 795 | Accidental Poisoning 3,435 | Accidental Poisoning 6,230 | Chronic Lwr. Resp. Dis. 15,614 | Alzheimer's 62,814 | Diabetes 74,219 | Chronic Lwr. Resp. Dis. 4% (1,486,130) |
| 6 | Septicemia 278 | Exposure to Smoke/Fire 169 | Homicide 113 | Heart Disease 248 | Heart Disease 450 | Heart Disease 633 | Heart Disease 3,250 | HIV 5,340 | Chronic Liver Disease 13,894 | Influenza/ Pneumonia 57,670 | Influenza/ Pneumonia 65,163 | Perinatal Period 3% (1,110,448) |
| 7 | Nephritis/ Nephrosis 181 | Heart Disease 159 | Heart Disease 93 | Accidental Drowning 209 | Accidental Drowning 309 | Accidental Drowning 223 | HIV 1,588 | Homicide 3,110 | Suicide 10,324 | Diabetes 54,919 | Alzheimer's 63,457 | Suicide 3% (1,104,339) |
| 8 | MV Traffic Crashes 144 | Influenza/ Pneumonia 141 | Influenza/ Pneumonia 79 | Exposure to Smoke/Fire 140 | Congenital Anomalies 241 | Congenital Anomalies 171 | Diabetes 657 | Chronic Liver Disease 3,020 | MV Traffic Crashes 9,700 | Nephritis/ Nephrosis 35,254 | MV Traffic Crashes 43,340 | Diabetes 3% (1,067,600) |
| 9 | Stroke 101 | MV Nontraffic Crashes[4] 101 | MV Nontraffic Crashes[4] 43 | MV Nontraffic Crashes[4] 120 | MV Nontraffic Crashes[4] 108 | HIV 131 | Stroke 583 | Stroke 2,460 | Accidental Poisoning 6,804 | Septicemia 26,445 | Nephritis/ Nephrosis 42,453 | Homicide 2% (827,103) |
| 10 | Meningitis 77 | Septicemia 77 | Septicemia 35 | Chronic Lwr. Resp. Dis. 114 | Accidental Falls 106 | MV Nontraffic Crashes[4] 117 | Congenital Anomalies 426 | Diabetes 2,049 | HIV 5,959 | Hypertension Renal Dis. 18,657 | Septicemia 34,069 | Accidental Poisoning 2% (749,593) |
| ALL[3] | 28,025 | 4,205 | 2,558 | 6,555 | 16,141 | 16,030 | 41,300 | 89,461 | 439,300 | 1,804,373 | 2,448,288 | All Causes 100% (37,485,508) |

[1]When ranked by specific ages, motor vehicle crashes are the leading cause of death for age 3 and each age 5 through 33.

[2]Number of years calculated based on remaining life expectancy [2002 data from CDC] at time of death; percents calculated as a proportion of total years of life lost due to all causes of death.

[3]Not a total of top 10 causes of death.

[4]A motor vehicle nontraffic crash is any vehicle crash that occurs entirely in any place other than a public highway.

**Source:** National Center for Health Statistics (NCHS) CDC, Mortality Data 2003.

**Note:** The cause of death classification is based on the National Center for Statistics and Analysis (NCSA) Revised 68 Cause of Death Listing. This listing differs from the one used by the NCHS for its reports on leading causes of death by separating out unintentional injuries into separate causes of death, i.e., motor vehicle traffic crashes, accidental falls, motor vehicle nontraffic crashes, etc. Accordingly, the rank of some causes of death will differ from those reported by the NCHS. This difference will mostly be observed for minor causes of death in smaller age groupings.

not driving after drinking (or riding with those who do), and observing traffic rules. Although overall deaths in traffic have been declining since 1966, motor vehicle traffic crashes remain the leading cause of death in the age group 19–34 (see Table 1.1).

At the same time, people in this age group would be wise to establish preventive lifestyle habits to serve them as they grow older. Foremost is to be a nonsmoker (Chapter 13). Smoking is a universal risk factor for heart disease, lung disease, and several types of cancer. Abstaining from other psychoactive drugs (Chapter 12) and using alcohol in moderation, if at all, go a long way toward preserving health and prolonging life. Other preventive measures are to

- Document your health history using the online tool "My Family Health Portrait" to predict increased risk for certain diseases and to develop prevention and early detection strategies (Chapters 7 and 8).

- Adhere to a sound diet in accordance with MyPyramid.gov (Chapters 9 and 10).

- Exercise properly to promote cardiovascular and overall health (Chapter 11).

- Practice safer sex (Chapter 6) and learn to extricate yourself from abusive and dangerous relationships (Chapter 4).

- Cultivate mental health (Chapter 2) and learn how to manage stress (Chapter 3).

- Conduct medical maintenance by seeing a medical professional regularly (Chapter 15), doing applicable self-exams (Chapter 7), keeping up on your immunizations (Chapter 6), and avoiding environmental pollutants and practicing wise consumerism (Chapter 15).

**Age Group 40–64.** The preventive measures in the age group 19–39 should continue. Those listed below become even more important for people in the 40–64 age group.

- Keep exercising. People tend to gain weight most rapidly between ages 55 and 65. At the same time, muscle mass declines while fat increases (Chapter 10). Aerobic exercise (Chapter 11) is highly beneficial to the cardiovascular system, lowers cholesterol, helps to lower blood pressure, and offers protection against diabetes and some cancers (Chapter 7). Strength training (also covered in Chapter 11) preserves bone density (which works against osteoporosis—see Chapter 14) and contributes to general health.

- Continue to eat nutritionally (Chapter 9). The diet, however, may change somewhat in this age group. Menopausal women, for example, may need more calcium and should consider the benefits of hormone replacement therapy (Chapter 14).

- Pay even more attention to medical maintenance. In this age range people tend to require more frequent attention from medical professionals. Also, some new tests have been introduced to detect the presence of certain conditions that, if caught early, can be treated more successfully. Essential tests are blood pressure screening, cholesterol tests (Chapter 8), Pap tests (Chapter 5), and sigmoidoscopy and diabetes screening (Chapter 7), among others.

**Age Group 65 and Older.** Deconditioning, more than age, is responsible for most problems later in life. The following considerations are important.

- Keep exercising. Maintain a mix of aerobic and strength-training exercise, and add stretching and balance activities if they are not already part of the regimen.

- Adjust the diet, if necessary, following the advice of medical professionals. This may mean increasing the calcium intake (for women). Most dietary recommendations, however, remain the same.

- Step up medical maintenance as the risk for diseases continues. The same screening tests as done in the previous age group should continue, perhaps more often. Be wary of solving maladies through over-the-counter drugs (Chapters 12, 14, and 15), which usually just mask symptoms.

- Preserve mental health. Depression is common among people in this age group. Some people begin to feel they have outlived their usefulness and need social support (Chapter 4) more than ever. Some depression

## FYI | ADD 10 YEARS TO YOUR LIFE

If you want to add years to your life, you can begin today. One of the determinants of health is behavior. By making the decision to do something about living longer, you can add 10 years (really, 9.9 years) to your life by engaging in the following activities.

| Years added | How to do it |
| --- | --- |
| 2.4 | Eat a vegetarian-style diet |
| 2.1 | Exercise vigorously three times a week |
| 2.9 | Eat nuts five times a week |
| 1.5 | Maintain a healthy weight (body mass index [BMI] below 25) |
| 1.0 | Take hormone replacement therapy (HRT) at perimenopause (if advised by a physician) |

*Source:* Joan Quinn, "Add 10 Years to Your Life," *Prevention*, January 2002, p. 37.

**TABLE 1.2 ▶** Comparison of Leading Medical Problems and Causes of Death in the United States by Age Group

| AGE GROUP | | |
| --- | --- | --- |
| **AGES 19–39**<br>**LEADING MEDICAL PROBLEMS** | **AGES 40–64**<br>**LEADING MEDICAL PROBLEMS** | **AGES 65 AND OVER**<br>**LEADING MEDICAL PROBLEMS** |
| ■ Nose, throat, and upper respiratory infections<br>■ Injuries<br>■ Viral, bacterial, and parasitic infections<br>■ Acute urinary tract infections<br>■ Eating disorders<br>■ Violence, rape<br>■ Substance abuse | ■ Osteoporosis and arthritis<br>■ Nose, throat, and upper respiratory conditions<br>■ Orthopedic deformities and impairments of back, arms, and legs<br>■ Cardiovascular diseases<br>■ Hearing and vision impairments | ■ Nose, throat, and upper respiratory conditions<br>■ Osteoporosis and arthritis<br>■ Hypertension<br>■ Urinary incontinence<br>■ Cardiovascular diseases<br>■ Injuries<br>■ Hearing and vision impairment |
| **LEADING CAUSES OF DEATH** | **LEADING CAUSES OF DEATH** | **LEADING CAUSES OF DEATH** |
| ■ Motor vehicle accidents<br>■ Cardiovascular diseases<br>■ Homicide<br>■ Coronary artery diseases<br>■ AIDS<br>■ Breast cancer<br>■ Cerebrovascular diseases<br>■ Cervical and other uterine cancers | ■ Cardiovascular diseases<br>■ Coronary artery diseases<br>■ Breast cancer<br>■ Lung cancer<br>■ Cerebrovascular diseases<br>■ Colorectal cancer<br>■ Chronic obstructive pulmonary disease<br>■ Ovarian cancer<br>■ Diabetes | ■ Cardiovascular diseases<br>■ Cerebrovascular diseases<br>■ Pneumonia and influenza<br>■ Chronic obstructive pulmonary diseases<br>■ Colorectal cancer<br>■ Breast cancer<br>■ Lung cancer<br>■ Diabetes<br>■ Accidents |

*Source:* Harvard Medical School, Health Publications Group, August 1997.

is a result of the natural grieving following loss, but, according to the Harvard Medical School Health Publications Group, nonspecific depression can be treated successfully about 80% of the time. The same organization says the single most important factor in successful aging is connectedness. People who have more friends have fewer colds because being connected to others bolsters the immune system (Chapter 3).

The leading medical problems and causes of death by the three age groups presented here are summarized in Table 1.2.

## THE FUTURE

Health issues are at the forefront in contemporary life. Advances in medicine and research are continuing. The problems, as well as many of the solutions, have been identified. In large measure these solutions entail lifestyle changes. People can do their part to reverse the rising financial, physical, and emotional costs of health care by taking charge of their personal health instead of depending on the health care community to deal with health problems after they have developed. With these kinds of changes, the 21st century might well be proclaimed "the era of health."

## Summary

■ The most widely accepted definition of health, by the World Health Organization, is "a state of complete physical, mental, and social well-being, not merely the absence of disease or infirmity."

■ Wellness has been defined as "the adoption of healthy lifestyle habits that will enhance well-being while decreasing the risk of disease."

■ The components of wellness are physical, mental/ intellectual, emotional, social, environmental, and spiritual.

■ The three levels of prevention are primary (prevention), secondary (early detection and treatment), and tertiary (treatment after becoming ill).

■ The leading causes of death at the beginning of the 20th century were largely infectious diseases.

■ Today, the leading causes of death—heart disease, cancer, stroke, and chronic lung disease—are the result of lifestyle choices/behavior.

■ A documented family health history is an important tool in determining disease risks and planning prevention strategies.

■ The health belief model (HBM) is one theory that is used to explain the likelihood of a person taking the

- recommended action when health is compromised or threatened.

- Hidden killers include tobacco, poor diet coupled with inactivity, alcohol, and unsafe sexual practices.

- People in the United States are living longer, and men are starting to close the longevity gap that women have held. Life expectancy for blacks is increasing. However, white females and white males live more than 5 years longer than black females and black males.

## Personal Health Resources

ThomsonNOW™ Visit the ThomsonNOW website at http://thomsonedu.com/thomsonnow for valuable resources that will:

- Help you evaluate your knowledge of the material.

- Guide you through tutorials to help you understand and apply the material.

- Allow you to take an exam-prep quiz to better prepare for class tests.

Healthy People 2010 This site has information, from *Healthy People 2010: Understanding and Improving Health,* that represents the ideas and expertise of a diverse range of individuals and organizations concerned about the nation's health. The project goals (increase quality and years of healthy life and eliminate health disparities) and the supporting objectives in 28 focus areas that were developed by experts from federal agencies under the U.S. Department of Health and Human Services can be accessed. The full text of *Healthy People 2010* (volumes I and II) is available on the website. 1-877-696-6775

**www.health.gov/healthypeople**

National Center for Chronic Disease Prevention and Health Promotion (NCCDPHP) This site offers information aimed to prevent death and disability from chronic disease and includes statistics about risk behaviors, specific populations, maternal and infant health, to include more than 15 programs and campaigns, such as Global Health, Healthy Youth, and WISEWOMAN.

**www.cdc.gov/nccdphp/**

National Health Information Center (NHIC) This site offers a health information referral service to professionals and consumers with health questions and puts them in touch with organizations best able to provide answers. 1-800-336-4797

**www.nhic-nt.health.org/**

National Highway Traffic Safety Administration (NHTSA) This site offers information and statistics on transportation issues such as highway accidents, seat belt usage,

alcohol-related accidents, states with highest rates of accidents, and crash fatality rate trends. 1-800-424-9393

**www.nhtsa.dot.gov/**

## It's Your Turn for Study and Review

1. Name the four factors that influence your health. Describe an experience (personal, family, or acquaintance) that you can associate with each of these factors.

2. Prevention is a key component of wellness. Using the information that you described in review item #1, indicate if each situation is applicable to a primary, secondary, or tertiary prevention. If the situation is applicable to tertiary prevention, indicate a primary or secondary prevention strategy that could have been employed in the situation.

3. List the top five leading causes of death of adults in the United States. Go to the website of the National Center for Health Statistics at www.cdc.gov/nchs and find the leading causes of death for persons aged 15–24 and 25–44. Compare the data.

4. Using your age group, indicate at least three risk factors other than heredity that influence your health.

5. Find a news article that describes in detail a disease or health condition. Applying the constructs of the health belief model, write your analysis of the news article.

## Thinking about Health Issues

Family Health History—"I encourage all families to take time to collect important health history information that can benefit all family members. Even with all the high-tech tests, medicines, and procedures available in today's modern health-care setting, family health history remains the cornerstone of our efforts to prevent disease and promote personal health. It's clear that knowing your family history can save your life." U.S. Surgeon General Richard H. Carmona, M.D., M.P.H., February 2006.

1. Access the Web-based family history tool—"My Family Portrait"—www.familyhistory.hhs.gov/ (English) or www.familyhistory.hhs.gov/spanish (Spanish), enter your family health information, print the results, and share them with a family member (a first or second degree relative, if possible).

2. Bring your "My Family Potrait" to your personal health class. Make a report to your classmates that summarizes the data and includes three changes in behavior (short-term and long-term) that you can take to reduce your risk of developing health problems (premature death) that "run in your family."

3. One of the components of wellness is social health. One way to enhance your social health is to begin to advocate for family and community health. Choose a health issue and advocate for people who are not able to speak for themselves. For a selection of health issues arranged by the months of the year, turn to Appendix A of this text—"2007 National Health Observances: The Year 2007 at a Glance." (www.healthfinder.gov/library/nho/nhoyear.asp?year=2007)

## Selected Bibliography

"Age Is Only a Number." *Essence*, January 2002, pp. 81, 123–124.

Begley, S. "Shaped by Life in the Womb." *Newsweek*, September 27, 1999, pp. 50–57.

Berg, E. "Getting It Write." *Health*, January/February 2001, pp. 82–89.

Carmona, R. H. & D. J. Wattendorf. "Personalizing Prevention: The U.S. Surgeon General's Family History Initiative." *American Family Physician*, January 1, 2005, 71 (1), pp. 36, 39.

Evans, K. "Journey of the Spirit." *Health*, April 2001, pp. 118–123, 178–179.

Finch, Steven. "To See Your Future, Look into Your Past." *Health*, October 1996, pp. 92–96.

Glanz, K., F. M. Lewis, and B. K. Rimer (Eds.). *Health Behavior and Health Education: Theory, Research, and Practice*. San Francisco: Jossey-Bass, 1997.

*Harvard Women's Health Watch*, August 1997, 4 (12), pp. 2–3.

"Health Disparities Experienced by Black or African Americans—United States." *Morbidity and Mortality Weekly Report*, January 14, 2005.

Hoeger, Werner, W. K., L. W. Turner, and B. A. Hafen. *Wellness: Guidelines for a Healthy Lifestyle*, 3rd edition. Englewood, CO: Morton Publishing, 2002.

McCarty, S. "You Don't Have to Grow Old." *Health*, November/December 2000, pp. 96–101.

McDowell, M. A., J. P. Hughes, & L. G. Borrud. "Health Characteristics of U.S. Adults by Body Mass Index Category: Results from NHANES 19992002." *Public Health Reports*, January/February 2006, 121 (1), pp. 67–73.

"Most U.S. Adults at Risk of Becoming Overweight or Obese." *FDA Consumer*, November–December 2005, p.7.

National Center for Health Statistics. "Deaths—Leading Causes." www.cdc.gov/nchsfastats/lcod.htm. Accessed April 2006.

"Online Version of 'My Family Health Portrait' Available in English and Spanish." *FDA Consumer*, May-June 2006, pp. 16–17.

Quinn, Joan. "Add 10 Years to Your Life." *Prevention*, January 2002, pp. 36–37.

Shute, N. "Where We Come From." *U.S. News and World Report*, January 29, 2001, pp. 36–41.

Spake, A. "You Owe Your Family So Much—Even Your Illness." *U.S. News and World Report*, March 12, 2001, pp. 74–76.

"Special Report: Do Just 1 Thing! And You Can Live a Longer, Healthier Life." *Prevention*, September 2001, pp. 121–181.

National Highway Traffic Safety Administration–National Center for Statistics and Analysis. Subramanian, Rajesh. MotorVehicle Traffic Crashes as a Leading Cause of Death in the United States, 2003. www.nhtsa.dot.gov. Accessed April 2006.

U.S. Census Bureau. *Statistical Abstract of the United States: 2000*, 120th edition. Washington: DC: U.S. Government Printing Office, 2000.

U.S. Department of Health and Human Services. *Healthy People 2010: Understanding and Improving Health*. Washington, DC: U.S. Government Printing Office, January 2000.

U.S. Department of Health and Human Services. *Healthy People 2010 Midcourse Review*. www.healthypeople.gov/data/progrvw/. Accessed March 2006.

U.S. Department of Health and Human Services. *U.S. Surgeon General's Family History Initiative*. www.surgeongeneral.gov. Accessed January 2006.

Yoon, P. W. M. T. Scheuner, M. Gwinn, M. J. Khoury, C. Jorgensen, S. Hariri, and S. Lyn. "Awareness of Family Health History as a Risk Factor for Disease—United States, 2004." *Morbidity and Mortality Weekly Report*, November 12, 2004, 53 (44), pp. 1044–47.

**Name** _____   **Course** _____

**Date** _____   **Section** _____

To assess how well you measure up in each of the areas covered in this book, place a checkmark in front of each item that is applicable to you. Add the number of checkmarks for each chapter. The higher the subtotal, the stronger you are in that area. Lower subtotals indicate areas needing improvement. By comparing your subtotals, your relative strengths and weaknesses will become apparent, and you can pinpoint those areas of knowledge or behavior that you may choose to work on.

## Chapter 1   Introduction to Personal Health

_____ **1.** I exercise for 20 to 30 minutes at least three times a week.

_____ **2.** When there is a choice, I walk, run, or ride a bike instead of driving or taking public transportation.

_____ **3.** I read a newspaper or listen to or watch the news daily.

_____ **4.** I like to hear others' views on a topic.

_____ **5.** I consider myself an optimist, not a pessimist.

_____ **6.** I do not hold grudges or harbor long-standing feuds.

_____ **7.** I enjoy participating in groups and like to meet new people.

_____ **8.** I have at least one good friend whom I trust and who freely confides in me.

_____ **9.** I believe in a power higher than myself.

_____**10.** My behaviors generally conform to and reflect my beliefs and values.

**Subtotal**

## Chapter 2   Personality and Emotional Health

_____ **1.** When I get angry, I get it out of my system and let it go.

_____ **2.** I have a sense of control in my life and do not consider myself a victim of outside circumstances.

_____ **3.** I like myself most of the time.

_____ **4.** I am flexible and adapt to change easily.

_____ **5.** I have a sense of direction and general plan for my life.

_____ **6.** When I get the blues from time to time, they are brief and I bounce back with my usual energy and enthusiasm.

_____ **7.** When I feel down, I have someone in whom I feel comfortable confiding.

_____ **8.** I look at problems as challenges and face them instead of running away.

_____ **9.** I am not overly hard on myself, and when I do make mistakes, I look upon them as learning experiences.

_____**10.** I get satisfaction from helping others and giving of myself to others.

**Subtotal**

## Chapter 3    Stress and Health

_____ **1.** When I feel stressed, I take a break and relax.

_____ **2.** I do not get sick often, and when I do, it does not last long.

_____ **3.** I am committed to my goals and work toward them.

_____ **4.** I willingly face the challenges in my life.

_____ **5.** I have no trouble going to sleep and I get plenty of rest.

_____ **6.** I am able to manage my time so I am not constantly doing last-minute cramming for an exam or racing to get an assignment in on time.

_____ **7.** I watch very little television.

_____ **8.** I do not consider myself a procrastinator.

_____ **9.** I have developed or learned some ways to relax after a stressful time.

_____ **10.** I let off steam by doing some strenuous activity.

**Subtotal**

## Chapter 4    Personal Relationships

_____ **1.** I almost never feel lonely even when I am alone.

_____ **2.** I have fostered close relationships that have endured over time.

_____ **3.** I am comfortable with my sexual self.

_____ **4.** I respect the people I date and expect the same from them.

_____ **5.** I do not attempt to control or dominate other people.

_____ **6.** I feel free to express my feelings and communicate readily in an intimate relationship.

_____ **7.** I am able to trust others and am trustworthy myself.

_____ **8.** I consider marriage a lasting, committed bond.

_____ **9.** I believe that having children is a lifelong responsibility.

_____ **10.** I believe that relationships do not just happen; I have to work on them.

**Subtotal**

## Chapter 5    Human Sexuality, Contraception, and Reproduction

_____ **1.** I can describe the changes to the human body that occur during puberty.

_____ **2.** I am able to label the parts of the male and female reproductive systems and describe their functions.

_____ **3.** I am familiar with the various forms of birth control, their advantages and disadvantages.

_____ **4.** I understand the sexual response cycle and the physical process of conception.

_____ **5.** I can explain the stages in the birth process.

_____ **6.** I can describe some of the symptoms of premenstrual syndrome (PMS) and how to alleviate this condition.

_____ **7.** I can name some of the complications of pregnancy and birth.

_____ **8.** I have regular physical exams, including of the reproductive system.

_____ **9.** I do breast self-exams (females) and testicular self-exams (males) regularly.

_____ **10.** I have good hygiene and do not engage in risky sexual behaviors.

**Subtotal**

# Chapter 6    Communicable Diseases

_____ **1.** I can explain the difference between communicable and noncommunicable diseases.

_____ **2.** I have been inoculated for the childhood diseases as recommended by the American Academy of Pediatrics.

_____ **3.** I can explain the concepts of immunity and autoimmune diseases.

_____ **4.** I am able to name the classifications of pathogens.

_____ **5.** I understand the routes of invasion by pathogens and the body's defense mechanisms against them.

_____ **6.** I have an understanding of the most common sexually transmitted diseases and their symptoms.

_____ **7.** I understand the dynamics of HIV and AIDS and the particular risks for contracting this virus.

_____ **8.** If I have an STD, I intend to meet my responsibilities toward my sexual partners in preventing its spread.

_____ **9.** I am willing to be a support person for someone else with an STD by providing hot-line numbers and encouraging the person to seek help.

_____**10.** I can cite the trends in STD and AIDS infection.

**Subtotal**

# Chapter 7    Noncommunicable Diseases

_____ **1.** I am taking lifestyle steps to reduce my risk for developing cancer some time during my life.

_____ **2.** I can name seven warning signs of cancer.

_____ **3.** I periodically check my body for signs of skin cancer, especially if I am fair-skinned and have had at least one severe sunburn.

_____ **4.** I refrain from tanning (sun and artificial) and protect my skin from damage.

_____ **5.** I understand how allergies occur and what to do to combat them.

_____ **6.** I can explain the differences between Type I and Type II diabetes and how they are managed.

_____ **7.** I am aware of the deleterious effects of tobacco and do not use it or have taken steps to quit.

_____ **8.** I am familiar with the most prevalent blood disorders, their symptoms, diagnosis, and treatment.

_____ **9.** I am aware of the common skin conditions and how they are treated.

_____**10.** If I get tension headaches from stress, I am able to alleviate them through relaxation techniques.

**Subtotal**

# Chapter 8    Cardiovascular Diseases

_____ **1.** I am conversant on the trends in cardiovascular diseases over the years.

_____ **2.** I understand the role of lifestyle in cardiovascular disease.

_____ **3.** I am able to explain the heart and its functioning.

_____ **4.** I can cite the major risk factors for cardiovascular diseases.

_____ **5.** I am taking nutritional steps to lower my risk for developing heart disease.

_____ **6.** I can name some disorders of the heart, their symptoms, diagnosis, and treatment.

_____ **7.** I have had my blood pressure checked recently.

_____ **8.** I participate in aerobic exercise regularly to reduce the risk for incurring cardiovascular disease.

_____ **9.** I avoid cigarette smoking or, if I smoke, am taking steps to quit.

_____**10.** I stay within the guidelines for recommended weight.

**Subtotal**

## Chapter 9     The Basics of Nutrition

_____ **1.** I can cite the six basic nutrients.

_____ **2.** I understand the types of cholesterol and their roles in the body.

_____ **3.** I can explain the different types of fats and their effects on health.

_____ **4.** I know the role of protein and its major nutritional sources.

_____ **5.** I understand why water is considered the most valuable nutrient and drink plenty of it.

_____ **6.** I know the difference between fat-soluble and water-soluble vitamins and include each in my diet accordingly.

_____ **7.** I include sources of minerals in my diet.

_____ **8.** When shopping, I read and heed food labels.

_____ **9.** I use MyPyramid as my guide in eating a balanced diet.

_____**10.** I avoid fast-food restaurants most of the time.

**Subtotal**

## Chapter 10     Weight Management

_____ **1.** I understand the concepts of body composition and metabolism.

_____ **2.** I can explain setpoint theory.

_____ **3.** I know the differences between overweight and obesity.

_____ **4.** I refrain from fad diets and yo-yo dieting in favor of lifestyle habits including proper nutrition and exercise.

_____ **5.** I am not obsessed with being thin to the point where it jeopardizes my health.

_____ **6.** I can assess my body composition generally through the waist-to-hip ratio technique.

_____ **7.** I am able to calculate my caloric needs according to the basal metabolic rate (BMR) factor.

_____ **8.** I do not succumb to the lure of over-the-counter diet pills and short-cut exercise equipment to lose weight.

_____ **9.** If calipers are available, I am able to determine my body composition through the skinfold technique.

_____**10.** I recognize that weight management is a lifelong proposition and am developing habits toward that end.

**Subtotal**

## Chapter 11     Physical Activity and Health

_____ **1.** I can recite several physical and psychological benefits of exercise.

_____ **2.** When exercising, I always warm up and cool down sufficiently before and after.

_____ **3.** I know how to take my pulse and determine my maximal heart rate accordingly.

_____ **4.** I am able to determine my recovery heart rate.

_____ **5.** I can estimate how hard to exercise using the rate of perceived exertion.

_____ **6.** When exercising, I include stretching in the workout.

_____ 7. My exercise program balances cardiorespiratory and strength training.

_____ 8. I do not and would not take anabolic steroids.

_____ 9. I dress properly, including the correct shoes, when I exercise.

_____10. I am familiar with the most common exercise-related injuries and how they are to be treated.

**Subtotal**

## Chapter 12    Psychoactive Drugs and Medications

_____ 1. I do not use tobacco (either smoking or smokeless) or am taking steps to quit.

_____ 2. I am familiar with the health effects of using tobacco.

_____ 3. I am knowledgeable of current laws dealing with tobacco use.

_____ 4. If I drink alcohol at all, I do so in moderation.

_____ 5. I am aware of the chronic effects of alcohol on the body.

_____ 6. I never drive after drinking.

_____ 7. If someone else has been drinking in my presence, I offer to give him or her a ride instead of allowing him or her to drive.

_____ 8. I can go to a party and still have fun without drinking.

_____ 9. If I have even one drink, I do not take any medications.

_____10. I am aware of organizations dealing with alcoholism to which I can refer a friend if need be.

**Subtotal**

## Chapter 13    Tobacco and Alcohol

_____ 1. I understand the process by which drugs in general affect the brain.

_____ 2. I am able to debate the pros and cons of drug legalization.

_____ 3. I can describe the different routes by which drugs enter the body.

_____ 4. I am able to define and identify the various classifications of drugs and give examples of each.

_____ 5. I can identify the trends in drug use and can give some possible reasons.

_____ 6. I do not use marijuana.

_____ 7. If I drink coffee, I do so in moderation.

_____ 8. I do not use stimulants to stay awake and study for tests or finish assignments.

_____ 9. I follow the instructions when using over-the-counter and prescribed medications.

_____10. I have no difficulty saying no when drugs are offered to me.

**Subtotal**

## Chapter 14    Aging, Dying, and Death

_____ 1. I am able to discuss the trends and demographics of aging in the United States.

_____ 2. I can identify some of the impacts of aging on the body.

_____ 3. I am developing lifestyle habits now to counteract the ill effects of aging.

_____ 4. I do not smoke.

_____ **5.** If I use alcohol, I do so in moderation.

_____ **6.** I am looking ahead and planning financially for the future.

_____ **7.** When I have to face a loss, I recognize the stages of grief and do not hide from my feelings.

_____ **8.** I have a viable will.

_____ **9.** I am able to debate the pros and cons of doctor-assisted suicide.

_____**10.** I am sensitive to the needs of elderly people with whom I come in contact and help them in some way whenever the need presents itself.

**Subtotal**

## Chapter 15    Consumerism and Environmental Health

_____ **1.** I am a wise consumer, able to make wise purchases and not be fooled by fraudulent claims and products.

_____ **2.** I know how to access health care if I need it.

_____ **3.** I do not overuse over-the-counter medications.

_____ **4.** I have regular dental checkups.

_____ **5.** I avoid environmental pollutants when I can.

_____ **6.** I am aware of the effects of secondhand smoke and avoid smokers when I can.

_____ **7.** I do not abuse my ears by subjecting them to high-decibel music.

_____ **8.** I am cautious in using food additives and food products that may pose health risks.

_____ **9.** When I am sick, I consult a physician or clinic instead of trying to self-medicate.

_____**10.** I check expiration dates on products and do not use any whose date has expired.

**Subtotal**

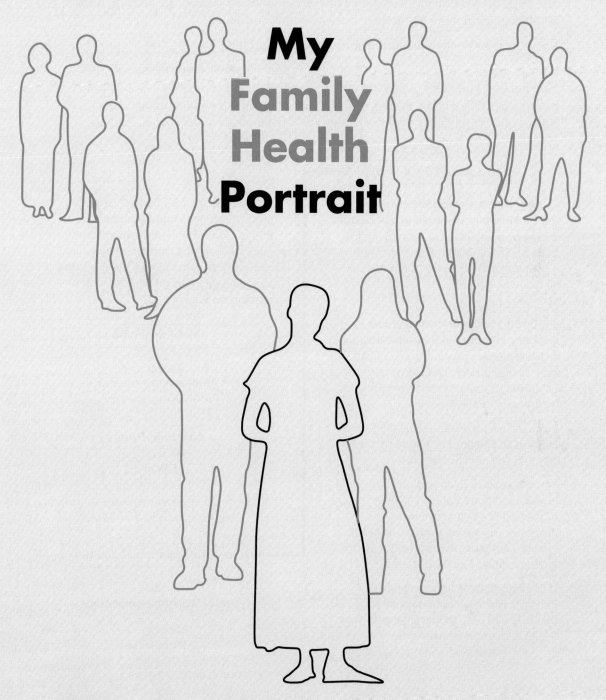

# My Family Health Portrait

# The Surgeon General's Family History Initiative

# THE SURGEON GENERAL'S FAMILY HISTORY INITIATIVE
## HOW TO CREATE MY FAMILY HEALTH PORTRAIT

The Surgeon General has launched a national initiative to encourage all American families to learn more about their family health histories.

Knowing your family's medical history can save your life.

With a copy of your family health history, you and a health care professional can individualize your care to prevent and screen for conditions for which you may be at higher risk. Family events, such as Thanksgiving or family reunions, offer a great chance to gather the information for "My Family Health Portrait."

### WHOM SHOULD I TALK WITH?

To get the most accurate health history information, it is important to talk directly with your relatives. Explain to them that their health information can help improve prevention and screening of diseases for all family members.

Start by asking your relatives about any health conditions they have had—including history of chronic illnesses, such as heart disease; pregnancy complications, such as miscarriage; and any developmental disabilities. Get as much specific information as possible.

It is most useful if you can list the formal name of any medical condition that has affected you or your relatives.

You can get help finding information about health conditions that have affected you or your family members—living or deceased—by asking relatives or health care professionals for information, or by getting copies of medical records.

If you are planning to have children, you and your partner should each create a family health portrait and show it to your health care professional.

Knowing your family health history is a powerful guide to understanding risk for disease. However, keep in mind that a family history of a particular illness may increase risk, but it almost never *guarantees* that other family members will develop the illness.

### Most Important

Parents
Brothers and Sisters
Your Children

### Also Important

Grandparents
Uncles and Aunts
Nieces and Nephews
Half-Brothers and Half-Sisters

### Obtain Information If You Can

Cousins
Great Uncles and Great Aunts

The "My Family Health Portrait" form will help you collect and organize your family information. No form can reflect every version of the American family, so use this chart as a starting point and adapt it to your family's needs.

First write each of your relatives' names in the designated boxes and circle whether they are male (M) or female (F). On the next line, write the name of any health conditions they have had. If you know the age at which they were diagnosed with a condition, write that in parentheses after the condition. For example: "diabetes (diagnosed—age 37)."

If family members have died, write "deceased" and the age at which they died. For example: "heart attack (deceased—age 63)."

For twins, write "twin" on the first line for both individuals. If the twins are identical, write "identical twin" on the first line for both.

If your family includes half brothers or half sisters, write "half brother" or "half sister" on the first line and note "different father" or "different mother" on the next line.

Some conditions are more common in people with a shared background or ancestry. It is important to record the ancestry of your relatives and be as specific as possible. For example, if you know that your grandmother is Hispanic and her family comes from Mexico, write "Mexican" underneath her name. Likewise, if your family is from Africa, Asia, Europe, or South America, note the country they came from, if possible.

Once you complete "My Family Health Portrait," take it to your health care professional so that he or she can better individualize your health care. Be sure to make a copy for your records and update it as circumstances change or you learn more about your family's health history.

Congratulations on taking this step toward a longer, healthier life! "My Family Health Portrait" can be an effective way to improve your health—today and in the future.

**CUT OUT AND ADD TO CHART AS NEEDED**

M
F

M
F

M
F

M
F

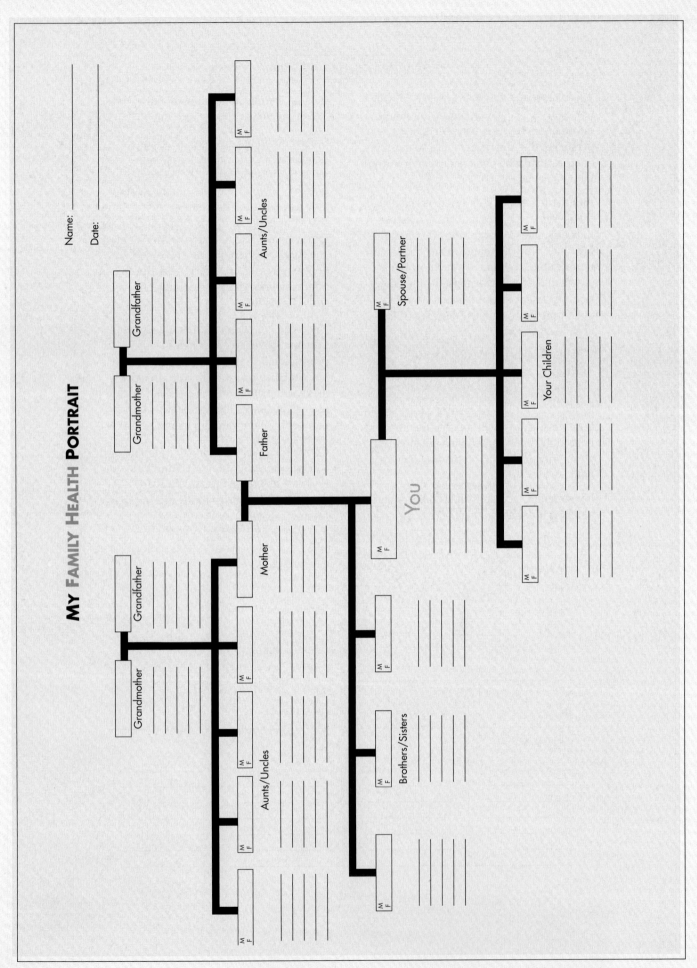

MY FAMILY HEALTH PORTRAIT

Name: _____

Date: _____

Grandfather

Grandmother

Aunts/Uncles

Father

Grandfather

Grandmother

Aunts/Uncles

Mother

You

Brothers/Sisters

Spouse/Partner

Your Children

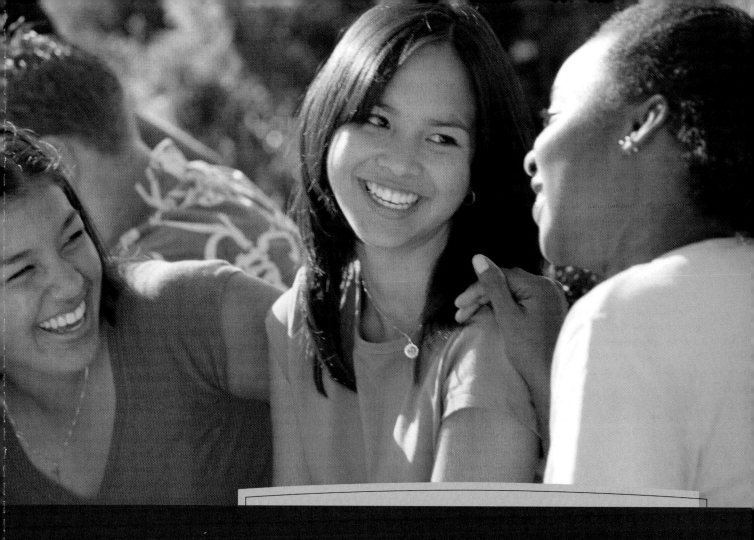

© SW Production/Brand X Pictures/Jupiterimages

# Chapter Two Personality and Emotional Health

**OBJECTIVES** ■ Define personality. ■ Explain psychoanalytic theory. ■ Identify the main premise of developmental psychology. ■ Describe the cultural differences in interpersonal needs. ■ Identify the levels in Maslow's hierarchy of needs. ■ Identify the personality types and their relation to emotional health. ■ Explain the toxic core and its components. ■ Cite the attributes of emotional health. ■ Describe various emotional disorders. ■ Differentiate the health practitioners who diagnose and treat emotional and mental disorders. ■ Identify barriers to seeking diagnosis and treatment. ■ Identify one reliable source for information about depression that offers depression screening.

ThomsonNOW™ Log on to ThomsonNOW at http://thomsonedu.com/thomsonnow to access and explore self-assessments, interactive tutorials, and practice quizzes.

Humans are all alike in many ways, yet each person is uniquely different, with a distinct personality. Each individual is the author of his or her life's performance, or production. People develop not just biologically but also through their interaction with physical, social, and spiritual environments. Each day is different from the day before, and each interaction is a learning experience. Interactions allow individuals to meet their physical and emotional needs.

**Personality** includes all the traits—mental processes, feelings, and behaviors—that influence how a person deals with the realities of the world. More than 100 personality variables (predispositions to behave and respond in certain ways to certain situations) have been identified. Personality is not static. It is influenced by many internal and external factors, including environment, culture, heredity, and socialization by institutions including family, church, school, and peer groups.

## Theories of Personality

Various theories have been set forth in an attempt to explain why people are the way they are. Among these theories are psychoanalytic, behavioral, developmental, and humanistic.

### PSYCHOANALYTIC THEORY

Sigmund Freud is the father of psychoanalytic theory, or **psychoanalysis,** a branch of **psychology** based on the concept of the human **psyche.** These terms are derived from Greek mythology, in which Psyche was a princess loved by Cupid. In Greek, psyche means "soul."

Freud defined three facets of the psyche: the **id,** the **ego,** and the **superego.** He emphasized early childhood events and the **libido** as major forces propelling a person throughout life. Freudian theory has had a major influence on professional disciplines including medicine, through its branch of psychiatry; education; and sociology and social work, among others.

### BEHAVIORAL PSYCHOLOGY

With the advent of **behavioral psychology,** the field of psychology branched off in a different direction. In the view of its originator, B. F. Skinner, all behavior is learned. Human actions can be explained in terms of **stimuli.** Through conditioning, desired behaviors can be learned through rewards, and undesirable behaviors can be extinguished through punishment.

Behavioral psychology, then, explains behavior as being a product of external forces, not a consequence of processes in the mind. It relies on tangible, quantifiable measures instead of subjective interpretations. For example, in attempting to reduce the number of a child's tantrums, a behaviorist might count the number of tantrums in a given time and note the increase or decrease in tantrums as measured against aversive (negative) reinforcement.

### DEVELOPMENTAL PSYCHOLOGY

Another branch of psychology focuses on the stages in life and the necessity of completing certain **developmental tasks** to achieve a complete personality and emotional health. Among adherents of this theory was Erik Erikson. From the psychoanalytic theory of his mentor, Freud, he advanced a broader social and cultural perspective. He also emphasized successful psychological development as opposed to the abnormal personality, as Freud did.

Erikson postulated that human development throughout the life span proceeds through eight stages, each characterized by a crisis to be resolved. Successful resolution of the conflict enables the person to advance to the next stage. Erikson's stages are shown in Figure 2.1.

From birth to age one the conflict to be resolved is trust versus mistrust. An infant who is fed and comforted will more likely develop trust than one who is not. In the toddler stage the dilemma centers on the need to explore and gain independence, offset by frequent self-doubt. This conflict is well illustrated by the "terrible twos." During the preschool stage the child develops a conscience, alternating between taking initiative and harboring guilt. During the elementary school ages the child develops a newfound appreciation for accomplishment, often negated by feelings of insecurity when he or she does not succeed.

Adolescence is marked by identity confusion: Who am I? Ideally resolved by adulthood, this crisis is replaced by one involving the balance of needs for intimacy and for "my own space." By middle age the person is conflicted by altruistic motivations in being a parent and doing community work versus maintaining one's own creativity, which essentially requires self-centeredness.

Toward the end of the lifespan, if the person has advanced developmentally through each of the previous phases, the task to be resolved centers on integrity versus despair, a time when the person has to affirm the value of life and its ideals. People at this stage reflect on their life and assess what they have done. Successful resolution of this stage brings a sense of contentment and fulfillment.

Sometimes a person becomes stuck at a stage. For example, a certain amount of self-love, or narcissism, is healthy, but if a person does not develop empathy or the ability to give of self, he or she may not be able to develop satisfying intimate relationships. According to Erikson, then, to be psychologically healthy means resolving issues successfully at each of the eight stages.

**FIGURE 2.1 ▶** Erikson's Developmental Conflict Stages

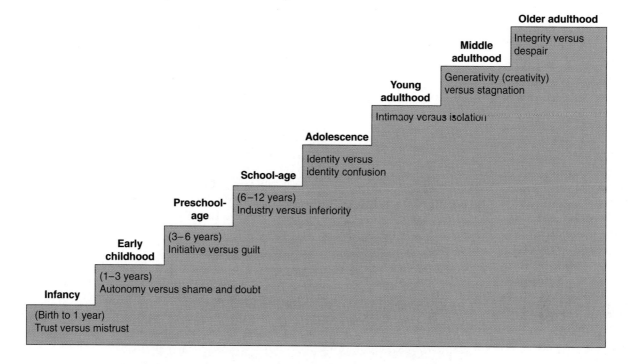

**Older adulthood**

Integrity versus despair

**Middle adulthood**

Generativity (creativity) versus stagnation

**Young adulthood**

Intimacy versus isolation

**Adolescence**

Identity versus identity confusion

**School-age**

(6–12 years)
Industry versus inferiority

**Preschool-age**

(3–6 years)
Initiative versus guilt

**Early childhood**

(1–3 years)
Autonomy versus shame and doubt

**Infancy**

(Birth to 1 year)
Trust versus mistrust

## HUMANISTIC PSYCHOLOGY

**Humanistic psychology** is based on humanism, a philosophy that asserts the dignity and worth of individuals and their capacity for self-realization. One well-known contributor to humanistic psychology was Carl Rogers, through his **client-centered therapy.** The person most often associated with this branch of psychology, however, is Abraham Maslow.

**Maslow's Hierarchy of Needs.** Maslow developed the hierarchy of needs depicted in Figure 2.2. Like Erikson, Maslow proposed a series of stages, each building on the previous one. Unlike Erikson, however, Maslow saw a person's climb toward the top as less age-related and as fluctuating between stages depending on the circumstances in the person's life.

The first level of needs, according to Maslow, is physiological. These needs include air, water, food, shelter, sleep, sex, and survival. Once these needs are fulfilled, the person develops a need for safety and security; that is, to be protected from harm. After those needs have been met, the person looks for social acceptance and belonging, love and affection. Positive self-esteem (or ego fulfillment in the Freudian schema) hinges on these needs being met. The ultimate level is **self-actualization.** People at this stage accept reality, themselves, and others; are both independent and creative; appreciate people and the world around them; and have vitality.

### KEY TERMS

**Personality** the total of all individual characteristics that make each person unique

**Psychoanalysis** literally, "analyzing the psyche"

**Psychology** the study of the human psyche

**Psyche** all conscious and unconscious mental functions (Freud)

**Id** the part of the psyche that seeks pleasure and satisfaction of basic drives

**Ego** the part of the psyche that controls and regulates basic drives

**Superego** internal voice or conscience; determines acceptable and unacceptable behavior

**Libido** sex drive

**Behavioral psychology** theory holding that all behavior is learned

**Stimuli** external agents that incite responses

**Developmental tasks** work to be done at various stages in a person's life (Erikson)

**Humanistic psychology** theory that behavior is motivated by a desire for personal growth and achievement

**Client-centered therapy** a focus on clients and their beliefs and needs as more important than the counselor's (Rogers)

**Self-actualization** fulfillment of one's potential

**FIGURE 2.2** ▶ Maslow's Hierarchy of Needs

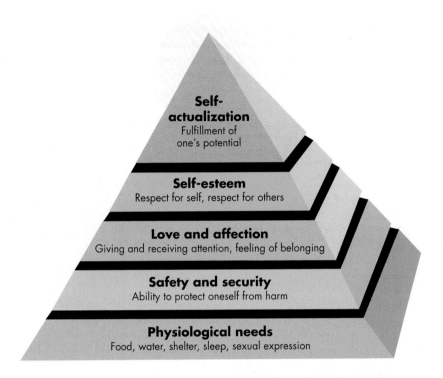

**Schutz's Interpersonal Needs.**    Psychologist William Schutz theorized that every person has three categories of **interpersonal needs** that can be met only through interaction with other people. Whereas Maslow's categories included physical needs, Schutz addressed only psychological needs. In his schema they are inclusion, control, and affection.

The inclusion need emphasizes the drive to establish and maintain satisfactory relationships. The control need is met by attaining influence, power, leadership, authority, intellectual superiority, high achievement, and independence. The need for affection goes beyond inclusion and refers to intimacy, a topic explored further in Chapter 4. Schutz developed the FIRO-B (Fundamental Interpersonal Relations Orientation-Behavior) scale to measure the extent to which these three needs are being met in a person.

Cultural differences appear in Schutz's interpersonal needs. According to intercultural expert Donald Klopf, Americans have much stronger inclusion needs than the Japanese, Koreans, Chinese, Micronesians, and Australians. One reason may relate to family life. The Asians, Micronesians, and Australians maintain stronger family bonds, and family relationships are close, satisfying their needs for inclusion, control, and affection. Americans are acculturated to be more independent. Children are encouraged to leave home sooner and are trained to assume larger roles in society. Therefore, Americans are more likely to have unmet interpersonal needs and look for nonfamily individuals and groups to fulfill these needs.

## Personality Types

In recent years the connection between personality and health has received much attention. Most researchers now seem to accept the concept of an **immune-competent personality.** Likewise, researchers continue to investigate the **disease-prone personality.**

### TYPE A, TYPE B, AND TYPE C PERSONALITIES

During the 1950s Dr. Meyer Friedman and Dr. Ray Rosenman studied risk factors that could lead to coronary heart disease. These doctors coined the term **Type A personality** to describe people who were impatient, quick-tempered, hard-driven, aggressive, and ambitious. Type As developed heart attacks in greater numbers than people without that constellation of traits.

More recent research by Duke University researcher Redford Williams and others identified one facet of the Type A personality—antagonistic hostility—as the factor most associated with risk for heart disease. The other characteristics, such as competitiveness and impatience, seem to be less dangerous.

Stemming from this finding is the concept of the **toxic core,** a group of traits that are most poisonous to physical health. The most toxic traits are believed to be

1. Cynical beliefs that others are bad, selfish, mean, and untrustworthy.

---

**Tips for Action** How to Blow Off Anger the Healthy Way

■ Recognize anger for what it is. Do not be afraid of it or try to suppress it.

■ Figure out what made you so angry—then figure out whether it is worth being so upset about.

■ Stop before you act. Calm down first. Take a deep breath. Then get ready to deal with the anger.

■ If you are angry at another person, stay calm while explaining why. Try to negotiate.

■ Try to understand where the other person is coming from.

■ When all else fails, forgive the other person. Everyone makes mistakes, and carrying a grudge will hurt you more than anyone else.

---

2. Frequent angry feelings when these negative feelings arise.

3. Aggressive acts toward others when these angry feelings arise.

Type As may be at greater risk for heart disease because their bodies make unusually small amounts of high density lipoprotein (HDL) cholesterol ("good cholesterol"), according to Dr. Michael Miller, director of preventive cardiology at the University of Maryland. He cautions, however, that the association between these variables does not prove a cause-and-effect relationship.

Anger and hostility are not the same. Everyone experiences **anger.** It is a temporary emotion that can range from exasperation to intense rage. In contrast, **hostility** is an ongoing accumulation of irritation, a chronic form of anger. The Latin term *hostis* means "enemy." For hostile people, enemies seem to be everywhere—in the classroom, on the elevator, in the supermarket checkout line, on the freeway, in the next apartment. Hostility is marked by lack of trust in people in general and the belief that others are "out to get me."

Because of the health-damaging effects of hostility, people become their own worst enemy. The mechanism that translates emotions into physical problems is

explained in Chapter 3, along with the physical consequences of stress-related hostility.

Researchers have identified two other personality types: a **Type B personality** and a Type C personality. Type Bs are calm, casual, relaxed, and easy-going. The term "laid-back" is often applied to them. They take one thing at a time, are not bothered by pressures, and do not get agitated. The **Type C personality,** also known as the cancer-prone personality, describes people who are likely to have had hostile relationships with one or both parents, a bleak childhood, and feelings of loneliness and isolation.

---

**VIEWPOINT** *Are You Type A, Type B, or Type C? Which personality type do you think you are? Are you satisfied with your personality? Do you believe personality types can be changed? Why or why not?*

---

**KEY TERMS**

**Interpersonal needs** a theory proposing that all humans have three basic psychologial needs—inclusion, control, and affection

**Immune-competent personality** personality that enables a person to handle pressure without becoming ill

**Disease-prone personality** personality that tends toward illness

**Type A personality** characterized by being impatient, aggressive, ambitious, hot-tempered, and hard-driving; has higher risk for heart disease

**Toxic core** group of personality traits most detrimental to physical health; cynicism, frequent anger, and aggression

**Anger** temporary emotion that combines physiological and emotional arousal; can range from mild irritation to intense rage

**Hostility** chronic form of anger characterized by lack of trust in others

**Type B personality** characterized by being calm, casual, and relaxed

**Type C personality** characterized by those who are easily distressed but do not express their hostility

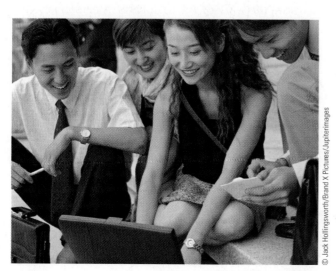

© Jack Hollingsworth/Brand X Pictures/Jupiterimages

▲ *The drive for achievement is a strong interpersonal need*

## Tips for Action How to Boost Your Optimism

- Surround yourself with optimistic people so you will begin to catch their attitude.
- Try to genuinely like all sorts of people, regardless of ethnic and cultural differences.
- Be patient with yourself.
- Get past disappointments and look at these as challenges.
- Set small, attainable goals. Reward yourself when you meet those goals.

- Look beyond yourself. Become other-centered.
- Gather all the facts before you form a conclusion. Be open-minded. Stretch your thinking.
- Face your problems and develop strategies for solving them instead of trying to escape them.
- Have fun and relax. Learn to laugh at yourself, enjoy yourself, and respect yourself.

**TABLE 2.1 ▶** Comparison of Type A, Type B, and Type C Personalities

| TYPE A | TYPE B | TYPE C |
|---|---|---|
| Is hard-driving | Is easy-going | Is passive |
| Is highly competitive | Is cooperative | Acquiesces readily |
| Tends to interrupt others | Listens well | Is apologetic |
| Is hurried, impatient | Is content to wait | Is overly nice, accepting |
| Tends to anger quickly | Is laid-back | Is overanxious, painfully sensitive |

These individuals often have made one or more strong emotional commitments to someone or something, only to be disappointed or rejected. They are overly anxious to please, unassertive, and overly cooperative. A consistent descriptor is "too nice." Some studies have shown a link between the Type C personality and cancer. Among several theories is one suggesting that how a person copes with cancer has a bearing on its outcome. People who face cancer with determination to beat it tend to outlive those who accept the prognosis and acquiesce—that is, the Type C. The personality types are compared in Table 2.1.

### EXPLANATORY STYLE

**Explanatory style** is a habitual way of thinking. The two major styles are pessimistic and optimistic. The pessimistic explanatory style has three thought patterns.

1. Assuming that a problem is never-ending; it will never go away.
2. Believing the problem affects everything and is not just an isolated incident.
3. Internalizing everything ("It's my fault"), often placing the wrong blame at the wrong time.

Explanatory style has an extremely powerful influence on health and wellness. A negative explanatory style affects both emotional and physical well-being, and it can lead to anxiety, depression, guilt, anger, and hostility.

In contrast, an optimistic explanatory style promotes emotional and physical health. Optimistic people tend to have a sense of personal control. They also have outgoing personalities. In study after study, **extroverts** report greater happiness and satisfaction with life than **introverts.** Extroverted people are more involved with people. They have a larger circle of friends.

### LOCUS OF CONTROL

The concept of **locus of control** originated several years ago with the work of Julian Roberts. A person is somewhere along a continuum. At one end of the continuum is the external locus of control. At the opposite end is the internal locus of control (see Figure 2.3). People with an external locus of control believe that the things that happen to them are unrelated to their own behavior and, therefore, are beyond their control. People with an internal locus of control believe that negative events are a

**FIGURE 2.3 ▶** Locus of Control Continuum

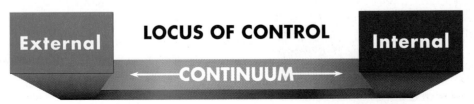

**Tips for Action** How to Overcome Shyness

■ Improve your social skills by introducing yourself at a party. Then ask questions of the other person and let him or her do most of the talking. Listening is a valued skill.

■ Take part in discussions with small groups of people with whom you are comfortable. This should enable you to gain confidence so you eventually can branch out to other discussion groups.

■ Take an assertiveness-training class or a public-speaking course.

■ Join a club in which you are interested, and volunteer to be on a committee.

■ Always try to think positively about yourself.

consequence of personal actions and thus potentially can be controlled.

The results of a host of studies show the importance of control. As a whole, people with greater sense of control are at less risk for illness. Scientists are realizing that an internal locus of control has an even more profound role in protecting health than they once thought.

Former *Saturday Review* editor Norman Cousins, renowned for his work linking attitudes and health, maintained that, in general, "anything that restores a sense of control to a patient can be a profound aid to a physician treating serious illness." That sense of control is more than a mere mood or attitude. It may be a vital pathway among the brain, the endocrine system, and the immune system (see Chapter 3).

## SHYNESS

Shyness is a personality trait. It may have its roots in low self-worth, lack of social skills, or even heredity. Shy people usually avoid speaking up in public and in social gatherings. They avoid attention. Although it should not mistakenly be assumed that all shy people are unhappy or maladjusted, shyness in some cases can lead to loneliness or depression.

## Assessing Personality

Sometimes an assessment of personality is helpful when personality variables are being related to other areas, such as education, counseling, and career satisfaction. One such scale was developed by Andrew L. Comrey. The Comrey Personality Scale is a self-administering instrument consisting of 180 items, 20 per scale, for each of eight personality dimensions. These are trust versus defensiveness, orderliness versus lack of compulsion, social conformity versus rebelliousness, activity versus lack of energy, emotional stability versus neuroticism, extroversion versus introversion, masculinity versus femininity, and empathy versus egocentrism.

Another widely used personality scale is the Myers-Briggs Type Indicator. Katherine Briggs and, later, Isabel Briggs Myers and her husband, Clarence Myers, expanded Carl Jung's theories of people's inclinations and preferences for dealing with life. Their 16-box matrix consists of the personality variables of extroversion versus introversion, sensing versus intuition, thinking versus feeling, and judging versus perception. Combining the four preferred modes, the result is a person who is, for example, introverted, intuitive, feeling, and perceptive in style. Each of these styles can be related to work environments, optimal relationships, and learning style, among other practical applications.

## Emotional Health

Emotional health has been described as the capacity to live life to its fullest in ways that enable a person to realize his or her own potential. Emotional health begins with a person's true understanding of how he or she feels about himself or herself.

Emotionally healthy people have high **self-esteem.** A person with high self-esteem has confidence, a sense of positive self-regard, and belief in self. Self-esteem has been called the blueprint for behavior, as it guides what a person thinks he or she can do and thus a person's striving toward goals.

## KEY TERMS

**Explanatory style** the way people perceive the events in their lives— optimistic or pessimistic

**Extrovert** an outgoing personality

**Introvert** a reflective, inner-centered personality

**Locus of control** a concept in personality theory based on a person's perception of control, whether internal or external factors are more controlling

**Self-esteem** a way of looking at oneself; may be high or low

**VIEWPOINT** *Norman Cousins, former editor of the* Saturday Review *and member of the University of California at Los Angeles medical faculty, twice intrigued the medical community and the public alike by overcoming a massive heart attack and a degenerative spinal disease. Cousins followed his physician's regimen each time but also surrounded himself with positive people, positive emotions, and laughter. He was healed by modern medicine as well as by love, hope, faith, confidence, and a tremendous will to live. How can emotions and laughter heal a person?* **What is your opinion?**

Much research attests to the value of healthy self-esteem to overall health, both mental and physical. It can boost the immune system, protect against disease, and aid in healing. It often has a bearing on whether people do or do not get sick and, if they do, how long they stay sick. Some evidence, for example, shows that recovery from mononucleosis is related to ego strength; the higher the self-esteem, the more rapid the recovery.

Emotionally healthy people are constantly reassessing their identity through life. They develop a sense of the vast opportunities and liberties available to them to fulfill their needs and aspirations. On the one hand, they have the capacity to love. On the other hand, they have the ability to deal with loss. At the forefront of emotionally healthy individuals is to feel good about themselves, their relationships with others, their vocation, and their recreational activities. On many occasions emotionally healthy people experience happiness and fulfillment to a height of ecstasy. At other times they experience heartaches, pain, sadness, disappointments. Emotionally healthy people are better equipped to pull themselves out, to bounce back, or get over a bad experience.

Furthermore, emotionally healthy people take responsibility for their behaviors, their feelings, and their actions. They work at solving problems with a positive attitude. They do not dwell on negative aspects of the past, other than to learn from them. These individuals solve problems as they arise and also make long-range plans, accept new experiences, make individual and independent decisions, and set realistic goals for themselves.

Underpinnings of emotional health include

- A true perception of reality
- Adaptation to change
- Social relationships
- Job satisfaction
- Recreational satisfaction
- Spirituality

## A TRUE PERCEPTION OF REALITY

Emotionally healthy people are able to face reality whether it is pleasant or unpleasant. They cope with the problems they encounter instead of escaping and retreating to drug misuse and abuse or overindulgence in food or sex.

## ADAPTATION TO CHANGE

Emotionally healthy people realize that nothing is absolute or unchangeable. Adaptable people deal with life as they find it and do not expect it to change at a whim. Though individuals often become secure in familiar situations and environments, emotionally healthy people adapt to changing circumstances when necessary. They have a continuous and positive interest in what goes on around them. They realize that the world is a special place to inhabit—even though it can stand some improvement.

## SOCIAL RELATIONSHIPS

People learn early that much satisfaction is derived from communicating and associating with other people. Most people want the approval of other people. They have a strong need for love and acceptance. Social relationships range from familial relationships to romantic and sexual unions to platonic acquaintances and classmates. In keeping with Maslow's theory, people have a strong need and desire for love and belonging. The ability to form satisfying relationships develops early in life. Ideally, children receive love and acceptance from their parents, relatives, and other caring, giving adults. From this they learn how to develop positive social relationships.

## VOCATIONAL SATISFACTION

To be productive and efficient in one's chosen vocation is another indicator of emotional health. When setting vocational goals, young people often have difficulty recognizing attainable career goals. Each person should take into consideration his or her abilities and limitations. Further, each person should realize that he or she must expend effort to reach goals. The constantly changing workplace demands continuous professional growth and flexibility.

## RECREATIONAL SATISFACTION

A prime indicator of emotional health is the enjoyment of constructive activities other than work. Recreational activities may consist of sports, traveling, hunting and fishing, dancing, cooking, reading, gardening, enjoying music and other art forms, and many others. Recreation can play a vital role in a person's life. If done with others, it allows people to meet, know, understand, and appreciate others. Involvement in outdoor recreation promotes physical health and heightens appreciation of the environment.

The World Health Organization (WHO) is often known as the international agency with the mission to eliminate, or at least control, communicable diseases around the world. According to research conducted by WHO, mental and neurological disorders, including Alzheimer's disease, epilepsy, anxiety disorders, and depression, affect 400 million people worldwide, and the numbers are rising. In an effort to reverse this trend, WHO in 2001 developed a yearlong campaign called "Stop Exclusion—Dare to Care." According to José Caldas de Almeida, Ph.D., coordinator of mental health programs for the Pan American Health Organization, the campaign is designed to reach people around the world to raise awareness (about mental health and the effective drug treatments and interventions that are available) through political initiatives, speeches, and cultural activities. The goal is to erase the stigma of mental illness so that people will seek the appropriate intervention.

## SPIRITUALITY

**Spirituality** is not just a covenant, doctrine, ritual, or ceremonial activity in a church, storefront church, synagogue, mosque, temple, altar, or place of worship. It is an extremely individual thought, feeling, or personal experience. Spirituality grows out of individual needs, often during times of crisis—sickness, sorrow, despair, failures, injustices. Spirituality teaches respect for one's existence, respect for others, and allows people to align what is best in them against what is worst in them. It is tied to forgiveness, altruism, volunteerism, hope, faith, empathy, and love.

Faith and spiritual belief can nurture a person throughout life—from the modest beginning to the complex end. Spirituality can bestow wisdom and strengthen virtue. It can surround one with effective tools for protection. Although belief in a higher power can offer positive and helpful support, spirituality can leave many questions unanswered and many needs unmet. Spirituality does not make people certain, comfortable, and sure about everything. It does not relieve people from the duty of thought. Spirituality leads an individual to ask questions and think about actions and consequences. It empowers the individual, boosts creative energy, and fosters inner peace and harmony.

A person's spiritual state can contribute to emotional health and help a person to deal with health problems. Spirituality plays an important role in the way an individual responds to illness and other stressors. Meditation and prayer are demonstrably effective tools for managing stress and anxiety. Faith may provide the boost of emotional strength a person needs in difficult situations.

## Mental/Emotional Disorders

According to the National Mental Health Association, 54 million individuals have mental health disorders. Approximately 50,000 to 60,000 people reside in mental hospitals, and other people with emotional disabilities are found among the nursing home and homeless populations. Although precise numbers are not obtainable, the recorded statistics provide some indication of the prevalence of emotional disturbances at any given time. These numbers ebb and flow, as emotional disturbance is not a static condition.

The American Psychiatric Association (APA) has classified and updated its definitions of emotional disorders in the *Diagnostic and Statistical Manual of Mental Disorders* (DSM–IV). The representative categories discussed here are

- Schizophrenia and Other Psychotic Disorders
- Anxiety Disorders
- Mood Disorders

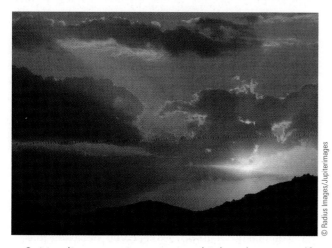

▲ *Spirituality recognizes a power higher than oneself*

© Radius Images/Jupiterimages

### KEY TERMS

**Spirituality** a belief in a power higher than oneself and a faith that affirms one's life

**VIEWPOINT** *Mental illness is the second leading cause of disability in the United States. One out of five Americans experiences a mental disorder. Why is there such a stigma attached to mental illness? What can you do to promote your personal mental health and advocate for others?*

## SCHIZOPHRENIA

Deterioration in functioning is a mark of **schizophrenia.** The person's thought processes are disorganized, and conversations may seem illogical and hard to follow. Social relationships, performance at school and work, and personal appearance may decline noticeably. The schizophrenic person may exhibit inappropriate facial expressions or emotions and display psychomotor disturbances such as rapid pacing or rocking movements. Thought disturbances include delusions of being grand, important, or able to save the world. Perceptual disturbances encompass auditory, visual, and tactile hallucinations.

Theories as to the cause of schizophrenia include a congenital or stress-induced biochemical imbalance, family environment, prenatal infection, and a family history of mental illness. A study published in *Schizophrenia Bulletin* reports evidence showing that the condition is linked to infections of the fetus. In one finding, 20% of the members of a cohort in New York City whose mothers had German measles (rubella) were diagnosed with adult schizophrenia (a 10- to 20-fold increased risk). Exposure to influenza during the first and second trimesters was associated with a three-fold increased risk of schizophrenia and a seven-fold risk if the prenatal exposure occurred during the first trimester. Prenatal exposure to the protozoa that causes toxoplasmosis was associated with a 2½-fold increase in risk. Other research published in this journal reports genetic links to schizophrenia and bipolar disorder.

Schizophrenic disorders range from mild to severe and may affect up to 2 million Americans. These disorders should be diagnosed and treated promptly and professionally by a psychiatrist. This may be done on an outpatient basis, or it may require hospitalization. Treatment may consist of antipsychotic medications and support therapy for the affected person as well as family members.

## ANXIETY DISORDERS

**Anxiety disorders** are characterized by alarm, fear, or even terror that certain circumstances evoke in a person. If a circumstance poses a serious threat or a real danger, being afraid is a natural response. The human life span would be shorter if people did not learn what situations or circumstances were dangerous and take action to avoid

them. Individuals with anxiety disorders, however, experience feelings of fear or anxiety in the presence of things or situations that do not cause anxiety for most people. To reduce the anxiety the perceived threat causes, these people tend to avoid the situation that precipitates it. Examples of anxiety disorder are phobias, panic disorder, obsessive compulsive disorder (OCD), and post-traumatic stress disorder (PTSD). Recent research suggests that anxiety disorders are related to abnormal activation of a small structure of the brain (the amygdala) that coordinates the fear response.

**Panic Attack.** The **panic attack** as described by the DSM-IV is an individually distinct period of intense discomfort or fear with four or more specific symptoms that develop without warning and peak (usually) within 10 minutes. Panic attacks may occur within the context of the other anxiety disorders described in this section. People who have had panic attacks sometimes describe their feelings as claustrophobic. The person may sense impending doom and the need to escape. Physical and mental symptoms include sweating, feeling dizzy, rapid heartbeat, breathing difficulties (as if one is suffocating or choking), chills or hot flashes, fear of losing control, and mental confusion.

These episodes can occur while shopping at the grocery store or mall, while driving or riding in a car, or even when the person is alone. Some people can anticipate the onset of a panic attack and avoid the situations that most likely will trigger it; others cannot. The most common age of onset is the late teen years and early twenties. According to the National Institutes of Mental Health, only one in every three people with panic attack is diagnosed and treated correctly.

**Obsessive Compulsive Disorder.** The USA Network television private investigator Adrian Monk (portrayed by actor Tony Shalhoub) is the personification of **obsessive compulsive disorder (OCD).** However, unlike Monk, most people with OCD do not have an assistant to help them with their recurrent obsessions and compulsions, which are so time consuming that they take more than an hour a day and affect the person's productivity. At this point obsession becomes a problem, causing distress and impairment. Common obsessions include repeated thoughts of contamination (becoming contaminated by shaking hands), repeated doubts (wondering if the car door is locked), the need to place things in a particular order (becoming anxious or distressed if objects are not symmetrical or in order by color), and aggressive impulses (screaming profanity at a funeral) or horrific impulses and thoughts. Extreme obsessive thoughts might be to think repeatedly of killing or hurting a dearly loved or highly respected person, for example.

Compulsive behavior is repeated behavior that is engaged by a person to reduce anxiety or stress. The

The World Health Organization (WHO) is often known as the international agency with the mission to eliminate, or at least control, communicable diseases around the world. According to research conducted by WHO, mental and neurological disorders, including Alzheimer's disease, epilepsy, anxiety disorders, and depression, affect 400 million people worldwide, and the numbers are rising. In an effort to reverse this trend, WHO in 2001 developed a yearlong campaign called "Stop Exclusion—Dare to Care." According to José Caldas de Almeida, Ph.D., coordinator of mental health programs for the Pan American Health Organization, the campaign is designed to reach people around the world to raise awareness (about mental health and the effective drug treatments and interventions that are available) through political initiatives, speeches, and cultural activities. The goal is to erase the stigma of mental illness so that people will seek the appropriate intervention.

## SPIRITUALITY

**Spirituality** is not just a covenant, doctrine, ritual, or ceremonial activity in a church, storefront church, synagogue, mosque, temple, altar, or place of worship. It is an extremely individual thought, feeling, or personal experience. Spirituality grows out of individual needs, often during times of crisis—sickness, sorrow, despair, failures, injustices. Spirituality teaches respect for one's existence, respect for others, and allows people to align what is best in them against what is worst in them. It is tied to forgiveness, altruism, volunteerism, hope, faith, empathy, and love.

Faith and spiritual belief can nurture a person throughout life—from the modest beginning to the complex end. Spirituality can bestow wisdom and strengthen virtue. It can surround one with effective tools for protection. Although belief in a higher power can offer positive and helpful support, spirituality can leave many questions unanswered and many needs unmet. Spirituality does not make people certain, comfortable, and sure about everything. It does not relieve people from the duty of thought. Spirituality leads an individual to ask questions and think about actions and consequences. It empowers the individual, boosts creative energy, and fosters inner peace and harmony.

A person's spiritual state can contribute to emotional health and help a person to deal with health problems. Spirituality plays an important role in the way an individual responds to illness and other stressors. Meditation and prayer are demonstrably effective tools for managing stress and anxiety. Faith may provide the boost of emotional strength a person needs in difficult situations.

## Mental/Emotional Disorders

According to the National Mental Health Association, 54 million individuals have mental health disorders. Approximately 50,000 to 60,000 people reside in mental hospitals, and other people with emotional disabilities are found among the nursing home and homeless populations. Although precise numbers are not obtainable, the recorded statistics provide some indication of the prevalence of emotional disturbances at any given time. These numbers ebb and flow, as emotional disturbance is not a static condition.

The American Psychiatric Association (APA) has classified and updated its definitions of emotional disorders in the *Diagnostic and Statistical Manual of Mental Disorders* (DSM–IV). The representative categories discussed here are

- Schizophrenia and Other Psychotic Disorders
- Anxiety Disorders
- Mood Disorders

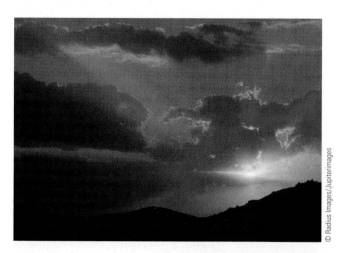

© Radius Images/Jupiterimages

▲ *Spirituality recognizes a power higher than oneself*

### KEY TERMS

**Spirituality** a belief in a power higher than oneself and a faith that affirms one's life

person using these behaviors (checking, hand washing, ordering) or mental acts (counting, praying, repeating a mantra) does not derive pleasure or gratification from them. People who are compulsive are driven emotionally to repeat acts that other people view as unnecessary and a waste of time. Classic examples of compulsive behavior are repeated hand washing and an intense need for order and cleanliness. Returning many times to the dormitory to ensure that the door to the room is secured and locked is another example of compulsive behavior.

**Post-Traumatic Stress Disorder.** In the wake of September 11, 2001 ("9/11"), and the devastation caused by hurricanes Katrina and Rita in 2005 to the city of New Orleans and the Gulf Coasts of Louisiana, Mississippi, and Alabama, post-traumatic stress disorder is an emotional health condition that is experienced by thousands of people and their families. According to the National Mental Health Association, 5.2 million American adults (18 to 54 years old) have the condition **post-traumatic stress disorder (PTSD)** during the course of a year.

A person with post-traumatic stress disorder replays a traumatic event again and again in his or her mind. The person may have been a victim, for example, of rape, incest, or some other type of sexual assault. Survivors of natural disasters, combat (30% of Vietnam War veterans, 8% of Persian Gulf War veterans, and 26% of soldiers returning from Iraq and Afghanistan), automobile accidents, as well as rescue personnel and people who witness a traumatic event may develop PTSD. Victims of social violence such as physical assault, car-jackings, gay bashing, or cross burning may develop this condition. These individuals keep reliving the traumatic event and dream about the trauma. When encountering a situation, being in an environment similar to the one involved in the trauma, or on the anniversary of the traumatic event, the person may become mentally and physically distressed, experience "flashbacks," and have nightmares. Other symptoms include problems sleeping, irritability, and depression. To cope, he or she avoids conversations that remind him or her of the traumatic event.

In response to the needs of soldiers who have participated in Operations Enduring Freedom and Iraqi Freedom (returning from the war in Afghanistan and Iraq), as well as their families, friends, and employers, the National Mental Health Association, the Department of Veterans Affairs, AMVETS (American Veterans), and the Reserve Officers Association (ROA) have partnered to establish the program *Operation Healthy Reunions*. This program distributes educational materials on reuniting with spouses and adjusting after the war, depression, PTSD, and toll-free telephone numbers and Web addresses to immediately access health resources.

PTSD may be diagnosed if the symptoms last for more than one month. Treatment of PTSD may include cognitive-behavior therapy, group therapy, exposure therapy, and medications.

## FYI | RISK FACTORS FOR DEPRESSION

The causes of depression vary from one person to another. Any of the following could contribute to developing the disorder.

- Stressful life changes
- Susceptibility to biochemical imbalance
- Family history of depression
- Pessimistic outlook on life
- Excessive alcohol or drug use
- Painful childhood experiences

## MOOD DISORDERS

A **mood disorder** involves emotional extremes that are persistent and interfere significantly with a person's ability to function. There are three main types of depressive disorders. Alternating highs and lows could be a sign of **bipolar disorder** (manic-depressive illness), which is characterized by sudden, dramatic shifts in emotion (abnormally and persistently elevated mood or irritability), seemingly without relation to external variables. Symptoms include overly inflated self-esteem, racing thoughts, physical agitation, decreased need for sleep, and excessive risk taking. In the manic, or high, phase, the person experiences ecstasy, bursts of energy, and hyperactivity. This phase usually is followed by severe depression, the low phase. Between cycles—which last days, weeks, or months—the person can have normal moods. An accurate diagnosis of bipolar disorder is extremely important.

## KEY TERMS

**Schizophrenia** a psychological disorder characterized by severe disturbances in perceptions, thoughts, moods, and behaviors

**Anxiety disorders** psychological conditions characterized by exaggerated fear

**Panic attack** a condition in which a person is overwhelmed by feelings of anxiety and loss of control

**Obsessive compulsive disorder** an anxiety disorder in which a person has constant unpleasant and unacceptable thoughts and performs repetitive acts that are unnecessary

**Post-traumatic stress disorder** a condition in which a person mentally reexperiences a violent event

**Mood disorder** a condition characterized by emotional extremes without apparent reason

**Bipolar disorder** a mood disorder characterized by sudden, dramatic, and alternating shifts in emotion; manic-depressive disorder

## Tips for Action How to Beat Depression

Depressive disorders make you feel exhausted, worthless, helpless, and hopeless. These thoughts and feelings make some people feel like giving up. Instead, if you feel depressed:

■ Do not set difficult goals or take on a great deal of responsibility right now.

■ Do not make major life decisions.

■ Break large tasks into small ones, set some priorities, and do what you can as you can.

■ Do not expect too much from yourself too soon, as this will only increase feelings of failure.

■ Try to be with other people; it usually is better than being alone.

■ Participate in activities that may make you feel better.

■ Do mild exercise.

■ Go to a movie or a ballgame.

■ Participate in religious and social activities.

■ Do not overdo it or get upset if your mood is not greatly improved right away. Feeling better takes time.

■ Do not expect to snap out of your depression. People rarely do. It is a gradual process.

■ Do not accept negative thinking. It feeds the depression.

---

More common is **major depressive disorder** or **depression.** During their lifetimes, about 25% of American women and 10% of American men will be depressed. The results of a study conducted by the World Health Organization (WHO), Harvard University School of Public Health, and the World Bank determined that by the year 2020, "depression will be second only to heart disease as a cause of medical and physical disability." Depression has been linked as a risk factor for physical conditions such as heart attack, stroke, diabetes, preeclampsia, and premature labor. In other words, depression is a disease that makes it difficult to treat and control certain physical illnesses.

Chronic depression is characterized by a sad mood; symptoms include loss of interest in activities that the person once enjoyed, change in appetite or weight, difficulty sleeping or oversleeping, feelings of worthlessness, difficulty concentrating, and recurrent thoughts of death or suicide. Research has shown that in depression, the regulation of critical neurotransmitters is impaired. In some cases stressful life events, such as the death of a family member, may trigger major depression in susceptible persons.

The third type of depressive disorder is called dysthymic disorder, which is chronic but less severe than major depressive disorder. This condition is diagnosed when the depressed mood persists for at least two years with at least two other symptoms of depression.

Sometimes a person may feel sad or unhappy (feel blue) and present an aura of gloom. However, some people hide the problem so well that even those who are close to them are not aware of it. Symptoms of the blues include at least some of the following.

■ Pessimistic attitude

■ Trouble concentrating

### FYI | SYMPTOMS OF DEPRESSION

If you know someone with five (or more) of the symptoms below, encourage him or her to talk to a physician.

■ A profoundly down mood for at least two weeks

■ Diminished interest or pleasure in activities

■ Appetite loss or increase

■ Problems sleeping; insomnia

■ Feelings of guilt, worthlessness, hopelessness, pessimism

■ Low energy

■ Difficulty thinking or concentrating

■ Agitation or lethargy

■ Recurring thoughts of death or suicide

*Source:* American Psychiatric Association, *Diagnostic and Statistical Manual of Mental Health Disorders* (DSM-IV) (Washington, DC: APA, 1994), p. 327.

■ Temporary withdrawal from family and friends

■ Apathy (an "I don't care" attitude)

■ Episodes of sadness and crying

■ Temper flare-ups

■ Low energy

Because of beliefs that a depressed person should be able to shake off the symptoms or "get over it," a person with depression may not realize that she or he has a treatable disorder. Symptoms of any of the depressive disorders should not be ignored. If they persist, a competent

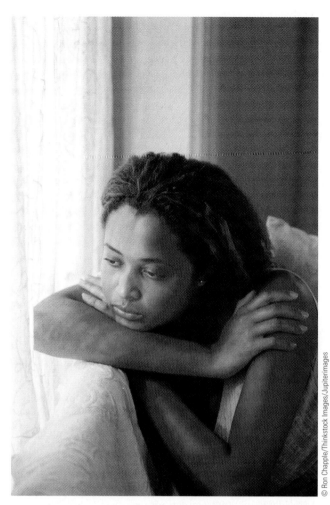

© Ron Chapple/Thinkstock Images/Jupiterimages

▲ *Depression can range from a mild form of the blues to severe clinical depression.*

medical professional should be consulted. Depression can be treated with medication, psychotherapy, or both. If the depression stems from a physical health problem such as an underactive thyroid or a chemical imbalance in the brain, called **clinical depression,** specific medication might resolve the problem. If this is not the case, a referral can be made to a competent psychiatrist. Depression is a medical condition that is treatable with medication in about 80% of all cases.

**Antidepressant Drugs.** The newest antidepressant drugs are in the class of selective serotonin reuptake inhibitors or SSRIs. The most prescribed brands include Zoloft, Lexapro, and Paxil. It may take up to eight weeks before the person notices improvement. Therefore, it is important to take the medication as prescribed. These antidepressants affect the brain's neurotransmitter serotonin to control depression by

- Curbing feelings of rage and calming depressed people who are angry.
- Making people less sensitive to minor slights.

- Improving mental concentration, thereby rendering people more effective and functional.
- Turning on the pleasure center, which makes people more open to meeting people and doing things.
- Instilling a sense of hope that life is within one's control.

**Seasonal Affective Disorder.** One form of depression that became recognized by the American Psychiatric Association in 1987 is **seasonal affective disorder (SAD).** It arises from less exposure to sunlight during the winter months. Up to 10% of people living in the northern United States may have this disorder, contrasted with less than 2% in the southern states, reflecting the differences in sunlight hours.

People with SAD are irritable and apathetic, sleep more, and are less active than normal. Women are about four times more susceptible to SAD than men are, and it seems to be most prevalent in the 20- to 40-year age range. This disorder also tends to run in families.

Some scientists believe SAD is related to a malfunctioning hypothalamus gland. The most beneficial treatment (for about 80% of patients) is light therapy, in which a person is exposed for a time each day to a light source that mimics the sun. Treatments also considered might be dietary changes, stress management techniques, exercise, and prescribed antidepressants.

Winter blues, a milder form of SAD, affects millions of people, mostly in northern climates. It can be eliminated or at least minimized by taking walks in the daylight, exercising, and taking in fresh air.

## Suicide

Most people think about suicide at one time or another. Persistent thoughts of this nature should be taken seriously. A person may express feelings of being trapped or that life has no purpose. Some people feel that the pressures in their lives are so intolerable that suicide is the only alternative. Suicide usually is planned and premeditated. Most suicidal individuals give some possible

### KEY TERMS

**Major depressive disorder** or **depression** a serious medical condition that is characterized by depressed mood or loss of interest or pleasure in nearly all activities, including the ability to function on a day-to-day basis

**Clinical depression** extreme emotional low stemming from a physical problem such as a chemical imbalance in the body

**Seasonal affective disorder (SAD)** form of depression caused by lack of exposure to sunlight during the winter

---

## Tips for Action How You Can Help

Most people who threaten suicide are really asking for help, and many of them respond positively when they receive human contact and support. Some of the following suggestions may help.

■ Ask the person if he or she is really thinking about suicide.

■ Reassure the person of his or her strong qualities, attributes, and importance, but do not try to analyze the person's behavior.

■ Listen to the person, and show genuine interest. Show strength, stability, and firmness.

■ Reassure the person that you are going to do everything possible to help him or her remain alive.

■ Seek professional help as quickly as possible.

■ Never make challenging statements such as, "You won't kill yourself!" or "Go ahead—I don't believe you'll do it." This person needs support.

Colleges, universities, and other institutions, agencies, and organizations are prepared and equipped to help people who are at their wits' end. Various on-campus and off-campus emergency services are available. The counseling center, health services center, local mental health centers and private mental health organizations, campus police department, and religious support services are just a few services available.

---

warnings or signs of their intent. Common signals include the following.

■ Dramatic mood changes (unexplained high mood after a period of depression)

■ Giving away personal possessions and getting affairs in order

■ Loss of appetite

■ Anxiety, agitation, unusual periods of sleeplessness or sleepiness rage, uncontrolled anger, seeking revenge

■ Engaging in risky or reckless activities

■ Other psychological changes such as withdrawal and overt sadness

■ Constant talk (or writing about death, dying, or suicide) of death or suicide threats

■ Seeking access to firearms or other means (medications or poisons) to commit suicide

According to data from the National Center for Health Statistics (NCHS), suicide took the lives of 31,484 Americans in 2003 (latest official data available). For

**FIGURE 2.4 ▶** Rate, Number, and Ranking of Suicide for Each State

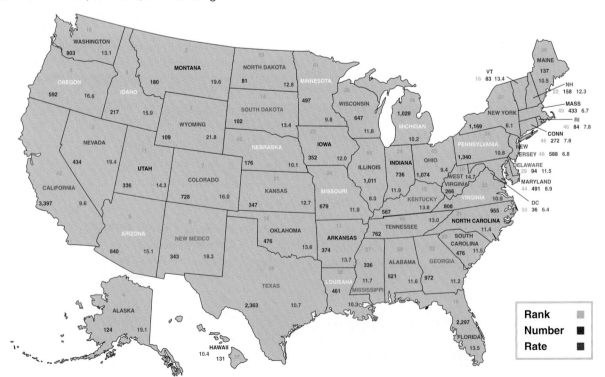

adults, suicide ranks as the eleventh leading cause of death in the United States. On average, one person every 16.7 minutes commits suicide. It is estimated that when a person commits suicide, the tragedy "intimately affects" at least six other people (family, friends, colleagues). Although females are more likely to attempt suicide, males are at least four times more likely to die from suicide.

Many people may experience one or more risk factors for suicide and are not suicidal. However, the following are some of the risk factors for suicide.

- One or more diagnosable mental or substance abuse disorders
- Family history of suicide
- Family violence, including physical or sexual abuse
- Prior suicide attempt
- Firearm in the home (16,907 of the suicides annually involve firearms)
- Exposure to the suicidal behavior of others, including family, peers, or in the news or fiction stories

Together, white males and females account for 90% of all suicides. Of the ethnic groups, American Indians have the highest suicide rate, though wide tribal differences exist. The lowest suicide rates for all racial and gender groups are among African-American females. Figure 2.5 compares the white and non-white suicide rates, and Table 2.2 gives the rates by age group. The highest rate is among the elderly, an issue that will be explored further in Chapter 14.

The statistics for children, teens, and young adults are grim. In the four decades between 1952 and 1992, the incidence of suicide in adolescents and young adults

**FIGURE 2.5** ▶ Comparison of White and Non-white Suicide Rates in United States by Gender

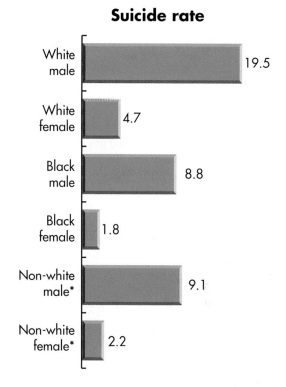

nearly tripled. Between 1980 and 1997, the rate of suicide increased 109% for 10- to 14-year-olds and 11% for 15- to 19-year-olds. Presently, for young people 15 to 24 years of age, suicide is the third leading cause of death, behind unintentional injury (accidents) and homicide. The risk for suicide in young people is highest for young Caucasian

**TABLE 2.2** ▶ U.S. Suicide Rates by Age, Gender, and Racial Group, 1994–2003 (Rates per 100,000 population)

| AGE AND GROUP | 1994 | 1995 | 1996 | 1997 | 1998 | 1999 | 2000 | 2001 | 2002 | 2003 | AGE AND GROUP |
|---|---|---|---|---|---|---|---|---|---|---|---|
| 5–14 | 0.9 | 0.9 | 0.8 | 0.8 | 0.8 | 0.6 | 0.8 | 0.7 | 0.6 | 0.6 | 5–14 |
| 15–24 | 13.8 | 13.3 | 12.0 | 11.4 | 11.1 | 10.3 | 10.4 | 9.9 | 9.9 | 9.7 | 15–24 |
| 25–34 | 15.4 | 15.4 | 14.5 | 14.3 | 13.8 | 13.5 | 12.8 | 12.8 | 12.6 | 12.7 | 25–34 |
| 35–44 | 15.3 | 15.2 | 15.5 | 15.3 | 15.4 | 14.4 | 14.6 | 14.7 | 15.3 | 14.9 | 35–44 |
| 45–54 | 14.4 | 14.6 | 14.9 | 14.7 | 14.8 | 14.2 | 14.6 | 15.2 | 15.7 | 15.9 | 45–54 |
| 55–64 | 13.4 | 13.3 | 13.7 | 13.5 | 13.1 | 12.4 | 12.3 | 13.1 | 13.6 | 13.8 | 55–64 |
| 65–74 | 15.3 | 15.8 | 15.0 | 14.4 | 14.1 | 13.6 | 12.6 | 13.3 | 13.5 | 12.7 | 65–74 |
| 75–84 | 21.3 | 20.7 | 20.0 | 19.3 | 19.7 | 18.3 | 17.7 | 17.4 | 17.7 | 16.4 | 75–84 |
| 85+ | 23.0 | 21.6 | 20.2 | 20.8 | 21.0 | 19.2 | 19.4 | 17.5 | 18.0 | 16.9 | 85+ |
| 65+ | 18.1 | 18.1 | 17.3 | 16.8 | 16.9 | 15.9 | 15.3 | 15.3 | 15.6 | 14.6 | 65+ |
| Total | 12.0 | 11.9 | 11.6 | 11.4 | 11.3 | 10.7 | 10.7 | 10.8 | 11.0 | 10.8 | Total |
| Men | 19.8 | 19.8 | 19.3 | 18.7 | 18.6 | 17.6 | 17.5 | 17.6 | 17.9 | 17.6 | Men |
| Women | 4.5 | 4.4 | 4.4 | 4.4 | 4.4 | 4.1 | 4.1 | 4.1 | 4.3 | 4.3 | Women |
| White | 12.9 | 12.9 | 12.7 | 12.4 | 12.4 | 11.7 | 11.7 | 11.9 | 12.2 | 12.1 | White |
| Nonwh | 7.2 | 6.9 | 6.7 | 6.5 | 6.2 | 6.0 | 5.9 | 5.6 | 5.5 | 5.5 | Nonwh |
| Black | 7.0 | 6.7 | 6.5 | 6.2 | 5.7 | 5.6 | 5.6 | 5.3 | 5.1 | 5.1 | Black |

**Objectives for Mental Health**

- Reduce the suicide rate.

- Reduce the proportion of homeless adults who have serious mental illness.

- Increase the proportion of adults with mental disorders who receive treatment.

---

males, although the rates increased most rapidly in young African-American males.

The National Center for Injury Prevention and Control (NCIPC) is working to raise awareness of suicide as a serious public health problem and to institute long-term prevention strategies to reduce attempts and actual suicides. Low and declining suicide rates in some states and population groups offer hope that legislation and environmental and cultural changes can reduce the incidence of suicide. Examples of such changes include preventing inappropriate access to firearms (53.7% committed with a firearm) and other deadly methods such as drugs (17.3% poisoning), community support, and teaching better coping skills.

## COLLEGE AND SUICIDE

Suicide is the second leading cause of death among college-age students, approximately 1,100 deaths per year. The Jed Foundation is a not-for-profit organization (founded by Donna and Phil Satow after their son, a college sophomore, committed suicide in 1998) dedicated to assisting colleges and universities in promotion of the emotional well-being of their students. The foundation recognizes that suicide and suicidal behavior demand solutions that are "multifaceted and collaborative." The foundation has identified 12 essential services necessary to address suicidal behaviors on college campuses, to include screening and targeted educational programs, stress-reduction programs, on-site counseling and off-campus referrals, on-site medical services, and emergency services. Additionally, an assessment profile ("A Checklist for Your Institution") is available at www.jedfoundation.org. This document is a valuable tool for you and for any director of student services to inventory existing campus services and to make recommendations for additional services needed to address suicidal behaviors on your campus.

## Mental Health Professionals, Facilities, Organizations, and Equal Access to Health Insurance

At times daily activities and other events may overwhelm people and affect their state of mind. During these times they are advised to take mental health breaks to restore equilibrium to their psyche. These activities include meditating, taking a long walk, getting engrossed in a hobby, exercising, or talking with a close friend or family member.

Mental health problems sometimes become too serious to be left to self-diagnosis and treatment. In these cases, professional intervention should be sought before the problem becomes unmanageable. If anxiety or depression begins to interfere markedly, causing problems at school, at work, and with interpersonal relationships, the person should see a mental health professional. Any person who has attempted or dwells on the notion of suicide should be seen immediately.

A psychiatrist is a physician (M.D.) or an osteopathic physician (D.O.) who specializes in the diagnosis and treatment of mental disorders, using psychotherapy as well as medication. Because psychiatrists are physicians, they have the expertise to make a medical diagnosis.

A clinical psychologist holds a Ph.D. or Psy.D. in psychology and diagnoses and treats psychological problems with various psychological testing and psychotherapies. Clinical psychologists are not physicians and generally may not prescribe medications for treatment.

The psychiatric registered nurse is responsible for the nursing care of patients in the hospital or other clinical settings. The psychiatric registered nurse (R.N. or B.S.N.) has additional clinical training in nursing and mental health problems.

The psychiatric social worker is responsible for coordinating available resources for the patient or client and family. This professional assists in making the transition from treatment to community as smooth as possible. The psychiatric social worker usually holds the degree of Master of Social Work (M.S.W.).

A variety of facilities and organizations specialize in diagnosing and treating mental health problems or provide mental health services. They are categorized as:

- Psychiatric hospitals (public or private)

- Community mental health centers, which may be supported in some part by taxes and grants

- Voluntary agencies such as the National Mental Health Association, with local chapters in major cities throughout the United States

Rap music evolved in the 1970s and 1980s and is a significant influence on other forms of music as well as on media, art, and the social development of young people nationally and internationally. "African-American children born in the early eighties can be considered the offspring of the rap and hip hop era," says clinical psychologist Don Elligan. Rap music has influenced socialization processes of African-American youth in the areas of clothing, posture (the cool pose), and language. Realizing its impact, one approach in psychotherapy that has proven successful for some young African-American men is the use of rap music in mental health treatment. In the *Journal of African-American Men*, Elligan reported positive results using Rap Therapy in the treatment of an African-American male teen who had problems with grief and anger management after his father was murdered. Elligan reported that using rap music as a tool to reach young African-American males is "sensitive to both culture and developmental issues of young African-American men and is easily integrated into a cognitive behavioral model of treatment." Using five phases of Rap Therapy (assessment, alliance, reframing, role play with reinforcement, and action and maintenance), Elligan was able to use his young patient's love of rap music (the patient had memorized lyrics of his favorite rap songs and written rap lyrics) to encourage him to write about his anger and grief using rap lyrics. As a result of the Rap Therapy, the patient was able to talk to his mother and the therapist about his father's death, his anger management skills improved substantially (classroom outbursts decreased), and he was more compliant in doing his schoolwork.

## COMPREHENSIVE HEALTH INSURANCE PARITY

Unfortunately, people with comprehensive health insurance assume that emotional and mental illnesses are covered by their plans just as other medical and surgical health problems. According to the National Mental Health Association (NMHA), the best mental health parity legislation covers all (no exemptions) mental health and substance abuse disorders under a private insurance plan.

Only 34 states have enacted laws that require some type of health insurance parity for mental illnesses. Additionally, many of the states' statutes require severe mental illness (SMI) to be covered but not mental illness such as PTSD and the eating disorders. As many as 13 states have mental health mandates but not parity; two states have no mental health mandates and no parity. After the Mental Health Parity Act of 1996 was passed in Congress, it became unlawful for companies with more than 50 employees to set annual and lifetime dollar limits on mental health care but exempt medical and surgical care from these limits. Loopholes in the law have allowed some employers and insurance companies to set limits on the number of outpatient office visits and inpatient care and require higher insurance copayments related to mental health benefits. Where does your state stand on comprehensive health insurance parity, and what is being done to eliminate this discrimination? To find out, go to www.nmha.org.

Anyone is subject to stresses that can cause temporary emotional instability. Emotionally healthy people usually are able to adjust, solve the problem, and get on with life. If emotional problems become more complex or disabling, however, do not delay in seeking professional intervention.

## Summary

- Among the various psychological theories that have been proposed to explain the personality are psychoanalytic, behavioral, developmental, and humanistic.

- Erik Erikson postulated that human development proceeds through eight crisis stages, each of which must be resolved successfully to maintain emotional health.

- Abraham Maslow's hierarchy has five levels of needs that humans must meet on their way to self-actualization.

- Personality types and physical health are related, as exemplified by the toxic core of the Type A personality, which carries risk for heart disease and other illnesses, and the Type C, or cancer-prone, personality.

- Whether a person has a pessimistic or an optimistic overall way of thinking has an effect on physical health.

- Locus of control ranges along a continuum from external ("factors outside of myself determine my lot in life") to internal ("many things in life are in my control").

- Emotional health is based on a true perception of reality, adaptability to change, satisfying interpersonal relationships, job satisfaction, recreational activities, and spirituality.

- Mental and emotional disorders range from mild, such as occasional blues, to severe disorders in which the person loses touch with reality, such as schizophrenia.

- Anxiety disorders include panic attacks, obsessive compulsive disorder, and post-traumatic stress disorder.

- Seasonal affective disorder and winter blues are related to external factors such as lack of sunlight and weather conditions.

- Suicide is a serious consideration of many young people with warning signs that beg for professional help.

- Psychiatry is the medical specialty that diagnoses and treats mental illness.

- Most comprehensive health insurance plans limit benefits for mental illnesses to include PTSD and substance abuse (health insurance parity).

## Personal Health Resources

**ThomsonNOW** Visit the ThomsonNOW website at http://thomsonedu.com/thomsonnow for valuable resources that will:

- Help you evaluate your knowledge of the material.

- Guide you through tutorials to help you understand and apply the material.

- Allow you to take an exam-prep quiz to better prepare for class tests.

Centers for Disease Control and Prevention (CDC), National Center for Injury Prevention and Control (NCIPC). This federal agency works to reduce illness, disability, and death and the costs associated with injury. Fact sheets are available on violence, unintentional injury, and suicide.

**www.cdc.gov/ncipc/ncipchm.htm**

The Jed Foundation's U-Lifeline Endorsed by the American College Health Association (ACHA). This interactive site has valuable resources and support for college-age students in times of crisis or doubt. The site can be customized to the needs of a college's (mental) health center and offers the ability to screen for suicide risk and depression.

**www.ulifeline.org**

National Alliance for the Mentally Ill (NAMI). A not-for-profit organization that supports mental health through advocacy, education, and promotion of public policy related to mental health and mental illness. Information available on this site includes, for example, facts on various topics, news and hot topics (responding to trauma and terrorism), and discounts on books and other materials for members at the NAMI store. Spanish language resources available.
800-950-NAMI (6264)

**www.NAMI.org**

National Institute of Mental Health (NIMH). Part of the National Institutes of Health, this agency has current information on mental health and mental illness. Information available includes fact sheets on a variety of conditions (PTSD, depression, and anxiety disorders), research news, and links to other sites related to mental health. Depression awareness, recognition, and treatment can be accessed at this site.
800-421-4211

**www.nimh.nih.gov/**

National Mental Health Association (NMHA). The nation's oldest not-for-profit organization, it is dedicated to the promotion of mental health through advocacy for the 54 million persons with mental disorders, education, and research. Information is available on a variety of topics related to mental health and mental illness, including depression screening and tips for the young, seniors, and college students, and a "find a therapist" directory. Operation Healthy Reunions (a partnership among NMHA and leading military organizations) is the first-of-its-kind program that targets the mental health and mental illness concerns of military personnel involved in Operations Enduring Freedom and Iraqi Freedom and their families. The site also has news summaries, a calendar of events, and legislative alerts.
800-969-NMHA (6642)

**www.NMHA.org**

## It's Your Turn for Study and Review

1. Describe the attributes of personality Type A, Type B, and Type C. Choose one of your favorite movies or television shows, identify one character that represents each personality type, and explain the attributes of that character that caused you to make your decision.

2. Identify the six characteristics of emotional health. Choose one that you would like to improve and list four actions that you plan to take to make the improvement.

3. Booker T. Washington said, "Success is to be measured not so much by the position that one has reached in life as by the obstacles which he has overcome while trying to succeed." Describe Abraham Maslow's hierarchy of needs based on your personal experiences and Booker T. Washington's quote.

4. Differentiate among schizophrenia, anxiety, and mood disorders by citing an example and signs of each.

5. You have noticed that one of your friends has displayed at least three of the warning signals of suicide discussed in this chapter. What will be your response? Find the telephone number of the suicide or crisis intervention hotline in your area. Do you know if your campus offers this type of service

through the student health center or student counseling service?

6. Differentiate between a psychiatrist and a clinical psychologist by degree and scope of practice.

## Thinking about Health Issues

Can positive emotions and laughter help improve your health?

Trisha Yeager, "Laugh Your Way to Better Health," *American Fitness*, March 2000, p. 26.

1. How are medical professionals and humor specialists utilizing the healing benefits of laughter?

2. What are five health benefits of humor?

3. How can a person add humor to his or her daily routine?

4. What is the relationship between humor and self-esteem? What is the relationship between humor and the immune system?

## Selected Bibliography

American Psychiatric Association. *Diagnostic and Statistical Manual of Mental Disorders* (DSM–IV). Washington, DC: APA, 1994.

Brown, A. S. "Prenatal Infection as a Risk Factor for Schizophrenia." *Schizophrenia Bulletin*, 32:2, April 2006, pp. 200–202.

Burrell, D. "This Year's International Mental Health Agenda: Erasing the Stigma of Mental Illness." *Psychology Today*, May/June 2001, p. 24.

Carney, R. M., et al. "Major Depressive Disorder Predicts Cardiac Events in Patients with Coronary Artery Disease." *Psychosomatic Medicine*, 50, 1988, pp. 627–633.

Comrey, A. L. *Comrey Personality Scales*. San Diego, CA: Educational and Industrial Testing Service, n.d.

Craddock, N., O'Donovan, M. C., and Owen, M. J. "Genes for Schizophrenia and Bipolar Disorder? Implications for Psychiatric Nosology." *Schizophrenia Bulletin*, 32:1, January 2006, pp. 9–16.

Elligan, Don. "Rap Therapy: A Culturally Sensitive Approach to Psychotherapy with Young African-American Men." *Journal of African-American Men*, 5, Winter 2000, pp. 27–36.

Freidman, H. S. *The Self-Healing Personality*. New York: Henry Holt and Co., 1991.

Glied, S. and Cuellar, A. "Better Behavioral Health Coverage for Everyone." *New England Journal of Medicine*, 354:13, March 10, 2006, pp. 1415–1417.

Goldman, H. H., et al. " Behavioral Health Insurance Parity for Federal Employees." *New England Journal of Medicine*, 354:13, March 10, 2006, pp. 1378–1386.

Hyman, S. E. and Rudorfer, M. V. "Depressive and Bipolar Mood Disorders." In *Scientific American Medicine*, vol. 3, edited by D. C. Dale and D. D. Federman. New York: Healtheon/Web MD Corp., 2000, Section 13, Subsection II, p. 1.

Jung, C. *Psychological Types*. New York: Harcourt Brace, 1923.

Klopf, D. W. *Intercultural Encounters*. Englewood, CO: Morton Publishing, 1991.

Lehmann, C. "Racism Often at Root of Misdiagnosing Minority Patients." *Psychiatric News*, 29, December 16, 1994, p. 9.

Maslow, A. *Motivation and Personality*, 2nd ed. New York: Harper and Row, 1970.

McKinnon, D. "The Development of Personality." In *Personality of the Behavior Disorders*, edited by M. V. Hunt. New York: Ronald Press, 1994.

Mozure, C. M., et al. "Adverse Life Events and Cognitive-Personality Characteristics in the Prediction of Major Depression and Antidepressant Response." *American Journal of Psychiatry*, 157:6, 2000, pp. 896–903.

Myers, I. B. *The Myers-Briggs Type Indicator*. Palo Alto, CA: Consulting Psychologists Press, 1962.

Rodgers, J. E. "Extreme Psychology." *Psychology Today*, 39:4, July/August 2006, pp. 86–93.

Rosenman, R. "Do You Have Type 'A' Behavior?" *Health and Fitness*, 1987, supplement.

Satcher, D. "Mental Health." *Psychology Today*, January/February 2000, pp. 32–36.

Schutz, W. *FIRO-B*. Palo Alto, CA: Consulting Psychologists Press, 1967.

Simon, G. "Treating Bipolar Disorder: Present and Future." *Psychology Today*, November/December 2001, p. 87.

"Spirituality and Women's Health." *Journal of Obstetric, Gynecologic and Neonatal Nursing*, 24, March/April 1995, p. 3.

Suinn, R. M. "The Cardiac Stress Management Program for Type A Patients." *Cardiac Rehabilitation*, 5, 1975, pp. 13–15.

Szalavitz, M. "Should I Drop My Antidepressant?" *Psychology Today*, 39:2, March/April 2006, p. 59.

Szegedy-Maszak, M. "Reason to Be Happy." *U.S. News and World Report*, 140:19, April 10, 2006, pp. 41–43.

White, J. and Cones, J. *Black Man Emerging: Facing the Past and Seizing a Future in America*. New York: Freeman and Company, 1999.

**Name** _____     **Date** _____

**Course** _____     **Section** _____

Check any symptoms you have had for two weeks or more:

☐ Loss of interest in things you used to enjoy.

☐ Feeling sad, blue, or down in the dumps.

☐ Feeling slowed down or restless and unable to sit still.

☐ Feeling worthless or guilty.

☐ Changes in appetite or weight loss or gain.

☐ Thoughts of death or suicide; suicide attempts.

☐ Trouble concentrating, thinking, remembering, or making decisions.

☐ Trouble sleeping or sleeping too much.

☐ Loss of energy or feeling tired all of the time.

☐ Feeling pessimistic or hopeless.

☐ Being anxious or worried.

If you have had five or more of these symptoms for at least two weeks, you may have major depression. See your health care provider. Even if you have only a few depressive symptoms, your health care provider can be of help.

*Source:* Adapted from U.S. Department of Health and Human Services, *Depression Is a Treatable Illness, A Patient's Guide* (Washington, DC: U.S. Government Printing Office, 1994).

Name _____     Date _____

Course _____     Section _____

AA = Almost Always     O = Occasionally     R = Rarely     N = Never

| | | | | | |
|---|---|---|---|---|---|
| **1.** | Do you find yourself bragging or exaggerating the importance of your role? | AA | O | R | N |
| **2.** | Are you jealous of the possessions, opportunities, or positions of others? | AA | O | R | N |
| **3.** | Do you find yourself judging your behavior by other people's standards or expectations rather than your own? | AA | O | R | N |
| **4.** | Are you possessive in your relationships with friends or family members? | AA | O | R | N |
| **5.** | Is it difficult for you to acknowledge your own mistakes? | AA | O | R | N |
| **6.** | Do you resort to bullying and intimidation in your dealings with others? | AA | O | R | N |
| **7.** | Do you put people down so that you can feel one up? | AA | O | R | N |
| **8.** | Are you a perfectionist? | AA | O | R | N |
| **9.** | Must you be a winner in recreational activities to have fun? | AA | O | R | N |
| **10.** | When faced with new opportunities, do you feel inadequate or insecure? | AA | O | R | N |
| **11.** | Do you have difficulty accepting compliments? | AA | O | R | N |
| **12.** | Do you refrain from expressing your feelings and opinions? | AA | O | R | N |
| **13.** | Do you shy away from trying new things for fear of failure or looking dumb? | AA | O | R | N |
| **14.** | Do you neglect your own needs to respond to others' needs? | AA | O | R | N |

"Almost Always" or "Often" answers to any of these questions may indicate that your self-esteem needs attention.

*Source:* Reprinted with permission from *Structured Exercises in Stress Management, Volume 2,* © 1984, 1994. Donald A. Tubesing. Published by Whole Person Associates, 210 West Michigan, Duluth, MN 55802–1908, 218–727–0500.

Name _____     Date _____

Course _____     Section _____

Each question describes a specific or general situation that you probably have encountered. If you haven't, imagine as vividly as you can how you would react in the situation.

Following each description are two responses, A or B, describing how that situation might affect you, or how you might behave under those circumstances. In some instances neither response may seem to fit, or both may appear equally desirable. Go ahead and answer anyway, choosing the single response that is more likely for you in that situation. Choose only one response for each situation described.

Take as much time as you need to make your choice for each item, but remember, what seems right at first glance—your "gut reaction"—usually represents your true position.

1. A teenager drives by my yard with the car stereo blaring acid rock.
   A. I begin to understand why teenagers can't hear.
   B. I can feel my blood pressure starting to rise.

2. The person who cuts my hair trims off more than I wanted.
   A. I tell him or her what a lousy job he or she did.
   B. I figure it'll grow back, and I resolve to give my instructions more forcefully next time.

3. I'm in the express checkout line at the supermarket, where a sign reads: "No more than ten items please!"
   A. I pick up a magazine to pass the time.
   B. I glance ahead to see if anyone has more than ten items.

4. Many large cities have a visible number of homeless people.
   A. I believe that the homeless are down and out because they lack ambition.
   B. The homeless are victims of illness or some other misfortune.

5. There have been times when I was very angry with people.
   A. I was always able to stop short of hitting them.
   B. I have, on occasion, hit or shoved them.

6. The newspaper contains a prominent news story about drug-related crime.
   A. I wish the government had better educational/drug programs, even for pushers.
   B. I wish we could put every drug pusher away for good.

7. The prevalence of AIDS has reached epidemic proportions.
   A. This is largely the result of irresponsible behavior on the part of a small proportion of the population.
   B. AIDS is a major tragedy.

8. I sometimes argue with a friend or relative.
   A. I find profanity an effective tool.
   B. I hardly ever use profanity.

9. I'm stuck in a traffic jam.
   A. I usually am not particularly upset.
   B. I quickly start to feel irritated and annoyed.

10. There is a really important job to be done.
    A. I prefer to do it myself.
    B. I'm apt to call on my friends or co-workers to help.

11. Sometimes I keep my angry feelings to myself.
    A. Doing so can often prevent me from making a mountain out of a molehill.
    B. Doing so is usually a bad idea.

12. Another driver butts ahead of me in traffic.
    A. I usually flash my lights or honk my horn.
    B. I stay farther back behind such a driver.

13. Someone treats me unfairly.
    A. I usually forget it rather quickly.
    B. I'm apt to keep thinking about it for hours.

14. The cars ahead of me on an unfamiliar road start to slow and stop as they approach a curve.
    A. I assume that there's a construction site ahead.
    B. I assume someone ahead had a fender bender.

15. Someone expresses an ignorant belief.
    A. I try to correct him or her.
    B. I'm likely to let it pass.

16. I'm caught in a slow-moving bank or supermarket line.
    A. I usually start to fume at people who dawdle ahead of me.
    B. I seldom notice the wait.

17. Someone is being rude or annoying.
    A. I'm apt to avoid that person in the future.
    B. I might have to get rough with the person.

18. An election year rolls around.
    A. I learn anew that politicians are not to be trusted.
    B. I'm caught up in the excitement of pulling for my candidate.

19. An elevator stops too long on a floor above where I'm waiting.
    A. I soon start to feel irritated and annoyed.
    B. I start planning the rest of my day.

20. I'm around someone I don't like.
    A. I try to end the encounter as soon as possible.
    B. I find it hard not to be rude to the person.

21. I see a very overweight person walking down the street.
    A. I wonder why this person has such little self-control.
    B. I think the person might have a metabolic defect or a psychological problem.

22. I'm riding as a passenger in the front seat of a car.
    A. I take the opportunity to enjoy the scenery.
    B. I try to stay alert for obstacles ahead.

23. Someone criticizes something I've done.
    A. I feel annoyed.
    B. I try to decide whether the criticism is justified.

24. I'm involved in an argument.
    A. I concentrate hard so I can get my point across.
    B. I can feel my heart pounding, and I breathe harder.

25. A friend or coworker disagrees with me.
    A. I try to explain my position more clearly.
    B. I'm apt to get into an argument with him or her.

26. Someone is speaking very slowly during a conversation.
    A. I'm apt to finish his or her sentences.
    B. I'm apt to listen until he or she finishes.

27. If they were put on the honor system, most people wouldn't sneak into a movie theater without paying.
    A. That's because they're afraid of being caught.
    B. It's because it would be wrong.

28. I have strong beliefs about rearing children.
    A. I try to reward mine when they behave well.
    B. I make sure they know what the rules are.

29. I hear news of another terrorist attack.
    A. I feel like lashing out.
    B. I wonder how people can be so cruel.

30. I'm talking with my mate, boyfriend, or girlfriend.
    A. I often find my thoughts racing ahead to what I plan to say next.
    B. I find it easy to pay close attention to what he or she is saying.

31. There have been times in the past when I was really angry.
    A. I have never thrown things or slammed a door.
    B. At times I have thrown something or slammed a door.

32. Life is full of little annoyances.
    A. They often seem to get under my skin.
    B. They seem to roll off my back unnoticed.

33. I disapprove of something a friend has done.
    A. I usually keep the disapproval to myself.
    B. I usually let my friend know about it.

34. I'm requesting a seat assignment for an airline flight.
    A. I usually request a seat in a specific area of the plane.
    B. I generally leave the choice to the agent.

35. I feel a certain way nearly every day of the week.
    A. I feel grouchy some of the time.
    B. I usually stay on an even keel.

36. Someone bumps into me in a store.
    A. I pass it off as an accident.
    B. I feel irritated at the person's clumsiness.

37. My mate, boyfriend, or girlfriend is preparing a meal.
    A. I keep an eye out to make sure nothing burns or cools too long.
    B. I either talk about my day or read the paper.

38. A boyfriend or girlfriend calls at the last minute to say that he or she is "too tired to go out tonight," and I'm stuck with a pair of $15 tickets.
    A. I try to find someone else to go with.
    B. I tell my friend how inconsiderate he or she is.

39. I recall something that angered me previously.
    A. I feel angry all over again.
    B. The memory doesn't bother me nearly as much as the actual event did.

40. I see people walking around in shopping malls.
    A. Many of them are shopping or exercising.
    B. Many of them are just wasting time.

41. Someone is hogging the conversation at a party.
    A. I look for an opportunity to put him or her down.
    B. I soon move to another group.

42. At times I have to work with incompetent people.
    A. I concentrate on my part of the job.
    B. Having to put up with them ticks me off.

43. My mate, boyfriend, or girlfriend is going to get me a birthday present.
    A. I prefer to pick it out myself.
    B. I prefer to be surprised.

**44.** I hold a poor opinion of someone.
   **A.** I keep it to myself.
   **B.** I let him or her know it.

**45.** In most arguments I have, the roles are consistent.
   **A.** I'm the angrier one.
   **B.** The other person is angrier than I am.

**46.** Slow-moving lines often can be found in banks and supermarkets.
   **A.** They are an unavoidable part of modern life.
   **B.** They often are because of someone's incompetence.

*Source: Anger Kills,* © by Redford Williams and Virginia Williams, 1993. Reprinted with permission of Times Books, a division of Random House.

| SCORING KEY | |
|---|---|
| CYNICISM | _____ |
| ANGER | _____ |
| AGGRESSION | _____ |
| TOTAL **HOSTILITY** | _____ |

To score your Cynicism level, turn back to the test and look at the following items and responses: 3(B), 4(A), 7(A), 10(A), 14(B), 18(A), 21(A), 22(B), 27(A), 30(A), 34(A), 37(A), 40(B), 43(A), and 46(B). Give yourself one point every time your answer agrees with the letter in parentheses after each item number. Thus, if your answers matched the letters in the parentheses for 8 of the 15 Cynicism questions, your Cynicism score would be 8.

Enter your Cynicism score on the appropriate line at the end of the test.

- If your score is 0 to 3, your Cynicism level is very low.

- If your score is 4 to 6, your Cynicism level is probably high enough to be of some concern.

- If your score is 7 or more, your Cynicism level is very high.

To score your Anger level, give yourself one point for each answer that agrees with the letter in parentheses after these items: 1(B), 6(B), 9(B), 13(B), 16(A), 19(A), 23(A), 24(B), 29(A), 32(A), 35(A), 36(B), 39(A), 42(B), and 45(A). Enter the total on the line marked "Anger" in the scoring key.

- If your score is 0 to 3, your Anger level is very low.

- If your score is 4 to 6, your Anger level is probably high enough to deserve your attention.

- If your score is 7 or higher, your Anger level is very high.

To score your Aggression level, give yourself one point for each answer that agrees with the letter in parentheses after these items: 2(A), 5(B), 8(A), 11(B), 12(A), 15(A), 17(B), 20(B), 25(B), 26(A), 28(B), 31(B), 33(B), 38(B), 41(A), and 44(B). Write the total on the "Aggression" line of the scoring key.

- If your score is 0 to 3, your Aggression level is very low.

- If your score is 4 to 6, your Aggression level is borderline and you may want to consider ways to reduce it.

- If your score is 7 or more, you probably need to take serious steps to reduce your Aggression level.

Your Total Hostility score is the sum of the three aspects you have just scored. Add your Cynicism, Anger, and Aggression scores and enter the total on the "Total Hostility" line of the scoring key. Any score above 10 is high enough to increase your risk of health problems.

Name _____     Date _____

Course _____     Section _____

Try the following tips to help plan a week that will leave you feeling good, inside and out. If you are receiving treatment for a mental health problem, these tips can help you manage your illness and support your treatment and recovery.

## SUNDAY

**Relax.** Try meditating, taking a walk in a natural setting, or reaching out spiritually or through prayer. Quiet reflection, alone or in the company of others, can improve your state of mind, strengthen your sense of self and community, and give you time away from a hectic schedule to collect your thoughts and re-energize for the week ahead.

## MONDAY

**Make a plan.** Decide what tasks you need to complete for the week and make a plan for when and how to do them. If you are overscheduled, decide what can wait a week or two. If you don't have much on your schedule, plan some activities you'll look forward to.

## TUESDAY

**Surround yourself with supportive people.** Make plans with family members and friends, or seek out activities at which you can meet new people, such as a club, class or support group. Reconnect with someone you have lost touch with and create new memories.

## WEDNESDAY

**Take care of your body.** Taking care of yourself physically can improve your mental health. Be sure to eat nutritious meals, avoid cigarettes, drink alcohol only in moderation, drink plenty of water, get enough sleep and exercise regularly.

## THURSDAY

**Give of yourself.** Volunteer your time and energy to help someone else. You'll feel good about doing something tangible to help someone in need—and it's a great way to meet new people who share your interests and compassion.

## FRIDAY

**Broaden your horizons.** Create a change of pace or expand your interests. Explore a new hobby, plant a garden, plan a road-trip, try a new restaurant, take dance lessons, or learn to play an instrument or speak another language.

## SATURDAY

**Value yourself.** Treat yourself with kindness and respect, and avoid self-criticism. Take stock of the qualities you like about yourself, your accomplishments and abilities. Take some time every day to relax, reflect and rejuvenate.

**To learn more, contact your local Mental Health Association, or call the National Mental Health Association at 800-969-NMHA (6642) or visit www.nmha.org.**

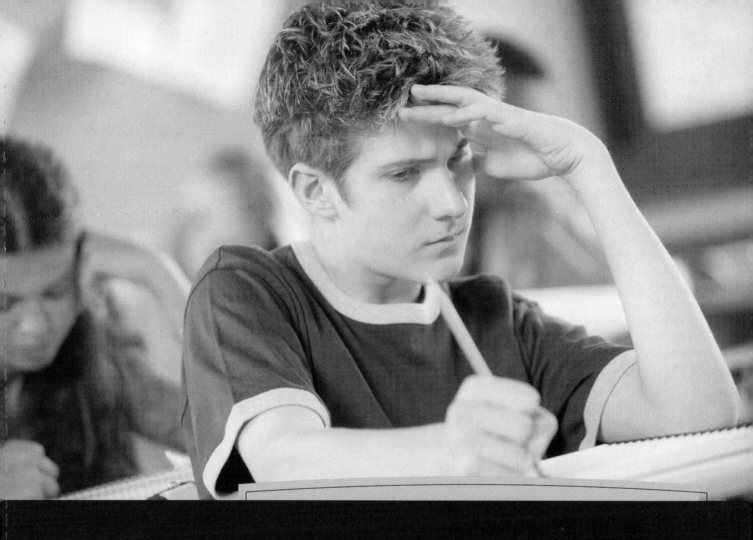

# Chapter Three  Stress and Health

**OBJECTIVES** ■ Define stress and identify its characteristics. ■ Describe the relationship between stress and illness. ■ Contrast distress and eustress. ■ Explain the general adaptation syndrome. ■ Describe the fight-or-flight response. ■ Enumerate some physical and emotional signs of stress. ■ Apply a variety of strategies for managing stress. ■ Explain the importance of nutrition and exercise in reducing stress.

ThomsonNOW™  Log on to ThomsonNOW at http://thomsonedu.com/ thomsonnow to access and explore self-assessments, interactive tutorials, and practice quizzes.

Stress is a normal part of our daily lives. Our bodies respond to stressful situations and events that we think pose a threat. Each person reacts to stress differently. Some people will be extremely stressed about situations that do not affect others. All persons must learn to cope with stress, because prolonged stress affects the body, causing headaches, hair loss, hypertension, skin problems, and chronic heart conditions including heart attacks.

An understanding of stress has improved since it was associated with heart disease at the 1949 Conference on Life and Stress and Heart Disease, sponsored by the National Heart Institute. With this recognition came a broader awareness of the influence of all emotions, including stress, on chronic diseases. A growing body of evidence indicates that virtually every illness known in contemporary times is impacted, for good or bad, by emotions. The link between the mind and the body is the immune system.

## The Science of Psychoneuroimmunology

The term **psychoneuroimmunology (PNI)** was coined in 1964 by Dr. Robert Adler, director of the division of behavioral and psychosocial medicine at the University of Rochester. PNI is based on the knowledge that emotions such as stress send chemical messages to the brain. These messages alter involuntary physiologic responses, which affect the way the brain responds to messages from the immune system in the presence of disease.

Although some controversy and skepticism still surround PNI, the theories behind this science are not new. More than 4,000 years ago, Chinese physicians noted that physical illness often followed episodes of frustration. Some of the world's greatest physicians and philosophers—Hippocrates, Galen, and Descartes, among others—believed in the link between the body and mind. Today, evidence abounds on the neurological connection to the immune system. Some cases in point follow.

- After conducting a long-term analysis of thousands of hospital patients, University of Rochester researcher George L. Engel and his colleagues found that the majority of people hospitalized for a physical illness had a psychological upset shortly before they got sick.

- A research team from several London hospitals gave questionnaires to more than 200 middle-aged men who were registered patients at a general practice clinic. The questionnaires helped the research team identify emotions such as worry, sadness, anxiety, and depression. Based on those questionnaires alone, and not on the men's medical condition or history, the researchers predicted

### FYI | STRESS AND DISEASE: A PANDORA'S BOX

As research continues into the link between stress and the immune system, scientists have come up with a veritable shopping list of conditions caused or aggravated by stress.

| | |
|---|---|
| Allergies | Hypertension (high |
| Angina | blood pressure) |
| Arteriosclerosis | Irritable bowel syndrome |
| Asthma | Kidney disease |
| Cancer | Lupus |
| Chronic backaches | Migraine headaches |
| Chronic tuberculosis | Multiple sclerosis |
| Cold sores | Myasthenia gravis |
| Coronary thrombosis | Pancreatitis |
| Diabetes | Psoriasis |
| Eczema | Raynaud's disease |
| Epileptic attacks | Respiratory ailments |
| Epstein-Barr syndrome | Rheumatoid arthritis |
| Gastritis | Shingles |
| Heart disease | Stroke |
| Herpes viruses | Ulcerative colitis |
| Hives | Ulcers |

which men were most likely to have a heart attack within a year. They were 81% accurate in their predictions.

- The Health Insurance Plan of Greater New York did a follow-up study of 2,000 men who had suffered a heart attack. They found that those men who were under a great deal of emotional stress were four times more likely to have a second, fatal heart attack. The telling factor was stress. The researchers determined that the hormones released during stress had crippled or damaged the heart.

## Stress in a Nutshell

Austrian-born Hans Selye, considered the father of stress research, defined **stress** as "the nonspecific response of the human organism to any demand placed upon it." Stress results from a physical, emotional, social, or spiritual event or condition that causes people to adapt—to adjust to a certain situation. Simply stated, stress occurs whenever something changes and people are forced to adapt to change.

What Selye says in his definition of stress is critical to understand: The body reacts to stress the same way regardless of the event that precipitates the response. Your heart may pound and your stomach may churn with

- Increase quality and years of healthy life.
- Increase the number of persons seen in primary health care who receive mental health screening and assessment.
- Increase the proportion of adults with mental disorders who receive treatment.

- Increase the number of states, including the District of Columbia, and territories with an operational mental health plan that addresses cultural competence.

excess acid whether you just received a new set of "wheels" or got caught cheating on an exit exam.

Further, stress is no respecter of persons or situations. No one can escape it, wish it away, or even live without it. The only way to be completely free of stress is to be dead. The American Institute of Stress claims that 90% of all American adults experience high levels of stress once or twice a week and a fourth of all American adults are subject to crushing levels of stress nearly every day. It can happen at home, in the classroom, on the job, in families, and between friends. It can even be between people and their surroundings, in the form of extreme heat or cold, noise, pollution, or overcrowding. Stressors (and examples) can be

- Physical (fatigue or a bacterial infection)
- Emotional (pent-up anger or hostility)
- Social (rejection or embarrassment)
- Intellectual (confusion)
- Spiritual (guilt)

The very process of living entails change. Therefore, people of all ages, both sexes, all races, every culture, and every socioeconomic group, are susceptible to stress. The problem occurs with unremitting stress—the kind that requires constant adaptation to chronic change. Unremitting stress can become a threat to health, because maintaining lifelong wellness is difficult when much of the body's energy is channeled into coping with stress.

Researchers at the American Institute of Stress estimate that 75% to 90% of all visits to health care providers result from stress-related disorders. The National Council on Compensation Insurance reports that stress-related

## KEY TERMS

**Psychoneuroimmunology (PNI)** a science focusing on how the mind affects the immune system and physical condition

**Stress** demands that place physical and emotional strain on an individual

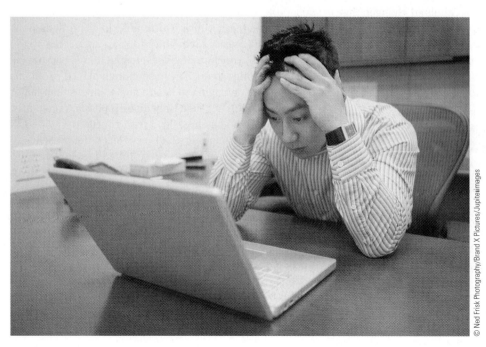

◄ *Many people encounter stress on the job*

claims account for almost one-fifth of occupational diseases. Fully one-fourth of all worker compensation claims are for stress-related injuries, and researchers estimate that 60% to 80% of all industrial accidents in the United States are related to stress.

Stress is not limited to what goes on in a person's thoughts. Stress is a nonspecific, automatic biological response to demands made upon an individual. Scientifically speaking, stress is any challenge to **homeostasis.** Stress is a biological and biochemical process that begins in the brain and spreads through the **autonomic nervous system,** causing the release of hormones and exerting eventual influence over the immune system.

Stress is not necessarily negative. Hans Selye used the term **distress** to denote detrimental stress—too much stress in a short time, chronic stress over a long time, or a combination of stressors that throw the body out of balance.

Selye coined the term **eustress** to describe the stress that keeps life interesting and provides opportunity for growth. Positive stress is associated with happy occasions such as family gatherings, class reunions, graduations, victorious athletic competitions, weddings, births, and baptisms. Other good stressors may be getting a driver's license, buying the first car, landing the first job, or moving into the first apartment. Eustress is a challenging force that helps a person feel successful, loved, secure, accepted, and protected.

Some stressful situations are challenging, stimulating, and rewarding. Competitive sports are excellent examples. To gear up for any competitive sport, worry about winning, and exert extreme amounts of skill and energy for long periods of time is extremely stressful, both physically and emotionally. The athletes who do it believe the rewards and thrills are well worth the stress—and millions of fans could not agree more.

Distress is associated with the kinds of changes that disrupt homeostasis. For example, leaving home for the first time brings with it many sources of distress—interacting with unfamiliar people, missing the established social support system, having too little money, and experiencing conflicts in social relationships.

## Sources of Stress

Stress can be psychological, environmental, physiological, and psychosocial. Psychological stress can come from almost anywhere—missing a bus, not having enough money to make ends meet, having an argument with a friend. Environmental stressors range from the relatively common (air pollution, temperature extremes, overcrowding, unsanitary conditions, lack of security, water pollution) to the catastrophic (a hurricane like Katrina, tornado, tsunami, earthquake). Although stressors such as forest fires are certainly dramatic, they are not necessarily the most damaging in the long term. Chronic exposure to

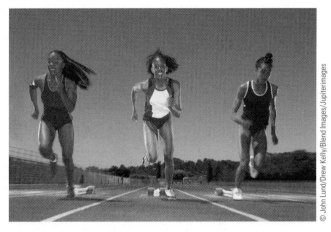

▲ *Positive stress can occur on happy occasions such as an athletic competition*

noise or the threat of living in a high-crime neighborhood, for example, could have much greater long-term effects than one-time exposure to a disaster.

Physiological stress could stem from injury, illness, surgery, genetic weaknesses, prolonged exercise, physical disabilities, or inadequate nutrition.

Psychosocial stressors are those that arise from interpersonal relationships, from living, working, and playing with other people. Some examples are stress from the expectations imposed by others, discriminatory behavior from others, intense social interactions, and social isolation. Possibly the most common is **conflict,** the stress that results from two things in opposition.

Some of the most pervasive stressors are the **hassles** of everyday living—for example, losing car keys, getting stuck behind a disorganized shopper in the supermarket line, forgetting about an important exam, waking up to a miserable snowstorm, being kept waiting for an appointment, getting stuck in a traffic jam. In his now-famous book *Future Shock*, Alvin Toffler listed, among the 10 top hassles, rising consumer prices, losing items, and having too many things to do. These seemingly trivial problems may be more damaging to health and wellness than major stressors, partly because they disturb people constantly, piling up with no end in sight.

Although researchers had recognized the presence of stress decades earlier and even linked it specifically to disease, not until early in the 1950s was anyone able to categorize specific contributors to stress. During the early 1950s, University of Washington psychiatrist Thomas Holmes noted that the most common denominator for stress was significant change in the life pattern. He began to search for specific links between disease and what he called social "life events," the things in life that call for the greatest adjustment. He discovered that the more major life events a person was subjected to within a brief period, the more likely the person was to become ill—in essence, to be depleted by the exhaustion of stress.

**FIGURE 3.1 ▶** Stressors throughout the Life Span

### Children
separation from a parent
death of a parent
divorce of parents
lack of adult supervision
inferior day care
struggles to become independent
socialization
birth of a sibling
anxieties about school
bullies
changing schools
conflicts with teachers
dares by classmates
parental pressure to achieve
lack of parental interest in achievements
discrimination (relating to race, weight, hair color, disability)

### Adolescents
physical changes during puberty
heightened sexual awareness
peer pressure
the desire to be independent
the need to establish identity
lack of supportive relationships
changing relationships with parents and siblings
divorce or loss of parents
confusing sexual messages
low self-esteem

### College students
academic pressure
course overload
career decisions
self-doubt
feelings of anonymity
financial struggles
measuring up to expectations (from self and others)
loneliness and isolation
intimidation
separation from parents and established social networks
dramatic changes in environment
developing sexual intimacy with a partner

### Adults
marriage
parenthood
family planning, responsibility for others (including aging parents)
changing roles within the family, career challenges
dual-career marriage
loss of a job
financial struggles
marital stress
divorce
death of a spouse or other family member
complex interpersonal relationships

### Elderly
retirement
memory loss
physical deterioration
loss of independence, financial struggles
death of a spouse or other family member or friends
loneliness
boredom

Holmes teamed with his colleague Richard Rahe to develop what they called the Social Readjustment Rating scale. More commonly known as the Holmes-Rahe scale, it assigns a numerical score to the four dozen or so life changes that most increase the risk for disease. By adding the scores assigned to each life event that happens within a year, the likelihood of someone developing a stress-related illness may be predicted.

Not all the items on the Holmes-Rahe scale are negative. Marriage, an outstanding personal achievement, and a vacation are positives. Some of the items on the scale can be either negative or positive. The key word is *change.* Each item on the Holmes-Rahe scale describes a change in social routine—a need to adapt.

A significant source of stress for students is pressure—moving out of home, exams, relationships and arguments, working too hard, a job interview, natural disasters, and the death of someone close. These kinds of pressures often come from the people around them: parents, mates, friends. More commonly, however, it comes from within, from the fear of what others may think, from a desire to achieve important goals, or from a host of expectations people place on themselves.

Every period of life presents different challenges. Some of the stressors during various life stages are set forth in Figure 3.1.

## The General Adaptation Syndrome

When the body becomes stressed, regardless of the source of the stress, it undergoes the stress response, or **general adaptation syndrome (GAS).** This is the same response that primitive people used when facing the various threats

### KEY TERMS

**Homeostasis** the body's internal sense of balance

**Autonomic nervous system** the portion of the nervous system that controls involuntary bodily functions, especially the glands, smooth muscle tissue, and the heart

**Distress** negative stress

**Eustress** positive stress

**Conflict** the stress that results from two opposing and incompatible goals, demands, or needs

**Hassles** various minor annoyances that occur daily

**General adaptation syndrome (GAS)** the body's attempt to react and adapt to stressors

K. Kendler, L. Thornton, and C. Prescott reported the relationship between stress and recurrent depression after interviewing male-male, female-female, and male-female twins. Each interview assessed the occurrence, to the nearest month, of 18 personal and social network classes of stressful life events and episodes that were followed by the onset of major depression. Women reported more interpersonal whereas men reported more legal and work-related stressful life events. Women consistently reported higher rates of housing problems, loss of confidants, crises and problems getting along with individuals in their proximal network, and illness of individuals within their distal networks. Men reported higher rates of job loss, legal problems, robbery, and work problems. Women were more sensitive to the depressogenic effects of problems with getting along with individuals in their proximal network; men were more sensitive to the depressogenic effects of divorce or separation and work problems.

in their environment, called **fight or flight.** It consists of the physiological changes that occurred in rapid-fire succession when a cave dweller was confronted by a saber-toothed tiger. The body systems sped up, and hormones started surging into the bloodstream. The senses sharpened, and energy levels heightened. Everything combined to enable cave dwellers to either conquer their enemies or run for their life. While society has become more civilized, the human body has not. A student giving an oral presentation to critical peers has the same physiological response as the cave dweller who faced the saber-toothed tiger.

The general adaptation syndrome occurs in three general stages: alarm, resistance, and exhaustion. These are depicted in Figure 3.2.

## ALARM

The stress response begins the second the brain perceives any kind of stress or threat. An alarm sounds inside the body. Immediately the sympathetic branch of the autonomic nervous system—the same complex set of nerves that operates independently of conscious thought to control heart rate, digestion, breathing, and other automatic body functions—takes over. Control centers in the brain act with split-second speed and accuracy in a chain reaction.

- The hypothalamus directs the pituitary gland to release **adrenocorticotropic hormone (ACTH).**
- ACTH stimulates the adrenal glands to release **cortisol** and other key hormones.
- Sympathetic nerves stimulate the adrenal glands to release **epinephrine** and **norepinephrine.**
- In case of injury, the brain releases **endorphins.**

The custom mixture of hormones surging through the bloodstream triggers a rapid and immediate series of changes throughout the body, shown in Figure 3.3.

- The mucous membranes in the nose and throat shrink to widen the air passages; the air sacs in the lungs dilate so more air can enter the lungs.
- The heart pumps harder and faster to circulate more oxygen throughout the body; blood pressure increases dramatically, and the spleen releases red blood cells to increase the blood's oxygen-carrying capacity.
- Digestion stops so much-needed blood will not be diverted to the stomach; as part of that process, the mouth gets dry, digestive juices from the pancreas diminish, and muscles in the intestines relax.
- Blood vessels in the skin constrict, and goosebumps arise on the skin.

**FIGURE 3.2** ▶ Stages in General Adaptation Syndrome

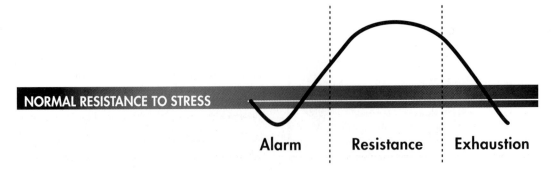

NORMAL RESISTANCE TO STRESS

Alarm          Resistance          Exhaustion

**FIGURE 3.3** ▶ The Alarm Reaction

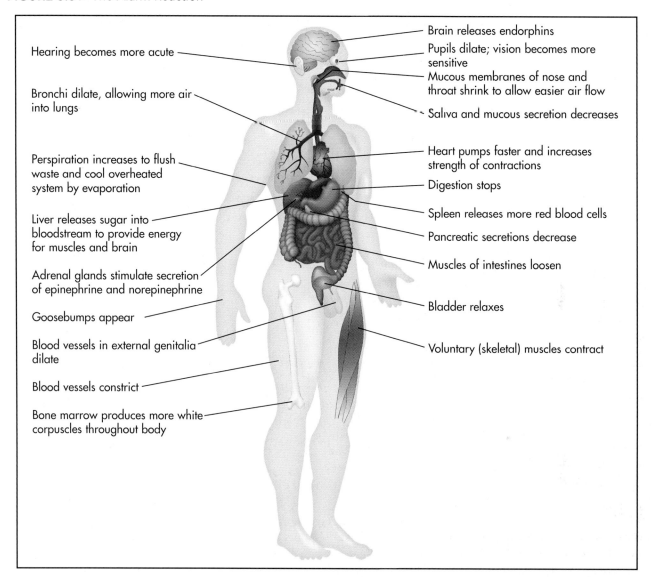

- Brain releases endorphins
- Pupils dilate; vision becomes more sensitive
- Mucous membranes of nose and throat shrink to allow easier air flow
- Saliva and mucous secretion decreases
- Heart pumps faster and increases strength of contractions
- Digestion stops
- Spleen releases more red blood cells
- Pancreatic secretions decrease
- Muscles of intestines loosen
- Bladder relaxes
- Voluntary (skeletal) muscles contract

- Hearing becomes more acute
- Bronchi dilate, allowing more air into lungs
- Perspiration increases to flush waste and cool overheated system by evaporation
- Liver releases sugar into bloodstream to provide energy for muscles and brain
- Adrenal glands stimulate secretion of epinephrine and norepinephrine
- Goosebumps appear
- Blood vessels in external genitalia dilate
- Blood vessels constrict
- Bone marrow produces more white corpuscles throughout body

- The liver releases sugar into the bloodstream to provide instant energy.
- Perspiration increases; the palms get sweaty.
- The muscles get tense, prepared for a workout.
- The senses—sight, hearing, smell, taste, and touch—become acute, ready to identify any danger.

During the alarm stage a person can have superhuman strength. The physiological reactions of the alarm stage are what enable a small woman to lift a car weighing several tons off the chest of a toddler.

## RESISTANCE

The alarm and resistance stages of the stress response evoke more than 1,400 known physiochemical reactions. During the resistance stage, the person meets the perceived

### KEY TERMS

**Fight or flight** series of physiological changes that stress evokes: alarm, resistance, and exhaustion

**Adrenocorticotropic hormone (ACTH)** hormone released by the pituitary gland that stimulates the adrenal glands to release other hormones in the initial stage of stress

**Cortisol** hormone released by the adrenal glands in the first stage of stress

**Epinephrine** hormone released by the adrenal glands during the first stage of stress, affecting metabolism, the muscles, and circulation

**Norepinephrine** hormone released by the adrenal glands during the first stage of stress that affects circulation

**Endorphins** natural painkillers released by the brain

challenge. The adrenal glands continue to release adrenaline, the thyroid gland pumps out hormones, and the hypothalamus releases endorphins. The adrenal glands also inhibit the release of sex hormones (to prevent the possibility of any diversion). Glucose and cholesterol enter the bloodstream, providing instant energy and endurance. Heart and breathing rates become more rapid to boost the oxygen supply to the body. The blood thickens, and the skin crawls and sweats.

Once the perceived challenge passes, the parasympathetic branch of the autonomic nervous system signals the alarm reaction to stop. The body tries to adapt—to achieve the homeostasis that existed before the stress occurred.

That is a substantial challenge. The body maintains its vital functions (such as heartbeat) within a very narrow range considered normal. The dynamic physical reactions to stress push the body to the limit. During resistance, then, the body is on guard, trying to resist the ill effects of the stress and return the body to normal. The body quickly repairs any damage that occurred during the alarm phase.

The resistance stage of the stress response is ideally suited to meeting the challenges of short-term stress. If the stress is short term, the body usually is able to adapt and return to a state of balance. If the stress becomes chronic, however, the body eventually loses its ability to adapt.

## FYI | DEFENSE MECHANISMS FOR COPING WITH STRESS

People learn to cope with stress in various ways—some of them healthy, some not. The more common defense mechanisms include the following.

- Daydreaming about pleasurable situations
- Repression—purposely or selectively forgetting unpleasant experiences
- Denial—flat refusal to believe or recognize that a stressful situation is real
- Rationalization—coming up with socially acceptable justifications for behaviors or situations
- Reaction formation—adopting behaviors and attitudes that are the opposite of how the person feels
- Projection—placing the blame for one's weaknesses or problems on someone else
- Displacement—redirecting socially unacceptable behavior from the true source to a less threatening substitute
- Regression—reverting or retreating to childish or childlike behaviors
- Isolation—detaching oneself from the underlying cause of a stressor

## EXHAUSTION

Most people experience the alarm and resistance stages of the stress response frequently. Only those under chronic stress, however, experience exhaustion, a stage in which the body's resources are depleted and its adaptive abilities are lost. Exhaustion occurs when the body is traumatized by one stress after another for a prolonged time.

During the exhaustion stage, many of the events of the alarm stage recur as the body attempts to adjust to higher levels of stress, but the resulting wear and tear knocks out the immune system and injures body systems and organs. The exhaustion stage sets in when long-term effects of stress emerge. The incredible series of physiological reactions involved in the alarm and resistance stages demands vast stores of energy. When this energy is sapped and the body is no longer able to adapt, the results are disease and premature death.

## Chronic Stress on the Body

With more than a thousand physical reactions taking place within a few minutes, stress and the general adaptation syndrome impact most body systems. The brain is the first to recognize a stressor. It immediately instructs the rest of the body how to adjust to the stressor. The brain continues to stimulate the stress reaction as long as 72 hours following a stressful incident.

The brain is not a discriminator of stressors. It reacts the same whether the stress is physical (almost having a car accident) or emotional (finding out while walking into class that you studied the wrong material for the exam). The resulting deluge of hormones and brain chemicals takes its toll. Elevated levels of stress hormones destroy vitally important brain cells.

The brain is not the only organ that suffers from chronic stress. The endocrine system works overtime, pumping out excess hormones that increase blood pressure, damage the lining of the heart and blood vessels, inhibit vitamin D activity, deplete calcium, increase the risk of diabetes, and suppress the immune system.

Stress affects every part of the digestive system. The mouth stops producing saliva. The regular rhythmic contractions of the esophagus are disrupted, so swallowing becomes difficult. Stomach function slows down. The stomach is bathed in gastric acid and its lining becomes fragile and engorged with blood. The liver overproduces glucose, and the pancreas becomes chronically inflamed. Production of hydrochloric acid increases, and normal peristaltic (wavelike) action is disrupted throughout the intestinal tract.

**TABLE 3.1 ▶** Symptoms of Stress

**COMMON SYMPTOMS OF STRESS**

Headache
Rapid heart beat
Stiffness in neck and shoulder muscles
Backache
Rapid breathing
Sweaty palms, hands
Sweating
Nausea, upset stomach, vomiting
Diarrhea
Irritability and "jumpy"
Irritated, frustrated
Intolerant of minor disturbances
Lose temper more than usual
Yell at others for no apparent reason
Tired more often
Worry too much about things not important
Doubts abilities

**CHRONIC STRESS PROBLEMS**

Cardiovascular
  High blood pressure
  Abnormal heartbeat (arrhythmia)
  Problems with blood clotting
  Hardening of the arteries (atherosclerosis)
  Coronary artery disease
  Heart attack
  Heart failure

Muscle Pain
  Neck, shoulder, low back pain
  Stress affects rheumatoid arthritis

Stomach and Intestinal Problems
  Stress may be a factor in gastro-esophageal reflux
  disease (GERD)
  Peptic ulcer disease
  Irritable bowel syndrome

Reproductive Organs
  Painful menstrual periods
  Decreased fertility
  Erection disorders/problems

Lungs
  Worsens asthma
  Worsens chronic obstructive pulmonary disease
  (COPD)

Skin Problems
  Worsens acne
  Worsens psoriasis
  Causes shingles to flare

Immune System
  Body more vulnerable to illness (colds and minor
  infections to major diseases)
  Worsens symptoms of chronic illness such as AIDS

**ACUTE STRESS PROBLEMS**

Abnormal heartbeat (arrhythmia)
Heart attack
Acute stress disorder
Post-traumatic stress disorders (PSTD)

*Source*: WebMD Health and Balance Effects of Stress
WebMD Medical Reference from Healthwise (June 2, 2005).

In the cardiovascular system the heart speeds up, blood pressure rises, serum cholesterol levels increase, and the blood thickens. Over time these effects seriously impair body functioning.

Because of the physical responses to stress, certain behavioral signs characteristically accompany stress. Changes in appetite are manifested in overeating or undereating. Sleep disturbances may be demonstrated by either insomnia or excessive sleep. Other common behavioral responses include inability to concentrate, lack of creativity, loss of memory, sexual problems, and impulsive behavior. Many people turn to tobacco, alcohol, and other drugs for relief.

Common emotional signs and symptoms include nervousness, forgetfulness, severe mood swings, anxiety, tearfulness, emotional instability, depression, difficulty completing tasks, and irritability. Table 3.1 summarizes the physical and emotional signs of stress.

## Burnout

Stress, especially chronic stress, can lead quickly to **burnout.** The physical signs and symptoms of burnout can include headache, indigestion, fatigue, and muscle soreness. Emotional symptoms can include depression, apathy, or loss of enjoyment in life.

## Hardiness

Some people seem incapacitated by seemingly minor stresses, and others seem to endure enormous strains and pressures. Suzanne Ouellette Kobasa, a psychologist, conducted a number of pioneering studies leading to her concept of **hardiness.** Hardiness is what spells the difference between getting sick from stress and being resilient to stress. According to Kobasa, hardiness comprises three personality traits: commitment, control, and challenge.

### COMMITMENT

**Commitment** is a value embedded in the personality. A person might be committed, for example, to an ideal greater than himself or herself, or the commitment may be to a certain philosophy, to political reform, or even to something as simple as a hobby.

---

**KEY TERMS**

**Burnout** physical and mental exhaustion caused by chronic stress

**Hardiness** a set of personality traits characteristic of people who are resistant to stress

**Commitment** a deep and abiding interest and dedication to something

## CONTROL

Believing that one can **control** the outcome of life events is another aspect of hardiness. It is the refusal to be victimized. Control is not the belief that one can control one's environment. Instead, it is the knowledge that one can control one's reaction to the environment.

## CHALLENGE

People who are not hardy look at change with feelings of helplessness and alienation. Healthy, hardy people face change as a **challenge,** responding with confidence, self-determination, eagerness, and excitement. Change becomes an eagerly sought-after challenge, not a threat.

## What to Do about Stress

One's ability to handle stress depends not only on inherent qualities but also on specific coping strategies, such as eating right, getting plenty of exercise, and managing time effectively. Dealing with stress successfully does not just happen. It requires planning and work. Sometimes it involves changing attitudes, ideologies, values, or goals. It may require making gradual but significant lifestyle changes to eliminate sources of stress. Managing stress entails strategies developed ahead of time, strategies that will improve one's physical and emotional condition and give one an edge in meeting stressful situations when they do arise.

## MEDITATION AND RELAXATION

**Meditation and relaxation,** which have been practiced for over 2,000 years, render powerful health benefits. Meditation reduces stress and changes the way a person perceives it (relaxation of the mind); relaxation is the reduction of stress in the body. It allows one's mind to positively affect the relaxing and healing processes.

As the body relaxes, blood flow to the arms and legs increases, which helps ease muscle tension. Laboratory studies have shown that people who meditate have fewer blood enzymes associated with stress and anxiety. More than 700 studies have proven that meditation induces the **relaxation response** and alleviates the harmful effects of stress.

The most essential element of meditation is something on which to focus, a **mantra** (meaningful word or phrase said silently). The goal is to train the brain to associate the mantra with calmness. Praying serves as a very powerful meditation/relaxation exercise in which one focuses on a power higher than oneself. To be effective, meditation has to be done in a comfortable position in a quiet place, free of distractions. No specific posture is required for meditation. A mantra can be used anywhere and at anytime.

To achieve the best effects from meditation, the person should avoid any stimulants (cigarettes, coffee, tea, cola drinks) for an hour or two before meditating. The best times to meditate and relax are early in the morning (before breakfast) and before dinner. Eating a meal just before meditating diverts blood to the stomach and inhibits the relaxation response. With regular meditation and relaxation, there are reductions of cholesterol levels and blood pressure. There is an increase of quality of life, intelligence levels, and longevity.

## STRESS AND YOUR DIET

Overeating, undereating, or eating the wrong foods can upset the body's balance, making all body systems more likely to suffer the ill effects of stress. An unbalanced diet makes a person more susceptible to disease in general and more vulnerable to the negative effects of stress in particular. Certain foods can even exaggerate stress by making a person uptight.

The battering that the body takes from stress can change its nutritional requirements. Chronic stress may

- Deplete important vitamins and minerals
- Increase the need for protein
- Increase the amount of fats in the bloodstream
- Boost caloric needs

Stressed people should eat foods that are low in fat, high in fiber, and rich in vitamins and minerals. Most of the calories should come from complex carbohydrates, such as whole-grain breads, rice, pasta, fruits, and vegetables. People under chronic stress should boost their protein intake with the leanest sources of protein possible: fish, poultry, lean cuts of beef, and low-fat or skim dairy products. Nutrition is discussed in depth in Chapter 9.

Experts advise against nutritional supplements touted as stress remedies or anti-stress formulas. The vitamins in these products are generally 70 or 80 times the U.S. Daily Values, which can produce mild to severe side effects. Research has even linked deaths to amino acid supplements advertised as remedies for anxiety, stress, depression, and premenstrual syndrome.

## REGULAR EXERCISE

Exercise, discussed further in Chapter 11, is a natural antidote to stress. Regular exercise will

- Ease muscle tension caused by stress
- Reduce the amount of adrenaline circulating in the bloodstream

## Tips for Action Stress-Fighters

Along with long-term strategies, try these quick fixes to fight stress.

- Confide in someone.
- Get a massage.
- Listen to some soft, relaxing, mellow music.
- Take a 20-minute nap.
- Lie down and put a warm compress on your eyes.
- Stand up and stretch.

- Luxuriate in a nice, long soak in a tub filled with hot water.
- Have a good cry—followed by a good laugh.
- Read a few pages in a good book.
- Listen to a tape of birds chirping, the wind whistling, or the waves lapping on the shore.
- Close your eyes and gently massage your temples.

---

- Decrease the intensity of stress
- Lessen the effects of stress
- Reduce the amount of time necessary to recover from stress
- Minimize the physiological reactions of the stress response
- Reduce the risk of getting sick, even for those under severe or chronic stress
- Increase resistance to stress-induced illness
- Minimize the symptoms of illness (such as headache)

### SLEEP

In coping with stress, getting enough sleep is a must. When the body is deprived of sleep, physical, mental, and emotional processes gradually deteriorate. The person who lacks sleep has difficulty concentrating, making decisions, recalling, and utilizing full intellectual abilities. Lack of sleep itself is a significant source of stress. Severe sleep deprivation can even cause psychosis.

Most people need six to eight hours of sleep a night to function well and feel refreshed. This requirement varies from one person to another. Some need more and some need less.

Almost everyone has **insomnia** at some time in life. Insomnia can be caused by stress. Other common causes are medical problems (respiratory conditions) and various lifestyle factors (overloading on caffeine within a few hours of bedtime). Short-term, temporary insomnia usually is not a serious problem. Long-term insomnia can cause serious medical problems and can contribute to chronic stress.

### MASSAGE

The Touch Research Institute at the University of Miami reports that **massage therapy** relieves stress, depression, and anxiety by affecting the body's biochemistry.

When researchers measured the stress hormone cortisol in participants before and after massage, they found that massage therapy lowered levels by up to 53%. (Cortisol can increase blood pressure and blood sugar levels and suppress the immune system.) Massage therapy increases two neurotransmitters—serotonin and dopamine—that aid in reducing depression.

### VISUALIZATION/IMAGERY

A technique that may work for some individuals is **visualization** or using your imagination. Using imagery or visualization involves focusing in on a mental image: a most comforting place in your mind. With the use of your senses of smelling, tasting, seeing, hearing, and feeling, you may be able to reach a spiritual place and find peace and relaxation within the mind and the body.

---

### KEY TERMS

**Control** the belief that one can influence the effects of life experiences on oneself

**Challenge** the capacity to see change as an opportunity for excitement and growth

**Meditation and relaxation** relaxation of the mind and body

**Relaxation response** an inborn bodily reaction that counteracts the harmful effects of stress

**Mantra** a word or phrase repeated silently during meditation

**Insomnia** prolonged and usually abnormal inability to obtain adequate sleep

**Massage therapy** increases serotonin and dopamine that aid in reducing stress

**Visualization** focusing in on a mental image that one is comfortable with

**Tips for Action** Move to Beat Stress

To get the most benefits from exercise:

■ Choose a form of exercise you like.

■ Find an activity suited to your personality. Do you want something that will let you daydream or something that involves a partner?

■ Consider how much equipment the exercise requires. Walking requires nothing more than a good pair of shoes. Golf requires a set of clubs, a handful of tees, and plenty of fresh balls.

■ Consider where you can exercise. You can walk or bicycle almost anywhere, unlike golfing, skiing, or playing racquetball and tennis.

■ Do not feel limited to what you can do already. If you think fencing sounds like fun, take a class.

■ Consider team sports. They provide social support—a proven stress buster.

## MANAGING YOUR TIME

One of the most common stressors is simply having too much to do in too little time. A fast-paced society coupled with the speed at which people move can be a significant stressor. Learning to manage available time can alleviate stress and reduce anxiety.

A key to effective time management is to determine how time is spent. The following steps might be taken to begin the process.

> Learn to prioritize, and be mature in setting priorities. Not every demand is a top priority. You usually can split tasks into those that are essential, important, and unimportant or trivial. Spend your time and attention on the things that are essential or important. If you have time left over, you can go for the trivial things.

> Use a daily planner to help organize commitments. Various kinds are available on the market. Look for the one that includes everything needed under one cover—a place to write addresses, phone numbers, references, appointments, tasks, and goals.

1. Judge realistically how long a task will take. Most people underestimate by about 50%, so get into the habit of adding 50% to the time you think it will take. Once you learn how to estimate realistically the time needed to complete different tasks, you can stop overcrowding your day with too much to handle.

2. Keep a diary for two weeks. You might be stunned to find out how much time you are spending on the phone or in front of the television. You cannot outline realistic goals until you know how you are spending your time.

3. Try to figure out your peak time. Are you a morning person, or do you get your second wind when most people are quitting for the day? Plan your most demanding tasks—studying, working—for the time you are at your peak. If you have to take a particularly

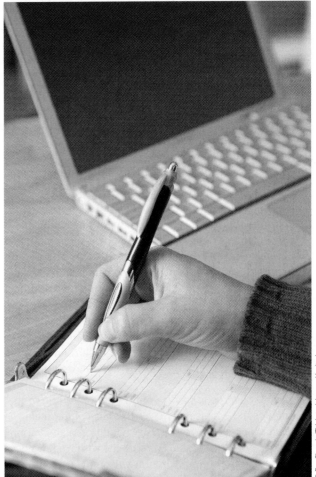

▲ *A daily planner is a helpful time-management tool*

challenging class and are generally sluggish in the morning, try to schedule it for the afternoon or find out if it is offered at night.

4. Before you go to bed at night, assess what went on that day. Did you meet all your goals? Were you able

**Tips for Action** A Good Night's Sleep

To find out how much sleep you need, go to sleep at the same time every night, then sleep until you awaken. (It will take a couple of weeks to determine what you need.)

■ Establish a sleep pattern: Go to bed at the same time every night and wake up at the same time every morning—even on the weekends when you can.

■ If you take a nap, limit it to 20 minutes; longer naps will interfere with sleep at night.

■ Do not exercise, use caffeine, or smoke late in the day. These stimulate the body.

■ Have a light snack before bedtime. You will sleep more soundly if you are not hungry.

■ Use your bed and bedroom only for sleeping. Do not watch television, study, eat, read, or do work in bed.

■ Deal with worries and pressures before you go to bed. Take notes on possible solutions, then forget about your problems until morning.

■ Take a warm bath an hour before bedtime. It will slow down your metabolism.

■ If you do not fall asleep within 20 minutes, get up, leave the bedroom, and do something quiet and relaxing until you feel sleepy. Do not toss and turn in bed, getting more and more stressed because you cannot fall asleep.

---

to accomplish all your top priorities? If not, pinpoint what went wrong, and then develop a strategy for change.

5. Write down your schedule for tomorrow. Include several periods to do what you want to do—soak in a hot tub, read a good book, watch a sports event on television, or talk to a friend. Knowing you can look forward to a few breaks can help you face the more stressful times.

You can do only so much in a single day or week. If you start to get overwhelmed, back off. Do not feel guilty if you have to say no to something or someone. Going to the movie with friends might be fun, but not if you have to stay up half the night to study for an exam in exchange for a good time.

## ADJUST ATTITUDES

The way a person thinks often determines what happens. Under stress, an **attitude adjustment** can help change the way stress impacts the body. Persons who express mostly positive emotions live longer and are more resilient than those who tend to remain emotionally negative. Emotionally negative people can cultivate skills that will help them to be more positive and optimistic.

1. Listen carefully to the words you use to describe yourself and your situation. Are they positive or negative? Listen for a few weeks. If you need to, use different phrases and descriptions.

2. Role play, either by yourself or with a friend. Start by relating a stressful situation you have experienced lately. Tell how you reacted. Then come up with different ways in which you could have reacted. If you are role playing with a friend, ask for feedback or

**FYI** TIME KILLERS

In every schedule you will find things that eat up your time. Necessary activities such as eating and sleeping can become time killers if you overdo them. Other time killers are not necessary. Try to eliminate them.

| | |
|---|---|
| Indecision | Watching television |
| Procrastination | Lengthy talking on the phone |
| Worry | Interruptions |
| Confusion | Too much socializing |
| Perfectionism | Browsing World Wide Web |
| | Computer games |

suggestions. Next, imagine some plausible stressful situations and outline how you would handle them. Concentrate on positive responses.

3. For one week look for the good in every person and every situation you encounter. You always can find something. This exercise conditions you to change your attitude over time.

4. Avoid words that signal defeat: always, never, should have, ought to. Replace them with more benign choices that reflect joy, thankfulness, and optimism.

---

## KEY TERMS

**Attitude adjustment** changing the way a person thinks about things

---

**Tips for Action** Time Management

To get the most out of your time:

■ Tackle one thing at a time. If you have a long list of things to do, move through the list calmly, one item at a time. Do the more complicated tasks first. Do not move on to the next item until you have finished the first one.

■ Set realistic goals; break long-term goals down into short-term ones.

■ Delegate the tasks that other people can do for you instead of trying to do everything yourself.

■ If you are faced with a difficult task, rehearse it mentally first. You will approach it with less stress and apprehension if you have something concrete in mind.

■ Take advantage of little chunks of time that crop up in your schedule; plug in a handful of short tasks.

■ Stay flexible, and plan for disruptions. Never schedule anything so tightly that something that is unexpected will throw off everything.

■ Reward yourself often.

■ Protect yourself against boredom; set a satisfying, realistic goal, then do something toward it every day.

---

## JOURNALING

Keeping a journal (**journaling**) can make one feel creative, imaginative, and unique and can give one a sense of purpose and competence. Recording your experiences can help you to understand and clarify your feelings. Journaling is a way of becoming more familiar with the self, by spending time alone in one's personal, private place and by expressing feelings in black and white. These private notes allow you to record your feelings, help you to make sense of your emotions, express your perceptions, release tensions, better understand various interactions, and laugh at yourself.

## MUSIC THERAPY

Music has been a strong and influential force in the psychological, sociological, physiological, and emotional aspects of individuals and cultures. **Music therapy** reduces stress and anxiety and causes one to enjoy a calm and relaxed state. Positive change has been brought about in some people with health or educational problems.

## HOBBIES

**Hobbies** provide various methods of relaxing and unwinding. Reading, listening to or making music, writing, painting, cooking, engaging in sports—active or spectator—can be excellent ways of reducing stress while enjoying a favorite hobby. Find the activity that fascinates you and makes you want to do "this thing" as often as you possibly can.

## PROGRESSIVE RELAXATION

**Progressive relaxation** is a stress reduction technique pioneered by Edmund Jacobson. Being a physician, he wanted to help patients who had tensed muscles associated with stress. His three-step technique is simple.

1. Contract (tense) a small muscle group.
2. Relax the muscle group.
3. Concentrate on determining how different the two sensations felt.

The progression can be from head to toes or from feet to head. It does not matter as long as all major muscle groups in the body are involved and eventually relax.

When doing progressive relaxation, the person first should tense the muscles as hard as possible, and then relax them. With a little practice, this becomes effortless and the muscles can be relaxed without having to contract them first.

Unlike meditation, in which the person should not think about what is happening to the body, progressive relaxation requires the person to concentrate on what is happening to the muscles. Acute awareness of the relaxed condition of the body yields the best results.

## BIOFEEDBACK TRAINING

Through **biofeedback training** a person can measure physiological functions of which he or she normally is not aware, such as skin temperature, heart rate, and blood pressure. This information is converted into something meaningful so the responses can be controlled.

## Tips for Action  Attitude Adjustments

To get the most from your thoughts:

■ Get rid of unimportant details. Keep your mind uncluttered so you can concentrate on what is really important.

■ While you are at it, let go of the past. Everyone makes mistakes; if you are going to spend time remembering, concentrate on your victories and pleasures, not your defeats and miseries.

■ Choose your worries. Stop worrying about things you cannot change. Concentrate instead on worrying about the things that matter.

■ Galvanize your worries into action. Figure out how to solve the problem, then tackle the steps one at a time.

■ Learn to laugh. A good laugh is great for your mental outlook, and it gives your whole body a workout.

■ Stop beating yourself. Think of yourself as a winner, a person who can handle stress.

■ Stop worrying about what everyone else thinks of you or wants out of you. The most important person you need to please is yourself. "Be your own best friend."

---

Unlike some other forms of relaxation exercises, people cannot learn biofeedback training on their own. It requires monitoring by extremely sensitive equipment, then teaching people to regulate their own physiological responses. Biofeedback training is extremely valuable as a stress management technique because it allows people to control physical responses to stress. Most people can learn effective biofeedback techniques in a few sessions from a trained therapist using monitoring devices.

## YOGA

**Yoga** is an ancient exercise that reduces the biological effects of stress. Yoga improves strength, flexibility, and endurance and changes the responses of the body and mind. When yoga is practiced, there is better control of blood pressure, pulse, respiratory rate, and body temperature.

People cannot design their own technique or routine in yoga, unlike in other relaxation exercises. Yoga is composed of precise postures done in a specific sequence combined with an exact breathing rhythm aimed to reduce tension and rigidity.

The yoga postures are difficult and complex, and they require training and practice. Few people can assume the postures at first, and many are not able to complete the sequence properly for as long as three months. A number of good yoga instruction books are available in the marketplace, and yoga classes might be taught at your college, university, or recreation center.

## HUMOR THERAPY

A good laugh is extremely healthy. Laughter increases endorphins (chemicals in the body that make you feel good). "Humor is good for whatever ails you." Laughing causes a dramatic deduction in stress-related chemicals and actually boosts the immune system.

## AROMATHERAPY

Various oils and plant extracts have been proven to promote relaxation. This may be explained by the association of nerves with smell and their link to the limbic system, which influences the endocrine system. The impact on the endocrine system affects moods, therefore promoting relaxation. Oils are used in baths, massages, and skin compresses, whereas scented candles are burned in many environs.

---

### KEY TERMS

**Journaling** recording personal occurrences, experiences, situations, and observations

**Music therapy** instrumental and vocal sounds for listening and relaxing pleasure

**Hobbies** chosen activities that one enjoys doing for relaxation

**Progressive relaxation** exercise to relieve stress, involving tensing and relaxing muscle groups

**Biofeedback training** method of measuring physiological functions controlled by the autonomic nervous system

**Yoga** exercise done to calm and stimulate the mind

**Humor therapy** laughing increases endorphins, which decreases stress

**Aromatherapy** relaxation from scents of oils, plant extracts, and candles

**Tips for Action** Steps in Meditation

Find a quiet room as free from distraction as possible. Turn off the phone. Regulate lights and temperature so you are comfortable.

1. Loosen your clothing if it is tight, especially at the wrists, neck, and waist. Sit in the most comfortable position for you. Place your feet flat on the floor. Rest your hands in your lap.
2. Inhale slowly and deeply, through your nose, hold your breath briefly, then exhale slowly. As you begin to breathe deeply, let the tension flow out of your body.
3. If you are concentrating on an object, close your eyes partially so the object appears blurred. If you are

focusing on a mantra, begin repeating it silently and rhythmically as you breathe in and out.

4. Gradually focus all your attention on that one thing.
5. Continue meditating for approximately 20 minutes.
6. When you are finished, give yourself time to readjust. Open your eyes, focus on various objects around the room, and gradually return to your normal breathing rate. While still seated, stretch your arms, legs, back, shoulders, and neck. Finally, stand up slowly.

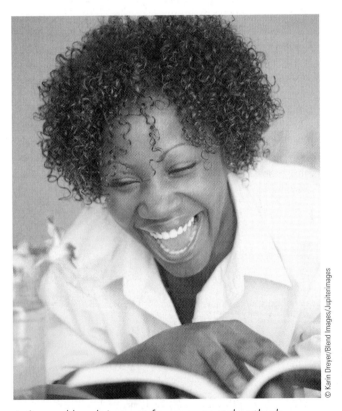

▲ *A good laugh is great for your mental outlook*

© Karin Dreyer/Blend Images/Jupiterimages

## Summary

- The science of psychoneuroimmunology studies the link between activity in the brain, the immune system, and health or disease.
- Stressors can be physical, emotional, social, intellectual, or spiritual. Stress can range from mild to

severe and can be positive and desirable (eustress) or negative and undesirable (distress). Seemingly minor stresses, or hassles, can have negative effects in the long term if they are unremitting over time. Stresses are different throughout the life span.

- The three stages of the general adaptation syndrome are alarm, resistance, and exhaustion.
- Hardiness has three components: commitment, control, and challenge.
- Signs of burnout include headache, indigestion, fatigue, and muscle soreness, as well as depression and loss of enjoyment for living.
- Stress management components include a balanced diet, regular exercise, sufficient sleep, and wise use of time.
- Techniques for stress reduction include reframing thoughts and relaxation techniques such as meditation, progressive relaxation, biofeedback training, yoga, and tai chi.

## Personal Health Resources

ThomsonNOW™ Visit the ThomsonNOW website at http://thomsonedu.com/thomsonnow for valuable resources that will:

- Help you evaluate your knowledge of the material.
- Guide you through tutorials to help you understand and apply the material.
- Allow you to take an exam-prep quiz to better prepare for class tests.

Healthfinder. Sponsored by the federal Office of Disease Prevention and Health Promotion, this website offers

## Tips for Action Progressive Relaxation

Regardless of the routine used for progressive relaxation, follow these guidelines:

- Lie on your back in the most comfortable position possible.
- Take off your shoes, and loosen any restrictive clothing.
- Close your eyes, rotate your ankles outward, and place your arms at your sides.
- Make sure you move all major muscle groups in the body. Do not forget your face, including your forehead, eyes, nose, mouth, cheeks, and tongue.

- As you move each muscle group, contract the muscles as tightly as you can, and hold the contraction for 30 seconds.
- If you experience pain or cramping during a contraction, release the contraction immediately.
- Concentrate on the dramatic difference in feeling between a tensed muscle and a relaxed one.

---

links to health information, publications, and organizations on a wide range of health topics. 1-877-696-6775

**www.healthfinder.gov**

Office of Minority Health Resource Center (OMHRC). This is a free, government-sponsored resource and referral service on minority health issues. Services are offered in English and Spanish. 1-800-444-6472

**www.omhrc.gov/OMHRC**

Stress Less. Temple University offers a plethora of information on dealing with student stress, economic stress (financial), student and personnel burnout and stress, and other stress-related topics. 1-215-204-7182

**www.nimbus.temple.edu/~mlombard/stressless/**

Mental Health Net. This site includes information and news releases on mental health topics such as anxiety, depression, stress, treatment research and modalities, and more. 1-800-528-9025

**www.cmhc.com/**

## It's Your Turn for Study and Review

1. How does stress affect the body, especially the immune system?
2. Define stress and explain the general adaptation syndrome.
3. List some psychological, environmental, physiological, and psychosocial stressors.
4. List some emotional, behavioral, and physical symptoms of stress. What are some techniques that can be used to control stress?

## Thinking about Health Issues

- Can massage therapy improve overall health?
"Massage Your Mood. A Friendly Touch Eases Stress and Anxiety." Altshul, Sara, *Prevention*, August 2006.

1. How does massage therapy physiologically help improve health? Provide at least two examples of health conditions that can be improved by using massage therapy.
2. In terms of body function, how does massage therapy differ from other types of relaxation techniques?

## Selected Bibliography

Aaronson, L. "Make a Gratitude Adjustment." *Psychology Today*, March/April 2006, pp. 60–61.

AARP. The Magazine. "How to Build Your Own Luck." July/August 2005, p. 101.

Altshul, S. "Massage Your Mood." *Prevention*, August 2006, 58:8, p. 100.

Borysenko, J. "Stress First Aid: How to Find Inner Peace in Mere Minutes." *Prevention*, September 2005.

Borysenko, J. "Make Your Own Luck." *Prevention*, 58:7, July 2006, pp. 101–103.

Borysenko, J. "Staying Centered." *Prevention*, 58:8, July 2006, pp. 107–109.

Cooper, A. and Dodd, J. "Put Stress on Hold." *Health*, 20:6, July/August 2006, p. 151.

Dickerson, S. and Kemeny, M. "Acute Stressors and Cortisol Responses: A Theoretical Integration and Synthesis of Laboratory Research." *Psychological Bulletin*, 130:3, May 2004.

Fraser, L. "The Reluctant Meditator." *Health*, 20:1, January/February 2006, pp. 124, 125, & 196.

Gard, C. J. "Panic Attacks More than Being Nervous." *Current Health*, April/May 2001, pp. 26–27.

Gilbert, K. "Can Extreme Stress Turn Hair Prematurely Gray?" *Psychology Today*, 39:2, June 2006, p. 20.

Gorrell, C. "Alone against the World." *Psychology Today*, March/April 2001, p. 16.

Hafen, B. Q. and Hoeger, Werner W. K. *Wellness: Guidelines for a Healthy Lifestyle*, 3rd ed. Englewood, CO: Morton Publishing, 2001.

Hoskins, N. "Nurture Your Body Image with Yoga." *Health*, 18:1, January/February 2004, pp. 59, 60, 63.

Jesionowski, K. "Exercising through the Winter Is Key to Physical and Mental Fitness." *Partners*, 2004, pp. 22, 23.

Kendler, K. S., Thornton, L. M., and Gardner, C. O. "Genetic Risk, Number of Previous Episodes, and Stressful Life Events in Predicting Onset of Major Depression." *American Journal of Psychiatry*, 158:4, April 2001, pp. 582–586.

Kendler, K. S., Thornton, L. M., and Prescott, C. A. "Gender Differences in the Rates of Exposure to Stressful Life Events and Sensitivity to Their Depressogenic Effects." *American Journal of Psychiatry*, 158:4, April 2001, pp. 587–593.

Levine, S. B. "Reinvent Your Expectations." *More*, April 2006, pp. 104–105.

Matousek, M. "Quit Your Pain." *AARP The Magazine*, 49:3B, May/June 2006, pp. 46, 48, 118.

Meltzer, R. "Repeat After Me: I Am Less Stressed." *Prevention*, 58:7, July 2006, p. 44.

McGowan, K. "Relax—Everything Is Under Control." *Psychology Today*, 38:4, July/August 2005, p. 11.

Mann, D. "Take It Easy: Controlling Cortisol Production Is Key to Controlling Stress." *Better Nutrition*, January 1999, p. 38.

Murray, B. "College Youth Haunted by Increased Pressures." *American Psychological Monitor*, 29:12, December 1998.

National Center for Health Statistics. *Healthy People 2010 Review*. Hyattsville, MD.

Pengilly, J. W. and Dowd, E. T. "Hardiness and Social Support as Moderators of Stress." *Journal of Clinical Psychology*, 56:6, June 2000, pp. 813–820.

Pirisi, A. "Race: The Color of Pain." *Psychology Today*, July/August 2000, p. 22.

Selye, H. *Stress without Distress*. New York: Lippincott, 1974.

Siegel, B. S. *Love, Medicine and Miracles*. New York: Harper and Row, 1986.

Singer, B. W. "Laughter Lowers Stress, Reduces Pain, and Revs Immunity." *Health*, October 2000, p. 76.

Spiegel, D. "Healing Words: Emotional Expression and Disease Outcome." *Journal of the American Medical Association*, 281:14, April 14, 1999, p. 1328.

Stress at Work U.S. Dept. of Health and Human Services, Public Health Service Centers for Disease Control and Prevention National Institute for Occupational Safety and Health (NIOSH) DHHS (NIOSH) Publication No. 99-101.

Substance Abuse and Mental Health Services Administration. *Mental Health: A Report of the Surgeon General*. Rockville, MD: U.S. Department of Health and Human Services, National Institutes of Health, 1999.

Segerstrom, S. and Miller, G. "Psychological Stress and the Human Immune System: A Meta-Analytic Study of 30 Years of Inquiry." *Psychological Bulletin*, 130:4, July 2004.

Toffler, A. *Future Shock*. New York: Random House, 1970.

*Wellness for a Lifetime, A Woman's Book for Health and Well-Being*, 2004.

Woodbury, M. A. "Headache, Heartache: The Pinn's the Same." *Health*, 18:2, March 2004, p. 112.

Name _____  Date _____

Course _____  Section _____

The answer depends in part on what is going on in your life. But it also depends on some other factors, such as what your attitudes are about those events and how much control you feel over what happens.

The first step in managing stress is to identify it, and the test below will help you do that. It is simple: Read each question, then circle the number that most closely describes your situation or attitude. If you are completely neutral, circle 5; if a question does not apply to you at all, skip it.

Ready?

Sharpen your pencil, and go to work.

1. How often do you suffer stress-related physical symptoms, such as headaches, jaw pain, neck pain, back pain, indigestion, abdominal pain, diarrhea, loss of appetite, excessive perspiration, fatigue, or a pounding in your chest?

   Rarely or never                                    Every day

   1    2    3    4    5    6    7    8    9    10

2. Do you wash your hands before you eat?

   Always                                    Rarely or never

   1    2    3    4    5    6    7    8    9    10

3. Do you take measures to keep your food safe, such as cooking it adequately, storing it properly, and avoiding obvious contaminants?

   Almost always                                    Rarely or never

   1    2    3    4    5    6    7    8    9    10

4. How often do you eat fresh fruits, fresh vegetables, whole grains, and foods high in fiber?

   Every day                                    Rarely or never

   1    2    3    4    5    6    7    8    9    10

5. How often do you eat food high in fat or sugar, including candy, pastry, soft drinks, and food from fast-food restaurants?

   Occasionally                                    Every day

   1    2    3    4    5    6    7    8    9    10

6. How often do you exercise?

   Every day                                    Rarely or never

   1    2    3    4    5    6    7    8    9    10

7. How many hours of sleep do you get each day?

   Eight or more                                    Less than four

   1    2    3    4    5    6    7    8    9    10

8. How many cups of coffee or caffeinated soft drinks do you drink each day?

   None                                    Five or more

   1    2    3    4    5    6    7    8    9    10

**9.** How often do you use alcohol, tobacco, over-the-counter drugs, or prescription drugs to relieve stress?

Never                                    Every day

1    2    3    4    5    6    7    8    9    10

**10.** If you have a relationship with a significant other, how would you describe that relationship?

Mutually satisfying in many ways            Marked by jealousy or insecurity

1    2    3    4    5    6    7    8    9    10

**11.** How do you feel when you have to say no to a request for your time, energy, talents, or money?

Confident and at ease                          Anxious and guilt-ridden

1    2    3    4    5    6    7    8    9    10

**12.** How would you characterize your support system?

Broad-based, many sources                   Limited or no sources

1    2    3    4    5    6    7    8    9    10

**13.** What kinds of friendships do you have?

At least several close friends and confidants        No close friends

1    2    3    4    5    6    7    8    9    10

**14.** What do you do if you have a problem you cannot solve on your own?

Seek help immediately                         Suffer on my own

1    2    3    4    5    6    7    8    9    10

**15.** How many major changes (such as entering or ending an intimate relationship, the death of a family member, a change in your financial status, moving, starting a new job, a change in sleeping habits, a change in living conditions, or a change in the number of arguments you have with roommates) have occurred in your life during the last year?

None                                      Many

1    2    3    4    5    6    7    8    9    10

**16.** How do you react when confronted with a problem or stressful situation?

Put it aside to gain perspective,           Feel overwhelmed
then focus on solutions                       or panic-stricken

1    2    3    4    5    6    7    8    9    10

**17.** How often do you retreat temporarily when you start to feel overwhelmed by stress?

Most of the time                              Never

1    2    3    4    5    6    7    8    9    10

**18.** How do you normally feel at the end of the day?

I got the important things done         I did not accomplish anything

1    2    3    4    5    6    7    8    9    10

**19.** How many hassles do you have in a typical day?

A few                                      Many

1    2    3    4    5    6    7    8    9    10

**20.** How much noise are you exposed to every day?

Not very much                                    Most of the day is noisy

    1    2    3    4    5    6    7    8    9    10

**21.** How comfortable is your environment? (Consider temperature extremes, humidity, crowding, and environmental pollutants.)

Very comfortable                                    Very uncomfortable

    1    2    3    4    5    6    7    8    9    10

**22.** Overall, how satisfying is your life?

Very satisfying                                    Very disappointing

    1    2    3    4    5    6    7    8    9    10

## Scoring

Time to take a look at your stress level. This exercise will tell you two things: It will indicate your general stress level; then it will help pinpoint the specific things that are causing you stress.

First, total up your score by adding every number you circled. Now divide it by the number of questions you answered. This is one test on which you do not want a high score. The closer your average creeps toward 10, the higher your stress level is likely to be. (By the way, it is important to average your stress score this way; a high level of stress in a few areas will not cause your general stress level to skyrocket.)

Next, go back and isolate what is causing you problems. Look back through your responses. Find those in which you circled a number higher than 5. Simple—you have found your problem areas.

Finally, determine some stress-busting strategies. Check out your problematic question number; then find the corresponding number among the tips below. The rest is up to you.

## Stress-Savvy Tips and Key to "How Stressed Are You?"

1. Stress-related physical symptoms are just that—related to stress. The best way to get rid of them is to get rid of the stress that causes them. In the meantime, there are a few things you can do to manage your most troublesome symptoms. For headaches: Keep a headache diary; it will help you identify what triggers your headaches, a first step in prevention. Until you can do that, try deep breathing, relaxation, stretching muscles to relieve tension in your neck and jaw, or a warm bath. For back pain: Try deep breathing combined with gentle stretching exercises, soaking in a warm bath, or meditation. For irritable bowel syndrome: Stay away from high-fat foods, avoid caffeine (including chocolate), add fiber to your diet (eat plenty of whole grains), and try relaxation exercises. For indigestion: Eat smaller meals more often during the day; stick to foods that are mild and easy to digest. Watching what you eat can also ease fatigue—eat foods rich in vitamins, potassium, calcium, iron, and zinc.

2. Washing your hands before you eat dramatically reduces your chance of picking up an infection—an obvious stressor. Other simple things you can do: Keep your hands out of your mouth, do not share eating utensils or drinking glasses, avoid contact with people you know are ill, limit sexual contact and use safe sexual practices, and make sure your immunizations are up-to-date.

3. You can avoid the physical stress of food-borne illness by scrubbing fruits and vegetables thoroughly; preparing raw meat on surfaces that can be easily cleaned; preparing raw meats separately from other foods; avoiding raw or rare meats or fish; cooking hamburger until it is no longer pink; boiling canned foods before you eat them; refrigerating leftovers immediately; avoiding foods that contain raw eggs; avoiding foods that are spoiled; and avoiding wild nuts, berries, mushrooms, and plants unless you are certain they are edible.

4. Stress robs your body of certain nutrients. If you are under stress from any source, you need an extra shot of certain vitamins and minerals. Especially important are the B vitamins (found in nuts, seeds, beans, peas, meat, and whole grains), vitamin C (found in citrus fruits, green peppers, dark-green vegetables, strawberries, and tomatoes), calcium (found in milk and dairy products, citrus fruits, dark-green leafy vegetables, and dried beans), and protein (found in

meat, fish, poultry, dairy products, and eggs). Do not forget that you can get a complete protein by combining certain plant foods—rice with legumes, wheat with soybeans, or legumes with corn, rice, wheat, or oats, for example.

5. Stress robs your body of some vital nutrients, and sugars and fats speed up the process. Sugars tend to strip out certain B vitamins and make you more susceptible to stress. Concentrate on eating a balanced diet of foods low in fats and sugars, check labels, and steer clear of foods that list sugar in any form as the first or second ingredient. Avoid skipping meals; eat a hearty breakfast and light supper; drink plenty of water; and check with your physician about nutritional supplements if you are under considerable stress.

6. Research proves that regular exercise diminishes the effects of stress—even stress you cannot avoid. The best kind of stress-busting exercise is continuous, rhythmic, aerobic exercise; walking, running, bicycling, swimming, or cross-country skiing are good choices. To avoid injury, make sure you allow for warm-up and cool-down time. And if your joints are a little creaky from inactivity, start slowly and build up gradually. Wear light-colored clothing in the summer, and several light layers of dark-colored clothing in the winter. Drink plenty of fluid before and after you exercise. You should feel energized, not tired, when you finish exercising. You are pushing too hard if you feel a heaviness in your arms or legs, soreness in your muscles or joints, or extreme fatigue.

7. Sleep relieves stress. While you are asleep, you breathe more deeply, your heart slows down, your blood pressure drops, and your muscles relax. To get better sleep, review the suggestions earlier in this section. Try to relax for an hour or so before you go to bed, do your best to stick to a regular sleep schedule, avoid eating a big meal right before you go to sleep, and do what you can to make your sleep environment comfortable.

8. Caffeine increases your sensitivity to stress by stimulating the central nervous system, charging up the autonomic nervous system, and lowering your ability to tolerate stress. Avoid caffeine or use it only in moderation. Remember, too, that caffeine is found in more than just coffee and cola drinks. Cut back on chocolate, cocoa, and over-the-counter medications that contain caffeine. Try drinking decaffeinated coffee or switching to a soothing herbal tea.

9. Alcohol might relax you at first, but research shows that, over the long term, alcohol increases stress by causing your body to churn out stress-related hormones. Keep a diary of your alcohol intake for a few weeks. If you are drinking too much (more than an occasional drink, or more than 12 ounces of beer or 4 ounces of wine at a time), take measures to stop. Find some other ways to relieve stress, and try substituting another kind of drink for alcohol—exotic fruit juices or sparkling mineral water can be fun.

   And do not forget tobacco. Smoking causes a long list of health problems. What you may not know is that smoking combined with stress escalates the situation. Take measures to stop. Ask your doctor or the college health center about local programs that can help you quit.

10. The least stressful relationship is one in which your companion is also your friend—someone with whom you share your feelings, triumphs, disappointments, goals, and dreams. If appropriate, healthy sexual expression should be part of that relationship. Aside from being a way to communicate within a committed relationship, the physiological processes involved in sex work to relieve stress and tension. Finally, remember that no matter how well matched you are, no two people can fill every need for each other. Maintain separate friends and interests to avoid becoming too dependent on each other.

11. The ability to assert yourself means you usually meet your own needs without destroying interpersonal relationships. Assertive behavior allows you to protect your own rights, which is essential to avoiding stress. If you are not very assertive now, start by respecting yourself. You are responsible for yourself, and others need to live with your decisions. If you need to say no, just say it; do not feel obligated to offer excuses. And remember the nonverbals that go along with it. Speak in a firm, steady voice without hesitation, stand straight, and look at the other person directly in the eye.

12. The larger your network of support, the better you will be able to manage stress. Ideally, your network of support should be broad, stemming from your family, church, neighborhood, school, social and political organizations, and friends. Try organizing or joining a study group (students in a class or within a major area of study), service group, sports team, hobby group, campaign team, social group, or simply a group of friends who share a favorite activity—bicycling, kite-flying, or watercolors, for example. Remember, the most valuable type of social support from groups such as these often happens from the informal contacts, such as riding to a meeting with someone or getting together for dinner after the meeting.

13. Research shows that one of the best ways to prevent stress-related illness is to have good friends—people you can really talk to, people with whom you can share your joys, concerns, apprehensions, and love. If you need to expand

your circle of friends, start by expanding your contacts. In other words, go where the people are. Draw people into conversation, invite people to informal get-togethers, show people you care, and get involved with others.

14. An important part of social support—and stress reduction—is your willingness to seek help when you need it and the assurance that there are people who can help you. Close friends can act as confidants, but you should also know that there are others in your support network to whom you can turn—a clergyman, school counselor, or therapist.

15. Research has shown that your chance of developing a stress-induced illness increases with the number of life crises you have during any given time. (Check the list of specific crises cited earlier in this section.) Whenever you can, avoid too many changes at once. If you have just ended an important relationship, for example, do not move to a new apartment and start a part-time job, too. For the best coping strategy, try to anticipate likely changes, then slow down your pace, be gentle on yourself, avoid as many new commitments as you can, and stay flexible. Still another strategy is called stress-inoculation. In essence, you imagine—vividly—the worst thing that could happen, then map out how you would handle it. Then, no matter what happens, you know you can do something to cope.

16. Your ability to adapt to situations and problems directly affects your ability to manage stress. Boost your odds by trying the following: Put the problem aside long enough to get perspective. What long-range effects will it have? Who does it involve? Then focus in on what you can do to solve the problem, and try to come up with several different alternatives. (Having several different plans for confronting the situation gives you flexibility and removes the anxious possibility of your only plan failing.) Above all, relax and keep a sense of humor. And, when you have met the challenge, reward yourself for succeeding.

17. There is nothing wrong with retreat; it is a coping skill that can help you buffer the effects of stress. Do not run away from problems or avoid responsibility. But when you are feeling overwhelmed, buy yourself some breathing space by going for a long walk, taking in a new movie, putting together a challenging puzzle, going to lunch with a friend, reading a favorite book, or taking a nap. The key is to get a mini-escape or time-out—something that will divert your thoughts and recharge your batteries. You will go back to the problem renewed and strong enough to handle the challenge.

18. If you want to manage stress, learn to manage your time. There are some excellent pointers earlier in this section. One of the most important tactics is prioritizing: Figure out which tasks are most important; then do those things first. It helps to make a list of everything you need to do, and then assign each a priority (for example, **1** for things you must get done today if you want to avoid problems, **2** for things that must be done but that could wait, and **3** for things you would like to do but that are not essential). Start out with the things that are the highest priority; get them done first. Then move to the second category. If you have time left over, start on the last category—but, if not, no big deal. For maximum effectiveness, schedule your time, delegate things that someone else could do for you, limit the number of interruptions you have, and plan for some breaks.

19. Hassles are defined as the irritants and annoyances—most of them fairly minor—that everyone encounters on a daily basis. Simply stated, they are part of living. Hassles can include things such as having to wait for someone, getting caught in traffic, not being able to find a parking space, having to stand in lines, being bothered by a fly, not being able to find the book you need at the library, conflicts with a roommate, having to endure a boring professor, sleeping in and missing breakfast, or not having enough change to do laundry. One or two are not bad. But when your day gets filled with hassles, your stress skyrockets.

    There is not much you can do to prevent hassles, but you can work smart to defuse them. Think ahead; anticipate what you can. If you think you might get stuck in traffic, leave 15 minutes early. If you know the parking on campus is a nightmare, ride the bus, ride your bike, walk, or join a carpool. If it is laundry day, stop at the bank on the way home and get a couple of rolls of quarters. If you have had trouble finding resource materials for a paper, start early. For the rest—those things you cannot circumvent—try to change your expectations. Do not expect to avoid traffic problems; do not expect to get your groceries without standing in line. If you learn to look at things differently, you will be able to wait patiently, sit calmly, and think of something pleasant instead of getting uptight.

20. Everyone knows that noise is irritating. But did you know that noise increases stress? It boosts the heart rate, increases blood pressure, tenses the muscles, and causes the body to secrete stress-related hormones. At certain decibels (a jet plane engine, a pneumatic riveter, a guitar amplifier), noise can permanently damage hearing. If you are trying to concentrate on a difficult task, even a little noise can be stressful. The most stressful is noise that constantly changes in intensity, frequency, or pitch.

    You can reduce your stress from noise. If you can, choose an apartment away from a busy street, a convenience store, a fast-food restaurant, or an industrial area. Look for a carpeted apartment. You at least want carpet in the rooms that are directly adjacent to other units. Choose upholstered instead of hard-surfaced furniture, heavy drapes instead of aluminum blinds. Put a small foam pad under noisy appliances, such as blenders. Turn down the TV and the stereo. And, if you are exposed to chronic noise, use cotton or ear plugs to protect your ears and filter out some of the sound.

21. The environment you live in can either soothe you or add to your stress. You cannot control some things, such as air pollution, but you can clean up clutter, keep your room at the most comfortable temperature, and use adequate lighting, for example. Do whatever you can to limit your exposure to pollutants, insecticides, pesticides, food additives, gasoline exhaust, industrial wastes, and glazes or paints that contain lead.

22. You will do best at coping with stress if you are generally satisfied. That is, you feel some control over your life, you are able to set and meet goals, you have aspirations you believe you will fulfill, the people closest to you are affectionate and caring, you feel valued, and you are able to make a meaningful contribution. Generally, satisfaction leads to optimism—and optimists suffer fewer symptoms of stress. If you are not optimistic and satisfied, try to figure out why. Change the things you can. Work to accept the things you cannot change. Most important, learn to concentrate on your successes and use what you learned from them to meet your challenges head-on.

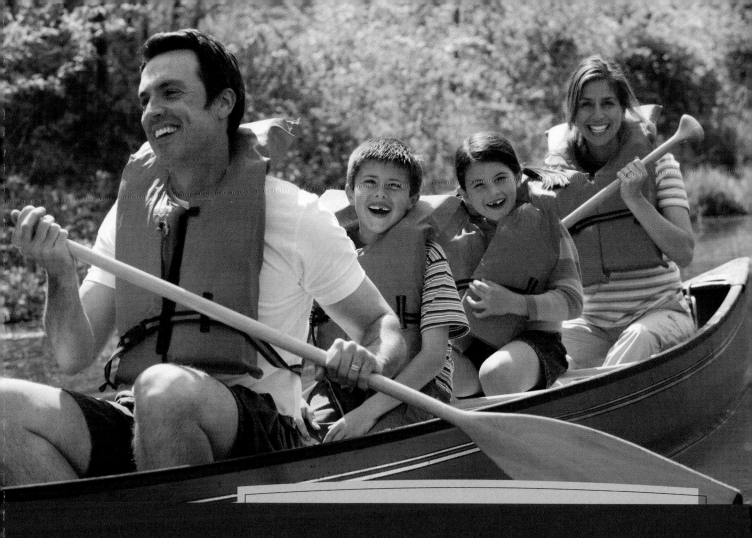

# Chapter Four  Personal Relationships

**OBJECTIVES** ■ Describe the role of personal relationships in health and well-being. ■ Name the qualities of friendship. ■ Discuss the risks involved in dating. ■ Name the various types of marriage. ■ Describe the forms in which families exist today. ■ Explain the dynamics of family and social violence—mate maltreatment and child maltreatment. ■ State short-term and long-term effects of child abuse. ■ Discuss the trends in violence in the United States.

ThomsonNOW Log on to ThomsonNOW at http://thomsonedu.com/ thomsonnow to access and explore self-assessments, interactive tutorials, and practice quizzes.

---

**Tips for Action** Building Better Friendships

■ **Create a tradition.** It could be a weekly walk or watching your favorite team's midweek game. Select something you both enjoy.

■ **Work together.** Side-by-side work provides a good opportunity to share thoughts and feelings about what is going on in your lives.

■ **Help someone heal.** Take time to be with a friend who is grieving or having problems.

■ **Say thanks.** Friends show their gratitude for favors, services, and thoughtfulness.

■ **Ask for help.** Both people in a friendship need to know the other will come through for them if needed.

*Source:* Alan Epstein, *How to Have More Love in Your Life* (New York: Penguin Books, 1996).

---

Healthy relationships are essential to physical and emotional health. They increase well-being and longevity. They begin with children bonding with their parents, then branching out to friends in the neighborhood and at school, and finally to the world at large. Relationships encompass social groups, work associates, and mates.

Relationships within the family are the foundation for future relationships. Some people believe the American family is in trouble because of the diminishing quality of parent-child relationships, manifested in divorce, single parents, and the two-parent working family. Children need the continuity of a loving, secure, constant environment in which to learn to trust and develop the self-esteem needed to thrive and eventually become autonomous.

## Friendships

The first relationships people form outside the family are friendships. Friendship is a vehicle by which people move out of themselves. They learn to share themselves with others and, in turn, discover others. Friendships are characterized by respect, trust, affection, and loyalty. Friends like to be together. In some cases, particularly when the family is absent or dysfunctional, friendships can assume a more important role than family.

Sometimes the absence of friends portends **loneliness.** Loneliness has been associated with higher rates of cancer and heart attack, among other diseases. Loneliness may compromise the immune system and leave lonely people vulnerable to various physical and mental illnesses.

Loneliness and being alone, however, are not the same thing. Being alone can be generative. After the loss of her husband, Charles, Anne Morrow Lindbergh wrote, in *Gift from the Sea:*

> I find there is a quality to being alone that is incredibly precious. Life rushes back into the void, richer, more vivid, fuller than before. It is as if in parting one did actually lose an arm. And then, like starfish, one grows it anew; one is whole again, complete and round—more whole, even, than before, when the other people had pieces of one.

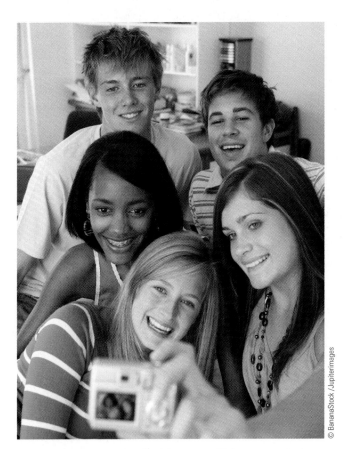

▲ *Friendships are a valuable part of life, particularly when family is absent*

Loneliness is associated with the quality, not the quantity, of relationships. It can stem from lack of attachments to others.

## Communication

Good communication is the basis for good relationships. Honest communication enables people to know each other and to grow close. In addition to verbal ways of communicating are the nonverbal ways, also called **body language.** Up to 95% of face-to-face communication is nonverbal.

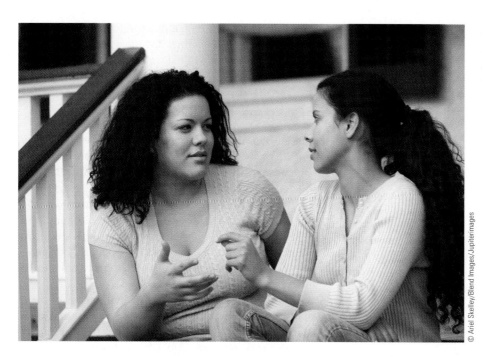

◀ *Friendships create a closeness in which two people share their feelings and thoughts*

© Ariel Skelley/Blend Images/Jupiterimages

Furthermore, communication has a profound influence on health and well-being. Most impacted is the cardiovascular system. During conversation, blood pressure increases. In contrast, the act of listening is relaxing. Paying calm attention to something outside oneself brings down blood pressure.

## Intimacy and Sexuality

Attachments to others require that the person have a capacity for **intimacy.** Many friendships have a sexual component or evolve into a sexual relationship. Physical attraction and romantic passion are stages of love that are driven by the brain neurotransmitters dopamine and serotonin. Conducting her research with the aid of an MRI, Dr. Helen Fisher (anthropologist at Rutgers University) has identified the brain's specific chemical pathways for passion. When people experience romantic love, the high dopamine levels create the intense energy, exhilaration, and the "can't be without you" feeling of attraction and romance. This form of intimacy will not last. Just as a person becomes desensitized to the effects of a psychoactive drug if it is used repeatedly (tolerance), the person becomes less responsive to the brain chemicals ("love potion") of romance. So what sustains long-term love relationships? Physiologically, scientists believe that the attachment to the one you love is driven by oxytocin. This hormone promotes feelings of bonding and connecting, which are essential for lasting love relationships such as monogamy.

Identity, sense of self, and roles all involve **sexuality.** Sexuality is present in a person from—and even before—birth. The components of sexuality include sexual orientation, biological sex, gender identity, and gender role.

From birth, both sexes have the capacity for orgasm, although many do not experience it. As they grow, some children discover orgasm through self-exploration, of which **masturbation** is a form of **autoerotic** behavior.

The first milestone in one's evolving sexuality is **puberty,** when boys and girls begin to show much more interest in the physical aspects of sex. Teenage boys begin to experience nocturnal emissions (wet dreams), and some girls have orgasmic dreams. At this stage teenagers are adults biologically. In psychological and social terms, however, they are still children and need at least five more years to reach a level of maturity commensurate with their physical status.

### KEY TERMS

**Loneliness** feeling of emptiness when a person's social network is significantly lacking in quality or quantity

**Body language** nonverbal communication; body positions, gestures, postures, and movements that send various messages to others

**Intimacy** a close association, contact, or familiarity with someone

**Sexuality** the total biological, psychological, emotional, social, environmental, and cultural aspects of sexual behavior

**Masturbation** self-stimulation of genitals or other erogenous areas

**Autoerotic** sexual behaviors aimed at self-stimulation

**Puberty** the stage in life ushering in adolescence, marked by major physiological changes dominated by increased production of sex hormones

**TABLE 4.1 ▶** Adolescents Having Sex

| AGES | FEMALES | MALES |
|------|---------|-------|
| 15 | 24% | 27% |
| 16 | 39 | 45 |
| 17 | 52 | 59 |
| 18 | 65 | 68 |
| 19 | 77 | 85 |
| 15–19 | 51 | +56 |

*Source:* Alan Guttmacher Institute, "Facts in Brief, Teen Sex and Pregnancy," 2003, www.agi-usa.org.

The percentages of boys and girls having sex are shown in Table 4.1. The latest data (2003) on teenage sexuality indicate that most teens begin having sexual intercourse in their mid- to late teens. The average age at first intercourse is 16.9 years for males and 17.4 years for females. More than half of 17-year-olds have had sexual intercourse. According to the National Center for Health Statistics, 50% of teens ages 15 to 19 have had sexual intercourse.

Each year approximately 1 million adolescent girls become pregnant (one in every 10 girls under age 20), and approximately 500,000 give birth. The United States has the highest adolescent childbearing rate in the industrialized world.

The Child Welfare League of America has gathered the following facts about teenage mothers.

- Adolescents age 17 and younger are twice as likely to deliver low birthweight babies (less than five and a half pounds at birth), who are 40 times more likely to die in the first four weeks of life than are newborns of normal weight.

- Teenage girls who give birth are less likely to complete a high school education than their nonparent peers.

- Only half of the females who have their first child at age 17 or younger will have graduated from high school by age 30.

- Teenagers who become mothers are disproportionately poor and dependent on public assistance.

Many parents, and teens themselves, believe teens are under too much pressure to have sex. TV, music videos, and movies promote sex without considering the consequences. Once teens know their friends are having sex, many follow their lead to avoid feeling left out. Girls often say they have sex to feel loved.

Love is a difficult concept because it means different things to different people at different stages in life. During adolescence, love tends to be romantic and synonymous with passion and intense feelings. Teens typically develop infatuations and fall in love. Although sex and love are different, they tend to become confused because they are new concepts at this developmental age, and they also may have different meanings for boys and girls. Sorting out these differences while developing intimate relationships is one of the tasks of adolescence.

## GENDER ROLE AND GENDER IDENTITY

Social norms are largely responsible for **gender roles.** Taking their cue from society in general, parents knowingly or unconsciously influence the formation of children's expected behavior based on their biological sex. This is done through the selection of toys (for example, dolls for girls, trucks for boys), color and types of clothing (pink and frilly for girls, blue and sturdy for boys), and the expectation of certain behaviors (girls should be gentle, kind, and submissive; boys should be tough, competitive, and aggressive).

**Gender identity** is each individual's sense of being female or male. Each person has a private, internal experience or sense of himself or herself as a male, a female, or some cross-gendered identity between the two. An individual who exhibits personality traits and behaviors that are associated both with males and with females is said to be **androgynous.**

## SEXUAL ORIENTATION

**Sexual orientation** is a component of sexuality characterized by emotional, romantic, or sexual attraction to persons of one or the other sex. Sexual orientation often becomes apparent during puberty, when hormonal changes are taking place in the body. A **heterosexual,** or straight, orientation is the most common. It means being attracted to persons of the opposite sex. **Homosexuals** are sexually attracted to members of the same sex. A homosexual male usually is referred to as gay; a homosexual female, a lesbian or gay. Homosexuality encompasses individuals of every socioeconomic level, educational background, ethnicity, and religious preference. In a third orientation, **bisexual,** individuals may have sexual attraction or relationships with members of both sexes.

A term often heard in regard to homosexuality is **homophobic,** which means a fear of homosexuals. Homophobia has led to discriminatory practices toward gays in employment, housing, and military services. As of 1974 the American Psychiatric Association stopped listing homosexuality as a psychosexual disorder in its *Diagnostic and Statistical Manual of Mental Disorders*. This was the first official step in continuing efforts by gay people to be accepted as equal members of society.

## SEXUAL DEVIATIONS

Some sexual behaviors fall outside societal norms for acceptability. Table 4.2 contains a listing of selected atypical sexual behaviors and their definitions.

## Focus on Diversity Sexual Differences in Communication Styles

One of the skills that is essential to keeping an intimate relationship strong and making it last is honest and open communication between the partners. Even though partners may be talking to each other, thay may not be communicating. Research suggests that women and men have different communication styles, and sometimes this hin ders their success in conveying information to each other. According to Julia Cole, who writes for *BBC Health and Fitness*, one key difference is that men do not talk or articulate the process they use in decision making. They tend to do this internally, and then announce the decision. Women tend to talk through the decision-making process and make any changes aloud before making the final decision. This difference in styles may cause a problem because the man perceives that the woman is always changing her mind. The woman perceives that the man did not consider her feelings and made a quick decision.

Cole makes the following suggestions so that partners will truly communicate and not just talk to each other.

- Set at least one hour aside to work though the decision-making process before making the decision.
- Let your partner know that when you are silent, you are thinking about what was said and not bored with what is being said.
- Do not jump to conclusions; find out if your partner's remarks are his or her final answer. Do not agree or disagree until you are sure.
- After the decision is made, allow time for it to settle in and to determine if you both are comfortable with it.
- Listen and talk to each other with respect. Remember-openness, honesty, and sincerity are foundations that will be eroded if you are disrespectful, cynical, and condescending.

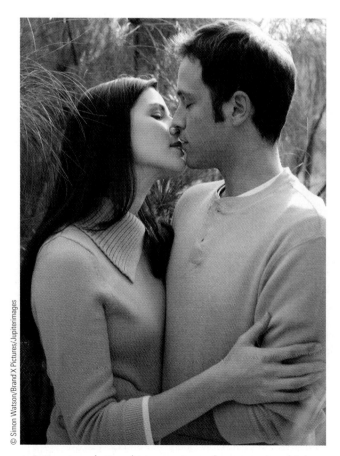

▲ *Intimate relationships create a closeness in which two people share their thoughts and feelings*

© Simon Watson/Brand X Pictures/Jupiterimages

## Dating

Dating usually begins during the teen years. Many times the partners explore several forms of intimacy such as kissing, hugging, and touching, which can easily lead to sexual intercourse. Too often teens emulate adult sexual

### KEY TERMS

**Gender roles** the different behaviors and attitudes that society expects of females and males

**Gender identity** a person's sense of being female or being male

**Androgynous** showing behaviors that are not gender-specific; they are identified with males and females alike

**Sexual orientation** one of the components of sexuality that is characterized by emotional, romantic, or sexual attraction to a person of a particular biological sex

**Heterosexual** having a physical attraction to the opposite sex

**Homosexual** having a physical attraction to the same sex

**Bisexual** having a physical attraction both to the same sex and to the opposite sex

**Homophobic** exaggerated fear of homosexuals

---

**Tips for Action** Do's and Don'ts After a Sexual Assault

DO:

■ Seek medical help as soon as possible.

■ Bring a change of clothes to the emergency room.

■ Get tested for sexually transmitted disease.

■ Inquire about emergency contraception.

■ Remember that what you say to medical personnel could be used in court.

DO NOT:

■ Shower, bathe, or brush teeth.

■ Douche.

■ Change clothes until after the exam.

■ Hesitate to call the police.

---

behavior without being aware of its responsibilities and consequences. In this day and age, sexual intimacy is a risky proposition because of the heightened chances of contracting sexually transmitted diseases, including AIDS—not to mention the potential for young girls' becoming pregnant.

## DATING VIOLENCE

Dating does not always go smoothly, and sometimes it is even physically dangerous. Further, violence in dating relationships tends to carry over into more permanent arrangements. Battered spouses often were battered dates. In the early teen years the perpetrators are more often girls than boys. As the boys become physically larger and stronger than girls, that statistic reverses itself, and males continue to be the perpetrators of violence more often than females in subsequent years. Dating abuse is defined as the physical, sexual, or psychological and emotional violence within a dating relationship.

Dating abuse data (2006) from the CDC (National Center for Injury Prevention and Control) reveal the following.

**TABLE 4.2 ▶** Atypical Sexual Behavior

| BEHAVIOR | DESCRIPTION |
|---|---|
| Exhibitionism | Showing one's genitals to unwilling observers and achieving sexual gratification by watching their responses |
| Fetishism | Becoming sexually aroused by inanimate objects (for example, brassieres, panties) or body parts (for example, lips, feet, hair) |
| Frotteurism | Obtaining sexual gratification by rubbing or pressing against an unwilling person's body |
| Incest | Sexual intercourse and other forms of sexual activities between close relatives such as father-daughter, mother-son, sister-brother (incest is illegal and prohibited in the United States) |
| Klismaphilia | Obtaining sexual pleasure from receiving enemas |
| Masochism | Experiencing sexual gratification while receiving physical or emotional pain and attendant suffering and humiliation at the hands of another (to include hypoxyphilia—sexual arousal by oxygen deprivation; blindfolding or sensory bondage) |
| Necrophilia | Obtaining sexual gratification by having sexual intercourse with a corpse |
| Paraphilia | A sexual disorder in which a person's sexual arousal and sexual gratification depend on unusual or atypical objects, arts, or imagery |
| Pedophilia | An adult's sexual attraction to children, which can include victimization of children for sexual gratification |
| Sadism | Being sexually gratified by inflicting physical pain or cruelty upon another |
| Sadomasochism (S&M) | Mutually participating in masochistic and sadistic acts |
| Telephone scatologia | Obtaining sexual gratification from making obscene telephone calls |
| Transsexualism | Feeling, thinking, and acting as a person of the opposite sex (this is not homosexuality); feeling trapped in the wrong body |
| Transvestism | Becoming sexually aroused by dressing in clothing worn normally by individuals of the opposite gender |
| Voyeurism | Obtaining gratification by secretly gazing at others as they dress, undress, or engage in sexual activities; variation is obscene phone calls, in which men (rarely women) are aroused sexually by anonymous communication and may masturbate during the phone call or immediately afterward |

## Tips for Action How to Diminish the Odds for Date Rape

- Develop clear lines of communication with the person you are dating. Communicate and clearly understand what each of you wants and expects from the date.

- Do not use psychoactive substances, including alcohol, in dating situations.

- Do not give clues or display body language that is flirtatious or indicates you are interested in having sex when you are not. For example, allowing a date to visit your bedroom or sit on the bed with you in your dorm room may send a clue that you are interested in becoming intimate.

- Do not be coerced into unwanted sexual activities.

---

- One in 11 adolescents reports being a victim of physical dating abuse.

- Dating abuse frequency among African-American students is 13.9%, 9.3% among Hispanic stuednts, and 7.0% among white students.

- Victims of dating abuse are at increased risk for injury, more likely to engage in binge drinking, suicide attempts, physical fights, and currently sexual activity.

If the cycle of abuse is to stop, it is imperative that teens learn to develop healthful and respectful relationships when dating. Mentors and even peers must continue to stress that abuse during dating is not the norm (despite what is portrayed in the media). Studies suggest that teens do not see the negative consequences of dating violence (31% of teens report having at least one friend who is in a violent relationship). Acceptance of dating abuse among friends is a link to future involvement in dating abuse.

The incidence of physical violence in college dating relationships is reported as 20% to 50%, varying from slapping and hitting to more life-threatening violence. The rate of severe violence among dating couples ranges from about 1% to 27% each year.

### DATE RAPE

A related phenomenon in modern dating is the frequency of **date rape,** or acquaintance rape. It is particularly widespread in college settings. Minnesota representative Jim Ramstad introduced in the U.S. Congress legislation entitled the Campus Sexual Assault Victims' Bill of Rights Act of 1991, which subsequently was enacted into law. He stated that more than 25% of college females have been raped by their date. In more than 70% of date rape cases, alcohol use—by cither or both the sexual abuser and the victim—has been a contributing factor. Jealousy is the other major cause.

Some perpetrators of date rape are using the drug Rohypnol, or roofies, on their victims. Because of the drug's sedative effects, unsuspecting victims under the influence of this drug are not able to defend themselves and often have no memory of the sexual assault.

The concept of date rape is complex. Frequently, individuals who come from homes where violence occurs between family members view violence as a normal part of relationships. Other date rape may be a result of miscommunication or differences in the way males and females interpret information concerning sex and invitations to participate.

## Marriage and Its Variations

The traditional nuclear family (married mother and father and their minor children living under one roof) is not as common as it was three decades ago. According to the U.S. Census Bureau (2004 data), there are 25,793,000 married couples living with their own children. Other household or family configurations are as follows: male householder with own children—1.93 million; female householder with own children—8.22 million; married couples with own household—57.71 million.

Some adults in the population are not married. According to the 2004 census data, 53.2 million persons 18 years old and over fall into the category "never married" compared to 48.2 million in 2000. The breakdown in this category for all races is 29.6 million males and 23.7 million females.

### COHABITATION

One popular adaptation of the traditional family unit is **cohabitation.** People who cohabit form what the U.S. Census Bureau terms the "unmarried-partner household." Its 2003 report (the latest figures available) indicated 5.6 million unmarried couple households in the United States, double the number in 1980. This is in comparison to 112 million households in the United States. The married couple household (57.7 million) is much more common than the unmarried couple household, but the trend toward living together

---

### KEY TERMS

**Date rape** sex without the consent of both of the dating partners

**Cohabitation** living together as spouses without being married

is rising. The two common unmarried-partner households are male householder/female partner (2.45 million) and female householder/male partner (2.41 million).

Many people do not perceive cohabitation as a novelty, as unmarried celebrity couples, such as Goldie Hawn and Kurt Russell, Beyonce Knowles and Jay-Z, or Oprah Winfrey and Stedman Graham have been readily accepted by society. Others, such as Eddie Murphy and Nichole Mitchell (now divorced), lived together for some time and started a family before deciding to marry. Among the reasons given for cohabitation is the need for freedom to dissolve the relationship without legal constraints if it does not work out. Some couples say their mutual love transcends the need for legal sanction.

"I don't wana' play house no more . . ." is one line of the lyrics of a popular song by the R & B artist Mary J. Blige that expresses the sentiments of some women who desire to move from cohabitation to marriage but the man does not. In dissolving a cohabitative relationship, problems do arise. In the case of couples not legally married, state laws that govern spousal and child support and the division of property usually do not apply. Of particular interest is the statistic that the divorce rate among couples who lived together before marriage is substantially higher than those who did not.

## TYPES OF MARRIAGE

**Marriage** should embody dedication, sharing, involvement, communication, and commitment. In the United States, only two individuals of the opposite sex are allowed to marry, known as **monogamy.** To date, Massachusetts is the only state that allows marriage for same-sex couples. Domestic partnership and civil union are recognized in the states of California, Connecticut, New Jersey, and Vermont. This legal status provides a range of benefits and privileges for same-sex couples that are similar to those for married couples. The federal government and most states do not recognize domestic partnership or civil union. In open-ended marriages one partner grants the other permission to have sexual intimacy with one or more others outside the marriage.

Another marital arrangement is **polygamy,** and its subtypes are **polyandry** and **polygyny.** Some cultures permit **communal marriage.**

Men and women still tend to marry people of their same race and ethnic background. Nevertheless, the percentage of Americans marrying outside their racial groups has been increasing over the past several decades. According to 1990 census data, interracial marriages increased about 550% between 1960 and 1990.

The current data available (2004) from the U.S. Census Bureau indicate that 2,157,000 married interracial couples (black,white, other race) reside in the United States. Of that number, 287,000 couples consist of black husbands with white wives; 126,000 couples consist of white husbands with black wives. In the category of Hispanics,

2,076,000 married couples consisted of a Hispanic and a person of another race.

Data for 2005 indicate that the median age at first marriage was 27.4 years for men and 25.8 years for women. Since the mid-1950s, when the median age at first marriage was at an all-time low (22.6 years for men and 20.2 years for women), adults have been waiting longer to marry.

## SEXUAL INTIMACY IN MARRIAGE

Married couples in their twenties are more sexually active than older ones. The former have sexual relations an average of three to four times a week. As couples become older, their frequency of sexual intimacy usually declines.

In the 1993 *Janus Report on Sexual Behavior,* at least 35% of married males and approximately 26% of married females admitted that they had been nonmonogamous. In most cases nonmonogamous activity is casual or recreational adultery. It has a low level of emotional involvement. Among the many reasons given for nonmonogamous relationships are the illness of a partner, a partner's lack of interest in sex, diminished passion, lack of love or respect, and boredom within the marriage. Conflicting interests and careers also can cause problems that may damage an otherwise stable relationship. Ultimately, the main reasons for infidelity are lack of love and commitment and unrealistic expectations of a partner.

Extramarital relationships can have devastating outcomes. A mate who finds out about the infidelity of

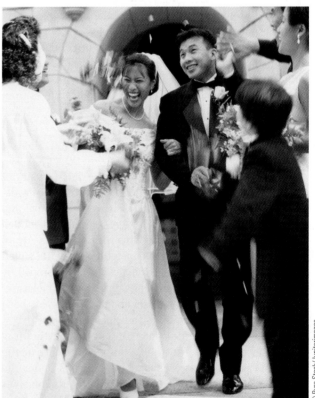

▲ *Keys to continued marital happiness include shared intimacy, marital respect, common values, and fidelity*

WHAT DOES "HAPPILY MARRIED" MEAN?

Ten characteristics of happily married people are the following.

1. They are giving people, meeting their emotional needs by doing for others—and they do not keep score.
2. They have a strong sense of commitment, do not take their happiness for granted, and are determined to make their marriages work.
3. They do not lose themselves in the relationship. Although they value their independence—the right to form their own opinions, make their own decisions, pursue their own goals—marital harmony is a top priority.
4. They have vigorous sexual drives. Sex plays a central and profoundly important role in the marriage.
5. They like to talk, sharing their thoughts about all sorts of subjects. They are open and direct, not manipulative.
6. They have a positive outlook on life.
7. They express appreciation and are generous with praise.
8. They have strong spiritual or religious convictions and commit themselves to a spiritual lifestyle, though they may not be affiliated with an organized church.
9. They recognize the needs of others, respect their differences, consider their feelings, and put themselves in the other person's shoes.
10. They are willing to grow, change, and work hard at their marriages. They know that a good relationship requires flexibility and effort to keep it alive.

COMMONALITIES IN A GOOD MARRIAGE

The best marriages tend to be ones in which the partners are similar in:

Ethnicity
Locality (geography; urban or rural)
Maturity (emotional and social)
Goals and ideals
Intelligence levels
Amount of education
Economic level and financial resources
Social strata
Value system
Religious beliefs

a formerly trusted partner feels a strong sense of betrayal. The resulting emotions can run the gamut of pain, anger, and depression, to fear of HIV/AIDS and other sexually transmissible diseases, to anxiety about emotional, physical, and financial abandonment.

In mature and responsible relationships, sexual intimacy is exclusive of others. It does not involve just a sexual act. It also includes showing appreciation for, sharing feelings with, having respect for, sacrificing for, and being loyal to the partner. Sexual intimacy is an important part of marriage. It can enhance and enrich a marital relationship through mutual enjoyment, love, companionship, commitment, and procreation.

## MARRIAGE AND HEALTH

The National Center for Health Statistics has reported that married people have fewer health problems than unmarried people. They are less likely to have high blood pressure, cancer, and heart problems. Research verifies that a happy marriage dramatically increases life expectancy. Death rates for single, divorced, and widowed individuals are significantly higher than the rates for married people. One postulated reason is that happy marriage helps keep the immune system strong.

What about unhappily married people? They may be the worst off in terms of good health and a long life. They have poorer health than their single counterparts, including divorced people. Dissatisfaction with one's marriage can lead to depression, high blood pressure, and reduced immune system functioning. After careful consideration, divorce may be the best solution in some circumstances.

## Loss of Relationships

Entering into relationships entails the risk of loss. It requires that a person be vulnerable to the hurt of loss. Two prevalent forms of loss are by divorce and by the death of someone with whom a person has had a close relationship.

### KEY TERMS

**Marriage** a legally and socially sanctioned union between a man and a woman

**Monogamy** marriage of a man and a woman

**Polygamy** a marriage simultaneously to more than two people

**Polyandry** a marriage in which one woman has more than one husband simultaneously

**Polygyny** a marriage in which one man has more than one wife simultaneously

**Communal marriage** a marriage of three or more individuals who share all family functions; also known as group marriage

**TABLE 4.3** ► A Comparison of Divorce for Selected Racial or Ethnic Groups, by Gender, in Millions

| RACE OR ETHNIC GROUP AND GENDER | 2000 | 2004 |
|---|---|---|
| African-American women | 1.7 | 1.9 |
| African-American men | 1.1 | 1.1 |
| White women | 9.3 | 10.3 |
| White men | 7.2 | 7.5 |
| Hispanic women | 1.0 | 1.2 |
| Hispanic men | 0.7 | 0.9 |
| Asian women | (NA) | 0.3 |
| Asian men | (NA) | 0.1 |

*Source:* U.S. Bureau of the Census, *Statistical Abstract of the United States: 2006,* 125th edition (Washington, DC: U.S. Government Printing Office, 2005).

## DIVORCE

In "Fairy Tales," Anita Baker sings of a relationship that has gone sour with the "knight in shining armor" bringing his love a "poison apple." Partners' expectations of marriage do not always mesh. Half of all marriages end in divorce. According to U.S. Census Bureau figures for 2004 (latest available), 21.8 million of all adults 18 years old and older who had ever been married were divorced.

The figures by racial group are given in Table 4.3. Marriages dissolve for many reasons, including infidelity; lack of financial support; sexual, social, or educational incompatibility; physical or emotional abuse; and disagreements about childbearing and childrearing.

## DEATH OF PARTNER

Sooner or later everyone likely will have to face the loss of a spouse, friend, or loved one. The most current U.S. Census data (2004) report that 13.8 million persons are widowed (11.1 million females compared to 2.6 million males). **Grief** is a way of responding to loss. Regardless of who has been lost, the stages of grief are the same. No two people react to grief in the same way, though. For some, grief becomes painful or debilitating. Others manage to cope reasonably well. The way in which a person handles grief tends to be a reflection of how the person copes with stress in general.

Even though the nature of each particular reaction depends upon the individual, the five general stages of grief are experienced the same way from one person to another.

1. **Shock and disbelief.** The initial reaction to news of a loss is shock and disbelief: "No way!" "I don't believe it!" Lasting from several minutes to several days, this stage is characterized by numbness and denial. The feeling of shock is a defense mechanism that allows the body time to gear up for coping with the stress of the loss.

2. **Awareness.** As the person becomes aware of the loss, he or she may cry, scream, become silent, want to be alone, or lash out in anger at others.

3. **Restitution.** During this third stage, the mourner relies on spiritual or religious beliefs, cultural traditions, or various other rituals that help him or her come to terms with the loss. Funerals, wakes, and memorial services help the mourner face the loss and accept its reality. The restitution stage also begins the long process of utilizing coping techniques. The survivor may begin to talk about the dead person and recall the person's personality, attributes, and mannerisms. By remembering things as simple as a gesture or a smile, the mourner begins to categorize the memories that eventually lead to healing.

4. **Idealization.** The mourner thinks constantly of the dead person's good qualities and may even try to emulate certain beliefs, behaviors, and attributes of the dead person. In this stage, which usually lasts several months to several years, the mourner gradually directs his or her feelings toward other survivors.

5. **Resolution.** At last the healing process is finished. The survivor reestablishes former contacts, readjusts to ordinary activities, establishes relationships other than those shared with the dead person, and accepts the environment without the dead person. The mourner still remembers the dead person's attributes and accomplishments but finally can also remember the deceased's failures and disappointments.

Even though grief is normal, natural, and necessary, it can cause illness because it involves intense emotions and is so inseparably connected to loss. A special kind of grief is **bereavement,** the process of disbonding from someone who played an important role in one's life and who is now gone. The intense grief involved in bereavement has been shown to pose significant health risks, ranging from immune system disorders to suicides, sudden deaths, and increased death rates from all causes.

## Parenting

The most prominent adults in children's lives—their parents—serve as their primary role models, conveying and directing most of the formative information the children receive. A child's behavior, attitudes, beliefs, and ideas—about responsibility, expectations, love, respect, commitment, and sex—are by-products of the adults who have reared them. Whether these attitudes, beliefs, and ideals are constructive or destructive, children most likely will utilize them. In most cases, these formative directives will serve as a road map for children as they become adults, form relationships, and become parents or guardians themselves.

---

**Tips for Action** Coping with Bereavement

To stay healthy while you grieve:

■ Keep things in your life as status quo as possible. The death of a loved one is a major source of stress so do what you can to cut down on other stressors (a new job, moving to a new house, going on vacation).

■ If you can, postpone making decisions that can wait until later.

■ Keep in touch with other people; social support is especially important now.

■ Avoid the temptation to use alcohol or drugs.

■ Get plenty of rest. Take naps if you need to, and try to maintain your normal sleeping pattern at night.

■ Eat a balanced diet.

■ Drink plenty of fluids, but steer away from alcohol, caffeine, and drugs.

■ Exercise regularly.

■ Create meaningful rituals (such as lighting a candle) around the life of your lost loved one to help keep him or her in memory.

---

Parenting is a continuous process. It demands considerable emotional and physical energies to create an environment for a child that is socially, emotionally, spiritually, and economically conducive to constructive growth and development. Parenting skills can be strengthened by utilizing resources offered by community groups, churches, and private organizations. Some local community agencies—schools, colleges, and universities—offer classes on parenting.

## SINGLE PARENTS

Single parents have a set of issues different from two-parent families. They are not able to divide the responsibilities of the household between adults. The single parent often has greater financial pressures. In addition, a single parent often wishes to develop a romantic relationship with someone, which can be more difficult when children are part of the mix. Children living with a single parent or adult are more likely to be in fairer or poorer health than those who are living with two parents.

Most single parents are mothers. In 2004 more than 60% of all African-American children under 18 years in the United States lived with a single-parent family headed by the mother. According to 1998 Census Bureau data, 3.1 million children are living with a single father. James Levine, director of the Fatherhood Project at the Families and Work Institute in New York, says judges are increasingly awarding custody to fathers, turning away from the "tender years doctrine" that decreed that young children should stay with their mothers. Those who study the American family are beginning to conclude that the absence of fathers in their children's lives deprives them of good male role models and is responsible for much of the increase in violence, crime, and gang memberships.

William Raspberry, syndicated columnist with the *Washington Post*, wrote in 1993:

We have never doubted that children need fathers.
Until now. We pay little attention to fathers as fathers,

even less to the fact that many of the men absent from their children's lives have been shoved aside, not just by mothers of those children but by the courts and social agencies, buttressed by the growing cultural notion of the superfluous father.

## STEPPARENTS

Another family unit that is becoming more prevalent is the blended family. In these families, previously divorced partners, one or both of whom have children, combine to form another family unit. Being a stepparent is a challenge for many. The children retain loyalties to the absent biological parent. They also may consider a parent's new relationship a threat to their own relationship with that parent.

Counselors usually suggest that the stepparent not try to assume the role of parent or become the child's primary disciplinarian. The biological parent must have the primary parental role. Stepparents cannot expect their stepchildren to love them immediately. Love must be earned, and it grows gradually over time. A stepparent, however, can listen to the stepchild and become a confidant, engendering rapport and, eventually, trust.

## Violence in Families

Not all families are functional. Many have serious problems. Some families become dysfunctional because of behaviors associated with alcohol and drug abuse (the topics of Chapters 12 and 13). Behavior patterns that

---

### KEY TERMS

**Grief** emotional reaction to a significant loss

**Bereavement** intense grief associated with the process of disbonding from a significant person who has died

## Tips for Action Twelve Ways to Build Strong Family Values

**1.** Eat together as a family as often as possible—certainly several full family dinners a week. Involve everyone (for example, younger children can set the table and older ones can clean up).

**2.** Hold weekly gatherings to plan family activities, trips, and vacations, and discuss immediate and persistent problems.

**3.** Schedule daily stress-reduction periods when the entire household is quiet—no TV or CDs. According to your family values, read, meditate, pray, exercise, or do whatever else works for your family.

**4.** Volunteer your time and talent to worthy causes in the church or community.

**5.** Participate in school. Become involved with teachers and administrators. Help with after-school and summer programs.

**6.** Do recreational activities as a family. Take walks, bike rides together.

**7.** Make or build things together. Share creative activities, and let children take the lead in some of these. Go for accomplishment, not perfection.

**8.** Take organized trips to sporting events, concerts, local fairs. Include everyone.

**9.** Bring children to work on occasion to let them see their parents' life away from home.

**10.** At least once a year travel away from home. Discuss vacation ideas with children.

**11.** Limit TV watching. Watch TV with children, monitor what they watch, and discuss what they see.

**12.** Stay involved. Keep informed about community and national issues that concern you and your children. Let children know your concerns and opinions, and listen to theirs.

*Source:* Benjamin Spock, *A Better World for Children* (New York: National Press Books, 1994), excerpted from the *Denver Post*, 1995.

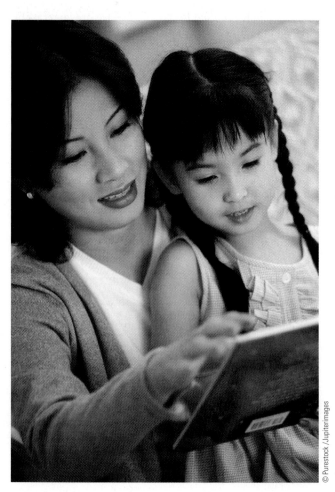

▲ *Parenting is a continuous process*

© Purestock /Jupiterimages

are part of children's lives, unfortunately, tend to be perpetuated from generation to generation unless the cycle is broken. Nowhere is this pattern more obvious than in family violence and abuse. Among ethnic groups, data from the National Violence Against Women Survey indicate that American Indian and Alaskan Native women and men, African-American women, and Hispanic women are at most risk for violence from spouses/partners. Social status and its indicators (education, income, occupation) may be more significant in that people of lower socioeconomic status are associated with higher numbers because they are reported more frequently by official agencies. The same survey found that young women and those women with incomes below poverty level are disproportionately victims of violence from a spouse/partner.

## INTIMATE PARTNER VIOLENCE

The country in the mid-1990s was mesmerized by coverage of the Lorena Bobbitt and the O. J. Simpson trials. (Bobbitt was accused of malicious wounding of her husband, John Wayne Bobbitt. She had severed his penis. Simpson was accused of murdering his ex-wife and her male friend.) Although these are extreme and highly publicized examples involving mate abuse, they are not isolated cases. Physical and emotional assault or intimate partner violence (IPV) is a fact of life for all too many victims. However, few cases are ever reported to police. As reported by CDC–National Center for Injury Prevention and Control (NCIPC), the estimate is that only 20% of IPV sexual assaults and 25% of physical assaults are reported.

## Tips for Action For Single Parents

■ Establish who has the power in the family. It is more difficult for one parent than two to have control—and it should not be the children.

■ Set fair ground rules, and discipline with love.

■ Be positive. Reward your child for good behavior.

■ Be practical. Inform the child that money to buy and do things will not be plentiful, if that is the case.

■ Give the child responsibility commensurate with his or her maturational level. Tell the child that he or she is part of the team. This will make the child feel wanted and needed.

■ In cases of divorce, do not badmouth the opposite parent or sabotage the child's time with the other parent. The child feels responsible for the divorce anyway, and

jeopardizing the child's relationship with the absent parent further conflicts the child.

■ Do not put your life on hold or become a martyr. Maintain a social life and keep your hobbies and interests. A happy parent is a better parent.

■ Enjoy your children. Children can be fun. If you are having a good time, they will have a good time, too.

■ Be a good role model for your child.

■ Stay physically fit. Exercise and eat right. The amount of energy you need as a single parent requires good nutrition and health.

■ Set goals that are realistic, yet flexible. Work toward those goals, and revise them as necessary. Elicit the child's input, and listen.

---

Nationally, 29% of women and 22% of men have experienced physical, sexual, or psychological IPV during their lifetime. Among U.S. women ages 18 and older, approximately 5.3 million incidents of IPV occur annually. The acts reported include grabbing, shoving, slapping, and hitting. According to Fox and Zawitz (2004), from 1976 to 2002, about 11% of homicide victims were killed by an intimate partner. In 2002, 76% of IPV homicide victims were female; 24% were male. Between 4% and 8% of pregnant women are abused at least once during the pregnancy. This increases the risk for birth defects and low birthweight babies. At highest risk of all are separated and recently divorced women.

Mate or spousal abuse is a potent and poisonous means of using force to control a victim, a complex phenomenon psychologically. Constance Dunlap, a Washington, DC, psychiatrist, says the primary problem is denial. Often both the woman and the man who is abusing her have grown up in homes where they have witnessed abuse or have been abused themselves. Consequently, they have a hard time seeing this behavior as abnormal (Table 4.4). These environments also do not nurture positive self-images or foster the development of social skills. Further, most mate abuse occurs in a context of abuse of alcohol or other psychoactive substances, which lessens inhibitions and distorts judgment.

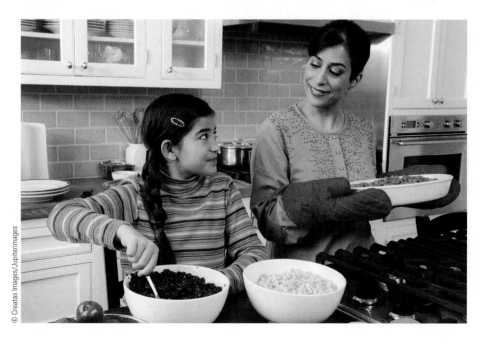

◄ *Parents should spend quality time with children*

---

**Tips for Action** How to Instill a Sense of Belonging in Children and Families

- Spend quality time with each other.
- Express love both verbally and nonverbally.
- Be open and honest.
- Set reasonable limits for children and take reasonable disciplinary measures when needed.
- Relate your own experiences and feelings with which family members can identify.
- Do not allow one child to verbally tear down a sibling.
- Make sure all members have specific responsibilities within the family.

- Do not show favoritism.
- Validate each family member's feelings.
- Do not be overly protective of any member.
- Deem all family members' opinions and values as worthy even though you may not agree with them.
- Maintain eye contact during communication whenever possible.
- Praise positive behaviors and attitudes.

---

**TABLE 4.4 ▶** Warning: This Relationship May Be Dangerous to Your Health

| WHAT YOU SEE | WHAT HE SAYS |
| --- | --- |
| Blaming | "I love you, but you make me hit you." |
| Hypermasculine behavior | "I make all the decisions in this family." |
| Emotional abuse | "You are so stupid. I don't know why I married you." |
| Isolation | "I don't like your friend Terri, and I don't want you going to the mall with her." "I know you have class, but call me before you leave the building." |
| Intimidation | "Just like I kicked that dog, I can kick you." |
| Coercion and threats | "If you don't do what I say, I'll leave you. You can't make it without me." |
| Economic abuse | "You don't need to make any more money. I can give you what you need when you ask me for it." |

Although domestic violence is predominately male-perpetrated, the Bobbitt case illustrates that men can be victims, especially when the woman is defending herself or retaliating for past abuse. Approximately 3.2 million incidents of IPV occur annually among men ages 18 and older. Women who assault men discover quickly that the partner is even more hesitant to report the abuse than women tend to be, often because of a macho orientation and also because the man does not tend to be believed. In some cases a man reporting abuse by a mate has been arrested and jailed himself.

Another complicating consideration arises from the differing values and practices of immigrants to the United States. For example, in many countries, women still are considered the property of men, as evidenced by dowries and arranged marriages. In many Asian countries, wives are expected to obey the husband as a duty to him. Women who do not are sometimes subject to beatings, many of which go unreported. In some South American countries, too, wives are considered as property or chattel.

Some warning signs of a potentially abusive relationship include verbal abuse, jealousy (constant calling, checking your car's mileage), and sudden mood swings of the abuser.

## CHILD MALTREATMENT– CHILD ABUSE

Abuse of children is a serious and widespread problem. Abused children often perpetuate the abuse or turn to other dysfunctional lifestyles to cope with it. In 2002, 906,000 children in the United States were confirmed by child protective service agencies as being maltreated. Of that number, the type of maltreatment experienced was 61%—neglect; 19%—physical abuse; 10%—sexual abuse; 5%—emotional or psychological abuse. In 2003 (latest data available) an estimated 1,500 children were confirmed victims of fatal maltreatment, according to the Department of Health and Human Services. The breakdown for child maltreatment mortality within and outside of the family unit is as follows.

- Physical neglect: 38%
- Physical abuse: 28%
- Multiple maltreatment types: 29%

Some of the childhood deaths for which the recorded causes are sudden infant death syndrome and natural causes may be the result of abuse.

The mortality figures do not reveal the total extent of child abuse. Although reliable statistics are difficult to obtain, the most comprehensive and methodologically sound report to date was by the U.S. Department of Health and Human Services. About two out of 1,000 children in the United States were confirmed by child protective service agencies as having experienced sexual assult in 2003. Furthermore, one in every two reported cases is unfounded. Irrespective of inaccuracy in reporting, abuse is a serious problem.

Child abuse may be physical, sexual, or psychological/emotional. Examples of **physical abuse** are hitting any part of the body with an instrument or object, scalding with hot water or caustic liquids, and burning a child's body with cigarettes.

**Sexual abuse** can include fondling, massaging, genital contact, intercourse, oral sex (fellatio and cunnilingus), and similar acts. **Incest** is a particularly damaging form of child abuse. **Psychological/emotional abuse** might take the form of shouting at a child: "You're no good"; "You're dumb"; "You're stupid"; "You'll never amount to anything." Nonverbal abuse might consist of ignoring a child or neglecting the child's physical and emotional needs. Some children never are told that they are doing well or that they are special. They are not hugged or touched—powerful means of making a child feel unloved and insecure.

Whether the abuse is physical, sexual, or psychological, the emotional pain is lasting and can do considerable and long-lasting harm to a child. Depending on the severity of physical abuse, long-term effects can be

- A higher rate of perceptual-motor deficiencies
- Lower scores on general intelligence tests
- Poorer academic achievement rates
- More social and behavior problems and adjustment difficulties
- Either extreme aggression or extreme withdrawal
- Defiance; nonconformity
- Drug use
- Delinquency

Long-term effects of child sexual abuse might include

- Compulsive masturbation, excessive curiosity about sex, adult behaviors, detailed information about sexual activity
- Bedwetting and soiling the bed
- Compulsive behavior
- Disturbed sleep patterns
- Disturbances in eating patterns
- Learning difficulties
- Artwork that reveals the sexual activity
- Stomachaches
- Skin disorders, particularly involving the genitalia

As a cautionary note, these are mere indicators and should not be taken as conclusive evidence of abuse. Some children who have not been abused may display the same symptoms.

Older children tend to cope by escaping, which can take the form of, for example, entering into an early marriage, becoming pregnant, running away from home, or committing suicide. Long-term consequences of childhood abuse in older children include

- Aggressive and violent behavior
- Conduct disorders
- Alcohol and drug use and abuse
- Emotional problems such as anxiety, depression, hostility, and schizoid disorders
- Suicide attempts and suicides
- Problems with interpersonal relationships
- Social incompetency
- Promiscuity
- Difficulties in the workplace
- Perpetuation of familial violence

The Child Abuse Prevention and Treatment Act, originally enacted in 1974 and subsequently amended and reauthorized, mandates that teachers and other specified professionals report suspected cases of abuse to the proper authorities. Abuse tends to revolve in a vicious cycle from generation to generation. About a third of abused children go on to abuse their own children. Children who grow up in an atmosphere of family violence are apt to think it is something to be expected, normal, and okay. As abused children become adults, they are more likely to engage in physical violence toward their family. Women who have been victims of child abuse are at greater risk for aggressive or defiant behavior from their mates than those who were not exposed to abuse. These females are more likely to socialize with, date, and marry men who have abusive backgrounds themselves. A large percentage of prostitutes are victims of abuse. Males who have lived in an environment of family violence are more apt to batter their mates than those who did not grow up in abusive homes.

---

## KEY TERMS

**Physical abuse** an act of physical harm intentionally inflicted on another

**Sexual abuse** unwanted and inappropriate sexually motivated acts toward another person

**Incest** sexual activity between close relatives—father-daughter, stepfather-stepdaughter, mother-son, brother-sister

**Psychological/emotional abuse** negative and hostile verbal or nonverbal treatment of another

## Societal Violence

Recognizing that violence often is the product of exposure to violence in the home and community, the high rate of violence in the United States is of increasing concern. Recent reports of children killing students or teachers at school have caused many parents, and society as a whole, to worry about school safety. In 2005 the Centers for Disease Control and Prevention's Youth Risk Behavior Survey reported the following:

- 33% of high school students reported being in a physical fight one or more times in the 12 months of the survey.
- 17% of high school students reported carrying a weapon (gun, knife, or club) on one or more of the 30 days preceding the survey.
- 6% of high school students reported not going to school on one or more days in the 30 days preceding the survey because they felt unsafe at school or on their way to and from school.

> **VIEWPOINT** *Pro- and antigun proponents are engaged often in heated debate over how far laws should go in controlling weapons in the United States. Advocates base their arguments on protections that they claim are provided by the Second Amendment to the Constitution. In defending stringent weapons control measures, opponents base their argument on safety. Which side are you on? How persuasive can you be in supporting your view?*

Reports of other forms of violence, such as intimate partner violence, gang violence, and sexual assault, cause everyone to think about personal safety. Assault (homicide) is the 13th leading cause of death in the United States.

Youth continue to be perpetrators and victims of violence. As reported in *Healthy People 2010: Understanding and Improving Health*, on an average day in the United States, 53 persons are victims of homicide, with disproportionate homicide rates for African American and Hispanic youth aged 15 to 24 years. Of the 5,570 homicides reported in 2003 among 10- to 24-year-olds, 86% were males and 14% were females.

When examining societal violence, suicide cannot be overlooked. Suicide trends for all youth have increased, but the rate for African-American youth aged 10 to 19 years increased from 2.1 to 4.5 per 100,000 population during 1980–1995. Since 1995, suicide is the third leading cause of death among African-American youth aged 15 to 19 years. Among African-American males aged 15–19 years, the suicide rate increased 146%, compared with 22% for white males.

*Youth Violence: A Report from the Surgeon General* (2001) has linked homicide rates with the health factors listed in Table 4.5. Among 10- to 24-year-olds, homicide

**TABLE 4.5** ▶ Health Factors Related to Homicide

| HEALTH FACTOR | CHARACTERISTICS |
| --- | --- |
| Physiology | Male, youth, biological dysfunction |
| Psychology | Commitment to violent lifestyle, impaired inhibitions against violence, repressed aggression, goal-oriented violence, reaction to provocative conditions |
| Environment | Depressed urban surrounding, diminished economic opportunities, socially disorganized neighborhoods, cultural acceptance of violence in United States, violence in the media |
| Lifestyle | Alcohol abuse, illegal drug use, lack of involvement in conventional activities, antisocial behavior, value system emphasizing violence |

is the leading cause of death for African Americans, the second leading cause of death for Hispanics, and the third leading cause of death for American Indians, Alaska Natives, and Asian/Pacific Islanders. Homicide is the leading cause of death in black males ages 15–44. The rate is more than seven times that of Caucasians. Black males have a lifetime chance of one in 21 of dying by homicide compared with one in 131 for Caucasian males. The rate of homicide for Hispanics is about two and a half times that for Caucasians. The high rate of homicide in the Hispanic population may reflect socioeconomic factors. Most Hispanics live in large cities, where homicide rates are high for all groups.

Although poverty is a strong correlate of homicides in blacks and Caucasians, it may not be the most important factor. The high black homicide rate might be attributed in part to anger, frustration, and low self-esteem resulting from racism, as well as society's historical disregard for violent crime against blacks. These issues may make blacks more aggressive in defending their integrity.

Violent ways of living are not inevitable or immutable. Some suggestions for preventing violence, set forth by the task force, are:

- *Informing and educating.* Media campaigns make the public aware of the enormity of the problem and convey the message that violence is not an acceptable way to deal with problems.
- *Building coalitions.* Consortia of civic, religious, political, youth, and community leaders could meet regularly to exchange ideas and develop programs.
- *Reducing television violence.* Various consumer, professional, and political groups are advocating reduction of violence as entertainment on television.
- *Reducing family violence.* Programs to assist in parenting and providing effective discipline that avoids excessive punishment should be developed.

- *Teaching nonviolence.* Health education curricula extending from elementary through high school should include teaching children how to manage hostility and aggression by nonviolent means. Good role models are needed in this effort.

- *Improving mental health programs.* Because aggressive and antisocial behaviors in children often are associated with later violence, improved and targeted mental health interventions are needed where appropriate.

- *Fighting chemical dependence.* Programs to reduce violence should include segments on the proper use of alcohol and drugs.

---

**VIEWPOINT** *Are some people "wired" to be violent? Andreas Meyer-Lindenberg (a neuroscientist) and his colleagues at the National Institute of Mental Health have identified genetic and neurochemical characteristics that may foster impulse violence. In the study that included 142 white adults (with no history of aggression or violence), the volunteers were identified with a weak-MAOA (monoamine oxidase A) gene or a strong-MAOA gene. Brain scans of the 57 men and women with the weak-MAOA gene displayed a "neural signature" or characteristics that hinder a person's ability to keep aggressive urges and impulses in check. Dr. Meyer-Lindenberg and his colleagues report that other influences (environmental and social) have a greater influence on impulsive violence. The weak-MAOA gene marker is just one small part of the mix. Would this research be useful to identify vulnerable young people so that early intervention strategies could be planned? What's your view?*

---

## CRIME AND VIOLENCE ON COLLEGE CAMPUSES

Institutions of higher learning are not immune to the trends in violence occurring in other segments of the community. As a result of the advocacy of the not-for-profit organization Security On Campus Inc. (SOC), the Student Right-to-Know and Campus Security Act of 1990 was enacted. It requires schools that participate in federal student aid programs to gather statistics of crimes reported to campus or local police departments and to publish them. In addition to murder, assault, sex offenses, and vehicle theft, the institutions must report illegal weapons possession, alcohol and drug violations, and referrals for campus disciplinary actions for these violations. The 2001 crime report that compares the years 1997 to 1999 shows that fewer crimes were reported on college campuses than their surrounding communities. Burglary was the most frequently reported crime followed by motor vehicle theft. In 1999 the reported cases of homicide were lower than in 1998, with 11 cases on campus compared with

24 reported cases in 1998. According to SOC, students are responsible for close to 80% of the criminal activity occurring on the campus, and alcohol and drugs are involved in approximately 90% of campus crime.

## VICTIMIZING BEHAVIORS

**Rape.** Unfortunately, rape is one of the most underreported crimes, and the data available underestimate the actual number of assults. The NCIPC reports the following:

- 9% of high school students reported that they have been forced to have sexual intercourse (12.3% African American, 10.4% Hispanic, 7.3% white).

- 20% to 25% of college women reported experiencing completed or attempted rape.

- Among adults nationwide, more than 300,000 women and more than 90,000 men reported being raped in the previous 12 months.

- Among the adults who report being raped, women experienced 2.9 rapes and men experienced 1.2 rapes in the previous year.

- In 80% of rape cases, the victim knows the perpetrator.

Most perpetrators are men. This is so when men are the victims of sexual violence. Seventy percent of rapes and 86% of physical assaults against males were by a male perpetrator. The underlying motivation in **forcible rape** is a need for power, induced by feelings of inferiority or insecurity. Legally, forcible rape is the carnal knowledge of another person forcibly and against his or her will. In contrast is **statutory rape,** which does not have the element of force. It often is applied to the case of an adult having sex with a person who has not reached the age of consent.

---

**VIEWPOINT** *Two schools of thought have formed regarding how to reduce crime and violence. One belief holds that criminals can be rehabilitated and can become productive citizens through professional counseling and related measures. The opposing view advocates punishment and incarceration for wrongdoers. A related controversy swirls around the issue of capital punishment. Do you believe in it? Develop arguments to defend whatever position you take.*

---

### KEY TERMS

**Forcible rape** unlawful sexual activity with a person without consent by force (to include substantial impairment of the victim with drugs) or threat of injury

**Statutory rape** unlawful sexual intercourse with an individual who has not reached the legal age of consent, regardless of whether it is against that person's will

## SEXUAL HARASSMENT AND STALKING

A key component in **sexual harassment** is that the sexual overture must be unsolicited and unwanted. Harassers are people in positions of power (for example, professors or employers) who give desirable things (for example, better grades or higher salaries) to underlings in exchange for sexual favors. They also might punish a person for not complying. For example, a student may have a grade lowered, or an employee may be refused a raise or even fired. Federal law now makes it easier for victims of sexual harassment to sue employers. Men are the more typical harassers because more men are in positions of power. Harassment, however, is gender-blind. The operative word is *power*. In Michael Crichton's novel *Disclosure*, and the movie based on it, the harasser is a woman.

A person can commit harassment by **stalking,** a relatively recent social concern. Stalking is the intent to harass, annoy, or alarm another person. Data from the NCIPC indicate that 97% of the stalking acts against women are perpetrated by men, and 65% of the stalking acts against men are perpetrated by men. Only about 50% of the incidents of IPV stalking directed toward women are reported. According to the law, it can consist of

- Repeated communications at inconvenient hours that invade the privacy of another and interfere in the use and enjoyment of another's home, private residence, or other private property.
- Repeated insults, taunts, challenges, or communications in offensively coarse language to another in a manner likely to provoke a violent or disorderly response.

## Summary

- Friendships are characterized by respect, trust, affection, and loyalty.
- Friendships are a valuable part of life, particularly when family is absent.
- Intimate relationships in contemporary times carry risks of sexually transmitted diseases and mate abuse.
- Communication is the basis of all relationships.
- Happily married couples are the happiest of all relationship categories.
- In addition to the traditional marriage and family, arrangements now include cohabitation, single parenthood, and stepparenthood.
- Abuses within relationships tend to be carried from generation to generation unless the cycle is broken.
- A person who suffers a loss normally goes through five basic stages of grieving.
- Societal violence is influenced by many factors, including problems in families.

- Violence stems in part from violence in the home and exposure to violence in the media and community.
- Victimizing behavior under the spotlight recently is intimate partner violence.
- Intimate relationships create a closeness in which two people share their thoughts and feelings.
- Keys to continued marital happiness include shared intimacy, marital respect, common values, and fidelity.
- Parenting is a continuous process.
- Parents should spend quality time with children.

## Personal Health Resources

**ThomsonNOW** Visit the ThomsonNOW website at http://thomsonedu.com/thomsonnow for valuable resources that will:

- Help you evaluate your knowledge of the material.
- Guide you through tutorials to help you understand and apply the material.
- Allow you to take an exam-prep quiz to better prepare for class tests.

Centers for Disease Control and Prevention, National Center for Injury Prevention and Control (NCIPC). This federal agency works to reduce and prevent illness, disability, and death due to injury. Information on intimate partner violence, unintentional injury, and suicide is available. 770-488-1506

**www.cdc.gov/ncipc/ncipchm.htm**

U.S. Department of Education, Office of Postsecondary Education provides access to the Campus Security Statistics website, the Education Department's report on college crime to Congress, and other links to information about criminal acts on college campuses. 1-800-USA-LEARN

**www.ope.ed.gov/security**

Security On Campus Inc. This not-for-profit organization advocates for improving safety on college campuses. It provides safety tips, current news, and information about legislation related to campus security. 1-888-251-7959

**www.campussafety.org**

Sexuality Information and Education Council of the United States (SIECUS). This not-for-profit organization develops, collects, and disseminates information and promotes comprehensive education about sexuality. In cooperation with the Centers for Disease Control and Prevention, Division of Adolescent and School Health, it sponsors the National School Health Education Clearinghouse. The site includes a variety of information on sexuality, including tips for

teens, parents, and other adults, religious institutions, and policy makers, as well as links to other sites.
212-819-9770

**www.SIECUS.org**

Planned Parenthood Federation of America Information is provided on reproductive health through news releases, newsletters, statistics, fact sheets and answers to frequently asked questions (FAQs), and a site map. This site is a resource on sexuality for parents, educators, and advocates.
1-800-829-7732

**www.ppfa.org/**

Birthright This not-for-profit organization offers women with unplanned pregnancies alternatives to abortion. Services include free pregnancy testing, emotional support, legal and medical advice, and site map.
1-800-550-4900 (United States and Canada)

**www.birthright.org**

## It's Your Turn for Study and Review

1. According to Blair Justice, University of Texas, people with strong friendships generally produce lower levels of stress hormones when they are faced with problems. Contrast the terms *intimacy* and *loneliness*. Identify at least three other benefits of intimacy.

2. Ana and Frederick are discussing the concept of personal identity when creating a fact sheet for the members of their health class. Ana says that sexuality should not be included on the fact sheet. Fred does not agree. With which one do you agree? Defend your response and include a description of the four components of sexuality.

3. Create a fantastic story using five of the atypical sexual behaviors (with their definitions) included in this chapter. The story should begin with, "Once upon a time," and it must have a G or PG13 rating.

4. Differentiate the types of marriage and variations of marriage. Identify two health benefits of marriage.

5. Identify by definition the types of violent and victimizing behavior addressed in the chapter. Identify at least four strategies to reduce violence in society.

## Thinking about Health Issues

What can be done to prevent domestic violence? Lynda Juall Carpenito, "Domestic Violence: None of Your Business?" *Nursing Forum*, 36:1, January/March 2001, p. 3.

1. What are some examples of domestic violence?
2. What are some signs manifested by a friend or a partner that is suggestive of abuse or potential future abuse?
3. What should parents of girls and parents of boys tell their children about domestic violence and rape prior to entering college?
4. What should you not tell a friend who is currently a victim of abuse? Why?

## Selected Bibliography

Andrinopoulos, K., Kerrigan, D., and Ellen, J. M. "Understanding Sex Partner Selection from the Perspective of Inner-City Black Adolescents." *Perspectives on Sexual and Reproductive Health*, 38:3, 2006, pp. 132–138.

Bohmer, C. and Parrot, A. *Sexual Assault on Campus: The Problem and the Solution*. New York: Lexington Books, 1998.

Bower, B. "Violent Developments: Disruptive Kids Grow into Their Behavior." *Science News*, 169:21, May 27, 2006, pp. 328–329.

Centers for Disease Control and Prevention, National Center for Injury Prevention and Control. "Facts about Violence among Youth and Violence in Schools." **www.cdc.gov/ncipc.**

Centers for Disease Control and Prevention. "Suicide among Black Youths—United States, 1980–1995." *Morbidity and Mortality Weekly Reports*, 47:10, 1998, pp. 193–196.

Centers for Disease Control and Prevention, National Center for Health Statistics. "Fast Stats A to Z." **www.cdc.gov/nchs.**

Centers for Disease Control and Prevention, National Center for Injury Prevention and Control. "Dating Abuse Fact Sheet." Accessed August 15, 2006. Available at **www.cdc.gov/ncipc/.**

Centers for Disease Control and Prevention, National Center for Injury Prevention and Control. "Intimate Partner Violence: Fact Sheet." Accessed August 15, 2006. Available at **www.cdc.gov/ncipc/.**

Centers for Disease Control and Prevention, National Center for Injury Prevention and Control. "Youth Violence: Fact Sheet." Accessed July 30, 2006. Available at **www.cdc.gov/ncipc/.**

Centers for Disease Control and Prevention. "Youth Risk Behavior Surveillance—United States, 2005." *Morbidity & Mortality Weekly Report*, 55:SS-5, 2006; p. 1–108.

### KEY TERMS

**Sexual harassment** unwanted sexual pressuring of someone in a subordinate, vulnerable, or dependent position by another in a position of power

**Stalking** repeated communications or actions with the intent of harassing, annoying, or alarming another person

Cole, J. "Men and Women Communicate Differently." *BBC Health and Fitness*, January 2002. **www.bbc.co.uk/health.**

Crosby, R., DiClemente, R., Wingood, G., et al. "Condom Failure among Adolescents: Implications for STD Prevention." *Journal of Adolescent Health*, 36, 2005, pp. 534–536.

Fohn, R. "Campus Security: Students and Families Can Now Check Colleges' Crime Reports Online." *U25*, 2001, pp. 24–27.

Goodwin, J. *Price of Honor.* Boston: Little, Brown, 1994.

Graves, G. "Does Divorce Run in Families?" *Health*, January/February 2001, pp. 54–55.

Johnson, P. "Silent Agreements: Are You Signing Up for Heartbreak?" *Essence Magazine*, June 2001, p. 108.

Jones, A. *Next Time She Be Dead: Battering and How to Stop It.* Boston: Beacon Press, 1994.

Jones, A. and Schecter, S. *When Love Goes Wrong: What to Do When You Can't Do Anything Right.* New York: HarperCollins, 1992.

Kantrowitz, B. "Gay Families Come Out." *Newsweek*, November 4, 1996, pp. 50–54.

Klopf, D. *Intercultural Encounters.* Englewood, CO: Morton, 1998.

Leland, J. "Shades of Gay." *Newsweek*, March 20, 2000, pp. 46–49.

Levy, B. *In Love and in Danger.* Seattle: Seal Press, 1998.

Lindbergh, A. M. *Gift from the Sea.* New York: Random House, 1991.

Marshall, E. "The Shots Heard 'Round the World." *Science*, July 2000, pp. 570–574.

Malinosky-Rummell, R. and Hansen, D. J. "Long-Term Consequences of Childhood Physical Abuse." *Psychological Bulletin*, 114, 1993.

Moir, A. and Jessel, D. *Brain Sex: The Real Difference between Men and Women.* New York: Lyle Stuart, 1989.

Mulvihill, G. (2007, February 20). Hundreds of couples granted civil unions in New Jersey. *The Montgomery Advertises*, p. A3.

Roiphe, K. *The Morning After: Sex, Fear, and Feminism on Campus.* Boston: Little, Brown, 1993.

Ryan-Wenger, N. M. and Copeland, S. G. "Coping Strategies Used by Black School-Age Children from Low-Income Families. *Journal of Pediatric Nursing*, 9:1, February 1994, p. 33.

Simons, R., et al. "Explaining Women's Double Jeopardy: Factors That Mediate the Association between Harsh Treatment as a Child and Violence by a Husband." *Journal of Marriage and the Family*, August 1993, pp. 713–723.

Slater, L. "Love." *National Geographic*, February 2006, 209:2, pp. 32–49.

Spock, B. *A Better World for Children.* New York: National Press Books, 1994.

"Think Twice Before Shacking Up." *Health*, October 2000, p. 24.

Thornhill, R. and Palmer, C. "Why Men Rape." *The Sciences*, 40, January/February 2000, pp. 30–36.

U.S. Bureau of the Census. *Statistical Abstract of the United States: 2006*, 125th Ed. Washington, DC, 2005.

U.S. Department of Health and Human Services, *Youth Violence: A Report of the Surgeon General.* Rockville, MD: HHS, 2001.

Wood, C. "Why Do Men Do It?" *Maclean's*, August 7, 2000, pp. 34–37.

# Self Assessment 4.1 Are You in an Abusive Relationship?

**Name** _____   **Date** _____

**Course** _____   **Section** _____

Check any of the questions below to which you can truthfully answer "yes."

- ☐ Are you afraid of your partner?

- ☐ Does your partner monitor your comings and goings?

- ☐ Does your partner control who you can and cannot talk to?

- ☐ Are you forced to have sex against your will?

- ☐ Are you told what you can and cannot wear?

- ☐ Are you verbally or physically abused for looking at another man (woman)?

- ☐ Has your partner threatened to harm your children?

A "yes" response to any of these questions signals trouble and the need to get help.

*Source:* Dr. Carolyn Ramsey, in an article by Laura B. Randolph, "Battered Women: How to Get and Give Help," *Ebony*, September 1994. Used with permission.

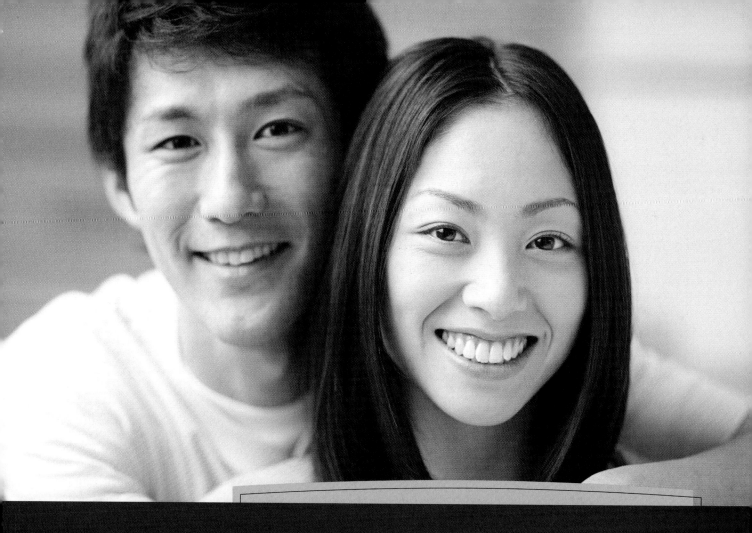

# Chapter Five Human Sexuality, Contraception, and Reproduction

**OBJECTIVES** ■ Explain the genetic difference between males and females. ■ Explain the menstrual cycle. ■ Identify the four phases of human sexual response. ■ Describe how conception occurs. ■ Identify the factors involved in prenatal care. ■ Differentiate the three stages of labor. ■ Identify complications associated with pregnancy and birth. ■ Explain the different methods of abortion. ■ Identify remedies for infertility.

ThomsonNOW™ Log on to ThomsonNOW at http://thomsonedu.com/thomsonnow to access and explore self-assessments, interactive tutorials, and practice quizzes.

Although people no longer need to follow their natural instincts, as they once did, to reproduce and thus ensure continuation of the species, the reproductive drive continues unabated. Further, humans' innate interest in sex is fueled by media bombardment of sexual images in which people leap from bed to bed with abandon, disregarding the present-day realities of sexually transmitted diseases (STDs), alarming rates of teen pregnancy, and sex crimes. Sex is not intrinsically bad, however. It can reflect the joy of mature love. It can result in new life that is anticipated with eagerness.

The sociological and psychological aspects of personal relationships are covered in Chapter 4. This chapter focuses on its physical facets, with the anticipation that awareness and understanding of the physiology of sex will contribute to its rational and satisfying expression.

## Male and Female Sexual Anatomy

**Sex** is determined early in prenatal development. Hormones and chromosomes are responsible for the formation of genitals that determine whether a person is male or female. The human sex organs serve two major functions: reproduction (procreation) and pleasure, including intimate personal communication.

Both males and females have a pair of **gonads.** The male gonads are called **testes,** and the female gonads are called **ovaries.** Gonads are responsible for the production of sex hormones and **gametes**—the **sperm** and the **ova.**

When a sperm and an ovum unite, as a result of sexual intercourse, conception occurs, creating new life. About eight weeks after conception the sex organs of this new life differentiate. How they do this depends upon genetic instructions dictated by the sex chromosomes X and Y. The father determines the sex because some of his sperm carry the X chromosome and some carry the Y chromosome. The mother's eggs are all Xs. If a sperm carrying an X chromosome fertilizes an egg, the combined XX will produce a female. If a sperm carrying a Y chromosome fertilizes an egg, the resulting child will be a male with the identifying XY chromosome. This concept is illustrated in Figure 5.1.

## THE MALE REPRODUCTIVE SYSTEM

**External Genitals.** The external male genitals are composed of the penis, glans, urethra, scrotum, and testes, as illustrated in Figure 5.2. **Semen** and urine both are expelled through the **penis.** These two processes cannot be accomplished at the same time, as they are controlled by muscular sphincters. The penis is constructed of spongy erectile tissue and many small nerves and blood vessels. At its tip is the **glans,** important in sexual arousal. During sexual arousal the spongy tissue becomes engorged with blood, causing the penis to become erect. **Erection** is necessary for sexual intercourse. Usually after **ejaculation** the penis returns to a flaccid position.

**FIGURE 5.1 ▶** Sex Determination

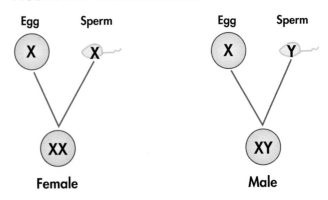

Female          Male

**FIGURE 5.2** ▶ External Male Genitalia

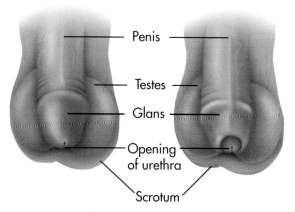

- Penis
- Testes
- Glans
- Opening of urethra
- Scrotum

**Circumcised        Uncircumcised**

The **urethra** is the long duct connected to the bladder, which runs through the center of the penis, carrying and releasing urine and semen from the body. The **scrotum** contains the testes, the epididymis, and the lower portion of the vas deferens. The major purpose of the scrotal sac is to protect the testes and to keep the testes at a stable temperature of at least 4°F to 5°F below that of the body's normal 98.6°F. This means that the temperature of the testes should be around 93.6°F for **spermatogenesis** to take place.

**VIEWPOINT** Same Sex, Safe Sex? *Women who have sex with women have a dangerous fantasy—that lesbian sex is safe sex. "Some women believe that a lesbian identity is like wearing a giant condom," says Greta R. Bauer, a researcher at the University of Minnesota School of Public Health who published a study on lesbian sexual health in the* American Journal of Public Health. *Yet it appears to be the total number of sexual encounters, not the gender of their partner, that most increases women's risk of sexually transmitted diseases (STDs).*

*Pregnancy aside, women who sleep with women expose themselves to the same risks—HIV, chlamydia, herpes, genital warts—as women who have sex only with men. "Many women get lulled into a false sense of security," says Caren Stalburg, an OB-GYN and a clinical assistant professor at the University of Michigan. "If they can't get pregnant, they figure the behavior is risk-free." It is what you are doing, not with whom you are doing it, that puts you at risk. All women should get an annual pelvic exam, Pap smear, and STD testing—no matter how they define their sexuality.*
**What is your opinion?**

**Internal Genitals.** As shown in Figure 5.3, the two testes (testicles) are almond-shaped glands. They produce the male gametes (sperm) and the male hormone **testosterone**. Each testicle is composed of sperm-producing **seminiferous tubules**. The production of testosterone, which begins in adolescence, stimulates the functioning of the male reproductive system and the development of secondary masculine characteristics. These characteristics include development of body hair, facial hair (beard and mustache), the formation of more defined muscles, and a deepening voice. Table 5.1 lists these changes.

**KEY TERMS**

**Sex** the quality of being male or female

**Gonads** sex glands, the primary reproduction organs

**Testes** almond-shaped male sex glands that produce sperm and testosterone

**Ovaries** almond-shaped female sex glands that produce eggs, or ova, and the hormones estrogen and progesterone

**Gametes** sex cells

**Sperm** male gametes

**Ova** female gametes; eggs

**Female genital mutilation (FGM)** or "female circumcision"; the practice of cutting away the entirity or parts of the female external genitalia (clitoris, labia)

**Clitoridectomy** excision of the clitoris

**Infibulation** the practice of fastening the prepuce or labia minora together with clasps, stitches, or other devices to prevent coitus

**Semen** thick, milky fluid containing sperm that is expelled through the urethra

**Penis** male organ of sexual activity

**Glans** sensitive tip of the penis

**Erection** the engorged, rigid state of the penis during sexual arousal

**Ejaculation** sudden discharge of semen from the penis as a culmination of the sexual response

**Urethra** long duct running through center of penis, which carries and releases urine as well as semen

**Scrotum** loose pouch of skin containing the testes

**Spermatogenesis** sperm cell production

**Testosterone** hormone produced by the testes that regulates male sexual development

**Seminiferous tubules** hollow, cylindrical structures that make up most of the testes and produce sperm

## FYI | MALE CIRCUMCISION

The medical procedure of circumcision has a cultural as well as a physical connotation. Worldwide, circumcised males are in the minority; only about 15% of the population practices circumcision—most prominently Jewish and Muslim peoples, for religious reasons. Most Europeans, Asians, Central and South Americans do not. Many Africans are Muslims or practice circumcision as a rite of manhood.

From the early 1940s to the mid-1970s, most parents in the United States had their newborn sons circumcised. In 1971, however, the American Academy of Pediatrics (AAP) came out against the procedure as being unnecessary, and this was followed by a drop in the rate of circumcision from 85% in 1974 to 60% by 1990.

Benefits of circumcision are cleanliness and prevention of infection resulting from bacteria being trapped under the foreskin. Research has shown further that uncircumcised infants have more urinary tract infections, which can lead to kidney damage. Circumcision also may reduce the spread of sexually transmitted diseases and cancer of the penis, the latter of which develops almost exclusively in uncircumcised men.

Drawbacks include pain to the infant (some compare it with female genital mutilation), and the risk of complications and surgical errors. Although the AAP now has taken a neutral stand, opponents of circumcision claim it is the leading unnecessary surgery in the United States.

**TABLE 5.1** ▶ Sex Changes Beginning at Puberty

| MALES | FEMALES |
|---|---|
| Growth spurt begins | Growth spurt begins |
| Oil and sweat glands become more active (if clogged, acne may develop) | Oil and sweat glands become more active (if clogged, acne may develop) |
| Testes start to grow | Breasts start to develop |
| Penis starts to grow | Menstruation begins |
| Body and facial hair starts to grow, stimulated by androgen | Secondary hair starts to grow (pubic region, under arms), stimulated by estrogen and progesterone |
| Genitalia produce mature sperm, often released during nocturnal emissions | Pregnancy becomes possible |
| Muscles become defined | Body becomes more curved |
| Skeletal system matures | Skeletal system matures |

The sperm cells mature in the **epididymis,** and the **vas deferens** convey the sperm from the epididymis up the ejaculatory duct. The fluid-producing glands include the seminal vesicles, the prostate gland, and the Cowper's glands. The **seminal vesicles** produce and secrete fluid for sperm to move in. The **prostate gland,** located directly below the bladder, produces the largest amount of seminal fluid that is released during ejaculation. The **Cowper's glands** produce a preejaculatory fluid into the urethra during sexual excitement. Secretions from the testes, seminal vesicles, prostate gland, and Cowper's glands together form semen, which contains the sperm cells discharged from the urethra upon ejaculation.

## THE FEMALE REPRODUCTIVE SYSTEM

**External Genitals.** The external female genitals, the **vulva,** are composed of the mons pubis, labia majora, labia minora, vaginal opening (introitus), clitoris, and perineum, as identified in Figure 5.4. During puberty (see Table 5.1) hair begins to grow on and eventually covers the **mons pubis.** The **labia majora** cover the labia minora, clitoris, urethral opening, and vaginal opening. Under it, the **labia minora** cover the **prepuce** or clitoral hood. Unlike the male urethra, the female **urethra** is not part of the genitals.

The **introitus** is the opening of the vagina leading to the internal genitals and the uterus. The **hymen** may cover the vaginal opening partially at birth; in some cases it is not intact. The **clitoris** is located at the upper end of the vulva above the urethral opening. When the female is stimulated sexually, the clitoris becomes engorged with blood. The area between the back of the vaginal opening and the anus is the **perineum.**

**Internal Genitals.** Internal genitals of the female, as shown in Figure 5.5, include the vagina, uterus and cervix, fallopian tubes, and ovaries. The **vagina** is the passage leading to the internal reproductive area. As one of the structures responsive to sexual arousal, the vagina is elastic enough to receive the erect penis and its ejaculate and to serve as the birth canal during vaginal delivery. It also carries menstrual blood outside the body.

The **uterus** (womb) is the organ within which the fetus gestates and develops. It stretches to accommodate the growing fetus. The **cervix** sometimes is called the neck of the womb. The **endometrium** builds during the early stages of the menstrual cycle so it may accommodate a fertilized egg. If fertilization does not occur, this lining is shed monthly through menstruation.

The **fallopian tubes,** or oviducts, connect the uterus with the two ovaries. The part of the tube closest to the ovary is called the **fimbriae,** responsible for pulling the egg cell into the fallopian tube. Lining the walls of the fallopian tubes are **cilia,** whose task is to move an egg down

**FIGURE 5.3 ▶** Internal Male Genitalia

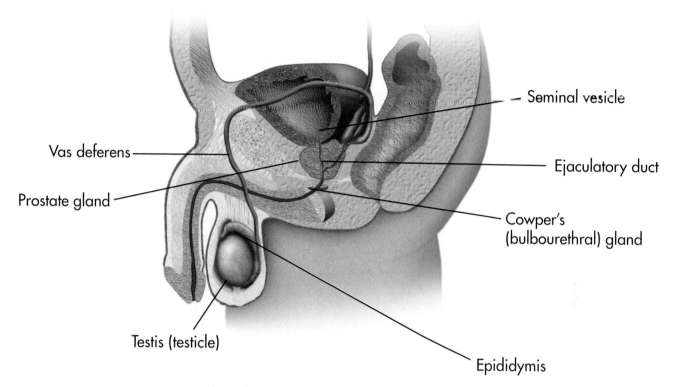

Vas deferens

Prostate gland

Seminal vesicle

Ejaculatory duct

Cowper's (bulbourethral) gland

Testis (testicle)

Epididymis

the fallopian tube to the uterus. Fertilization usually occurs in the lower third of the fallopian tube.

The ovaries are responsible for producing the female hormones estrogen and progesterone. **Estrogen** promotes the growth and function of the female sex organs and the development of female secondary sexual characteristics, such as breast development. This development begins at puberty (see Table 5.1). Estrogen is synthesized

## KEY TERMS

**Epididymis** storage structure along the top of each testicle where sperm cells mature

**Vas deferens** tubes that carry the sperm from the epididymis up the ejaculatory duct

**Seminal vesicle** glands that produce a fluid suitable for sperm motility

**Prostate gland** organ that produces seminal fluid

**Circumcision** surgical removal of foreskin of penis

**Cowper's glands** two pea-sized organs that produce preejaculatory fluid

**Vulva** outer female genitalia

**Mons pubis** mound of fatty tissue covering the pubic bone

**Labia majora** two outer folds of tissue covering vaginal opening

**Labia minora** two folds of skin within labia majora

**Prepuce** single fold of skin that covers the clitoris and the glans of uncircumcised penis

**Urethra** duct through which urine from the bladder is released from the body

**Introitus** vaginal opening

**Hymen** membrane partially covering the vaginal opening

**Clitoris** sensitive female sex organ, which becomes erect when sexually excited

**Perineum** the area between the back of the vaginal opening and the anus

**Vagina** three- to five-inch tubular passage leading to internal reproductive areas that connects with the uterus

**Uterus** pear-shaped, muscular organ within the pelvic cavity where the fetus develops; also called the womb

**Cervix** lower portion of the uterus that connects with the vagina

**Endometrium** interior lining of the uterus

**Fallopian tubes** four-inch tubular passage leading from upper portion of the uterus to each of the two ovaries

**Fimbriae** fingerlike projections at the end of fallopian tubes

**Cilia** hairlike projections inside of the fallopian tubes

**Estrogen** hormone produced by the ovaries that controls female sexual development

FIGURE 5.4 ▶ External Female Genitalia

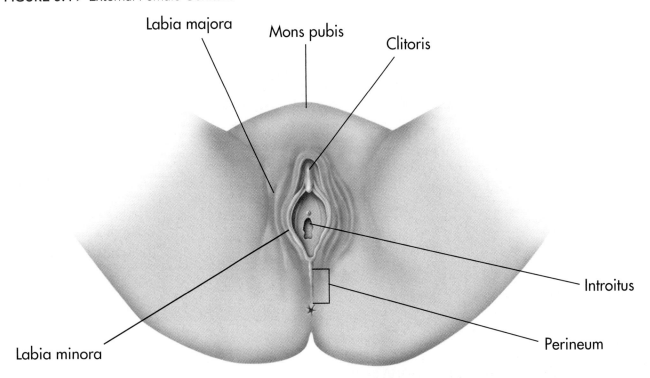

mainly by the ovaries. **Progesterone** promotes growth and maintenance of the uterine endometrium (lining), mammary glands, and placenta. If fertilization occurs, it sustains the endometrium throughout pregnancy and prevents the further release of eggs from the ovary. At puberty, these eggs start to mature, and usually one bursts from its **follicle** each month. In later life hormone production decreases, eggs no longer are released, and the woman enters menopause.

## Common Disorders of the Reproductive System

### MALE DISORDERS

Disorders of the male reproductive system most often involve the prostate gland. Aside from cancer, discussed in Chapter 7, the most common prostate condition is **benign**

FIGURE 5.5 ▶ Internal Female Genitalia

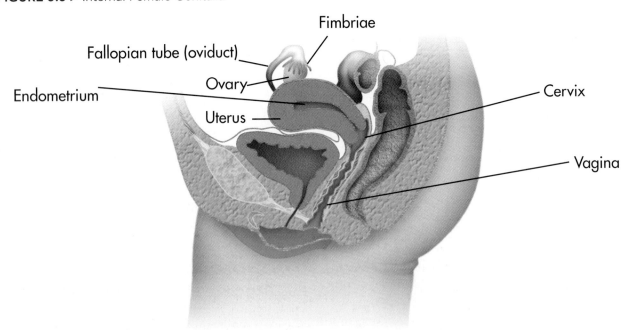

**prostatic hypertrophy (BPH)** or **enlargement.** Benign means that it is not cancerous. BPH rarely causes symptoms before age 40, but more than half of men in their sixties and as many as 90% of men in their seventies and eighties have this condition. Over time BPH can lead to urinary tract infections, bladder and kidney damage, and **incontinence.**

Symptoms of BPH vary, but the man typically has problems with or changes in urination, such as a hesitant, interrupted, weak stream; urgency and leaking or dribbling; and more frequent urination, especially at night. In some cases a man may find himself unable to urinate at all. This problem can be triggered by taking a decongestant drug. Urinary retention also can be brought on by alcohol, cold temperatures, or a long period of immobility.

Diagnosis involves, first, a rectal exam. If any cause for suspicion is found, an ultrasound test, which displays an image of the prostate gland on a screen, may be done. Sometimes the doctor will ask the patient to urinate into a special device that measures how quickly the urine is flowing; reduced flow often suggests BPH. Another test used to diagnose conditions of the urogenital tract is the intravenous pyelogram (IVP). A dye is injected into a vein, and then an x-ray is made. The dye reveals any obstruction or blockage in the urinary tract. A third test procedure is the cystoscopy, in which, after numbing the penis with a solution, the doctor inserts a small tube through the opening of the urethra. The tube contains a lens and a light system, which help the physician see the inside of the urethra and bladder.

A number of recent studies have questioned the need for early treatment when the gland is barely enlarged. The condition clears up without treatment in up to a third of all mild cases. Regular check-ups are suggested, however. Alpha blocker drugs may be prescribed to help relax muscles in the prostate. However, they do not cure the condition or reduce the need for future surgery. Drug treatments for BPH include the 5-alpha-reductase inhibitors finasteride (Proscar®) and dutasteride (Avodart®) and the alpha blockers that relax the smooth muscle of the prostate and bladder neck to improve urine flow. These include terazosin, which was developed to treat hypertension, and Flomax® or Uroxatral®, which were developed specifically to treat BHP.

When treatment is necessary, most doctors recommend removing the enlarged part of the prostate. In transurethral surgery no external incision is needed. It is done through the urethra, most often using a resectoscope inserted through the penis. If this procedure cannot be used, as is the case when the gland is greatly enlarged, an external incision may be the method of choice. Finally, endoscopic surgery (TURP) or a method using lasers (TUVP) is used to remove or vaporize the offending tissue.

Other disorders of the male reproductive system are listed in Table 5.2. Cancers of the male reproductive system are covered in Chapter 7.

## FEMALE DISORDERS

The most common disorders involving the female reproductive system are endometriosis, uterine fibroid tumors, vaginitis, and premenstrual syndrome (PMS). Others are outlined briefly in Table 5.3.

**TABLE 5.3 ▶** Selected Disorders of the Female Reproductive System

| DISORDER | DESCRIPTION |
|---|---|
| Amenorrhea | Absence of menstruation |
| Cystocele | Protrusion into the vagina of a portion of the urinary bladder |
| Dysmenorrhea | Painful menstruation |
| Dyspareunia | Pain during intercourse |
| Fibrocystic disease of the breast | Benign (noncancerous) lumps in the breast |
| Leukorrhagia | Abnormal white discharge from the vagina caused by any of several conditions |
| Menorrhagia | Abnormally long (more than 7 days) or heavy menstrual flow |
| Ovarian cyst | Abnormal swelling or saclike growth on an ovary |
| Pelvic inflammatory disease (PID) | Inflammation of the uterus and fallopian tubes |
| Polycystic ovarian disease (PCOD) | A set of conditions in which the ovarian function is disturbed; ovary may enlarge and produce many small cysts |
| Prolapse of the uterus | Collapse, descent, or other change in position of the uterus |
| Rectocele | A condition in which part of the rectum protrudes into the vagina as a result of a hernia |
| Vaginitis | Inflammation of the vagina |

**TABLE 5.2 ▶** Selected Disorders of the Male Reproductive System

| DISORDER | DESCRIPTION |
|---|---|
| Gynecomastia | Excessive development of the male breasts |
| Hydrocele | Abnormal collection of fluid around the testes |
| Prostatitis | Infection or inflammation of the prostate gland |
| Urethritis | Infection or inflammation of the urethra |

## KEY TERMS

**Progesterone** hormone that prepares uterus for pregnancy

**Follicle** egg sac in ovary

**Benign prostatic hypertrophy (BPH)** or **enlargement** noncancerous enlargement of prostate gland

**Incontinence** inability to control urination voluntarily

**Endometriosis.** The lining of the uterus, the endometrium, is supposed to stay in the uterus until it is shed monthly in the form of menstrual blood. In some women parts of the endometrium migrate to the fallopian tubes, the ovaries, or even the abdominal cavity. This condition, called **endometriosis,** affects more than five million women in the United States, 10%–15% of all women of childbearing age. Although the cause is unknown, it seems to be related to estrogen, as it rarely occurs before puberty and tends to disappear after menopause.

As the endometrium in the uterus responds to the hormones of the menstrual cycle by getting thicker and then bleeding, so does the endometrial tissue that is sticking to the other reproductive structures. These **implants** bleed, may form cysts that can rupture, and cause scar tissue or adhesions to form in the pelvic cavity.

**Signs and Symptoms.** The symptoms vary from woman to woman, but sharp pain, cramps, and heavy bleeding during the menstrual period are common. Some women have chronic pelvic pain or pressure during **coitus.** If the implants have migrated to the bladder or the intestines, the woman may have pain when she urinates or has a bowel movement, especially during the menstrual period. The urine or stool may contain blood. Those affected also may have fatigue and lower back pain.

**Diagnosis.** Endometriosis should be diagnosed as soon as possible so it can be treated in the early stages of development. The notion that this condition is not common in African-American women and teenagers is not accurate. Undiagnosed, endometriosis becomes progressively worse and may lead to fertility problems. Infertility affects about 30% to 40% of women with endometriosis. Women of any age should not ignore severe menstrual cramps, which is one of the first symptoms of endometriosis.

Definitive diagnosis of endometriosis is made by **laparoscopy.** In this minor surgical procedure the abdomen is distended with carbon dioxide gas and the **laparoscope** is inserted through a tiny incision in the abdomen near the navel. Looking through the laparoscope, the physician can see where the endometrial implants are and check the condition of the other organs in the abdomen.

**Treatment.** Objectives of the treatment are not only to relieve pain and stop more implants from growing but also to preserve reproductive functioning. The treatment for endometriosis varies. The woman may be advised to use one of several hormone or drug therapies (tablets, nasal spray, injection) that temporarily halt ovulation and the menstrual cycle. During this time the implants are supposed to shrink and the other symptoms disappear. Various drug treatment uses **GnRH analogs.** This six-month therapy induces menopause medically, sometimes with its attendant symptoms (hot flashes, vaginal dryness, bone loss). Other drugs being investigated are RU486 (the abortion pill), steroids, and drugs that affect the immune system.

The alternative treatment for endometriosis is some form of surgery. In conservative surgical treatment, laparoscopic surgery is used to remove or destroy the endometrial implants and scar tissue. In the most nonconservative surgery, the uterus, ovaries, and fallopian tubes are removed.

**Uterine Fibroid Tumors.** You may have heard your grandmother refer to fibroid tumors as "fireball tumors." Uterine fibroids are one of the most common noncancerous gynecological conditions appearing in women of reproductive age. Estimates are that more than one in every four or five women over age 50 is affected. African-American women are more than three times as likely as Caucasian women to develop fibroids. Fibroid tumors account for 30% of the hysterectomies performed annually in the United States.

**Signs and Symptoms.** A fibroid tumor, or **myoma,** can be smaller than a jelly bean or larger than a cantaloupe. The growth of fibroids is believed to be stimulated by the hormone estrogen. Small fibroids usually do not cause problems. As they grow larger, however, they typically produce unusually heavy menstrual bleeding and pressure or pain in the abdomen. In some cases the fibroid can grow so large that it presses against the bladder and uterus, causing frequent urination and other problems with the urinary tract. Medium to large fibroid tumors may cause a woman's abdomen to protrude to the point at which she looks like she is pregnant.

Fibroids are classified by their position in the uterus. A submucous fibroid grows inward from the uterine wall, taking up space within the uterus. This type of fibroid is more likely to cause heavy and prolonged menstrual flow, which can result in anemia (deficiency of hemoglobin in the blood). A pedunculated fibroid grows on a stalk or a stem. This type can cause severe pain if the stalk becomes twisted and cuts off blood supply to the fibroid.

**Diagnosis and Treatment.** Fibroids may be diagnosed in a number of ways, including the standard pelvic exam, ultrasound, computerized tomography, magnetic resonance imaging (MRI), x-ray, and laparoscopy. Options for treatment have to weigh the relief of symptoms against the need to preserve reproductive functioning. If the woman wants to have a baby, **hysterectomy** will be delayed. In some cases the fibroid is removed in a **myomectomy.** In extreme cases, complications of heavy blood loss and scarring may prevent the woman from being able to bear children, and in some instances the fibroid will grow back.

Because fibroids tend to grow more slowly and may shrink in menopause, short-term drug therapy options that stimulate menopause are available. Many gynecologists are prescribing GnRH analogs (as in endometriosis), which block the production of estrogen and in turn cause the fibroids to shrink. These medications produce the same side effects as menopause, such as hot flashes, vaginal dryness, and bone loss. The other drawback is that when the medication is stopped, the fibroids begin to grow again.

**Premenstrual Syndrome.** **Premenstrual syndrome** is a condition of physical discomfort that a female may experience prior to her menstrual period. It is characterized by nervousness, irritability, emotional disturbance, headache, and depression in some combination. The condition is associated with the accumulation of fluid in the tissues and usually disappears after menstruation begins. The female hormone progesterone is believed to be part of the cause, and a deficiency of essential fatty acids also has been observed.

Once a month, about two weeks before the menstrual period, estrogen and progesterone begin to amass and come into conflict. Estrogen levels may soar for one woman, making her anxious and irritable; or progesterone may predominate, dragging her into depression and fatigue. She might feel bloated and gain weight, have a headache, backache, acne, allergies, or tenderness in the breasts. Her mood may swing erratically from euphoria to depression. When the period finally arrives, symptoms leave. In 5% to 10% of females, PMS is so severe that the condition is termed premenstrual dysphoric disorder (PMDD). Symptoms include severe joint and muscle pain, headaches, breast tenderness, and fatigue. Research at the University of North Carolina at Chapel Hill found that females with PMDD may experience more severe pain during the PMS period due to lower levels of beta-endorphins (the pain-killing hormone produced by the body) than non-PMDD sufferers.

PMS is believed to affect between a third and half of all American women between ages 20 and 50, says Dr. Susan Lark, director of the PMS Self-Help Center in Los Altos, California. Certain factors, such as bearing several children, seem to promote PMS, says Dr. Guy Abraham, a former professor of obstetrics and gynecologic endocrinology at the University of California, Los Angeles, School of Medicine. The problem may be inherited, according to Dr. Edward Portman, a PMS consultant, researcher, and director of the Portman Clinic in Madison, Wisconsin.

Not all PMS sufferers have the same symptoms and the same intensity of discomfort. And PMS sufferers do not necessarily respond to the same treatments. Finding the best way to handle PMS may require some trial and error.

## Sexual Arousal and Response

Sexual excitement is derived from stimuli such as touching, masturbation, intercourse, oral sex, and other sexual acts. It is often said that "90% of sex is in the mind"—indicating the powerful role of psychological factors in sexual arousal and function. The physiological mechanisms involved are

- Vasocongestion, the increased supply of blood into the genitals during sexual excitement
- Myotonia, which causes increased muscular contractions during orgasm

## RESPONSE CYCLE

The human sexual response cycle has four phases.

1. **Excitement phase.** In the excitement phase the male's penis becomes erect. The testes begin to expand, and the scrotal skin tenses and thickens. In females the vagina increases in size and a natural lubricant prepares the vagina to receive the penis. The uterus increases in size and elevates into the pelvic cavity, and the breasts swell. In both sexes the nipples become erect.

2. **Plateau phase.** The plateau phase is more intense and extended than the excitement phase. In men the penis becomes larger and harder and the testes enlarge. The Cowper's glands secrete a preejaculatory fluid, and the testes become completely engorged with blood and fully elevated. In females the lower portion of the vagina enlarges, and lubrication of the vaginal wall increases beyond that of the excitement phase. The uterus continues to increase in size and is elevated completely into the pelvic cavity. In both sexes the heart rate doubles and breathing becomes more rapid.

3. **Orgasmic phase.** The orgasmic phase is characterized in males by intense rhythmic contractions in the pelvic region, penis, seminal vesicles, prostate glands, and urethra. At this point orgasm and ejaculation of semen

---

## KEY TERMS

**Endometriosis** a condition in which pieces of the endometrium migrate to fallopian tubes, ovaries, or abdominal cavity

**Implants** pieces of endometrium that have migrated to other areas

**Coitus** sexual intercourse by insertion of a penis into a vagina

**Laparoscopy** a procedure that uses an optical device (laparoscope) to view the abdominal cavity

**Laparoscope** a fiber-optic instrument inserted through the abdominal wall to give an examining doctor a view of the abdominal organs

**GnRH analogs** gonadotropin releasing hormone analogs; a drug treatment for endometriosis

**Myoma** a mass of muscle and connective tissue growing in the uterus; surgically removed by **myomectomy**

**Hysterectomy** surgical removal of the uterus

**Premenstrual syndrome (PMS)** a hormone-induced condition of physical discomfort occurring about 10 days before menstruation

## Tips for Action If You Have PMS

■ **Be positive.** A positive, confident attitude can help you cope and maybe even prevent future episodes of premenstrual syndrome (PMS). Recite some positive affirmations (for example, "I can handle stress").

■ **Eat a little often.** Poor nutrition does not cause PMS, but certain dietary factors can accentuate the problem. Eat small meals low in sugar several times a day.

■ **Avoid empty calories.** Stay away from low-nutrient foods such as soft drinks and sweets containing refined sugar.

■ **Decrease dairy foods.** Eat no more than one or two portions per day of skim or low-fat milk, cottage cheese, or yogurt. The lactose in dairy products can block the body's absorption of magnesium, which helps regulate the estrogen level and increases its excretion.

■ **Ferret out fats.** Replace animal fats such as butter and lard with polyunsaturated oils such as corn and safflower oils. Animal fats contribute to the high estrogen levels that may intensify PMS.

■ **Get your daily allowance of vitamins and minerals.** Take a nutritional supplement every day containing vitamins $B_6$, A, C, D, E, calcium, magnesium, and L-tyrosine.

■ **Restrict salt.** Go on a low-sodium diet for seven to 10 days before the onset of your period, to offset water retention.

■ **Eat plenty of fiber.** Fiber helps the body clear out excess estrogens. Eat plenty of vegetables, beans, and whole grains.

■ **Cut down on caffeine.** Consume limited quantities of coffee, tea, chocolate, and other caffeine-containing substances.

■ **Abstain from alcohol.** Alcohol is a depressant. It also can worsen PMS headaches and fatigue and cause sugar cravings.

■ **Do not take diuretics.** Some over-the-counter diuretics draw valuable minerals out of the body along with water.

Instead, stay away from substances such as salt and alcohol, which cause water retention.

■ **Exercise.** Walk at a fast pace in fresh air, swim, jog, take up ballet or karate. Increase your level of activity for the week or two before PMS symptoms set in.

■ **De-stress your environment.** Surround yourself with soothing colors and soft music.

■ **Breathe deeply.** Shallow breathing, which many people do unconsciously, decreases your energy level and leaves you feeling tense. Practice inhaling and exhaling slowly and deeply.

■ **Soak in a tub.** Indulge yourself in a mineral bath to relax muscles from head to toe, for at least 20 minutes.

■ **Get extra sleep.** Go to bed earlier for a few days before PMS tends to set in.

■ **Adhere to a schedule.** Set reasonable goals and schedules for each day to avoid feeling overwhelmed, even if this means cutting back your routine.

■ **Decline social obligations temporarily.** Postpone big plans such as holding a dinner party until a time when you feel you can handle it better.

■ **Talk.** Discuss your PMS problems with your mate, friends, or co-workers. This can be highly beneficial.

*Sources:* Guy Abraham, M.D., former professor of obstetrics and gynecologic endocrinology, University of California, Los Angeles, School of Medicine

Penny Wise Budoff, M.D., director of Women's Medical Center, Bethpage, New York

Susan Lark, M.D., director of PMS Self-Help Center, Los Altos, California

Edward Portman, M.D., PMS consultant, researcher and director of Portman Clinic, Madison, Wisconsin

Peter Vash, M.D., endocrinologist and internist on clinical faculty of UCLA Medical Center

Extracted from editors of *Prevention Magazine, The Doctor's Book of Home Remedies* (Emmaus, PA: Rodale Press, 1990). Adapted by permission.

occur. In females rhythmic contractions occur in the vagina, uterus, and entire pelvic region. Not all women experience an orgasm with penile insertion; some have an orgasm as a result of stimulation of the clitoris.

4. **Resolution phase.** The resolution phase is the resting, relaxation, or reversal stage. All changes beginning with excitement in male and female are reversed. The male's erection is lost because blood rushes out of the spongy, erectile penile tissue, the muscles relax, and the genital organs return to their original nonstimulated sizes and positions. At this

point the male enters a **refractory period.** Depending upon a man's age and health, the refractory period may last several minutes to several days. Women do not have a physical refractory period.

## SEXUAL PROBLEMS

The sexual response can be influenced by a variety of physical and psychological factors that usually are interrelated. Sexual problems may be caused by anxiety, worry, fatigue, alcohol or other drug consumption, relationship conflicts, lack of interest, and other physical or emotional sources.

### Problems in the Female

**Vaginal Dryness.** During sexual arousal a clear fluid emerges in the vaginal wall. One function of this fluid is to facilitate entry of the penis into the vagina. Some women do not produce enough lubrication. During intercourse this problem may cause pain, irritation, and tearing of the vaginal tissue. Vaginal dryness can result from anxiety, hormonal imbalance, aging, and the use of oral contraceptives, antihistamines, and other medications.

Remedies include more precoital stimulation (foreplay) and commercial vaginal lubricants (lubricating jelly) developed specifically to alleviate vaginal dryness temporarily. Vaginal lubricants are not contraceptives; they do not afford protection from pregnancy. Petroleum jelly should not be used as a substitute for a lubricating jelly as it can cause vaginal irritation in some women. Also, when a condom is being used, petroleum jelly can cause the condom to weaken and tear.

**Vaginismus. Vaginismus,** strong, involuntary contractions in the muscles of the lower vagina, makes intercourse difficult, if not impossible. A woman with vaginismus may have contractions during pelvic exams and may even feel extreme discomfort with the insertion of one finger. The fundamental cause of vaginismus usually is **dyspareunia,** induced by fear, sexual conflict, or unpleasant sexual feelings. Women with this condition should consult a gynecologist.

### Problems in the Male

**Erectile Dysfunction (ED). Erectile dysfunction** or impotence, is the inability to achieve and maintain an erection firm enough for intromission and coitus. ED may be caused by diseases, medication, the use of alcohol or other drugs, injuries, and other psychological and physiological disorders. ED after age 40 is more common than previously thought. In a survey of nearly 1,300 men aged 40 to 70 in Boston, 52% reported some degree of impotence. Contributing factors were high blood pressure, heart disease, smoking, diabetes, some medications, and extreme anger or depression.

**Premature Ejaculation. Premature ejaculation,** emission of semen and loss of erection within 30 seconds to two minutes of beginning coitus, understandably can be frustrating to both partners. Any man who has long-term problems with premature ejaculation or impotence should consult a urologist.

## Fertility Control

In today's world, when both men and women tend to work outside the home and financial needs are greater, couples are more likely to plan just when to have children. Many are opting to have children later in life when they are more established. Nowadays, a woman's getting pregnant after 40 is not the unusual occurrence it was in the past.

### KEY TERMS

**Refractory period** the time immediately following orgasm when a male cannot be sexually stimulated

**Vaginismus** strong, involuntary contractions in the muscles of the lower part of the vagina

**Dyspareunia** painful intercourse

**Erectile dysfunction (ED)** inability to obtain or maintain an erection for coitus; impotence

**Premature ejaculation** emission of semen and loss of erection within 30 seconds to two minutes of beginning coitus

- Increase the proportion of sexually active persons who use condoms.

- Increase the proportion of females at risk of unintended pregnancy (and their partners) who use contraception.

- Increase the proportion of young adults who have received formal instruction before turning age 18 on reproductive health issues, including all of the

following topics: birth control methods, safer sex to prevent HIV transmission, prevention of sexually transmitted diseases, and abstinence.

- Increase male involvement in pregnancy prevention and family planning efforts.

- Reduce maternal death.

- Reduce low birthweight and very low birthweight.

## CONTRACEPTION

**Contraceptives** encompass drugs, artificial devices, and surgical procedures used to prevent fertilization, ovulation, or implantation. Periodic abstinence also is considered a method of contraception. When considering each method, variations include safety (health risks), effectiveness, cost, ease of use, availability, maintenance, and convenience. No contraceptive is 100% effective or 100% safe. Each has advantages and disadvantages, which are summarized in Table 5.4. The user or prospective user should be knowledgeable of the pros and cons. Sound judgment and personal responsibility are vital. The choice of contraceptives as a birth control method is an extremely personal decision.

Barrier methods place physical barriers between the sperm and egg. They prohibit the sperm from entering the cervix. These methods include the male and female condom, diaphragm, cervical cap, and vaginal spermicide.

**Male Condom.** The **condom,** a prophylactic measure, and informally called a "rubber," is designed to cover the erect penis and prevent semen from entering the vagina. The latex rubber condom (Figure 5.6) is the most effective type of condom. When using a condom without a reservoir, one-half inch should be left at the tip to capture semen and prevent the condom from tearing at ejaculation.

The condom is placed over an erect penis before any vaginal contact and insertion, and it is removed

**TABLE 5.4** ► Summary of Birth Control and Contraceptives

| CHARACTERISTIC | MALE CONDOM | FEMALE CONDOM | SPERMICIDES USED ALONE | DIAPHRAGM WITH SPERMICIDE | CERVICAL CAP WITH SPERMICIDE |
|---|---|---|---|---|---|
| Estimated effectiveness | About 85% | 74%–79% | 70%–80% | 82%–94% | At least 82% |
| Risks | Rarely, irritation and allergic reactions | Rarely, irritation and allergic reactions | Rarely, irritation and allergic reactions | Rarely, irritation and allergic reactions, bladder infection; very rarely, toxic shock syndrome | Abnormal Pap test, vaginal or cervical infections; very rarely, toxic shock syndrome |
| Protection against sexually transmitted diseases | Latex condoms help protect against sexually transmitted diseases, including herpes and AIDS | May give some protection against sexually transmitted diseases including herpes and AIDS; not as effective as male latex condom | Unknown | None | None |
| Convenience | Applied immediately before intercourse; used only once and discarded | Applied immediately before intercourse; used only once and discarded | Applied no more than one hour before intercourse | Inserted before intercourse; should be left in place six to eight hours after last intercourse; additional spermicide must be used if intercourse is repeated | Can remain in place 48 hours; not necessary to reapply spermicide upon repeated intercourse; may be difficult to insert |
| Availability | Nonprescription | Nonprescription | Nonprescription | Prescription | Prescription |

immediately from the vagina after the male orgasm and ejaculation. A reliable way of removing a condom is to hold the rim of the condom against the base of the penis. This allows the penis to be removed from the vagina without spilling sperm into the vagina.

When used properly and consistently, condoms coupled with vaginal spermicide can be effective as a birth control method. Condoms, some of which are lubricated or treated with a chemical spermicide, may be purchased in stores without a prescription. They are relatively inexpensive and cause no serious adverse side effects to either sexual partner. The most widely reported disadvantage is that condoms reduce male sensations during intercourse. Also, when spermicide (nonoxynol-9) is added to condoms, it can cause the genitalia to become irritated.

**Female Condom.** The **female condom** (fc female condom™) is a soft, strong, loose-fitting plastic pouch that lines the vagina. It has a soft ring at each end. The ring at the closed end is used to put the device inside the vagina and holds it in place. The other ring stays outside the vagina and partly covers the lip area. Female condoms are costlier than male condoms, and both can be used only once.

One problem with the female condom is that the outer ring can be pushed inside the vagina during sex. Some women have also reported that the penis slipped to

**FIGURE 5.6 ▶** Male Condom with Reservoir Tip

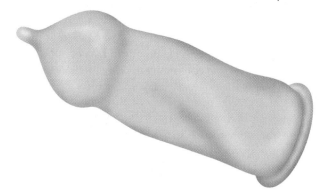

### KEY TERMS

**Contraceptives** any device, drug, or practice that prevents ovulation, fertilization, or implantation

**Condom** thin sheath placed over the penis that prevents semen from entering the vagina

**Female condom** sheath inserted into vagina to prevent fertilization and sexually transmitted diseases

**TABLE 5.4 ▶** Summary of Birth Control and Contraceptives *(Continued)*

| ORAL CONTRACEPTIVE PILL | INJECTION— DEPO-PROVERA® | INTRAUTERINE DEVICE | PERIODIC ABSTINENCE (NATURAL FAMILY PLANNING) | SURGICAL STERILIZATION |
|---|---|---|---|---|
| 97%–99% | 99% | 95%–96% | Highly variable, perhaps 53%–85% | Over 99% |
| Blood clots, heart attacks, strokes, gall bladder disease, liver tumors, water retention, hypertension, mood changes, dizziness, nausea; not for smokers | Amenorrhea, weight gain, other side effects similar to those with Norplant | Cramps, bleeding, pelvic inflammatory disease, infertility; rarely, perforation of the uterus | None | Pain, infection, and possible surgical complications in tubal ligation |
| None | None | None | None | None |
| Pill must be taken on daily schedule, regardless of frequency of intercourse | One injection every three months | After insertion, stays in place until physician removes it | Requires frequent monitoring of body functions and periods of abstinence | Vasectomy is a one-time procedure usually performed in a doctor's office; tubal ligation is a one-time procedure performed in an operating room |
| Prescription | Prescription | Prescription | Instructions from physician or clinic | Surgery |

**FIGURE 5.7 ▶** How to Insert Female Condom

 Inner ring is squeezed for insertion

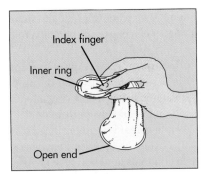

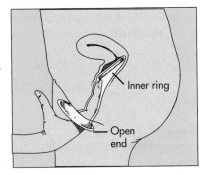

Sheath is inserted, similar to a tampon

Inner ring is pushed up as far as it can go with index finger

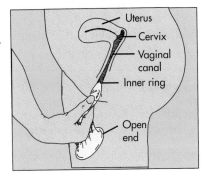

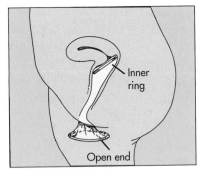 fc female condom in place

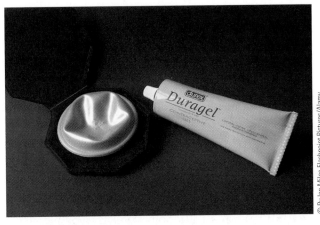

© By Ian Miles-Flashpoint Pictures/Alamy

▲ *Diaphragm and spermicide*

A health practitioner instructs the woman on how the diaphragm is to be inserted and removed. After applying a chemical spermicide containing nonoxynol-9 around the rim and inside the dome of the cup, it is inserted into the vagina and placed over the cervical opening no longer than an hour before intercourse. Before each act of intercourse, the woman must feel the diaphragm to determine whether it covers the cervical opening properly. The diaphragm must be left in place at least six hours after intercourse. If intercourse is repeated during this six-hour period, more spermicide must be added before each act of intercourse while the diaphragm is left in place.

Once the diaphragm is removed, it must be cleaned immediately with mild soap and warm water. After drying the device thoroughly and carefully, it should be placed in its container and stored in a cool, safe place.

Although the diaphragm may be difficult to insert at first, it is effective when used properly. It is even more effective when used in combination with the male condom. In cases of weight gain, weight loss, and childbirth, a diaphragm has to be refitted. Some women have reported occasional irritation and bladder infections when using the diaphragm. With normal use a diaphragm should be replaced every two years.

**Reversible Prescription Methods (Injectable Contraceptives).** A once-a-month injectable combination contraceptive (brand name Lunelle®) received Food and Drug Administration (FDA) approval in October 2000. Lunelle is administered intramuscularly in the arm, buttock, or thigh, and it prevents pregnancy primarily by inhibiting ovulation. Although the method is highly effective (failure rate is two per 100 women), it presents some common side effects such as weight gain, excessive bleeding, breast pain, menorrhagia, headache, acne, and dysmenorrhea.

The contraceptive **Depo-Provera®** is injected into the muscle of the arm or buttock for release into the bloodstream. Depo-Provera inhibits ovulation by suppressing the hormone secreted by the pituitary gland that stimulates release of the mature ovum. Each injection is effective for three months.

the side of the device entering the vagina. Other problems include difficulty inserting the fc female condom, minor irritation, discomfort, and breakage.

The female condom and the male condom should *not* be used at the same time. Figure 5.7 illustrates how to insert a female condom.

**Diaphragm.** The **diaphragm** is designed for premeditated sex, as it is available only after medical evaluation, including gynecological fitting and prescription.

The cost of the first visit and the initial injection depends on the female's physical examination and medical history. Each subsequent injection costs less. Side effects include breakthrough bleeding, amenorrhea, water retention, and weight changes. Women with a history of blood clots, undiagnosed vaginal bleeding, and breast cancer should not use Depo-Provera, nor should women who think they might be pregnant. Depo-Provera does not protect against sexually transmitted diseases.

**Etonogestrel Implant.** The single-rod subdermal implant releases etonogestrel for three years. It is a long-acting, reversible method and has proven to be highly effective in various European studies. It is associated with headaches, nausea, depression, bleeding, breast tenderness, and breast pain. Fertility status is restored quickly when the rod is removed.

**The Implanon®.** The FDA recently, approved the Implanon®, a matchstick-sized rod that is inserted under the skin of the upper arm. It is inserted in the health care provider's office with a local anesthetic. The Implanon® prevents pregnancy for up to three years, and it has been used since 1998 by over 2.5 million women throughout the world.

The Implanon® is said to be 99% safe, and when it is removed, the woman's fertility, usually returns to the level prior to using this method. Known side effects may include irregular bleeding; smoking cigarettes can increase the risk of severe heart conditions.

**Vaginal Ring.** The first hormonal vaginal contraceptive ring (brand name NuvaRing™) was approved by the FDA in 2001. Available by prescription only, the NuvaRing is a flexible polymer ring that is implanted in a woman's vagina for three weeks and removed and discarded during the fourth week of the menstrual cycle. It prevents ovulation by releasing a continuous low dose of the hormones estrogen and progestin. A new ring is inserted each month and must be used as directed by the manufacturer for maximum effectiveness.

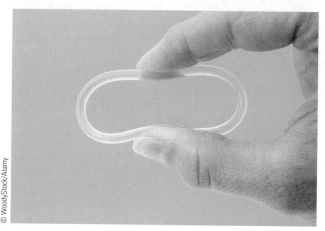

▲ *Vaginal ring*

**FIGURE 5.8** ▶ One Type of Intrauterine Device (IUD)

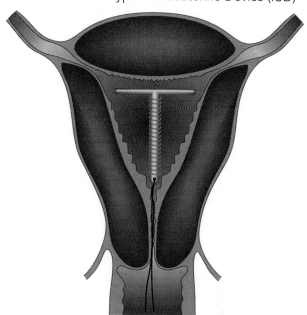

Some side effects of the NuvaRing include vaginitis, vaginal discharge, and vaginal irritation. It may increase the risk for stroke, heart attack, and blood clots. Smoking cigarettes while using the NuvaRing seriously increases the risk of cardiovascular disorders. It should not be used by women who have cardiovascular disease, blood clots, or certain types of cancer.

**Contraceptive Patch.** The contraceptive patch (brand name Evra™) provides a daily low-dose steroid. A sustained release device, it contains a progestin and an estrogen. The amount of the hormones released depends on the size of the patch prescribed. The patch is self-administered and worn for a period of three weeks.

**Intrauterine Devices.** An **intrauterine device** is inserted into the uterus by a health care specialist only after a medical examination, including a gynecological exam. The IUD must be inserted during a woman's menstrual period (usually the second day) while the cervix is dilated. It remains in place until a health care professional removes it.

The intrauterine device (IUD) system Mirena® was approved by the FDA in December 2000. The T-shaped IUD system, which releases a daily low-dose hormone

### KEY TERMS

**Diaphragm** rubber or plastic cup that fits over the cervix and prevents semen from entering the uterus and fallopian tubes

**Depo-Provera®** progestin contraceptive that is injected and lasts three months

**Intrauterine device (IUD)** small plastic contraceptive device placed in the uterus by a health care practitioner to prevent implantation

(levonorgestrel), is placed in the uterus to prevent pregnancy. The system contains a five-year supply of the hormone. It is very safe, about 99% effective at preventing pregnancy, makes the monthly period lighter and less painful, and can reduce anemia that heavy bleeding can cause.

Another IUD is the ParaGard (copper T-380). They are both T-shaped devices. The ParaGard shown in Figure 5.8 is partially wrapped in copper. Besides intensifying the inflammatory response, the copper is thought to have a chemical impact on the uterine lining, changing the normal levels of several enzymes. This creates an unfriendly environment for eggs and sperm to unite. The ParaGard is effective for up to 12 years.

Side effects include irregular bleeding or spotting in the first month, mood changes, acne, headache, nausea, and breast tenderness. The FDA cautions women to not use this method if they have a history of pelvic inflammatory disease or a previous ectopic pregnancy. It does not prevent sexually transmitted diseases.

Although the IUD is effective and relatively inexpensive, its use has declined in recent years. Problems attributed to the IUD include perforated uterus, pelvic infections, abnormally heavy menstrual bleeding, menstrual cramps, lower back pain, nausea, and breast tenderness. Other potential complications include ectopic pregnancy and pelvic inflammatory disease (PID), an infection of the vagina, uterus, and pelvic cavity. The IUD is thought to be spermicidal, creating an inflammatory response that kills sperm before they enter the fallopian tubes.

Females who never have been pregnant and may want to bear children someday may be advised against using an IUD. It increases the risks for infertility and repeated spontaneous abortions.

**Cervical Cap.** Like the diaphragm, the **cervical cap** must be prescribed by a health practitioner. Prior to insertion a chemical spermicide is placed in the cervical cap. An advantage of the cervical cap is that it may be inserted prior to intercourse and left in place two days (48 hours). Disadvantages of the cervical cap are that it may be difficult to insert and remove, some women have problems with proper fitting, and some women have reported discharges and unpleasant odors. Irregular Pap tests have been reported during the first six months of use with the cervical cap.

**FemCap.** FemCap is a precribed barrier cap that is used with a chemical spermicide and placed firmly with the precise fit over the cervix entirely. The FemCap is sold in three sizes—small for women who have never been pregnant, medium for women who have been pregnant, and a larger size for women who have delivered a baby/babies vaginally. Although FemCap is a barrier method, it does not protect from HIV/AIDS, HPV, and other sexually transmitted infections.

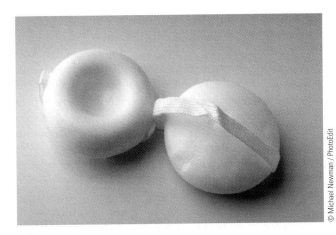

▲ *Vaginal sponge*

**Vaginal Sponge.** The **vaginal sponge** was pulled from the market in 1995. However, the Nonprescription Drugs Advisory Committee of the Food and Drug Administration voted in July 2001 to allow Allendale Pharmaceutical to resume marketing the Today Vaginal Contraceptive Sponge. The company must comply with specific labeling revisions such as warning consumers of increased risks for irritation when the sponge is worn for consecutive days, toxic shock syndrome, incidences of allergic reactions and infections, and removal difficulty.

When placed close to the cervix prior to intercourse, the sponge traps and absorbs sperm and the spermicide contained therein kills the sperm. After intercourse, it must remain in place according to directions, removed, and discarded.

**Chemical (Vaginal) Spermicide.** Chemical **spermicides** kill sperm before they enter the uterus. Spermicides have many different forms, including foams, creams, vaginal suppositories, jellies, and vaginal contraceptive film. The chemicals must be placed close to the cervix less than one-half hour before intercourse, and intercourse must take place within the hour. Chemical spermicides should

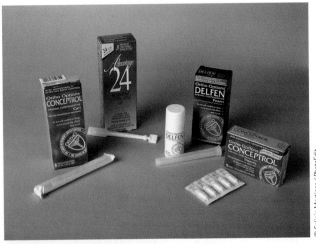

▲ *Chemical spermicides*

be applied before each act of intercourse. The chemicals lose their effectiveness after one use and after one hour.

An advantage is that spermicides are readily available. They may be purchased in stores without a prescription. Chemical spermicide always should be used with a condom for better protection against pathogens that cause sexually transmitted diseases. A disadvantage is that spermicides are messy. Also, they may irritate genital tissue in females and males. Symptoms include burning, a fine rash, and inflammation of genital tissue. The user may want to try another brand to see if it makes a difference.

**Oral Contraception. Oral contraceptives,** or birth control pills, are of two types: the combination pill and the progestin-only or minipill. All oral contraceptives are available to the female only after a gynecological examination and prescription. The examining health practitioner decides which type is best for the patient. The most common and effective—the combination pill—contains two hormones, synthetic estrogen and progesterone (progestin). Oral contraceptives are taken for 21 consecutive days, preferably at the same time each day. When taken as directed, the combination pill prevents ovulation.

The minipill contains a small amount of progesterone and no estrogen, and it must be taken daily without fail. When the minipill is taken as directed, it alters the mucus in the cervix (making it thick and tacky, and thus blocking sperm) and does not allow the endometrium to thicken. This prevents implantation of a fertilized egg.

The multiphasic pill is a different formulation of the combination pill designed to release variable doses, instead of constant doses, of estrogen and progesterone. This is more similar to the natural menstrual cycle. Like the other oral contraceptives, the multiphasic pill is taken for 21 consecutive days. Yasmin 28 contains two hormones (drospirenone, a progestin, and ethinyl estradiol, an estrogen). These hormones prevent ovulation and change the uterus and cervical mucus to make it more difficult for fertilization or implantation.

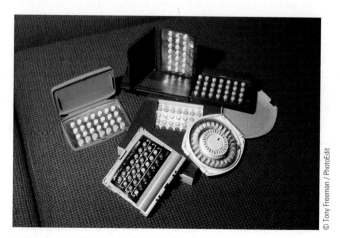

▲ *Oral contraceptives ("The Pill")*

© Tony Freeman / PhotoEdit

Some oral contraceptives are packaged with 28 tablets (21 pills are active and seven pills are inactive). The last seven tablets do not contain any hormones, although they may contain vitamins. The purpose of those tablets is to aid the woman in staying on schedule.

A major advantage of oral contraception is that it is highly effective in preventing ovulation. Also, the pill does not interfere with sexual activities. A major disadvantage is that it provides no protection against HIV and other pathogens that cause sexually transmitted diseases. Additional problems associated with the pill are *Candida* (yeast) infections, stomach cramping/bloating, weight gain, morning sickness (nausea), breakthrough bleeding between periods, irritability, headaches, vaginal discharge, acne, dark urine, and depression.

Women who smoke cigarettes should not take oral contraceptives. Women with any medical condition should discuss it with a health professional. The following medical conditions may prohibit use of oral contraceptives.

- Hypertension
- Stroke
- Diseases of the heart
- Gallbladder diseases
- Cancers of breast, cervix, vagina, and uterus
- Blood clots (history of blood clots in the leg)
- Severe headaches
- Diseases of the kidney and liver
- Family history of heart attack
- Diabetes
- Depression
- Epilepsy

Also, several medications may interfere with the effectiveness of oral contraceptives. These include various barbiturates (downers) and antibiotics. If a mother is nursing the baby, her gynecologist may recommend the progestin-only oral contraceptives (92% to 99.7% effective) since the estrogen in the "combination pill" decreases milk production.

## KEY TERMS

**Cervical cap** small rubber cap that fits firmly over the cervix and is used with a spermicide to prevent fertilization

**Vaginal sponge** foam sponge containing a spermicide, inserted in the vagina to prevent fertilization

**Spermicides** chemicals in the form of creams, foams, or jellies that are placed in the vagina and kill live sperm

**Oral contraceptives** hormonal tablets taken by women to prevent ovulation

## Tips for Action To Prevent Pregnancy

■ Do not get caught in the moment. The contraceptive technique "it won't happen to me this time" is not effective or reliable. The failure rate is 80% and often results in pregnancy.

■ Whether sexual intercourse is spontaneous ("it just happened") or planned in advance, the following basic precautions are important.

DO:

■ Prevent unintended pregnancy by using a reliable contraceptive at each act of intercourse and adhering to the manufacturer's directions for use.

DO NOT:

■ Use coitus interruptus. The partner who has no risk of pregnancy has little incentive to interrupt.

■ Use lotion, vaseline, or any other oil-based lubricant with a condom. These weaken the condom.

■ Use aerosol foam spermicides if coitus is to take place in a water environment (swimming pool or lake, bathtub, hot tub).

■ Douche after coitus.

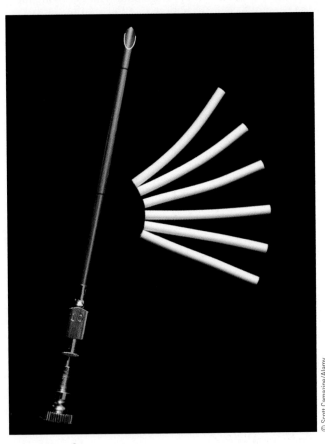

▲ *Norplant*®

**Implant (Progestin-Only Method).** Although **Norplant**® is no longer available, it is a contraceptive consisting of six flexible silicone tubes or capsules containing progestin. The capsules, each about the size of a matchstick, are inserted surgically just underneath the skin of the upper arm. Norplant is a long-lasting contraceptive that secretes progestin into the body slowly. While in place, it prevents pregnancy up to five years. If a woman

wishes to become pregnant, her health care provider can remove the capsules at any time. Women who are presently using Norplant may continue to do so.

## SURGICAL STERILIZATION

**Sterilization** is the most effective birth control method and should be considered permanent. It may be reversed in rare cases. A **vasectomy** (male sterilization) involves cutting and tying, or blocking off, the vas deferens (the two sperm-carrying ducts that transport the sperm from the testes to the ejaculatory ducts). Once the ducts have been blocked, sperm cannot get to the man's urethra. Figure 5.9 illustrates vasectomy. The surgical procedure lasts less than half an hour and is done on an outpatient basis. Occasionally, minor complications arise.

The male continues to produce sperm, which accumulate in the testicles and epididymis and are absorbed by body tissue. Immediately after surgery and for up to six to eight weeks, or until the man receives a negative semen analysis, the male is cautioned to use a reliable contraceptive when engaging in intercourse, to ensure protection in case viable sperm remain in the reproductive tract. As with any permanent procedure, males should think carefully about circumstances in which they may regret having had the vasectomy, such as divorce and remarriage with an accompanying desire for children.

**Tubal ligation** and Essure (female sterilization) involves the cutting and sealing of the fallopian tubes; **tubal occlusion** blocks the fallopian tubes. Figure 5.10 illustrates the cutting and tying method **(tubal ligation)**. A small incision is made near the navel with **laparotomy** and above the pubic hairline with **minilaparotomy.** A small, flexible telescope, a laparoscope, is inserted to locate the fallopian tubes. An instrument is threaded through the laparoscope to cut, tie, or block each tube commonly via electrical coagulation. This blocks the

**FIGURE 5.9 ▶** Surgical Sterilization of the Male (Vasectomy)

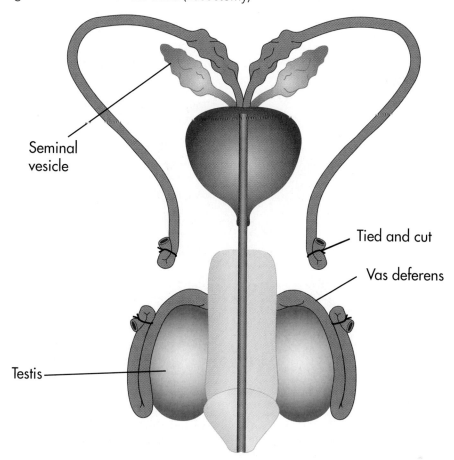

Seminal vesicle

Tied and cut

Vas deferens

Testis

sperm's passage to the egg. Tubal ligation is done with local anesthesia or general anesthesia. This surgery may be an outpatient procedure, or it may require hospitalization overnight or longer. A third procedure, the **colpotomy,** is done by going through the vagina and cervix. The colpotomy has a higher failure rate. **Essure** is a new sterilization procedure for women that is done when a physician goes through the vagina and places small microcoils into the fallopian tubes. These microcoils block the fallopian tube and prevent the sperm from reaching the egg (fertilization), granted the surgery was successful. A hysterosalpingogram (an x-ray) is used to check for complete blockage of the tubes. This method requires no anesthesia, no hospitalization, and approximately 24 hours of recovery. Other contraceptives must be used for at least three months after this procedure.

**Hysterectomy** usually is not done for contraceptive reasons. It is a major medical procedure to remove the uterus, which does render the female sterile, though the ovaries are left intact whenever possible. This surgery is performed on women who have serious gynecologic problems such as cancer, benign but harmful tumors, and severe menstrual problems.

### KEY TERMS

**Norplant®** long-lasting hormonal contraceptive implanted under the skin of upper arm by a health care practitioner to prevent ovulation

**Sterilization** surgical procedure that leaves a person infertile

**Vasectomy** male sterilization procedure in which vas deferens are cut and tied to block the transport of sperm

**Tubal ligation** female sterilization procedure in which the fallopian tubes are cut, sealed, or blocked to prevent sperm from reaching the ovary

**Tubal occlusion** a closing or shutting off of the fallopian tubes

**Laparotomy** female sterilization; a surgical procedure in which the fallopian tubes are cut or blocked

**Minilaparotomy** female sterilization; a procedure in which the fallopian tubes are cut or sealed

**Colpotomy** incision of the vagina with entry into the cul-de-sac

**Essure** permanent sterilization of the female

**Hysterectomy** total or partial surgical removal of the uterus

**FIGURE 5.10** ▶ Surgical Sterilization of the Female (Tubal Ligation)

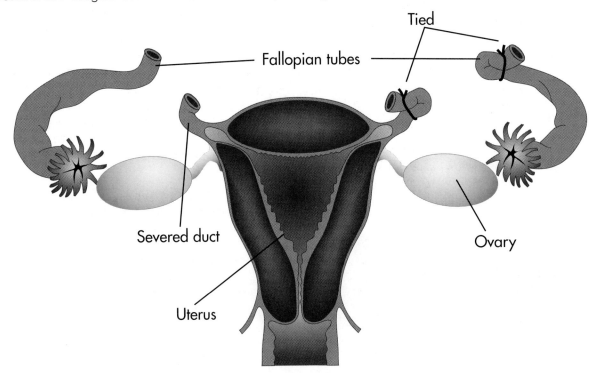

## FERTILITY AWARENESS-BASED METHODS (FAMS)

**Fertility Awareness-Based Methods (FAMs)**, sometimes called periodic abstinence and fertility awareness methods, are based on being aware of ovulation and fertility and avoiding coitus during the female's fertile period. None of the several FAM methods is reliable for women with unpredictable menstrual cycles and women whose pattern of intercourse is extremely spontaneous. These methods should not be used without extensive counseling from a gynecologist or family planning clinician.

The **calendar** or **rhythm method** requires the couple not to engage in sexual activity at the most fertile time of the menstrual cycle, ovulation. Two means have been developed to determine specifically when ovulation takes place: the basal body temperature (BBT) and cervical mucus methods.

**Basal Body Temperature.** The **basal body temperature method** is based on knowing that the female's body temperature drops slightly just prior to ovulation. Following ovulation, the temperature returns to normal. If a woman adheres to the instructions and learns her own pattern of temperature changes, she may be able to calculate her safe and unsafe times. Sometimes women who have infertility problems use BBT to try to become pregnant.

**Cervical Mucus Method.** The **cervical mucus method** also is known as the Billings method or ovulation method. A woman may be taught to detect changes in cervical mucus. Just prior to ovulation, cervical mucus increases and thickens, providing a fertile and safe environment for the viable sperm. Immediately following and prior to menstruation, the cervical mucus is dry. At

these times the woman is more likely to be infertile. When a woman uses this method along with BBT, it is called the sympto-thermal method.

**Standard Days Method (SDM).** A woman must keep a record of her menstrual cycle and refrain from unprotected intercourse on days eight through 19. This method can be used only if the woman has regular menstrual periods that are never shorter than 26 days and never longer than 32 days. Using a strand of colored beads, called Cyclebeads, each day the woman will move a marker ring one notch. When the ring sits on white beads (cycle days eight through 19) she is most likely to conceive and should refrain from sexual intercourse.

**Continuous Breast-Feeding-Lactational Amenorrhea Method (LAM).** The LAM is a form of fertility control that occurs when a woman aggressively breast-feeds (at least six times a day), which postpones ovulation for at least six months after a birth. When breast-feeding, the hormone prolactin (needed for milk production) is stimulated, thus inhibiting the release of gonadotrophin (hormone needed for ovulation). When ovulation does not occur, a woman cannot conceive.

## THE "EMERGENCY" CONTRACEPTION (EC)

EC or the "morning after" pill is an after-the-fact method. If a women thinks she may have become pregnant because of unprotected sex, EC can prevent fertilization and implantation. EC pills are taken up to 120 hours (and work best within the first 72 hours) after unprotected vaginal coitus. These pills may cause nausea, cramping, and vomiting and there should be a follow-up visit with the clinician within three weeks of use. EC reduces the risk of pregnancy by 75–89 percent when started within 72 hours. EC will not cause an abortion or affect an existing pregnancy. A woman should not use emergency contraception if she is pregnant.

In 1999, the Food and Drug Administration (FDA) approved the emergency contraceptive, Levonorgestral (Plan B) as safe and effective if taken within 72 hours of unprotected sex. Patients can either keep their prescription in-waiting or have the prescription filled and ready for use at their own discretion.

Be aware that despite a doctor's orders, a pharmacist can decide not to fill the prescription for Plan B based on his/her moral or religious beliefs. Alternative pharmacists (pharmacy) may have to be utilized in order to obtain the Plan B emergency method.

### Emergency IUD insertion.

The copper T 380 A IUD (Para Gard©) can be used for emergency contraception. A clinician must insert the IUD within five days of unprotected intercourse. Women at risk for sexually transmitted infections at the time of insertion or women who have been raped should not use the IUD for emergency contraception.

## TOTAL ABSTINENCE AND OUTERCOURSE

Total abstinence is a conscious personal decision to refrain from or postpone sexual intercourse. Among the reasons for this choice are moral and religious convictions, social maturity, awareness of the risks of contracting HIV/AIDS, HPV, and other STDs, and avoidance of pregnancy. For whatever reason, this is the most responsible choice. It demonstrates self-respect and respect for others. It enables young people to learn skills they need to evaluate and attain meaningful sexual relationships later on.

Outercourse is utilization of alternatives for sex play absent oral, vaginal, or anal intromission. Outercourse may include kissing, hugging, sexual body rubbing, utilization of sex toys, masturbatory activities, and baths/massages. If done safely, this technique prevents pregnancy, is effective against sexually transmitted infections, and could prolong virginity.

## COITUS INTERRUPTUS

In **coitus interruptus,** known commonly as withdrawal, the male removes his penis from the vagina just before ejaculation. This method, however, does not take into consideration that semen leaks from the penis prior to ejaculation and this fluid carries viable sperm. Thus, conception is possible even if the male does not ejaculate. Coitus interruptus is the oldest method of birth control and also is the least effective.

## ABORTION

Abortions are medical-surgical procedures. When they are performed under adequate medical conditions, they are considered generally safe. The earlier an induced abortion is done, the safer the procedure will be. Like any surgical procedure, however, abortions carry certain risks. Some

of the physical risks are bleeding, cramping, pain, and infection. Psychological consequences of considering and receiving abortions vary widely. Some women experience stress, guilt, remorse, fear, anger, and sadness.

Over 1.6 million abortions are done in the United States each year. The highest rates of abortion are with young, unmarried women who are less than 10 weeks pregnant. According to the National Abortion Federation, nearly 70% of the women who obtain abortions in the United States are Caucasians. African-American and Hispanic women, however, have high rates of abortions, as well as higher rates of childbirth.

**Legal Basis.** The 1973 *Roe v. Wade* Supreme Court case set specific standards to govern abortion decisions. It limited abortion as a pregnancy advanced past the first trimester.

In 1989 the Supreme Court handed down another abortion-related decision in *Webster v. Reproductive Health Services.* This decision did not overturn *Roe v. Wade,* as women still can abort within legal realms. Some restrictions remain, however. The Court forbade use of public facilities, resources, and personnel for abortion services, except in cases in which abortion is needed to save the woman's life, and required that doctors perform medical tests to determine the viability of the fetus whenever the doctor estimates the fetus is 20 weeks or older.

In June 1992, in *Planned Parenthood of Southeastern Pennsylvania v. Casey,* the Supreme Court continued to uphold the legal right to an abortion with advancing pregnancy limitations. But it gave a state more power to regulate abortions throughout the pregnancy, as long as the state does not place "undue burden" on the woman seeking an abortion. The most important restrictions in this case are the following:

1. A woman must receive information concerning embryo or fetal development and alternatives for aborting the pregnancy.

2. A woman must wait 24 hours after receiving information about fetal development and alternatives for ending pregnancy.

## KEY TERMS

**Fertility Awareness-Based Methods (FAMs)** any method of preventing pregnancy based on avoiding coitus during ovulation

**Calendar method** form of NFP that requires refraining from coitus during ovulation

**Basal body temperature (BBT) method** NFP method that uses a woman's temperature fluctuations to indicate when coitus is safe or unsafe

**Cervical mucus method** NFP that requires judging the thickness of cervical mucus to determine ovulation

**Coitus interruptus** withdrawal of the penis from the vagina before ejaculation

3. Minors must have written permission from parents or a judge.

4. Physicians are required to keep complete, detailed records that are subject to public disclosure.

**Two-Drug Abortion Method.** In September 1996, the Food and Drug Administration approved a Planned Parenthood study for the **two-drug induced abortion method.** In this method, a woman who is not more than seven weeks pregnant is injected with methotrexate, which stops the development of the embryo and placenta. Four to seven days after that, misoprostol tablets are inserted into the vagina, which cause the uterus to contract and expel the embryo and placenta.

Methotrexate and misoprostol have been approved by the FDA for some time. Methotrexate is used to treat cancer, arthritis, and psoriasis, and misoprostol is used to treat ulcers.

**Mifepristone.** Mifepristone (Mifeprex® and Early Option®), or **RU 486,** was approved by the Food and Drug Administration in September 2000. The abortion pill is an artificial steroid (menses inducer) that blocks absorption of the hormone progesterone. This prevents the lining of the uterus from supporting the developing embryo. It works only during the first nine weeks of pregnancy or up to 63 days from start of the last menstrual period. The entire medical procedure involves two or three visits to a physician. First the woman has a pregnancy test and pelvic examination. Then she takes three mifepristone tablets (600 milligrams) orally while in the physician's office. After 48 hours the woman visits the doctor again to receive a second drug, misoprostol (Cytotec). Misoprostol causes the uterus to contract and expel the embryo. This is accompanied by bleeding and mild to severe cramping for approximately five to six hours. About 2% of women using this method do not have to get the second drug because mifepristone alone causes the abortion. Seven to 14 days after the second visit, the physician checks to make sure the abortion is complete. (The manufacturer of Cytotec has warned doctors not to use this drug for abortions.)

As a sidelight, mifepristone seems to be a promising treatment for endometriosis, fibroid tumors of the uterus, glaucoma, and Cushing's syndrome, a disorder of the adrenal glands. It may be useful in treating cancers of breasts and ovaries, as well as meningioma, a type of brain tumor. It also is used as a morning-after contraceptive and to dilate the cervix.

**Vacuum Curettage or Aspiration.** **Vacuum curettage** or **aspiration** is the most commonly used method of abortion up to the 12th week of pregnancy. The cervix is dilated using **laminaria** (seaweed) or graduated dilators. The procedure utilizing laminaria is considered to be the gentlest. The laminaria absorbs the moisture from the cervix, which causes the cervical opening to expand.

Once the cervical opening is dilated enough (occasionally this can take up to 24 hours), a tube is inserted into the uterus. The tube is attached to a suction pump. This pump suctions the contents off the uterine wall—embryo or fetus, fetal tissue, and placenta or placental tissue. The procedure lasts approximately 10 to 20 minutes.

**Dilation and Curettage.** Through **dilation and curettage (D&C),** the embryo or fetus and placenta are removed from the uterus surgically. The woman's cervix is dilated, and a metal, spoon-shaped curette is used to scrape embryonic tissue off the wall. This procedure takes approximately 15 minutes and must be done by a qualified physician (obstetrician/gynecologist).

**Dilation and Evacuation.** The **dilation and evacuation (D&E)** abortion procedure is used between the 13th and the 15th weeks of pregnancy. Under local or general anesthesia the cervix is dilated and the fetus is removed with surgical instruments. An intravenous solution of oxytocin (a hormone) is given to encourage uterine contractions and limit loss of blood.

**Dilation and Extraction.** Dilation and extraction, so-called partial-birth abortion, is done during the late second and third trimester of pregnancy, when the fetus is almost fully delivered from the mother's birth canal. First the mother's cervix is dilated for three days. The physician turns the unborn baby into the breech position (feet first) and pulls the baby from the mother's uterus until all but the head is delivered. An opening is made at the base of the baby's skull and a large needle called a trocar is used to suction out the brain of the fetus before completing delivery.

**Prostaglandins.** **Prostaglandins** are naturally occurring substances in the body, or they may be refined chemicals. To induce abortion, prostaglandins are introduced into the amniotic sac via a needle inserted through the abdominal wall and uterus. This causes uterine contractions, which expel the embryo or fetus and placenta within 24 hours. This method is used between 16 and 20 weeks of pregnancy.

**Hysterotomy.** **Hysterotomy** is a major surgical procedure in which the fetus and afterbirth are removed from the uterus through the abdominal wall. It is done for abortion purposes on a limited basis during the second trimester of pregnancy.

# Reproduction

## THE MENSTRUAL CYCLE

A healthy female's reproductive organs begin to function at an average age of about 11 to 12 years. The trend has been toward earlier onset; age nine is no longer a rarity. The reproductive structures are intended to enlarge, mature, and become functional so the female can reproduce.

One of the first signs that these changes are occurring is the onset of the first **menstruation** or **menarche.**

During menstruation, the lining of the uterus or the endometrium is shed in the form of blood through the vagina. When a female menstruates, she is not pregnant and the reproductive organs are presumed to be working normally. If a female has not reached menarche by her 15th birthday, a gynecologist should be consulted to confirm that the reproductive system is developing normally.

The average length of each menstrual cycle is 28 to 32 days, although the cycle ranges from 21 to 42 days in the female population. (In many college-age women the menstrual cycle is irregular.) During this time several events are happening. Some can be seen; others are taking place behind the scene in the brain, the ovary, and the bloodstream. For the purpose of the discussion here, the length of this cycle will be considered to be 28 days, divided into four seven-day segments—menses, estrogenic, ovulation, and progestational, as illustrated in Figure 5.11.

During the first segment of the menstrual cycle, the menstrual period, the lining of the uterus is shed in the form of blood. The first day of bleeding marks the first day of the menstrual cycle and the menstrual period, which ranges from three to seven days. The endometrium is shed because hormone levels in the bloodstream have dropped. The hormone levels have dropped because implantation has not occurred.

At the end of the second seven-day segment of the menstrual cycle, another vital process—**ovulation**—occurs. It marks the middle of the 28-day menstrual cycle, occurring about the 14th day. The ovaries contain between 200,000 and 400,000 egg cells (ova), each housed in a tiny follicle. Upon chemical signals from the **pituitary gland** in the brain, **follicle-stimulating hormone (FSH)** and **luteinizing hormone (LH)** are activated. Usually only one egg cell matures and is released from the ovary during a menstrual cycle. The follicle secretes estrogen, which causes the pituitary to continue sending its signal of LH. The increase of LH and estrogen production causes the ovary to release from the activated follicle the egg cell or ovum that now is mature. The fimbriae of the fallopian tube or oviduct grab the egg and ferry it to the tube connected to the uterus. If no sperm are present, the egg degenerates after about 24 to 48 hours, and the menstrual cycle continues.

In the third seven-day segment of the menstrual cycle, the follicle from which ovulation originated becomes enlarged and is called the **corpus luteum,** Latin for "yellow body." This corpus luteum continues to make estrogen and secrete progesterone, another female hormone. Progesterone is the hormone that sustains the lining of the uterus in preparation for implantation of an anticipated fertilized ovum.

If the ovum does not implant, the fourth seven-day segment of the menstrual cycle ensues. In response to the high levels of estrogen and progesterone in the bloodstream, the pituitary gland stops producing FSH and LH. At this point the corpus luteum degenerates, estrogen and progesterone levels plummet, and the thickened layer of the endometrium is discharged through the vagina. The menstrual flow consists of blood, mucus, and endometrial tissue.

These four seven-day segments are supposed to occur in a continuous pattern. When the female menstruates again, this marks the first day of the next menstrual cycle. The process repeats itself until the female reaches menopause, which usually occurs between ages 35 and 55 or so. Menopause, the cessation of menstruation, is discussed in Chapter 14.

## CONCEPTION

When healthy spermatozoa are present in the fallopian tube at the time of ovulation, one of them may be successful in penetrating the egg cell and fertilizing it.

### KEY TERMS

**Two-drug induced abortion method** injection of methotrexate followed in several days by insertion of misoprostol into vagina to expel embryo

**RU 486** known as the abortion pill; mifepristone, a drug used to induce menstruation by preventing uterine lining from supporting embryo

**Vacuum curettage** or **aspiration** induced abortion procedure in which uterine contents are removed by suction

**Laminaria** wand made from dried seaweed used to expand the cervical opening as part of an abortion procedure

**Dilation and curettage (D&C)** surgical procedure that removes the embryo and placenta from the uterus by scraping

**Dilation and evacuation (D&E)** abortion procedure in which the cervix is dilated and the fetus removed by suction

**Prostaglandins** hormones that cause the uterus to contract; used to induce abortion

**Hysterotomy** surgical procedure in which the fetus and placenta are removed surgically through an abdominal incision

**Menstruation** monthly discharge of blood from the uterus through the vagina

**Menarche** the initial menstrual period

**Ovulation** release of a mature egg from the ovary in the middle of the menstrual cycle

**Pituitary gland** a pea-sized body in the brain, which releases hormones including follicle-stimulating hormone and luteinizing hormone

**Follicle-stimulating hormone (FSH)** a hormone that stimulates growth of the follicle in the ovary and spermatogenesis in the testes

**Luteinizing hormone (LH)** a hormone that stimulates ovulation in females and testosterone in males

**Corpus luteum** enlarged follicle that continues to secrete progesterone

**FIGURE 5.11 ▶** The Menstrual Cycle

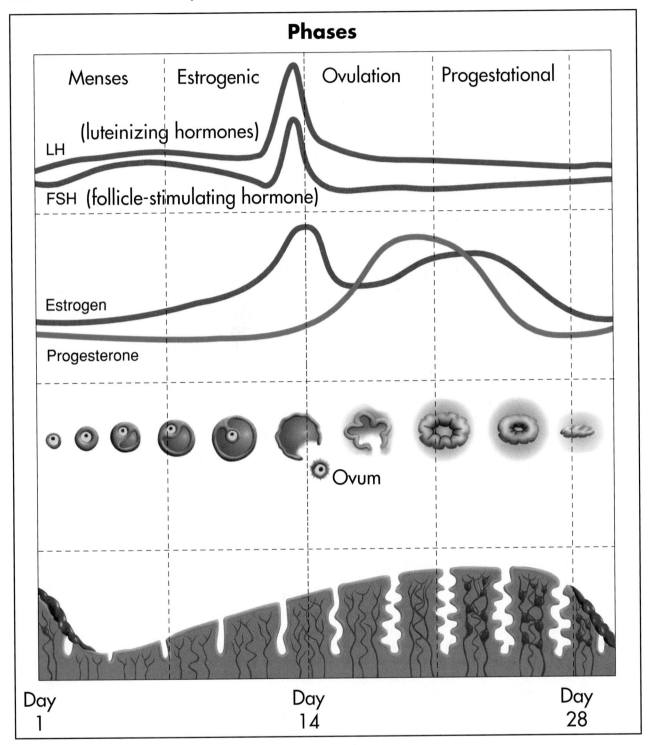

**Fertilization** normally takes place in the fallopian tube. The product is a **zygote.** This is the process of **conception.**

Usually one sperm and one egg unite to produce one baby. Two different scenarios, however, are possible.

1. A single fertilized egg divides into two cells that develop separately. Because the genetic material is the same, they are **identical twins.**

2. The woman's ovaries may produce two or more eggs upon ovulation. Each egg that is fertilized by a sperm cell will develop into a separate embryo—which eventually leads to the birth of twins, triplets, or more babies, termed a **multiple birth.** Twins who develop from this process are **fraternal twins.** They may be both boys, both girls, or one of each.

At fertilization the zygote moves in the fallopian tube toward the uterus. This journey takes about a week. Cell division and differentiation of the zygote occur during the trip. By the time this product of conception reaches the cavity of the uterus, it is referred to as an **embryo.** The embryo then sinks into the plush layer of the endometrial lining that has been prepared for it, called **implantation.** The implanted embryo continues to differentiate, and the developing placenta sends **human chorionic gonadotrophin (HCG)** through the mother's bloodstream to the pituitary gland, signaling it not to release FSH and LH. Thus, the hormones from the corpus luteum continue to secrete so the blood and mucous layer of the endometrium will remain intact to sustain the pregnancy.

## PREGNANCY

How does a woman know she is **pregnant?** Generally a woman experiences several symptoms that indicate life is growing inside her uterus. These signs vary from woman to woman. Some women claim they did not know they were pregnant until they went into labor. The first signs typically are

- Missed menstrual period
- Nausea and vomiting (morning sickness)
- Enlargement and tenderness of breasts and abdomen
- More frequent urination
- Sleepiness and fatigue
- Mood swings (resulting from hormonal changes)
- Increased secretions and discharge from vagina

A woman with any combination of these symptoms might suspect pregnancy. The usual course of action is to confirm these suspicions through a pregnancy test. The woman may have the test done at a health practitioner's office or may purchase one of the over-the-counter pregnancy test kits available at most pharmacies or retail outlets that sell feminine products. These tests all are designed to confirm the presence of the hormone HCG, which is in the urine and the bloodstream of the woman if she is pregnant. HCG can be detected in the blood before it is detectable in the urine. Following the manufacturer's instructions will reduce the chances of false positive or false negative results. The more definite signs of pregnancy begin to appear in the second trimester of pregnancy. When they do, there is no doubt that the woman has a fetus in her uterus. Confirmation is by

1. Fetal movement
2. Fetal heart sounds
3. Discovery of fetus by ultrasound or x-ray

Because radiation can damage the fetus, a pregnant woman should avoid x-rays and notify any health practitioner of her suspected or confirmed pregnancy if she is scheduled to be exposed to radioactive materials.

### FYI | HOME PREGNANCY TESTS

Over-the-counter pregnancy test kits have brought the diagnosis of a pregnancy from the doctor's office to the home. These tests are popular because they are relatively inexpensive, easy to use, and fairly reliable. Testing is not recommended until the first day of an expected period, primarily because testing too early can produce a false negative (an indication of no pregnancy when the woman is pregnant). Also, many pregnancies end in miscarriage early on. Because the hormonal levels take some time to revert, the result in this case could be a false positive (an indication of pregnancy when the woman no longer is pregnant). False negatives also may turn up if the urine collected has been sitting too long (usually a half hour or more) before the testing is done. Rarely, drinking considerable amounts of liquid shortly before testing can dilute the urine volume too much to measure.

Even though testing after the first day of a missed period is 98% accurate, the woman should see a physician for confirmation and continuing prenatal care. For example, the amount of human chorionic gonadotrophin the woman is producing should double every two days in normal fetal development, and the medical professional will want to monitor this.

*Source: "Polycystic Ovary Syndrome," Harvard Women's Health Watch,* November 1996, pp. 2–3.

## KEY TERMS

**Fertilization** union of egg and sperm cells; conception

**Zygote** fertilized egg

**Conception** the start of pregnancy, when a sperm cell fertilizes an egg cell

**Identical twins** two babies conceived at the same time as the result of a single fertilized egg that divides into two cells that develop separately

**Multiple birth** birth of twins, triplets, or more babies

**Fraternal twins** two babies conceived about the same time as the result of fertilization of two separate egg cells.

**Embryo** product of conception from weeks two through seven

**Implantation** attachment of embryo to lining of the uterus

**Human chorionic gonadotrophin (HCG)** a hormone produced by the placenta that signals the pituitary gland is not to release FSH and LH

**Pregnant** having a developing embryo or fetus in the uterus

## USE OF ANTIDEPRESSANT MEDICATION (SSRIs) DURING PREGNANCY

Approximately 10% to 20% of women experience depression during pregnancy. Depresssion during pregnancy has been linked to health problems in the mother and baby, to include preeclampsia, premature birth, low birthweight, and post-partum depression. In a study published in the *Archives of Women's Mental Health*, approximately 75% of the women who discontinued the use of their antidepressant prior to conception or during the first trimester relapsed into depression. A study published in the *Journal of the American Medical Asssociation (JAMA)* reported that of the 200 women who were taking antidepressants before pregnancies, 68% relapsed when they stopped taking their medicine after they became pregnant. In 2005, the Food and Drug Administration (FDA) issued a warning that the selected serotonin reuptake inhibitor (SSRI) antidepressant brand Paxil may cause fetal heart defects. So what should a pregnant woman do if she has a depressive disorder? It is

imperative that she discuss, early in pregnancy, alternatives to stopping the medication with her health care providers. These may include tapering the SSRI during the last trimester and using the lowest effective dose of the SSRI.

## PRENATAL CARE

Regular medical visits should be scheduled as soon as the pregnancy is confirmed. This scheduled maintenance of the woman and the expected baby is vital to their health. During these regular medical examinations the health of the mother and fetus is monitored. If any problems arise, they can be taken care of before they become serious and threaten the life of the mother, the survival of the fetus, or the health of the baby after delivery.

The National Center for Health Statistics in 1992 surveyed medical risk factors by race of the mother and found that major risks were higher for Native American women than for any other racial or ethnic group. For example, their incidence of pregnancy-related hypertension was four times as high as that for Chinese mothers (the lowest-incidence group for hypertension).

In prenatal care the mother receives periodic physical examinations, including blood and urine tests, to monitor her health status and development of the fetus. She also receives instructions and advice about nutrition and weight, exercise, and medications to enhance the chances of delivering a healthy baby. Nutrition is particularly important for both the mother and the developing fetus. For example, if the mother's diet is low in iron or calcium, the fetus takes most of it, resulting in a deficiency in the mother. The old axiom "You are eating for two" should not imply that the woman should eat twice as much. She instead has to make sure that her diet contains all the nutrients needed for both. Needs for protein, calcium, vitamins A, B, C, D, and E, iodine, iron, magnesium, and zinc increase as the fetus develops. Intake of folic acid should be doubled during pregnancy. A sensible, well-rounded diet for pregnant women will provide these nutrients, with the possible exception of iron, which often is prescribed to be taken orally.

Of the various health practitioners that provide prenatal care, foremost is the **obstetrician.** The **certified nurse-midwife** also has credentials to deliver prenatal care. The nurse-midwife can administer medication and deliver prenatal care for uncomplicated pregnancies. If medical problems arise during the pregnancy, the nurse-midwife has been educated to identify them and turn over the care of the patient to an obstetrician.

Childbirth classes are offered in most communities. Prospective mothers and fathers attend sessions to prepare these soon-to-be parents, training them in what to expect, how to ease the mother's pain, and how to facilitate the birth process. The mother practices a variety of techniques while the father coaches and serves as a support person, helping her breathe and relax.

**VIEWPOINT** *A doula is a woman experienced in childbirth who is trained and certified by a childbirth education organization, such as Doulas of North America, Birthworks, or the International Childbirth Education Association. Her function and focus is to provide continuous emotional support to the mother during labor and delivery and to manage the mother's pain without drugs. Research on doula support during labor conducted by Dr. John Kennell and his associates at Case Western Reserve University School of Medicine shows that continuous doula support decreased the need for epidurals, shortened labor, and reduced complications. Other benefits of doula-supported labor and delivery are reduction of stress and anxiety of the mother (mothers report a more positive labor and delivery experience); reduced need for forceps or cesarean section (C-section) in delivery; and mothers who are more likely to say "pass" when offered an epidural.*

*Health insurance in most states does not pay for a doula even though the medical benefits associated with doula-supported birth are documented. Fees for doulas range from $300 to $1,500. Certainly the cost of an epidural and a C-section, not to mention the risks of medical complications, would merit the use of a doula, when possible, as a cost-saving mechanism.*

*Considering the benefits to the mother, the baby, and even the insurance provider, should health insurance pay for doula-supported childbirth?*

Prospective parents should recognize the effects on the fetus's health of smoking, drinking alcohol, and taking other drugs. Table 5.5 contains a summary of the possible effects on the fetus of the mother's use of tobacco, alcohol, and other drugs during pregnancy.

## FETAL TESTS

Various tests can be done during gestation to gain information about the fetus.

1. **Ultrasound.** This technological device creates a **sonogram** of the fetus, showing the position, size, gestational age, and possible anatomic problems. Sonograms sometimes can reveal the sex of the fetus.

2. **Alpha-fetoprotein (AFP) screening.** High levels of AFP may indicate neural tube defects such as anencephaly (part or all of the brain is missing) and spina bifida. Low levels of AFP may indicate a chromosomal defect such as Down syndrome. This test usually is done between 15 and 20 weeks into the pregnancy.

3. **Amniocentesis.** Genetic analysis of the fetal cells in the fluid taken from the amniotic sac can reveal pos-

sible birth defects and sex of the fetus. It usually is done about 16 weeks into gestation.

4. **Chorionic villus sampling (CVS).** This more recent alternative to amniocentesis analyzes a tiny piece of chorionic villi containing fetal cells. CVS can be performed between the 9th and 11th weeks of pregnancy.

## GESTATION

Figure 5.12 traces fetal development. This period of **gestation** may be divided into **trimesters.** A full-term pregnancy has three trimesters.

**First Trimester (one to three months).** After fertilization, the egg divides in half within about 30 hours, the first of many divisions. On about the fourth day the cluster of cells reaches the uterus, and on the sixth or seventh day it is attached to the lining of the uterus. Just one week after conception the little mass of cells is considered an embryo. Between the second and ninth weeks all the major body structures are formed, and some—the heart, liver, testes—begin to function. This is a particularly vulnerable time for damage if the mother has an infection or uses drugs (discussed in Chapters 12 and 13). By the end of the second month, the embryo is considered a fetus and at the end of the first trimester is about four inches long and weighs about an ounce.

The three structures that are vital to survival of the fetus are the placenta (afterbirth), the amniotic sac, and

**TABLE 5.5 ▶** Effects of Tobacco, Alcohol, and Other Drugs on Fetus

| SUBSTANCE | POSSIBLE EFFECTS |
|---|---|
| Tobacco | Separation of placenta<br>Spontaneous abortion<br>Brain damage from reduced oxygen<br>Abnormal breathing<br>Sudden infant death syndrome<br>Ear, nose, and throat infections<br>Bronchitis<br>Pneumonia<br>Asthmatic attacks<br>Decreased lung efficiency |
| Alcohol | Miscarriage<br>Low birthweight<br>Contaminated breast milk<br>Fetal alcohol syndrome<br>Growth retardation<br>Facial abnormalities<br>Brain damage<br>Heart defects<br>Poor muscle coordination<br>Hearing impairment<br>Developmental delay (motor, social, language) |
| Other drugs (cocaine, heroin) | Separation of placenta<br>Spontaneous abortion<br>Low birthweight<br>Brain damage<br>Learning disabilities<br>Short attention span<br>Severe behavioral problems<br>Sudden infant death syndrome<br>Neonatal abstinence syndrome |

## KEY TERMS

**Obstetrician** physician who specializes in the care of women during pregnancy, delivery, and the period immediately following birth

**Certified nurse-midwife** registered nurse who is certified to care for women during pregnancy and delivery

**Ultrasound** a technology using high-frequency soundwaves to produce visual image of developing fetus

**Sonogram** visual image of developing fetus in uterus

**Alpha-fetoprotein (AFP) screening** a fetal testing procedure that analyzes AFP levels in a blood sample taken from the mother

**Amniocentesis** a fetal test in which fluid is removed from uterus through a long, thin needle inserted into abdominal wall and uterus into amniotic sac

**Chorionic villus sampling (CVS)** a fetal test of a tiny piece of chorionic villi containing fetal cells, removed from the cervix through a catheter

**Gestation** period from conception to birth (259–287 days)

**Trimester** a three-month period of pregnancy

▶ *Ultrasound testing can determine position of the baby, any abnormalities, and often the sex*

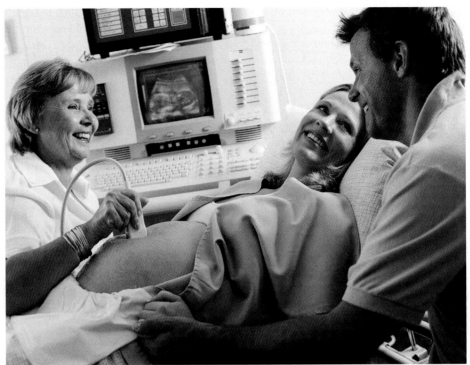

© BananaStock/Jupiterimages

the umbilical cord (navel cord). These structures must develop at the beginning of the first trimester.

1. The **placenta** is a structure about eight inches in diameter, attached directly to the endometrium. Through this structure nutrients, gases, and waste materials are exchanged from mother to fetus and fetus to mother. After delivery, the placenta is no longer necessary for the fetus to survive and, therefore, it is expelled. Its other name, afterbirth, is appropriate.

2. The **amniotic sac (amnion)** is filled with amniotic fluid and serves as a climate-controlled environment for the developing fetus. It cushions the fetus, protecting it from external bumps and jars. Cells that have sloughed from the skin of the fetus float in this amniotic fluid. To prevent the fetus from becoming waterlogged, mucus plugs the nose and throat, and the skin is covered by **vernix.**

3. The **umbilical cord** floats freely in the amniotic sac. One end of the umbilical cord is attached to the placenta and the other to the fetus's abdomen. Materials from the placenta pass back and forth through the cord from the mother to the developing fetus. After the child is born, the umbilical cord is tied, severed, and discarded along with the placenta, to which most of it still is attached.

**Second Trimester (four to six months).** At the beginning of the second trimester, the mother's abdomen is distended. She starts to show. Usually she can feel the fetus's movements between the 16th and 18th weeks. The fetus's hair is starting to appear, along with eyelashes and eyebrows, and the eyes are open. The fetus makes sucking movements. During this period of major growth, the fetus must receive adequate food, oxygen, and water through the placenta.

**Third Trimester (seven to nine months).** The fetus gains the most weight during the last three months, and in rare cases fetuses born at the beginning of this trimester have survived. By the 34th week the fetus probably can survive outside the uterus with proper care. The fetus's food intake must include calcium, iron, and nitrogen, derived from the food the mother eats. Mainly, the fetus is acquiring a fat layer and refining the respiratory and digestive organs, as well as gaining immunity from certain communicable diseases for a period after birth.

**Changes in the Mother's Body.** Figure 5.13 illustrates the changes that transform the mother's body during pregnancy. These can be summarized as

- Enlarged pituitary gland because of increased hormonal secretions
- Possible patches of pigmentation on the face
- Enlarged thyroid gland
- Slightly enlarged heart
- Raised diaphragm to allow the developing fetus more room
- Enlarged breasts and pigmented streaks on breast; darkened areola and enlarged nipples
- Enlarged cortex of adrenal glands

**FIGURE 5.12** ► Prenatal Development of the Fetus

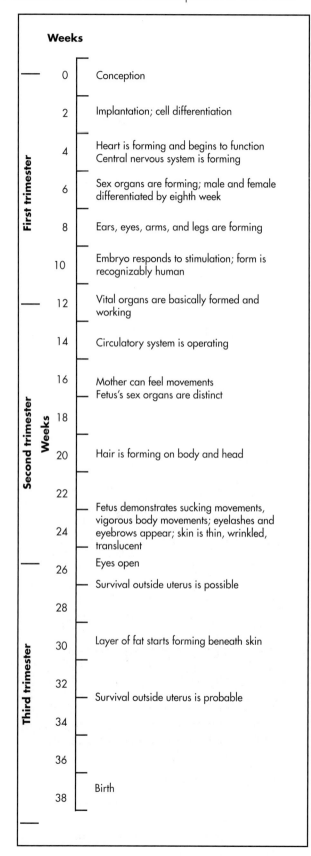

| Weeks | |
|---|---|
| 0 | Conception |
| 2 | Implantation; cell differentiation |
| 4 | Heart is forming and begins to function<br>Central nervous system is forming |
| 6 | Sex organs are forming; male and female differentiated by eighth week |
| 8 | Ears, eyes, arms, and legs are forming |
| 10 | Embryo responds to stimulation; form is recognizably human |
| 12 | Vital organs are basically formed and working |
| 14 | Circulatory system is operating |
| 16 | Mother can feel movements<br>Fetus's sex organs are distinct |
| 18 | |
| 20 | Hair is forming on body and head |
| 22 | |
| 24 | Fetus demonstrates sucking movements, vigorous body movements; eyelashes and eyebrows appear; skin is thin, wrinkled, translucent |
| 26 | Eyes open<br>Survival outside uterus is possible |
| 28 | |
| 30 | Layer of fat starts forming beneath skin |
| 32 | |
| 34 | Survival outside uterus is probable |
| 36 | |
| 38 | Birth |

First trimester (weeks 0–12), Second trimester (weeks 12–26), Third trimester (weeks 26–38)

- Stretch marks on abdomen and breasts
- Vertical brown line down the center of abdomen
- Uterus enlarged to 50–60 times its original size

Throughout pregnancy **Braxton-Hicks contractions** may occur. At the end of pregnancy, these may be confused with labor pains.

## BIRTH

Live birth, **parturition,** is accomplished through the process of **labor.** No matter how long it takes, labor is divided into three stages: dilation, delivery of the fetus, and delivery of the placenta (see Figure 5.14).

General anesthesia, once the norm, now is used rarely during childbirth. It slows contractions, causes sluggishness, and may precipitate respiratory problems in the baby. The common forms of anesthesia used today are as follows.

1. **Pudendal block.** A local anesthetic is injected through the wall of the vagina or the skin of the buttock to desensitize the pudendal nerve.

2. **Paracervical block.** A local anesthetic is injected around the opening of the uterus.

3. **Spinal anesthesia.** A solution containing a local anesthetic is injected into the fluid-filled sac surrounding the spinal cord. This blocks pain from below the waist.

4. **Epidural anesthesia.** The anesthetic is injected at the same place as the spinal anesthetic, but, instead

## KEY TERMS

**Placenta** organ through which fetus receives nourishment and empties waste via mother's circulatory system; the afterbirth

**Amniotic sac (amnion)** tough, transparent fluid-filled membrane that surrounds the fetus like a balloon

**Vernix** waxy, protective substance covering the fetus in the uterus

**Umbilical cord** attachment of tissue containing blood vessels connecting the fetus to the placenta, through which fetus receives nourishment

**Braxton-Hicks contractions** normal uterine contractions that occur periodically throughout pregnancy

**Parturition** live birth at end of pregnancy

**Labor** regular contraction of the uterus and dilation of cervix to expel the fetus

**Pudendal block** a local anesthetic that eliminates feeling from the lower vagina

**Paracervical block** local anesthetic injected around opening of the uterus to eliminate pain and feeling from lower vagina

**Spinal anesthesia** anesthetic to block pain, injected between fourth and fifth vertebrae of lower back

**FIGURE 5.13** ► Changes in Mother's Body During Pregnancy

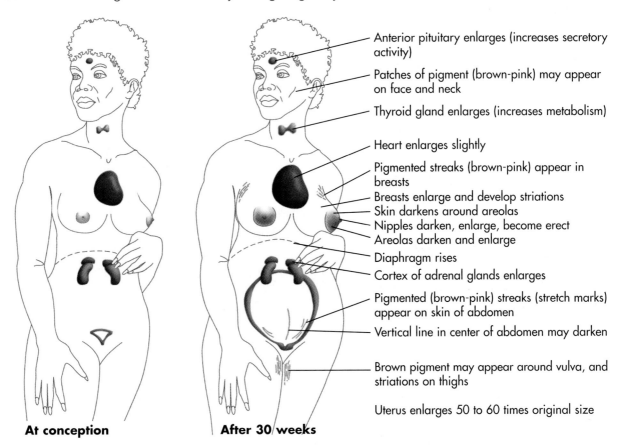

Anterior pituitary enlarges (increases secretory activity)

Patches of pigment (brown-pink) may appear on face and neck

Thyroid gland enlarges (increases metabolism)

Heart enlarges slightly

Pigmented streaks (brown-pink) appear in breasts

Breasts enlarge and develop striations

Skin darkens around areolas

Nipples darken, enlarge, become erect

Areolas darken and enlarge

Diaphragm rises

Cortex of adrenal glands enlarges

Pigmented (brown-pink) streaks (stretch marks) appear on skin of abdomen

Vertical line in center of abdomen may darken

Brown pigment may appear around vulva, and striations on thighs

Uterus enlarges 50 to 60 times original size

**At conception**         **After 30 weeks**

of a single injection, it is administered over a period of hours through a tiny plastic tube. Approximately 60% of women choose the epidural anesthetic to relieve or block pain during labor. The low dose administered today reduces the pain but does not hinder the mother from pushing during her contractions.

5. **Caudal anesthesia.** This method is the same as the epidural except that the tube is inserted at the tip of the spine.

Both caudal and epidural anesthesia can slow labor if administered too soon. Therefore, they are not given until the woman is in active labor.

Requests by women for regional anesthesia, especially epidural blocks, during labor and delivery have risen dramatically since the 1970s, when natural childbirth was in vogue. As reported in the July 1997 issue of *Anesthesiology*, both the American Society of Anesthesiologists and the American College of Obstetricians and Gynecologists endorse epidural and other forms of regional anesthesia because they allow the mother to remain alert and participate in the labor with less pain.

**Dilation.** The first stage of labor normally is the longest. During **dilation,** or **dilatation,** the uterus is contracting

and the opening to the cervix of the uterus also is getting wider to allow the fetus to emerge. The cervix has to dilate (open) 10 centimeters, or about 4 inches, while becoming thinner (**effacement**) for the fetus to pass through. The transition phase of this first stage of labor is most painful, and the mother may be nauseated and vomit. During transition the cervix dilates most rapidly, from about 7 centimeters until it reaches complete dilation.

Another event that may take place during the first stage of labor is a discharge from the widened cervix of a mucous plug or "bloody show" that serves as a stopper. This plug was held in place by the undilated cervix. In most women the amniotic sac or "bag of waters" ruptures during this stage of labor. Some first-time mothers mistake this liquid for urine. If the rupture occurs too soon before labor begins, the fetus is exposed to microorganisms in the vagina that may cause an infection.

**Delivery of the Fetus.** When the cervix is fully dilated, the fetus moves from the uterus into the vagina, which now serves as the birth canal. Upon **crowning,** some physicians perform an **episiotomy.** Other medical professionals believe this procedure need not be standard for every delivery. Before the delivery the woman should discuss with her physician the need for an episiotomy.

**FIGURE 5.14 ▶** Stages of Delivery

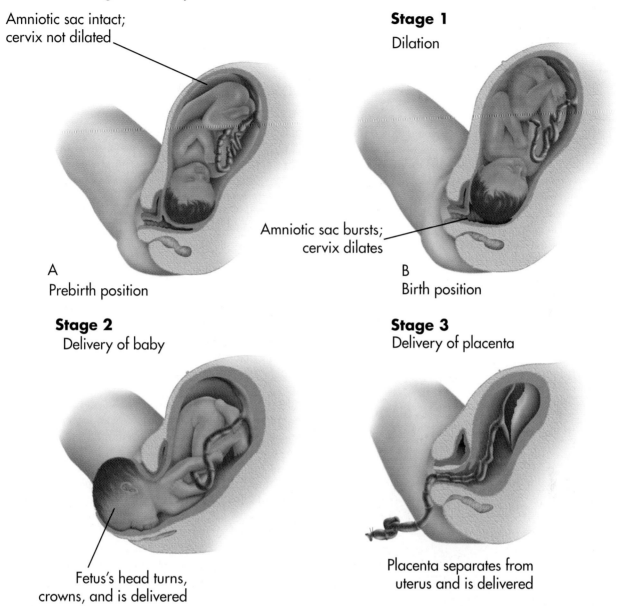

Amniotic sac intact;
cervix not dilated

**Stage 1**
Dilation

Amniotic sac bursts;
cervix dilates

A
Prebirth position

B
Birth position

**Stage 2**
Delivery of baby

**Stage 3**
Delivery of placenta

Fetus's head turns,
crowns, and is delivered

Placenta separates from
uterus and is delivered

During the second stage of labor, muscular contractions of the uterus should continue at regular intervals, and the mother is asked to push with each contraction. Strong contractions force the baby to be delivered, usually headfirst. After the head emerges, the baby's body rotates, and a continuing wave of strong contractions allows the shoulders and upper body to emerge. Additional contractions deliver the legs and feet. When the baby is out of the vagina, the mother's contractions subside for several minutes. During this time the umbilical cord is tied and cut.

The baby is wet and covered with vernix. The head usually is misshapen because of the narrow passageway it has traversed. The bones are flexible enough at this time to resume a normal appearance within a day or so. The birth process squeezes air out of the baby's lungs, but

**KEY TERMS**

**Epidural anesthesia** spinal anesthesia administered over a period of hours to desensitize lower back

**Caudal anesthesia** anesthetic injected through a tiny tube into the tip of the spine to dull sensation

**Dilation** or **dilatation** opening of the cervix to 10 centimeters; occurs during first stage of labor

**Effacement** thinning of cervix during the first stage of labor

**Crowning** the top of the fetus's head appearing at the vaginal opening during labor

**Episiotomy** procedure in which an incision is made from the bottom of the vaginal opening toward the anus to prevent tearing of vagina during birth

once the baby is born, the chest can expand and fill with air for the first time. The baby often announces this event by crying loudly. Between one and five minutes after birth, the baby's condition is assessed for heart rate, respiration, color, reflexes, and muscle tone. The resulting **Apgar score** provides a quick indication as to the infant's physical status.

**Delivery of the Placenta.** Following birth, the fetal materials left behind are no longer needed by either the baby or the mother. Contractions of the uterus are necessary to dislodge the placenta from the uterus. As it separates or peels itself from the uterus where it was attached, contractions push it and the umbilical cord attached to it out of the vagina. When this occurs, the third, and final, stage of labor is complete.

The uterus must stay contracted after the third stage of labor to prevent **hemorrhage.** This can be accomplished by massaging the mother's abdomen after delivery of the placenta. A natural way to stimulate uterine contractions is to allow the newborn to suckle. Either method encourages the uterus to contract and become firm so the

mother will not have complications from excessive bleeding after delivery. Failure of the placenta to be expelled completely can cause the mother to hemorrhage. Therefore, the delivered placenta is inspected carefully. If any piece from it is left behind, it has to be removed.

## POSTPARTUM PERIOD

The **postpartum** period may be difficult, physically and psychologically, for the mother. The uterus continues to contract for several days after the birth as it returns to its normal size. The woman's reproductive system requires about six to eight weeks to assume its prebirth condition. A bloody **lochia** may last several weeks after the birth. The psychological adjustment is more difficult to define, and it is specific to each woman and her circumstances. Nevertheless, it is real and merits attention.

Most mothers are overjoyed at the birth of their baby, but they may be overwhelmed with adapting to motherhood and the responsibilities of a new baby. About 80% of these new mothers experience the "baby blues" or a temporary period of sadness and crying for about 10 days after delivery. However, about 5% to 20% of mothers become depressed. This condition is called **postpartum depression (PPD)** and usually occurs within six months after giving birth. Postpartum depression is characterized by the symptoms of persistent feelings of anxiety, lack of motivation, problems with appetite and sleep, and, sometimes, thoughts of harming oneself or the baby. A far more severe form of this depression is termed postpartum psychosis (occurs in about 0.2% of women), which is characterized by hallucinations, delusions, thoughts of suicide or homicide. Postpartum depression is a medical condition that is treatable. If a new mother experiences persistent depression, medical attention should be sought immediately.

**Lactation** begins about three days following childbirth. Before that the breasts secrete **colostrum,** which contains antibodies that help the newborn ward off infectious diseases; it also is a source of protein. Breastfeeding is recommended over bottle feeding nowadays because breast milk is most suited to the baby's nutritional and digestive needs. Breastfeeding also stimulates contractions that help the uterus return to normal and may contribute to weight loss after pregnancy.

## COMPLICATIONS OF PREGNANCY AND BIRTH

Although most pregnancies are normal and progress to full term and delivery, complications can develop at any time (see Figure 5.15). Some of the problems are Rh incompatibility, eclampsia, heart problems, gestational diabetes, German measles, toxoplasmosis, sexually transmitted disease, ectopic pregnancy, spontaneous abortion, breech presentation, and cesarean section.

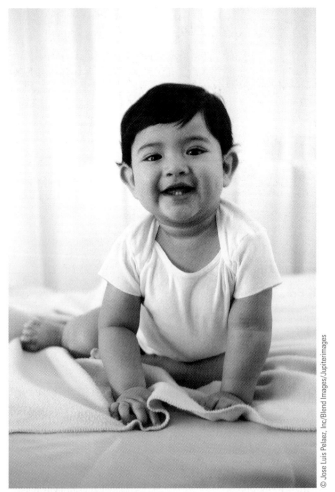

© Jose Luis Pelaez, Inc/Blend Images/Jupiterimages

▲ *A mother's proper self-care will help promote a healthy baby*

**FIGURE 5.15 ▶** Ten Leading Causes of Infant Mortality in the United States, 2002

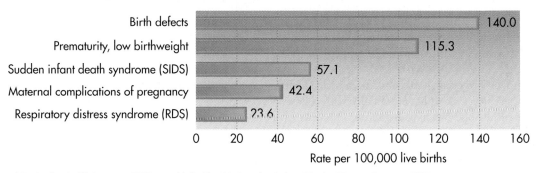

*Source:* National Centre for Health Statistics, 2002 period linked birth/infant death data, March of Dimes, Peristats, 2006.

**Rh Incompatibility.** Among the traits inherited from the mother and father is blood type, as well as the presence or absence of the rhesus factor, or **Rh factor.** About 85% of the population has inherited this chemical, and these individuals are designated Rh+. The remaining 15%, who do not have this chemical, are designated Rh–. If the mother is Rh– and the fetus she carries is Rh+, a problem could develop. Even though the circulatory systems of the mother and fetus are separate, small amounts of blood from the fetus may leak into the mother's circulatory system during the third trimester. The Rh– mother does not have this chemical, so her body responds by producing antibodies to protect her from the Rh+ chemical invasion. These antibodies, which protect the mother, pass through the placenta to her fetus. What protects the mother now becomes a health hazard to the fetus. The antibodies can destroy the fetus's red blood cells, causing jaundice, severe anemia, and other complications, which may lead to death of the fetus.

The Rh factor usually is not a problem in a first pregnancy because the mother does not produce enough antibodies to harm the fetus. If a subsequent fetus is Rh+, however, the mother's system is alerted to invading chemicals and quickly activates the antibodies, which can pose a serious threat to the health of the new fetus. Today, complications of Rh incompatibility are largely preventable. A dose of **RhoGAM** is administered to the Rh– mother between weeks 28 and 32 of pregnancy. Another dose is given within 72 hours after delivery. This vaccine eliminates any Rh+ chemical of the fetus from maternal circulation before the mother becomes sensitized and makes Rh+ antibodies that would harm the fetus.

**Eclampsia.** **Eclampsia** can result during the last trimester of pregnancy for unknown reasons. The first indicators, termed preeclampsia, are elevated blood pressure, sudden weight gain, protein in the urine, and edema (swelling from water retention), especially in the face, hands, and feet. About 5% of expectant mothers get preeclampsia during their first pregnancy, and 2% during later pregnancies. If uncontrolled, this condition may become more serious and progress to eclampsia. In eclampsia, convulsions accompany the symptoms of preeclampsia.

Risks to the pregnant woman include cerebral hemorrhage (burst blood vessel in the brain), damage to the liver or kidneys, and possible death. In addition, the risk to the fetus is premature labor and delivery. Women at greatest risk for developing preeclampsia are

- Teens
- Women over 35 years old
- Women with blood relatives who had the condition
- Women with inadequate nutrition (malnourished)
- Women who were hypertensive before pregnancy

Preeclampsia usually is treated by adjusting the diet. African-American women are at greater risk than others for this complication of pregnancy.

### KEY TERMS

**Apgar score** an evaluation of baby's health at birth based on heart rate, respiration, color, reflexes, and muscle tone; maximum score is 10

**Hemorrhage** excessive blood loss

**Postpartum** the first three months after childbirth

**Lochia** discharge of blood and mucus after childbirth

**Postpartum depression (PPD)** a psychiatric disorder consisting of severe depression that can affect a woman soon after giving birth

**Lactation** milk secretion from the breasts

**Colostrum** yellowish liquid secreted from the breasts preceding lactation; contains antibodies and protein

**Rh factor** chemical in bloodstream of most people that can cause complications during pregnancy when a mother who is Rh– (no Rh chemical) carries an Rh+ fetus

**RhoGAM** vaccine administered to counteract complications of Rh incompatibility

**Eclampsia** coma and seizures that may occur beginning about the 20th week of pregnancy associated with high blood pressure during pregnancy

**Complications from Maternal Heart Disease.** If a woman has a known heart condition before pregnancy, both mother and baby are at higher risk. Diet becomes particularly important, as well as not smoking or drinking alcohol. Any medications should be approved by a physician.

A woman who has congenital (present at birth) heart disease has a greater risk of having a baby with a heart defect. A fetal ultrasound test may detect this abnormality.

**Gestational Diabetes or Pregnancy-Induced Diabetes.** **Gestational diabetes** is diagnosed in about 3% to 5% of pregnant women in the United States. It differs from the other forms (discussed in Chapter 7) because it begins during pregnancy and disappears after delivery. Risk factors for gestational diabetes are

- Obesity
- Family history of diabetes
- Previous birth of a large baby, a stillbirth, or a child with a birth defect
- Excess amniotic fluid
- Women 25 to 30 years

A major problem affects the baby through an abnormality known as **macrosomia.** The fetus converts the extra glucose received from the mother. The resulting high blood glucose and high insulin levels result in large deposits of fat in the fetus. Sometimes the baby grows too large to be delivered vaginally and a cesarean section becomes necessary.

In addition, gestational diabetes increases the risk of hypoglycemia (low blood sugar) in the fetus immediately after delivery, when the body no longer receives sugar from the mother but retains the high insulin level. Other complications include congenital defects and stillbirth. African-American diabetic women, for some reason, are more likely than other diabetic women to lose their babies during and after birth.

The Council on Diabetes in Pregnancy of the American Diabetes Foundation strongly recommends that all pregnant women be screened for gestational diabetes (between the 24th and 28th week of pregnancy). The most common of the several tests is the 50-gram glucose test. Complications of gestational diabetes are manageable and preventable. The key is to control blood sugar through a diet prescribed by a qualified practitioner. The woman should use salt in moderation, cut down on caffeine intake, avoid sugars and fats in the diet, and emphasize complex carbohydrates, dietary fibers, iron, calcium, and protein. She also should avoid smoking and drinking alcohol.

**German Measles.** **German measles,** officially termed **rubella,** formerly was a common concern during pregnancy. Immunization at least three months prior to pregnancy can rule out this disease as a risk factor to the baby (it is relatively innocuous in adults). If a pregnant women has rubella during the first three months of pregnancy, the fetus has a 20% to 30% risk of damage to the eyes, ears, brain, or heart. This virus also can cause spontaneous abortion, low birthweight (LBW), or stillbirth. The best course of action is to become immunized before contemplating pregnancy.

**Toxoplasmosis.** **Toxoplasmosis** is caused by an organism that lives in the intestines of many mammals and birds. This disease tends to be mild in adults, but if a pregnant woman transmits the organism to her fetus, it may produce blindness or mental retardation. Precautions are simple: Thoroughly cook all meat, and wash your hands after handling pets and a cat's litter box.

**Sexually Transmitted Diseases.** Sexually transmitted diseases, discussed in Chapter 6, pose a real threat to developing fetuses and can leave lingering problems. Syphilis carries increased risk for miscarriage, and infected infants have greater risk for premature death, low birthweight, mental retardation, and chronic health problems. Untreated gonorrhea reduces a woman's chances of becoming pregnant, and if she does, it increases the risk for miscarriage. A woman who has active herpes at the time of delivery should have a cesarean section so the newborn will not be exposed to the virus in the birth canal. Infection in a newborn can cause blindness, mental retardation, neurological problems, and even death. Children born to HIV/AIDS-infected mothers tragically may have the disease also. Their symptoms and prognosis, like those of adults, paint a bleak picture for these children.

**Ectopic Pregnancy.** **Ectopic pregnancy** usually occurs in some portion of the fallopian tube, although the fertilized egg may attach itself to the ovary or within the abdominal cavity. At highest risk for this dangerous condition are women who have had a prior ectopic pregnancy, women who have had pelvic inflammatory disease as a result of gonorrhea or chlamydia, and women who use the intrauterine device contraceptive. The rates of ectopic pregnancy are increasing and may range from one in 65 to one in 200 normal pregnancies.

Signals of ectopic pregnancy include sweating, faintness and dizziness, rapid pulse, falling blood pressure, and abdominal pain. Because hormone production to prevent shedding of the endometrium is reduced, another symptom of ectopic pregnancy is vaginal bleeding in the form of spotting. The greatest risk to the pregnant woman is internal hemorrhage. A woman who suspects an ectopic pregnancy should seek medical attention immediately. The problem can be corrected by removing the contents of the affected fallopian tube surgically (possible in early diagnosis), by removing the entire fallopian tube, or, if necessary, by removing the uterus.

**Spontaneous Abortion.** Most **spontaneous abortions,** or **miscarriage** as it is commonly called, occur during the first trimester. The causes of spontaneous abortions are variable and may be related to a genetic defect of the fetus, infection, hormonal disturbances, alcohol intake, and even cigarette smoking. An estimated 10% to 40% of all pregnancies end this way. About 60% are attributed to chromosomal abnormalities in the fetus.

Signals for impending spontaneous abortion are vaginal bleeding and abdominal cramps. If the cervix continues to dilate, fetal and placental tissue passes into the vagina. Vaginal bleeding should be reported immediately to the health care provider. Bed rest and refraining from intercourse are the tried-and-true recommendations to stop an impending spontaneous abortion. If tissue is being passed, the process cannot be reversed. When the pregnant woman reports to the hospital, dilation and curettage is done to remove from the uterus all fetal tissues that were not expelled if the spontaneous abortion was incomplete. This is done to prevent further complications.

**Breech Presentation.** In a normal delivery the top of the baby's head emerges first. If the buttocks present (show) first, it is a **breech** position. About 3% of full-term pregnancies are breech. Breech presentations are more likely if the fetus is premature or if the mother is carrying more than one fetus in her uterus. To avoid complications for the mother and the fetus, a medical decision has to be made quickly whether to deliver the fetus in the breech position or to perform a cesarean section.

**Cesarean Section.** Occasionally the mother cannot deliver her baby through the vagina. When this situation arises, the fetus is removed through a **cesarean section (C-section).** Typically, cesarean delivery is performed under local anesthesia. Because this procedure involves surgery, it is more complicated than vaginal delivery. Cesareans typically are performed when the fetus's head is larger than the mother's pelvic girdle or when the fetus is in an unusual position. If the mother has health problems such as heart disease, diabetes, high blood pressure, or eclampsia, a C-section may ease the strain of a long labor and delivery. If the baby is in some sort of distress, such as having the umbilical cord pinched, or is subject to infection through vaginal delivery, a C-section may be indicated.

Critics of the growing reliance and possible overuse of cesarean section believe that many of these surgeries are done unnecessarily. Estimates of C-sections range from one in 10 of all births to as many as one in 4. The risk for maternal death from C-section is higher than that for vaginal delivery.

**Elective Cesarean Section.** Take the SUV in for service, pick-up the dry cleaning, schedule your C-section. The National Institutes of Health reports that about 33% of babies in the United States are delivered by cesarean

section and approximately 18% of those are elective C-sections (for nonmedical reasons). Since the "no pushing necessary" method of delivery is a surgical procedure, it increases the mother's risk for infection, and the average in-hospital recovery time is three to five days versus two days for vaginal delivery.

## Maternal and Infant Mortality

Some women die of maternal causes. These deaths occur to pregnant women due to complications of pregnancy, childbirth, and the **puerperium.** Minority women have a higher risk for maternal death than white women do. The rate for black and Hispanic women is highest of all—over three times the rate for white women.

The infant mortality rate (IMR) in 1999 was the lowest ever recorded in the United States. IMR is defined as the number of babies in every 1,000 born who die within the first year of life. Neonatal (newborn) mortality rates have declined over time for all racial and ethnic groups, although the declines have been more rapid for the white population. Internationally, the U.S. ranks 28 in IMR (7.0). The five countries with the lowest infant mortality rates are Hong Kong (2.3), Sweden (2.8), Singapore (2.9), and Finland and Japan at 3.0. Figure 5.15 gives the leading causes of infant mortality.

### KEY TERMS

**Gestational diabetes** form of diabetes (a metabolic disorder) that occurs only during pregnancy

**Macrosomia** literally, "large body"; refers to a condition in which fetus converts extra glucose from mother to fat

**German measles** or **rubella** viral infection that can damage eyes, ears, brain, or heart of the fetus during pregnancy if the mother contracts the disease

**Toxoplasmosis** parasitic disease resulting from exposure to uncooked meat or cat litter; can produce blindness or mental retardation in fetus

**Ectopic pregnancy** implantation outside of the uterus

**Spontaneous abortion** or **miscarriage** termination of pregnancy prior to 20th week

**Breech** positioning of fetus so buttocks are seen first at birth

**Cesarean section (C-section)** delivery of fetus through opening in abdomen and uterus created by a surgical incision

**Puerperium** 42-day period following childbirth when the uterus and vagina usually return to normal

**Congenital anomalies** defects that are present in a baby at birth

**Tay-Sachs disease** an enzyme deficiency occurring almost exclusively in children of Eastern European Jewish ancestry

The leading cause of infant mortality is a group of birth defects called **congenital anomalies.** Some of these are inherited. For example, **Tay-Sachs disease** occurs almost exclusively among children of Eastern European Jewish ancestry and relates to a genetic defect. Other congenital anomalies are induced by the mother's behavior during pregnancy (for example, smoking cigarettes, drinking alcohol, having nutritional deficiencies).

Ranking second in the IMR statistics are babies who die from **prematurity/low birthweight.** Low birthweight often is attributable to premature birth (about six months or less). Many low birthweight babies, however, are born at full term.

The major risk factors for having an LBW baby are drinking alcohol during pregnancy, an absence of health care, and teen pregnancy. Of particular concern is the teen birth rate.

**Sudden infant death syndrome (SIDS)** ranked third. Asian American babies seem to have the lowest risk, and African-American and American Indian babies have the highest risk. This tragic and mysterious disease may not have one single cause. Boys die from SIDS more often than girls do. SIDS tends to occur more than once in families. Some possible causes may be viral infections and allergies. Preliminary research done in the United States and Germany shows a link between crib death and newborns who have undiagnosed whooping cough (pertussis).

Cigarette smoking by the mother during pregnancy seems to be one of the biggest risk factors for SIDS. Another risk factor is the use of psychoactive drugs such as cocaine and heroin. Again for unknown reasons, more SIDS deaths occur in winter than in summer.

The Centers for Disease Control and Prevention, Office of Minority Health Resource Center reports that the death rate from birth to age one of black babies is approximately twice that of white babies. Pregnant black women are twice as likely as pregnant white women to receive absolutely no prenatal care or care beginning in the last trimester of the pregnancy, and three times as likely to have babies born with defects.

Social and economic factors contribute to the alarming disparity in the infant mortality rate between minority groups and white populations in the United States. Some of these factors are

- Low income and limited medical insurance
- Preexisting medical problems
- Poor nutrition
- Problems with transportation and child care that impede access to and use of services
- Lack of maternal education

## Infertility

According to the American Society for Reproductive Medicine, more than six million Americans have problems with fertility. Even though physical problems are associated with **infertility**, researchers have documented that emotional stress can cause men to produce less semen with fewer sperm cells that are less motile. In women, being depresssed is linked to low fertility.

Amidst rising birth rates and concern about overpopulation, the plight of one group may be overlooked. Approximately 15% of couples trying to become pregnant are frustrated and disappointed because they cannot conceive.

According to the American Fertility Society, in 40% of the couples who fail to conceive, the male is the sole contributing cause. In about a fourth of the cases, more than one factor is at work.

## CAUSES

Of the many factors that can cause male infertility, most of the problems relate to sperm production. In most cases the underlying cause is unknown, but some known causes are

- *Testicular disease*, which can result in *azoospermia*, or the complete absence of sperm in the semen
- *Mumps*, contracted after puberty
- *Hormone deficiencies*
- *Varicoceles*, or varicose veins above one or both testicles
- *Obstruction of the vas deferens*, because of infection by sexually transmitted disease, injury, or surgery

Treatments for male infertility include antibiotic therapy for infection, surgery to correct varicose veins in the scrotum or obstruction of ducts, and hormones to improve sperm production.

Female contributors to infertility include uterine abnormalities. About 10% to 15% of women with recurrent miscarriages have an abnormality in the structure of the uterus.

- *Incompetent cervix.* The cervix cannot support a pregnancy without surgical correction (which usually is successful).
- *Septate uterus.* The septum (ridge) protrudes into the uterine cavity. About 3% of the entire female population has this condition, but it does not cause a problem in half of these women.

A hysteroscopy or a special x-ray called a hysterosalpinogram (HSG) can identify abnormalities within the uterus. It also is used to determine if the fallopian tubes are open.

Another cause of female infertility is

- *Polycystic ovarian syndrome* (also called Stein-Leventhal syndrome or hyperandrogenism). Basically, **polycystic ovarian syndrome (PCOS)** involves overproduction of androgen and estrogen, which prevents ovulation and may result in ovarian cysts. The diagnosis is confirmed by measuring blood hormone levels, and an ultrasound may reveal the cysts. Some causes of PCOS are thought to be obesity (fatty tissue produces an excess of estrogen), overproduction of insulin, and dysfunctional adrenal glands. It may have a genetic link.

The treatment generally involves weight loss (if overweight), inducement of ovulation through injections of human menopausal gonadotrophin (HMG) drugs, and hormone treatments (low-dose oral contraceptives). In rare cases surgery is done.

Hormonal dysfunctions also may cause a woman to be infertile. These include

- *Luteal phase inadequacy.* The luteal phase of menstruation is crucial to implantation. If progesterone levels are low during this phase, infertility or miscarriage can result because the lining does not develop adequately for the embryo to implant securely. An endometrial biopsy can be used to assess problems related to the luteal phase, and disorders usually are treated by medical prescription.

- *Underactive or overactive thyroid gland.* Diagnosis is made through a simple blood test. Thyroid disorders usually can be treated with medication.

Additional reasons for pregnancy loss are

- *Genetic defects.* The embryo or fetus is found to be defective in an estimated 50% to 60% of first-trimester miscarriages. The most common genetic defect is an abnormal number of chromosomes. If the placenta or the fetus of a woman having her first miscarriage has the normal number of chromosomes, the second pregnancy has only a 50% chance of being abnormal. If the first pregnancy is genetically abnormal, the chance for an abnormal second pregnancy is greater.

Genetic causes may be diagnosed by a **karyotype** on the fetal tissue and on blood from both parents. A chromosomal analysis usually is recommended for all couples with a history of two or more early pregnancy losses. In about 5%, an abnormality in one parent explains the recurrent miscarriage.

- *Sexually transmitted diseases.* Although chlamydia has been linked to miscarriage, it is associated more clearly with infertility and tubal infection.

- *Immunologic causes.* The mother may have antibodies that cause blood clotting, which poses serious risks to the pregnant woman and inhibits fetal development. This usually leads to miscarriage.

Fertility in men and women alike declines with age, even though the man has the potential to father a child longer than a woman can conceive. Some women delay pregnancy during the times in their life when they are most fertile, only to have problems later. The infertility problem for other couples relates to timing. They are not having intercourse during the ovulation phase of the woman's menstrual cycle.

## SOLUTIONS

Charting basal body temperature throughout the woman's menstrual cycle reveals when ovulation occurs and, thus, when she has the best chance to conceive. The only equipment required is a thermometer. The woman takes her temperature upon waking every morning. If the basal body temperature has gone up for several days, ovulation has occurred. Figure 5.16 presents a BBT chart. The spaces with Xs indicate days of menstruation. Couples wishing to conceive should have intercourse at the time of ovulation.

According to a study published in the *New England Journal of Medicine*, a woman is more likely to conceive during the six-day period ending on the day of ovulation. There is a small probability of conception on the day before the six-day window and the day after ovulation.

Some other suggested solutions to infertility are

1. **Boxer shorts.** Men wearing jockey shorts may keep the groin area too warm and reduce sperm activity. Boxer shorts are an attested remedy for many.

2. **Hormone treatments (fertility drugs).** Clomid, Serophene, and Pergonal (equal parts of FSH and LH) stimulate egg production. Fertility drugs may be prescribed if one or both partners have a hormone imbalance. These drugs do have side effects, however, and some increase the probability for multiple births because of **superovulation.**

3. **Surgery.** In some cases microsurgery is done to remove scar tissue that is blocking the fallopian tubes in the female or the vas deferens in the male.

4. **Tubal ovum transfer.** The woman's eggs are retrieved and placed into the end of the fallopian tube

---

### KEY TERMS

**Prematurity/low birthweight (LBW)** weighing less than five and one-half pounds at birth

**Sudden infant death syndrome (SIDS)** death of a baby by an undetermined cause, usually while sleeping at night

**Infertility** inability to achieve pregnancy after trying for 12 months or six months for a woman 35 years old or older

**Polycystic ovarian syndrome (PCOS)** a female endocrine disorder characterized by irregular menstrual periods, infertility, and excessive body and facial hair

**Karyotype** photograph of a cell during cell division; shows chromosomes in order of size from largest to smallest; used to detect chromosome defects

**Superovulation** production and release of multiple ova as a result of taking fertility drugs

**FIGURE 5.16** ▶ Basal Body Temperature Chart

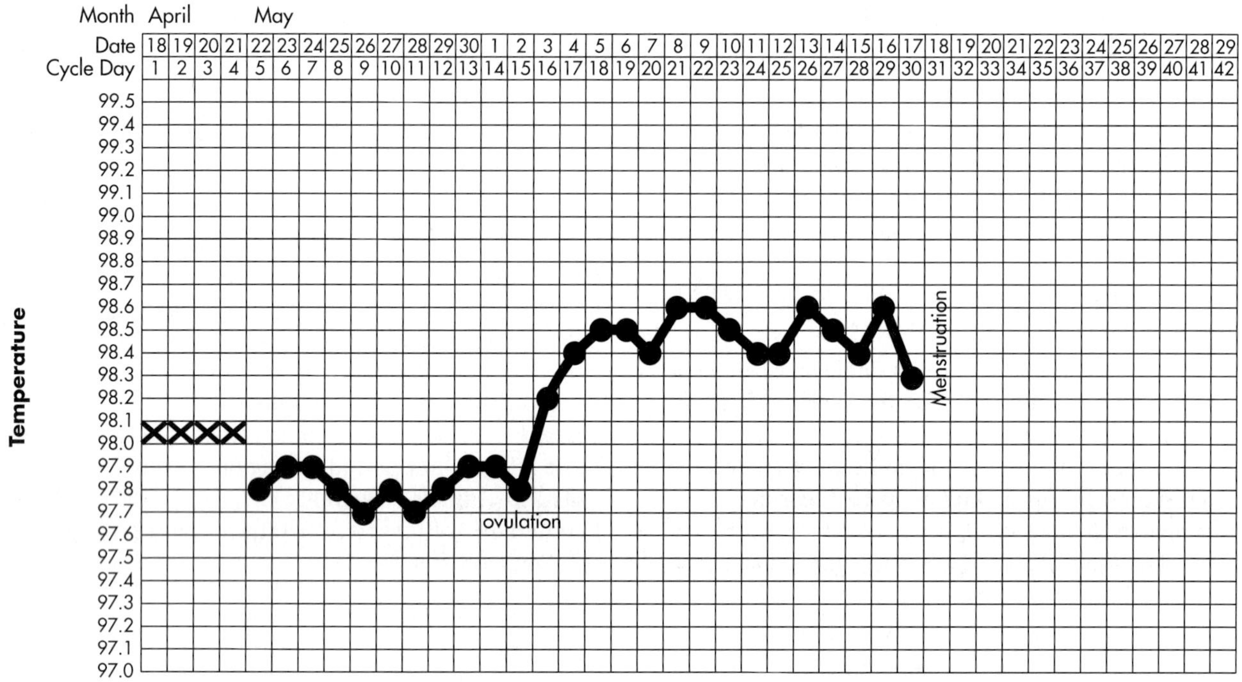

that opens to the uterus. The couple has intercourse or the woman is artificially inseminated.

5. **Artificial insemination.** The preferred term for this practice is **intrauterine insemination (IUI).** Three variations are

   a. **Gamete intrafallopian transfer (GIFT).** The sperm and eggs together are inserted into the fallopian tube. For this procedure to be successful, the fallopian tube must be healthy.

   b. **In vitro fertilization.** Fertilized eggs are implanted into the uterus. In 1978 Louise Joy Brown from England became the first "test-tube baby." Since that time, many more have been born.

   c. **Intracytoplasmic sperm injection (ICSI, pronounced "ick-see").** Developed in Belgium, this assisted reproductive technology (ART) has an advantage over in vitro fertilization for men with a low sperm count in that only one sperm, instead of many, is needed for fertilization.

## Adoption

A final option for those who want children is adoption. Agencies have different requirements concerning age, religion, race, and so on. Some variations on adoption are

- *Closed versus open.* In the past, **closed adoption** was the standard. The adoption records were closed to all the parties involved. More recently, **open adoption** is gaining acceptance with legal underpinnings. This

usually means limited exchange of information and contact between the birth parents and the adoptive parents. Some agencies allow the birth parents to choose the adoptive couple from preselected prospects.

- *Infant and older child adoption.* To adopt an infant usually requires that the adoptive adult be under a certain age, usually 35 to 45. Older couples are encouraged to adopt older children. Many agencies require at least 15 years between the age of the adoptive parents and the age of the child.

- *Interracial adoption.* Agencies differ in their requirements regarding adopting a child of a race different from the prospective parents'. Some hold that different races have different value systems, customs, and traditions and that interracial adoptions will encounter difficulties that would not be present in same-race adoptions. Recently, federal and state legislation has been introduced to promote interracial adoption.

- *Special needs adoption. Special needs* refers to a child who is not totally physically or emotionally healthy. Although adopting a special needs child requires a tremendous commitment of time and energy, the emotional rewards may be substantial.

## Summary

- Sperm have an X and Y chromosome, and eggs have one X; the male, therefore, determines the offspring's sex.

- Three common disorders of the female reproductive system are endometriosis, uterine fibroid tumors, and premenstrual syndrome (PMS).

- The sexual response has four phases: excitement, plateau, orgasmic, and resolution.

- Sexual problems include vaginal dryness and vaginismus in the female and impotence and premature ejaculation in the male.

- The typical menstrual cycle is 28 days, with four segments: menses, estrogenic, ovulation, and progestational.

- Various tests to gain information about the fetus include ultrasound, alpha-fetoprotein (AFP) screening, amniocentesis, and chorionic villus sampling (CVS).

- Types of anesthetic used during delivery are the pudendal block, paracervical block, spinal anesthesia, epidural anesthesia, and caudal anesthesia.

- Birth occurs in three stages: labor, delivery of the baby, and delivery of the placenta.

- A wide array of fertility control measures are available, each with constraints, advantages, and disadvantages.

- A variety of factors can contribute to infertility. Measures to correct infertility include basal body temperature (BBT) charting, fertility drugs, tubal ovum transfer, and forms of artificial insemination.

- Adoptions can be closed, open, interracial, older children, and children with special needs.

## Personal Health Resources

**ThomsonNOW** Visit the ThomsonNOW website at http://thomsonedu.com/thomsonnow for valuable resources that will:

- Help you evaluate your knowledge of the material.

- Guide you through tutorials to help you understand and apply the material.

- Allow you to take an exam-prep quiz to better prepare for class tests.

Planned Parenthood. This site provides information about birth control, pregnancy, sexually transmitted diseases, abortions, and the politics of each topic.
1-212-541-7800 (New York office)
**www.plannedparenthood.org**

Doulas of North America (DONA). This site provides information about doula-assisted childbirth and referrals to doulas in your area.
1-800-788-3662
**www.dona.com**

American College of Obstetricians and Gynecologists. Provides information on contraceptive techniques; information on reproductive health techniques, care, and research; and various reproduction-related documents.
**www.acog.com**

Centers for Disease Control and Prevention, Center for Health Promotion and Education. Provides health information, educational and resource materials, and epidemiological data compilations for health research.
**www.cdc.gov/**

Resolve. This organization provides in-person and online support groups for people with fertility problems.
**www.resolve.org**

## It's Your Turn for Study and Review

1. Outline the various changes that occur in women and men during the four phases of the sexual response cycle.

2. Outline six birth control methods and discuss the one your research favors over the other five.

3. Describe the concept of gender identity and gender role.

4. What are major sexual dysfunctions in men and women? What are ways to correct these problems?

5. How reliable is the condom? Discuss the issue fully.

6. Analyze the differences and the similarities in heterosexuals, homosexuals, and bisexuals.

7. Describe the main functions of the female and male sexual structures.

### KEY TERMS

**Intrauterine insemination (IUI)** a procedure in which sperm from a donor is placed in contact with one or more female ova; better known as artificial insemination

**Gamete intrafallopian transfer (GIFT)** eggs and sperm are collected, mixed, and inserted into fallopian tube

**In vitro fertilization** procedure in which a woman's eggs are placed in a glass dish and incubated with donor sperm

**Intracytoplasmic sperm injection (ICSI)** a procedure to induce conception by injecting a single sperm directly into an egg cell

**Closed adoption** adoption in which exchange of parental information is not allowed

**Open adoption** adoption in which some parental information is exchanged and some contact is allowed between the birth parents and the adoptive parents

## Thinking about Health Issues

Is circumcision necessary?
James W. Prescott, Marilyn Fayre Milos, and George C. Denniston, "Circumcision: Human Rights and Ethical Medical Practice," *The Humanist*, May 1999, p. 45 (1).

1. What are the principal findings and recommendations in the 1999 statement released by the American Academy of Pediatrics "that circumcision is unnecessary"?

2. From a purely medical standpoint, when is circumcision justified? From a medical ethics viewpoint, when is circumcision justified?

3. From a human rights standpoint, what do the authors say about circumcision? Compare and contrast their position with the recommendations of pediatricians.

## Selected Bibliography

Altshul, S. "Massage Your Mood." *Prevention*, 58(8), August 2006, p. 100.

Berman, L. "Do I Need to Stop the Pill Periodically." *Ladies Home Journal*, August 2005, p. 142.

Cohen, M. "How Not to Get Pregnant." *Prevention*, 57:9, September 2005, pp. 137–138.

Cohn, M. "To Push or Not to Push." *Prevention*, 58:4, April 2006, p. 128.

CVS Pharmacy, Drug Monograph Print, "Yasmin 28," July 30, 2006.

Dudones, G. "The Unkindest Cut." Ms. Magazine. Winter 2007; vol. 17, No. 1, p. 29.

Duenwald, M. "What You Need: Bridge Contraception." *More*, June 2005, p. 138.

"Emergency Contraceptive Pills," Women's Health Policy Fact Sheet, Kaiser Family Foundation, February 2004.

"Emergency Birth Control (Information from Your Family Doctor)." *American Family Physician*, 70:4, August 2004, p. 717.

"FDA Approves Mifepristone for Termination of Early Pregnancy," *FDA Consumer*, 34:6, November/December 2000, p. 7.

"FDA Consumer Special: NIH Review Confirms Condoms Effective against Transmission of HIV, Gonorrhea." *FDA Consumer*, 35:5, September/October 2001, p. 7.

Forman, G. "The Vagina Dialogues." *Seventeen*, June 2001, p. 88.

Graham, J. "Very Personal Health." *Redbook*, 207:2, August 2006, p. 53.

Green, R. *The Human Embryo Research Debate: Bioethics in the Vortex of Controversy*. New York: Oxford University Press, 2001.

Gregoire, A. "Assessing and Managing Male Sexual Problems." *British Medical Journal*, 318:7179, January 1999, pp. 315–317.

Jacoby, S. "Sex in America." *AARP The Magazine*, 48:4B, July/August 2005, p. 58.

Hanson, L. and Sassen, J. "Contraceptive Options." *American Family Physician*, 69:4, February 2004, p. 811.

Healy, B. "Ask and You Shall Receive." *U.S. News and World Report*, 140(19), May 22, 2006, p. 58.

Healy, B. "Birthing by Appointment." *U.S. News and World Report*, 140:22, June 12, 2006, p. 70.

Herndon, E. and Zieman, M. "New Contraceptive Options." *American Family Physician*, 69:4, February 2004, p. 853.

Janus, S. and Janus, C. L. *The Janus Report on Sexual Behavior*. New York: Wiley, 1993.

Kline, H. "Not in the Mood: Is the Pill Damaging Your Sex Life?" *Psychology Today*, November/December 2001, p. 30.

Liao, S. "Contraceptive Comeback." *Prevention*, 57:9, September 2005, p. 38.

Mohall, R. A. "The Truth about the Patch." *Prevention*, 58:4, April 2006, p. 38.

Murphy, S. T., et al. "Preaching to the Choir: Preference for Female-Controlled Methods of HIV and Sexually Transmitted Disease Prevention." *American Journal of Public Health*, 90:7, July 2000, pp. 1135–1137.

Olenick, I. "Levonorgestrel Is a Better Emergency Contraceptive than the Combination Pill." *Family Planning Perspectives*, 31:2, March 1999, p. 106.

Oliwenstein, L. "On Fertile Ground." *Psychology Today*, 36:6, November/December 2005, pp. 63–66.

"Polycystic Ovary Syndrome." *Harvard Women's Health Watch*, November 1996, pp. 2–3.

*Prostate Enlargement: Benign Prostate Hyperplasia*. National Kidney and Urological Disease Information Clearinghouse (NKUDIC), NIH. Accessed January 20, 2007. Available at kidney.niddk.nih.gov/kudiseases/a-z.asp.

Soares, C. "Why Human Clones Won't Work—Yet." *Discover*, January 2002, p. 64.

"Sterilization: Is Your Practice Up to Date?" *Contraceptive Technology Update*, 25:7, July 2004, p. 79.

Szalavitz, M. "Should I Drop My Antidepressant?" *Psychology Today*, 39:2, March/April 2006, p. 59.

U.S. Bureau of the Census. *Statistical Abstract of the United States: 2000*, 120th edition. Washington, DC: U.S. Government Printing Office, 2000.

U.S. Department of Health and Human Services. *Healthy People 2010: Understanding and Improving Health*. Washington, DC: U.S. Government Printing Office, 2000.

Vander Schaaf, R. "Helping Sperm Meet Egg." *Prevention*, 57:11, November 2005, p. 138.

Vander Schaaf, R. "Test Your Epidural Smarts." *Prevention*, 57:9, September 2005, pp. 139–140.

*Wellness for a Lifetime, A Woman's Book for Health and Well-Being*, 2006.

Weismiller, D. "Emergency Contraception." *American Family Physician*, 70:4, August 2004, p. 707.

Wilcox, A. J. "Timing of Sexual Intercourse in Relation to Ovulation." *New England Journal of Medicine*, 333, 1995, pp. 1517–1521.

**Name** _____     **Date** _____

**Course** _____     **Section** _____

Utilizing your knowledge of the material in this chapter, label the parts of the male external and internal reproductive system.

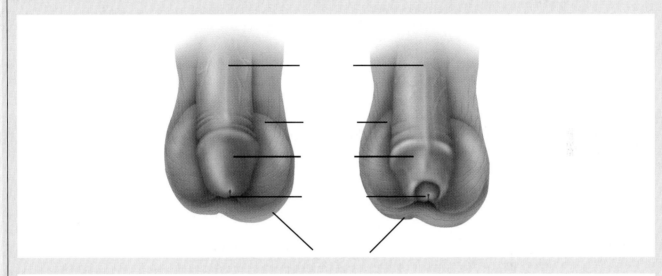

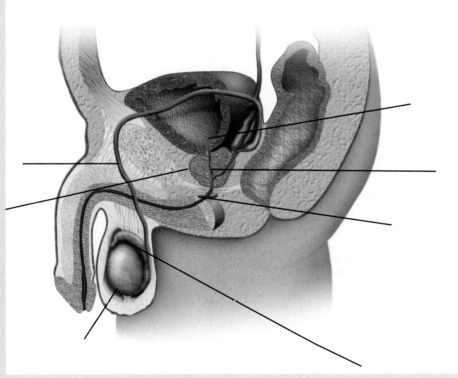

**Name** _____    **Date** _____

**Course** _____    **Section** _____

Utilizing your knowledge of the material in this chapter, label the parts of the female external and internal reproductive system.

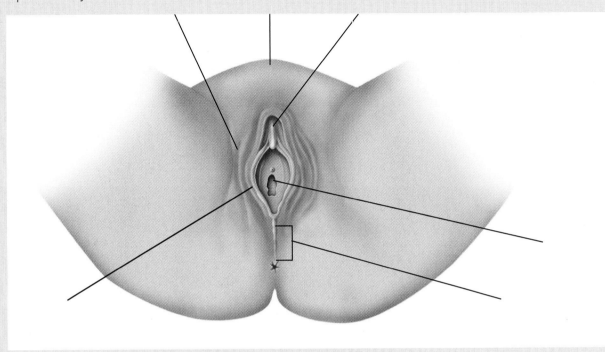

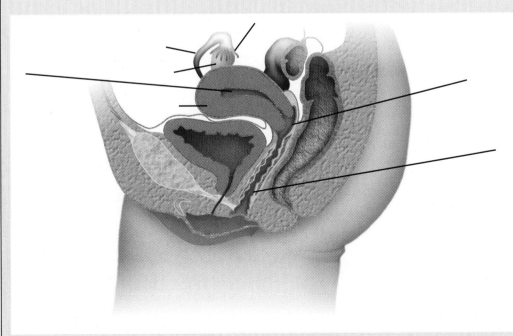

Name _____  Date _____

Course _____  Section _____

To choose the best method or methods of contraception or birth control, study each method carefully. Indicate if the method primarily prevents ovulation (O), fertilization (F), or implantation (I), and state advantages, disadvantages, and the rate of effectiveness of the most commonly used methods.

| Contraceptive or birth control method | Prevents | Advantage | Disadvantage | Effectiveness |
|---|---|---|---|---|
| Male condom | | | | |
| Female condom | | | | |
| Oral contraception (the pill) | | | | |
| Chemical spermicide | | | | |
| Diaphragm with chemical spermicide | | | | |
| Sterilization Tubal ligation Vasectomy | | | | |

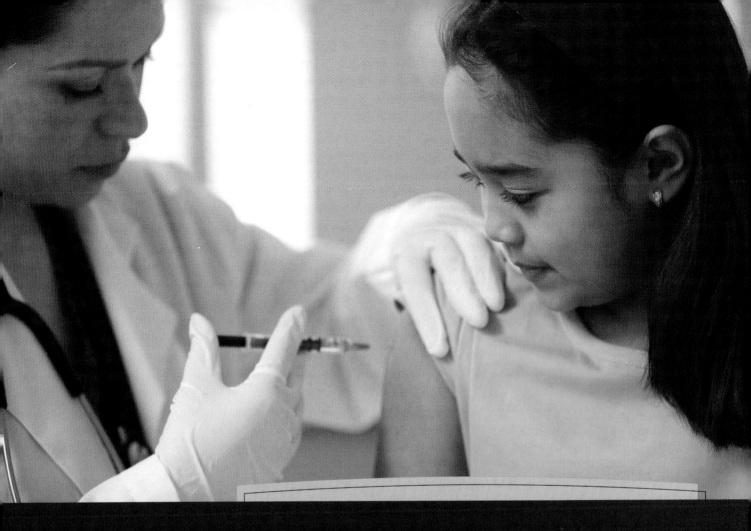

# Chapter Six  Communicable Diseases

**OBJECTIVES** ■ Define infectious or communicable disease. ■ Name the classifications of pathogens. ■ Describe the methods by which pathogens are transmitted. ■ Explain the course of infection. ■ Describe the mechanism involved in the immune response. ■ Name the communicable diseases for which immunizations are available. ■ Outline the demographics of HIV/AIDS. ■ Describe the symptoms and effects of common sexually transmitted diseases.

ThomsonNOW  Log on to ThomsonNOW at http://thomsonedu.com/ thomsonnow to access and explore self-assessments, interactive tutorials, and practice quizzes.

Many life forms that exist cannot be seen without magnification. Some are beneficial and some are not. The latter invade human bodies, make people ill, and sometimes even cause death. These sinister creatures are called pathogens. Their mission is to invade the body and then move silently to the next victim.

**Pathogens** are the causative agents of **infectious diseases.** These conditions also are called communicable or contagious diseases. Pathogens can be passed from person to person, **fomite** to person, or animal to person.

## Classes of Pathogens

Pathogens can be grouped into the following categories.

- Viruses
- Bacteria
- Fungi
- Protozoa
- Metazoa

Figure 6.1 depicts these classes of pathogens and lists conditions caused by each.

**Viruses** consist of genetic material protected by a protein shell. Examples of infectious conditions caused by viruses are the common cold, influenza (flu), and chickenpox. When comparing pathogens by size, the viruses are the smallest of the pathogenic organisms and often are airborne.

**Bacteria** come in three basic shapes: the spherical-shaped coccus, the rod- or club-shaped bacillus, and the spiral-shaped spirillum or spirochete. Among the diseases caused by bacteria are tuberculosis, strep throat, and syphilis. Some bacteria are carried in body wastes—a good reason for washing your hands, particularly before eating.

**Rickettsiae** once were believed to be closely allied with viruses but now are believed to be a small form of bacteria. Rickettsiae are transmitted by **vectors.** Two examples of rickettsial diseases are Rocky Mountain spotted fever, carried by a tick, and typhus, carried by lice, fleas, and ticks.

**Fungi** include mushrooms, molds, and yeast. Fungi like to grow in warm, dark, and moist environments. Common infectious diseases caused by fungi include athlete's foot, ringworm of the scalp (tetter), and yeast infection. (Human-invading yeasts are different from the yeasts used for making bread or beer.)

**Protozoa** live as parasites in humans. Some infectious illnesses caused by protozoa require a vector for transmission to humans. Malaria, African sleeping sickness, and the sexually transmitted disease (STD) trichomoniasis are caused by protozoa.

**Metazoa,** largest of the pathogens, can be seen without magnification. Intestinal roundworms and lice are

**FIGURE 6.1** ▶ Classes of Pathogens with Examples of Each

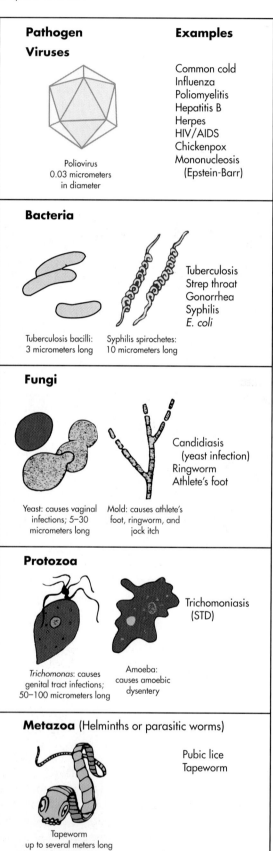

| Pathogen | Examples |
|---|---|
| **Viruses** | Common cold |
| | Influenza |
| | Poliomyelitis |
| | Hepatitis B |
| | Herpes |
| | HIV/AIDS |
| | Chickenpox |
| | Mononucleosis |
| | (Epstein-Barr) |

Poliovirus
0.03 micrometers
in diameter

**Bacteria**

Tuberculosis bacilli:
3 micrometers long

Syphilis spirochetes:
10 micrometers long

Tuberculosis
Strep throat
Gonorrhea
Syphilis
*E. coli*

**Fungi**

Yeast: causes vaginal
infections; 5–30
micrometers long

Mold: causes athlete's
foot, ringworm, and
jock itch

Candidiasis
(yeast infection)
Ringworm
Athlete's foot

**Protozoa**

*Trichomonas:* causes
genital tract infections;
50–100 micrometers long

Amoeba:
causes amoebic
dysentery

Trichomoniasis
(STD)

**Metazoa** (Helminths or parasitic worms)

Tapeworm
up to several meters long

Pubic lice
Tapeworm

Reduce the indigenous cases of the following vaccine-preventable diseases

- Diphtheria among people age 25 and younger
- Tetanus among people age 25 and younger
- Polio
- Rubeola

- Rubella
- Congenital rubella syndrome
- Mumps
- Pertussis

examples of conditions caused by metazoa. Tapeworms, for example, can be several feet long. Worm infestations usually come from contaminated food or drink, and their spread is controlled by good hygiene.

## The Course of Infectious Disease

For an infectious illness to occur, a pathogen and a "victim" must be present. In most cases the pathogen invades the person's body, multiplies, causes illness, and then dies. Death of the pathogen may result from the work of the infected person's immune system or from some medication the person takes to fight the condition. The course of most infectious diseases is fairly predictable, beginning with exposure and infection, followed by an incubation period, a prodromal period, the clinical stage, recovery or relapse, and termination.

### EXPOSURE AND INFECTION

First the person comes in contact with the pathogen as a result of exposure to infected persons, animals, or fomites. Upon exposure these pathogens invade the body through natural openings, breaks in the skin, or mucous membranes, such as in the nose. Once inside the body, the pathogens multiply and begin their destruction, which manifests itself as an infection. In some cases the infection is a **local infection.** If the pathogen moves to the circulatory and lymphatic systems and spreads to other regions or body systems, the condition is called a **systemic infection.** Systemic infections usually are more difficult to treat than local infections are.

### INCUBATION PERIOD

Upon exposure to pathogenic organisms, the symptoms of an infectious illness do not appear immediately. If this were the case, treatment would ensue immediately and responsible people would not expose others knowingly. During the incubation period the pathogens are working quietly but effectively and without the infected person's knowledge. The person is **asymptomatic.** Although he or she has no signs or symptoms of illness, the infected person is able to expose others to the pathogens he or she is carrying. The incubation period varies from one infectious disease to another—from a few days to a few weeks to several years.

### PRODROMAL PERIOD

The prodromal period is one of high communicability. During this stage the person becomes sick with nonspecific signs or warnings of illness that may include irritability,

### KEY TERMS

**Pathogen** disease-causing organism

**Infectious diseases** conditions in which a pathogen can be spread from person to person; also called communicable or contagious diseases

**Fomite** an object contaminated with a pathogen

**Viruses** microorganisms without their own metabolism that reproduce within the living cells of the person they invade

**Bacteria** a type of disease-causing microorganism

**Rickettsiae** microorganisms similar to bacteria that are transmitted to humans through insect bites

**Vector** insect carrier of pathogen

**Fungi** plantlike organisms that lack chlorophyll; some are pathogens

**Protozoa** one-celled animals that can live as parasites in humans

**Metazoa** multicellular animals that live as parasites in and on humans and animals

**Local infection** an inflammation that remains in the area of the body where the invasion of the pathogen occurred

**Systemic infection** an infection that spreads throughout the body via the blood or lymphatic system

**Asymptomatic** without signs of illness

a slight fever, or general aches and pains. Some type of treatment might help alleviate the symptoms during this phase of the disease.

## CLINICAL STAGE

At this point the specific symptoms of the illness manifest themselves and an accurate diagnosis usually can be made. In most cases the person is still contagious.

## RECOVERY OR RELAPSE

In the recovery stage the body's defenses or the medication overcomes the pathogen, the symptoms disappear, and the person gets well. The person may have a relapse, during which time the symptoms reappear, returning the person to the clinical stage.

## TERMINATION

The termination phase denotes victory. Because of the person's level of wellness or medical advances, he or she becomes well and may enter one of three states.

1. After an attack by certain pathogens, the person becomes protected for a lifetime and will not be able to contract the disease even if he or she is exposed to the pathogen again. Examples of this type of protection are found in the childhood diseases, such as measles (rubeola).

2. After having certain infectious diseases, the infected person does get well but may become ill again if reexposed to the pathogens. Acquiring German measles again is an example of **resusceptibility**.

3. Some individuals recover completely from an infectious illness but retain vestiges of the illness, which they can transmit to others. These people show no signs of illness but shed the pathogens of the disease that continue to take refuge in their bodies. They are asymptomatic carriers. An example of an infectious disease in which pathogens can be transmitted by an asymptomatic person or carrier is genital herpes.

## Routes of Invasion

Pathogens enter the body in four ways.

1. Skin or other body surfaces. Pathogens may enter directly through breaks caused by cuts, abrasions, burns, or punctures in the skin or other body surfaces. Some pathogens are absorbed through mucous membranes where no break exists. Other pathogens are able to penetrate intact skin.

2. Inhalation. Pathogens that are airborne may enter the body through the mucous membranes of the nasal passages or via the lungs.

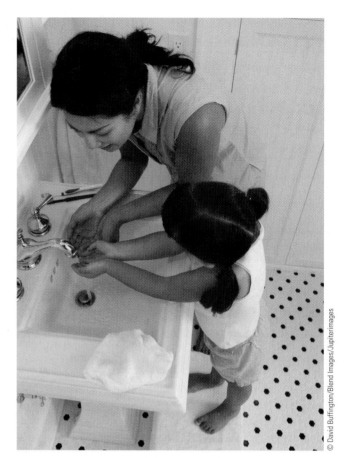

▲ *Washing the hands is one of the most effective means of preventing infectious diseases*

3. Contaminated food or water. People may expose themselves to pathogens by inadvertently eating or drinking something in which pathogens are living.

4. Fomites. Under certain conditions, exposure to objects such as used hypodermic needles and syringes, drinking glasses, or bed linens contaminated with pathogens can introduce the pathogen into the body.

## The Body's Defense Mechanisms

The human body has two fundamental means with which to defend itself from the marauding pathogens that assault it daily.

## THE FIRST RESPONSE

On the front line of defense is the **epidermis.** Without this protective covering humans would not survive long. By acting as a shield or cover, the epidermis stops most pathogens from invading the more vulnerable interior surfaces of the body. Often pathogens can be removed by washing with soap and water before they have the opportunity to enter through breaks in the skin.

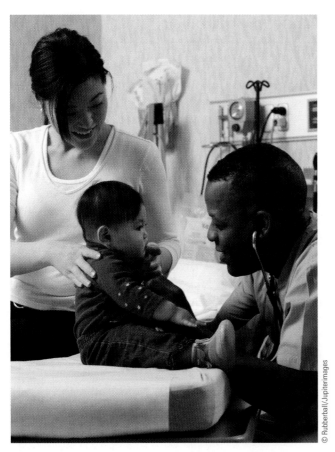

▲ *Regular medical examinations and scheduled immunizations are important for a child's good health*

**Mucous membranes,** although not as strong as the epidermis, help protect the interior surfaces from pathogenic invasion. The tissue is bathed with mucous secretions that trap particles and pathogens before they are able to establish infection. These secretions contain enzymes that inactivate pathogens. Mucous membranes line the digestive, respiratory, urinary, and reproductive tracts.

Other first-response defenders are tears and saliva, which contain antibacterial substances that dilute organisms or particles, rendering them ineffective. Cilia (specialized hairlike projections that line the bronchial tubes) sweep particles and pathogens from the lungs into the digestive tract, where they are killed by gastric secretions.

## THE SECOND RESPONSE

If the pathogenic raiders overwhelm the first-response systems that protect people initially, a second response comes from the body's immune system. The **lymphatic system** (Figure 6.2) consists of specialized vessels throughout the body containing **lymph nodes.** Lymph nodes are found in the head and neck, the armpits, the small of the back, and the groin, among other places.

**Macrophages** (phagocytes) and **lymphocytes** together fight pathogens. Macrophages are the Pac Man cells of the

immune system. They seek invading bacteria and foreign substances and then engulf and destroy them in a process called **phagocytosis.** Lymphocytes are made by bone marrow. These specialized cells work with the macrophages. Some lymphocytes stimulate the body to produce more lymphocytes as well as stimulate the production of antibodies.

When the body is invaded by pathogens, phagocytosis does not provide enough protection in some instances. A more elaborate mechanism of the immune system must be activated. The immune system senses the pathogen as a foreign substance, which now acts as an **antigen** in the body. At this point the lymphocytes come to the body's rescue to fight the infection. **B-cells** produce **antibodies** that are able to deactivate the invading pathogens so other body defenses can rid the body of these organisms. What is amazing about this process is that the antibodies produced are specific to the particular antigen for which they were created. People have many pathogen-specific antibodies in their immune systems.

Once activated by the antigen, the **T-cells** target the cells of the pathogen or the cells of the infected person

## KEY TERMS

**Resusceptibility** vulnerability to reinfection with a disease after having recovered from it

**Epidermis** top layer of skin

**Mucous membranes** moist tissues that help protect the interior surfaces of the body from invasion by pathogens

**Lymphatic system** specialized groups of vessels that network throughout the body and cleanse body tissues

**Lymph nodes** larger glands of the lymph system found in the head, neck, armpits, small of the back, and groin

**Macrophages** specialized white blood cells (phagocytes) that destroy pathogens

**Lymphocytes** specialized white blood cells produced in the bone marrow that identify pathogens and help macrophages fight pathogens

**Phagocytosis** the destruction of pathogens by macrophages

**Antigen** a substance that triggers the immune response

**B-cells** a type of lymphocyte that produces antibodies capable of deactivating invading pathogens

**Antibodies** protein substances that interact with antigens and form the basis of immunity

**T-cells** lymphocytes that activate additional B-cells, stop B-cell activity when the pathogen is destroyed, kill normal cells that have become cancerous, and attack pathogens

**FIGURE 6.2** ▶ The Lymphatic System

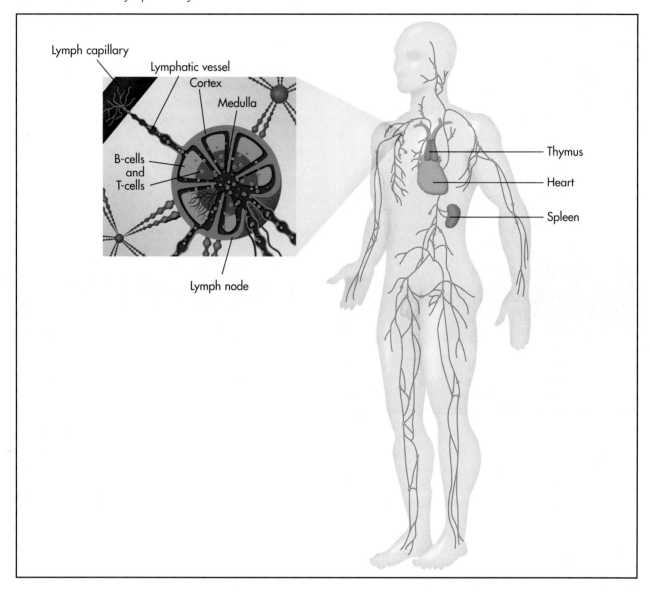

that the invading pathogens have penetrated. The T-cells then destroy these cells to protect the person.

**Immune Response.** The first exposure to the pathogen triggers the **immune response** (Figure 6.3), which may not have been strong enough to prevent the person from becoming ill at the first attack. If the person is reexposed to the same pathogen later, however, the memory T-cells and B-cells remember the specific antigen from the initial exposure. They then spring into action to protect the person from becoming ill from this new attack. The immune response on this occasion is much faster and stronger than it was on the first exposure.

The memory T-cells and B-cells do not leave the body; they remain in the person's lymphatic and circulatory system for many years—even for life in some instances. This type of **immunity** is called **acquired immunity.** The types of immunity are diagrammed in Figure 6.4.

Acquired immunity results from many of the so-called childhood diseases. Exposure to certain other pathogens does stimulate antibody production but does not confer protection to the person after subsequent reexposure and reinfection. This means that the person is resusceptible and may become ill with the same disease many times throughout the lifespan. This is true of many sexually transmitted diseases.

Also, because the various infectious diseases are caused by different and distinct pathogens, immunity to one does not confer immunity to another. And a person can be infected with more than one pathogen and have more than one communicable disease at one time.

## Tips for Action How to Keep Your Immune System Healthy

■ Eat a balanced diet including plenty of fresh fruits and vegetables for vitamin C and beta carotene, and meat, milk, and eggs for vitamin E.

■ Exercise moderately and often (but not when you are ill, as that can prolong recovery). Brisk walking at least five times a week for 45 minutes will benefit most people.

■ Develop close personal relationships, those in which you trust and can readily confide and vent frustrations. Stress is hard on the immune system.

■ Be sure to get enough sleep—six to eight hours a night—as lack of sleep leaves a person more vulnerable to infections and illness and sleep bolsters the immune system.

■ Do not smoke, as smoking lowers the level of some immune cells, and drink only in moderation, if at all.

■ Wash your hands with soap and water, as most viral diseases are spread by hand-to-hand contact.

■ Avoid contact with people who have diseases caused by airborne pathogens such as flu and chickenpox.

## IMMUNODEFICIENCY

Cancer, HIV infection, some congenital (present at birth) disorders, and a miscellany of other conditions are associated with **immunodeficiencies.** A unique disorder of the immune system is **autoimmunity.** Strictly speaking, HIV infection is not an autoimmune disease, although it does leave the body susceptible to many diseases. Autoimmune disorders such as rheumatoid arthritis and lupus erythematosus are noncommunicable. These are discussed in Chapter 7.

## Immunization

One of the success stories of modern times is the development of vaccines that have virtually eliminated many of the highly contagious diseases that formerly left their marks on many people, particularly children. For example, four decades after polio vaccines were first developed, the disease has been vanquished in the Western Hemisphere. The last case was in Peru in 1991.

Today, however, the health status of many Americans is being compromised by the return of some infectious diseases that were perceived as being no longer threats to health. Tuberculosis is on the rise. Public health departments are reporting more cases of rubeola (measles) and other childhood diseases. Immunizations have been developed to prevent these childhood illnesses (listed in Table 6.1). Reported cases are on the rise not because the vaccines are ineffective but, rather, because of parents' failure to immunize their children, as well as some scare tactics advising against immunization.

These tactics may explain why many children are not immunized for chickenpox. Prior to the development of a vaccine, there were about 4 million cases of chickenpox (*Varicella zoster* virus) and 150 deaths from complications annually in the United States, mostly in children ages 14

and younger. In 1995 the Food and Drug Administration (FDA) approved Varivax to immunize against the disease. The American Academy of Pediatrics, the American Academy of Family Physicians, and the Centers for Disease Control and Prevention (CDC) recommend that healthy children be immunized with the vaccine. The vaccine should not be given to children with a weakened immune system. Aspirin should not be given to a child for six weeks after the immunization. The concern of some parents and physicians was that 10% to 30% of children who are immunized still got chickenpox. Presently, the recommended immunization is two doses for better protection.

Most school districts require that children be immunized before they enter school. These regulations, however, do not protect children who are under five years old and not enrolled in an away-from-home educational program. More than half of U.S. infants are not getting all their recommended immunizations, according to *American Health* magazine. Figure 6.5 provides a schedule for immunizations.

A study done at the University of Washington, Seattle, reported that, in their first eight months, only 42% of

### KEY TERMS

**Immune response** body's reaction to first exposure to a pathogen

**Immunity** resistance to disease; may be natural or acquired

**Acquired immunity** protection from reacquiring an infectious disease because the first occurrence triggered specific antibodies against it

**Immunodeficiency** failure of the immune system to react to pathogens

**Autoimmunity** a disorder of the immune system in which the immune system attacks the body's own cells and tissues

**FIGURE 6.3** ▶ The Immune Response

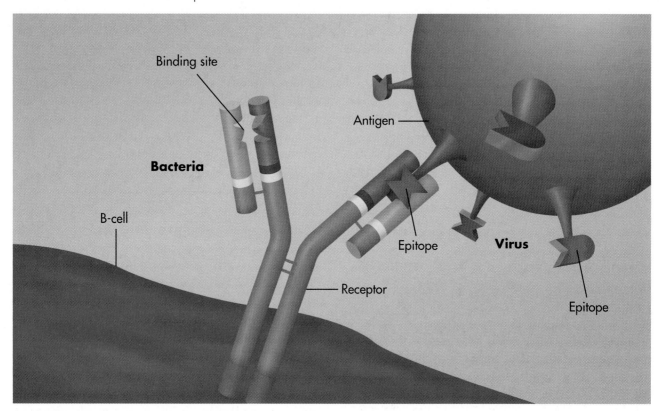

white infants and 29% of black infants received all their immunizations. Immunizations for preventable childhood diseases are available to everyone, regardless of ability to pay, at local branches of county public health depart-

ments. Table 6.2 presents a schedule of the childhood diseases for which immunizations have been developed. The schedule includes selected immunizations for adults in various situations.

**FIGURE 6.4** ▶ Types of Immunity

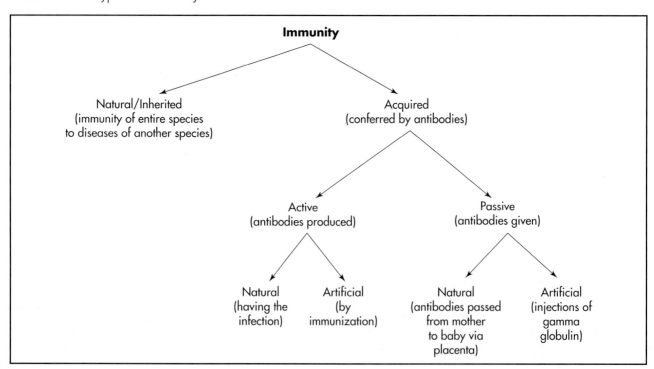

**Tips for Action** How to Avoid Colds and Cope with Colds

■ Wash your hands.

■ Keep your hands away from your eyes, nose, and mouth.

■ Avoid crowds.

■ Drink plenty of fluids. Drink at least eight ounces every two hours. Fluids, especially if hot, soothe the throat and help relieve congestion. Avoid alcoholic beverages because they tend to dehydrate the body.

■ Gargle with salt water. One teaspoon of salt in warm water every four hours is recommended. This helps to reduce swelling in the throat.

■ Get plenty of rest. Rest helps heal and restore.

■ Use disposable tissues instead of handkerchiefs. Handkerchiefs can harbor germs for up to several hours.

■ Inhale warm, moist air (steam). A vaporizer or humidifier, or pan of water on the stove, can be used. Take moderately warm to hot showers. These practices soothe inflamed mucous membranes.

■ Take medications only to relieve symptoms, and follow the advice on the label. Consult a physician if cold symptoms persist beyond a week.

*Source:* American Medical Security.

Even in America, pathogens remind us that being immunized for childhood diseases is still important and necessary for personal and public health. The mumps epidemic of 2006 was the largest reported in the United States since 1988. Since 2001, an average of 265 mumps cases are reported annually. However, from January 1 to May 2, 2006, 11 states (Illinois, Iowa, Kansas, Missouri, Nebraska, Pennsylvania, South Dakota, Wisconsin, Colorado, Minnesota, and Mississippi) reported 2,597 cases of mumps. The first cases in this outbreak were on a college campus in eastern Iowa (detected in December 2005). Are your immunizations up-to-date?

## Chronic Inflammation

When you "add insult to injury," the immune system responds with an -itis, the inflammatory reaction that alerts your body that all is not well. The body's classic responses to inflammation are redness and heat, tenderness and pain, and swelling. Although this chapter addresses conditions that cause inflammation, it is important to note that many noncommunicable, chronic health conditions are triggered by various "allergens" and produce inflammatory reactions in the body's major organs and systems. These conditions (acid reflux, arthritis, asthma, atherosclerosis, Crohn's disease, lupus) and the inflammatory responses related to them are addressed in Chapters 7 and 8.

## Common Infectious Diseases

With increased immunizations, as well as improved living standards, sanitation methods, and access to medical care, many infectious conditions are no longer considered threats to the public's health. Others, however, still undermine health, particularly in minority groups. Diseases thought to be eradicated have reemerged in some instances as health concerns.

## COMMON COLD

Of all human disease conditions, the cold, symptoms of which are depicted in Figure 6.6, is truly the most common. Most people have at least one cold a year, and as many as four may not be unusual. The **common cold** has been elusive in part because it can be caused by more than 200 different viruses. Colds are spread by droplets, such as are produced by sneezing. The virus enters the body through the mouth or nose. What differentiates a cold from other viral infections is the lack of high fever.

Symptoms of a cold appear one to three days after the person is infected. The first clues may be a scratchy throat or tickle in the throat, cough, tightness or dryness in the nose or throat, loss of appetite, and an out-of-sorts feeling. This is followed by additional symptoms such as a stuffy nose and sneezing. The illness usually is full-blown within 48–72 hours with teary eyes, runny nose, husky voice, difficult breathing, and dulled taste and smell sensations. Colds sometimes are accompanied by headache.

A cold typically lasts a week or two. Megadoses of vitamin C have been touted as a preventive measure, but many studies have shown no measurable effect. Antibiotics are not effective against colds.

### KEY TERMS

**Common cold** inflammation of the upper respiratory tract (nose and throat) caused by any of 200 or more viruses

**TABLE 6.1 ▶ Communicable Childhood Diseases**

| DISEASE | CHARACTERISTICS | DANGERS |
|---|---|---|
| Diphtheria | Bacterial disease usually affecting the throat and sometimes other mucous membranes and the skin. Sore throat, fever, and chills are the main manifestations. | Can make a child choke so badly that all breathing stops. Sometimes causes heart failure or pneumonia. |
| Hepatitis B | Blood-borne virus that damages the liver, passed to infant during pregnancy or birth. | Greatest danger is meningitis and also can cause pneumonia. |
| *Hib* or H-flu | Form of influenza. Children between six months and one year old are particularly susceptible. | Serious potential complication is meningitis. |
| Mumps | Swelling of salivary glands on one or both sides of the face, preceded by fever, headache, and vomiting. | Can cause deafness, diabetes, meningitis, encephalitis, and brain damage. In adult men can cause sterility. |
| Rubella (German measles) | Tends to be mild in children; greatest threat is to fetus of pregnant women in early pregnancy, when risk of deformed baby is up to 80%; miscarriage also common. Children usually receive vaccination (MMR) together against rubeola (measles) and mumps. | In a pregnant woman can cause miscarriage or lead to birth defects in the baby. |
| Rubeola (Red measles) | Symptoms similar to cold plus fever; affects respiratory system, skin, and eyes. Overt indication is the characteristic rash—small red spots on the body. | Can lead to pneumonia, blindness, ear infections and deafness, encephalitis, and brain damage. |
| Pertussis (Whooping cough) | Bacterial disease affecting mucous membranes lining the air passages. Cough for which it is named is a persistent, paroxysmal whooping that is the primary characteristic. | Can cause convulsions and brain damage. Pneumonia is a common complication. |
| Polio | Virus affecting central nervous system. Depending on the form, symptoms are flulike, affect respiration, involve muscle stiffness, weakness, and, in one variation, paralysis. No treatment is available, but development of vaccine in 1955 reduced incidence to near zero. | Often cripples and sometimes kills. If a child gets polio, little can be done. |
| Tetanus (Lockjaw) | Bacteria enter the body when something sharp such as a nail punctures or cuts the skin, or from abrasions or insect stings. Main characteristic is spasmodic contraction of muscles, first in the jaw and neck and later at other sites throughout the body. | High fever, convulsions, and pain are common. Can kill. |
| Varicella (Chickenpox) | Highly contagious viral disease that produces fever, nose and throat discharge, itching, pus-filled lesions on the body (sometimes on the scalp and in the mouth). | High fever, convulsions; before the vaccine (1995) annually—4 million cases, 13,500 hospitalizations, 150 deaths. |

Cold sufferers tend to rely on tried-and-true methods for relief from symptoms, the foremost of which are to get adequate rest, avoid chilling and extreme temperature changes, drink plenty of fluids (including juices), and eat nourishing foods. Commercial cold remedies on the market include the following.

- *Decongestants.* Shrink nasal blood vessels, relieving swelling and congestion, but may dry mucous membranes in the throat and worsen the condition.

- *Expectorants.* Stimulate the formation of respiratory secretions (phlegm), resulting in more but less viscous sputum. The Food and Drug Administration does not endorse expectorants, considering them ineffective.

- *Antitussives* (codeine and other drugs). Suppress coughing by blocking the cough centers in the brain. Their use may lead to failure to clear the lungs of phlegm and pathogens. Most appropriate for dry coughs.

- *Local anesthetics.* Suppress coughing. These throat lozenges and similar painkillers help relieve sore throat but are short-acting.

- *Analgesics* (aspirin, ibuprofen, acetaminophen). Help relieve muscle aches but may prolong the life of the cold. Even though **Reye's syndrome** is rare and is becoming even more uncommon, aspirin (or products containing aspirin) should not be administered to children who have colds or flulike symptoms or fever. Excessive long-term consumption of acetaminophen can lead to kidney failure.

Antihistamines are not used to treat cold symptoms. They are helpful only with allergies.

## INFLUENZA

**Influenza (flu)** can be mistaken for the common cold. Usually, however, it has more pronounced symptoms and more severe complications. Contrary to popular belief, flu

**FIGURE 6.5** ▶ Recommended Childhood Immunization Schedule, United States, 2006

## Recommended Childhood and Adolescent Immunization Schedule  UNITED STATES • 2006

| Vaccine ▾ / Age ▶ | Birth | 1 month | 2 months | 4 months | 6 months | 12 months | 15 months | 18 months | 24 months | 4–6 years | 11–12 years | 13–14 years | 15 years | 16–18 years |
|---|---|---|---|---|---|---|---|---|---|---|---|---|---|---|
| Hepatitis B[1] | HepB | HepB | | HepB[1] | | HepB | | | | | HepB Series | | | |
| Diphtheria, Tetanus, Pertussis[2] | | | DTaP | DTaP | DTaP | | DTaP | | | DTaP | Tdap | Tdap | | |
| Haemophilus influenzae type b[3] | | | Hib | Hib | Hib[3] | Hib | | | | | | | | |
| Inactivated Poliovirus | | | IPV | IPV | | IPV | | | | IPV | | | | |
| Measles, Mumps, Rubella[4] | | | | | | MMR | | | | MMR | MMR | | | |
| Varicella[5] | | | | | | Varicella | | | | Varicella | | | | |
| Meningococcal[6] | | | | | | | | | | MPSV4 | MCV4 | MCV4 / MCV4 | | |
| Pneumococcal[7] | | | PCV | PCV | PCV | PCV | | | | PCV | PPV | | | |
| Influenza[8] | | | | | Influenza (Yearly) | | | | | Influenza (Yearly) | | | | |
| Hepatitis A[9] | | | | | | | HepA Series | | | | | | | |

Vaccines within broken line are for selected populations

This schedule indicates the recommended ages for routine administration of currently licensed childhood vaccines, as of December 1, 2005, for children through age 18 years. Any dose not administered at the recommended age should be administered at any subsequent visit when indicated and feasible. ▮ Indicates age groups that warrant special effort to administer those vaccines not previously administered. Additional vaccines may be licensed and recommended during the year. Licensed combination vaccines may be used whenever any components of the combination are indicated and other components of the vaccine are not contraindicated and if approved by the Food and Drug Administration for that dose of the series. Providers should consult the respective ACIP statement for detailed recommendations. Clinically significant adverse events that follow immunization should be reported to the Vaccine Adverse Event Reporting System (VAERS). Guidance about how to obtain and complete a VAERS form is available at **www.vaers.hhs.gov** or by telephone, **800-822-7967.**

▢ **Range of recommended ages**   ▮ **Catch-up immunization**   ▮ **11—12 year old assessment**

*Source:* Centers for Disease Control and Prevention and the Advisory Committee on Immunization Practices (ACIP).

Note: Bars in the figure indicate ranges of recommended ages for immunization. Any dose not given at the recommended age should be given as a catch-up immunization at a subsequent visit when indicated and feasible. Additional vaccines may be licensed and recommended during the year.

viruses do not cause the nausea, vomiting, and diarrhea of the so-called stomach flu or intestinal flu. Those diseases are caused by other pathogens. Flu is an infection of the nose, throat, bronchial tubes, and lungs caused by specific influenza viruses. The disease is spread by droplets from sneezing and coughing.

Flu is caused primarily by two main types of viruses, the A virus and the B virus. Each has several strains named for their place of origin, such as the Hong Kong flu virus. Flu viruses are unique in that once a strain has spread in a population, its structure changes and it then is capable of causing a new form of flu because the antibodies produced to combat the original virus are not effective against the new form. An entirely new strain appears about every 10 years. Flu viruses may be particularly virulent because they are airborne viruses, which are easily transmittable.

Flu symptoms include high fever, chills, headache, muscle aches, and fatigue. Those infected also may have a dry cough and inflamed nasal passages. Flu usually has to run its course and is treated only by relieving the symptoms. Treatment is the same, in general, as that for colds. Some forms of flu are treated by aspirin substitutes, particularly amantadine hydrochloride.

By way of prevention, vaccines are administered to those who seek it, mainly aging people and those with chronic diseases. Vaccines are said to be 67% to 92% effective in preventing the flu. Because the strains of the flu virus are different each flu season, the flu vaccine should be taken annually.

## STREP THROAT

A sore throat may be a symptom of a cold or flu, or it may signal a more serious streptococcal infection, particularly if the sore throat is accompanied by fever, aching, and fatigue. To be on the safe side, the affected person should see a health professional.

### KEY TERMS

**Reye's syndrome** a disease that affects the brain of children ages two to 16 years following a viral infection; associated with aspirin

**Influenza (flu)** a viral infection of the nose, throat, bronchial tubes, and lungs

The only way to diagnose **strep throat** is through a throat culture, the results of which can be obtained in minutes. Strep throat is extremely contagious. Because it is caused by bacteria, it is treated by antibiotics to halt progression of the disease to possible rheumatic fever.

**FIGURE 6.6 ▶** Symptoms of the Common Cold

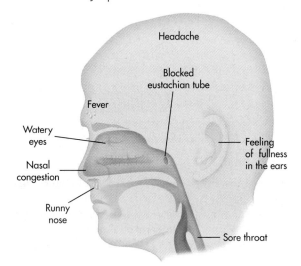

| FYI IS IT A COLD OR THE FLU? | | |
|---|---|---|
| **Symptom** | **Cold** | **Flu** |
| Fever | Rare | Characteristic, high (102°–104°); lasts three to four days |
| Headache | Rare | Prominent |
| General aches, pains | Slight | Usual; often severe |
| Fatigue, weakness | Mild | Can last up to two to three weeks |
| Extreme exhaustion | Never | Early and prominent |
| Stuffy nose | Common | Sometimes |
| Sneezing | Usual | Sometimes |
| Sore throat | Common | Sometimes |
| Chest discomfort, cough | Mild to moderate; hacking cough | Common; can become severe |

*Source*: Tamar Nordenberg, "Colds and Flu: Time Only Sure Cure," *FDA Consumer*, October 1996, pp. 15–18; table, p. 16.

**TABLE 6.2 ▶** Recommended Immunization Against Infectious Diseases—United States—2006

| IMMUNIZATION | CHILDREN | ADULTS |
|---|---|---|
| **Diphtheria, pertussis, tetanus combination (DTaP)** | 2, 4, 6, and 15–18 months and at 4–6 years (before or at school entry) | Not applicable |
| **Diphtheria, tetanus booster (Tdap)** | 13–18 years | Every 10 years |
| **Poliomyelitis (IPV)** | 2, 4, and 15–18 months and at 4–6 years | Those who might be exposed (those in health and sanitation occupations, travelers); normally no booster needed |
| **Measles (rubeola), mumps, rubella combination (MMR)** | 12–15 months and just before entering school | Adults under age 32 who received only one measles shot at one year of age or after; adults whose initial dose was given along with immunoglobulin—as routinely occurred from 1963 to 1975—should get two doses at least one month apart |
| ***Hib* type B** | 2, 4, 6, and 12–15 months | Not applicable |
| **Varicella, (chickenpox)** | 12, 15, or 18 months and 4–6 yrs | All adults without evidence of immunity to varicella (e.g., child care employees, teachers of young children, college students) |
| **Influenza** | Not applicable | Yearly, because of the changeability of viral strains |
| **Tuberculosis (TB)** | Those exposed to individuals with active tuberculosis | Those exposed to individuals with active tuberculosis |
| **Pneumococcal pneumonia (PCV)** | 2, 4, and 6 months | 65 years (1 dose); others as recommended |
| **Hepatitis B (Hep B)** | Birth | Those who may be exposed: indications – medical, occupational, behavioral, other (e.g., international travelers, clients of STD clinics, inmates of correctional facilities) |

*Source:* Centers for Disease Control and Prevention and the Advisory Committee on Immunization Practices (ACIP).

Diagnosis is obtained from blood samples. The best treatment is rest and plenty of liquids. Viruses do not respond to antibiotics. If mono is accompanied by strep throat, an antibiotic is prescribed to treat that condition. In severe cases, corticosteroid drugs are prescribed.

## CHRONIC FATIGUE SYNDROME

The cause of **chronic fatigue syndrome (CFS)** is still unknown to the medical community. Some professionals consider it to be a recurring form of mononucleosis and link it to the Epstein-Barr virus. The defining characteristic is found in its name—fatigue—and other symptoms are similar to mono, including aches and pains, swollen lymph glands, and low-grade fever. The symptoms may last from six months to several years, off and on.

According to one group of professionals, the Chronic Fatigue Immune Dysfunction Syndrome (CFIDS) Foundation in San Francisco, chronic fatigue syndrome seems to combine both autoimmune and immunodeficiency disorders. The immune cells act as if they are constantly battling a viral infection. The CFIDS Foundation says the disease affects about 1 million Americans, 70% to 85% of them women. Other estimates of incidence are as high as 3 million.

The British and Canadians call this disease myalgic encephalomyelitis; the Japanese call it low-natural-killer-cell syndrome; and some patients' groups call it chronic-fatigue-immune-dysfunction syndrome. No procedure is available yet to diagnose this condition. And, although analgesics, antidepressants, and complete rest have been tried, no specific treatment has been found to be effective for all patients. This mysterious disease continues to baffle the medical community.

## HEPATITIS

**Hepatitis** is a general term describing liver infections. Five types of viral hepatitis have been identified. All cause serious infections that can damage the liver, which can result in cirrhosis and the need for a liver transplant. Although it has missed the attention of many whose work is not related

---

| Characteristic | Strep | Cold |
|---|---|---|
| Onset | Rapid | Slower |
| Soreness | Marked | Less marked |
| Fever, aches, malaise | Marked | Mild |
| Respiratory symptoms | Present in half of cases | Present in most cases |
| Lymph nodes | Large and tender | No enlargement or tenderness |
| Complications | Rheumatic fever, streptococcal pneumonia, middle-ear infection, mastoiditis, nephritis | Bacterial sinusitis, middle-ear infection |
| Treatment | Antibiotics | Over-the-counter medications, gargling with salt water |

**FYI** — IS IT STREP OR A COLD?

*Source:* American Pharmaceutical Association and Dr. Jack Gwaltney, a cold expert at the University of Virginia School of Medicine in Charlottesville. Originally printed in *American Health*, December 1994.

Note: Any sore throat that lasts longer than 10 days or seems especially severe should be treated by a doctor.

## MONONUCLEOSIS

Infectious **mononucleosis,** better known as mono, is a contagious viral illness that attacks the lymph nodes in the neck and the throat, resulting in prolonged weakness, sore throat, swelling of the nodes, headache, fever, and nausea. Mono is caused by the Epstein-Barr virus and is spread by contact with droplets from the mouth and throat of a person infected with the virus. This has led to the descriptor "kissing disease." In addition, sharing drinking glasses and eating utensils or toothbrushes or touching something that has been in contact with the mouth of an infected person may transmit the virus.

Teens and young adults are the most susceptible to mono, although cases have been found in children less than a year old. It is rare in individuals over age 35. Most cases simply run a course over six to eight weeks, but sometimes it lasts as long as six months. Occasionally the infection spreads to the liver, causing jaundice (yellow-appearing skin and whites of the eyes), or to the spleen, which could burst.

### KEY TERMS

**Strep throat** an extremely contagious infection caused by a bacteria and treated with antibiotics

**Mononucleosis** a contagious viral illness that attacks the lymph nodes in the neck and throat; commonly called mono

**Chronic fatigue syndrome (CFS)** a viral illness that produces extreme fatigue and other symptoms similar to mononucleosis

**Hepatitis** inflammation of the liver caused by a virus; several types have been identified

to health care, the hepatitis C virus is responsible for a "liver-disease epidemic." In the United States, hepatitis C causes more infections than the virus that causes AIDS.

- *Hepatitis A.* The hepatitis A virus (HAV) lives in feces and can be transmitted through contaminated food, water, and bivalve mollusks such as oysters and clams. The major source of infection is personal contact with someone who has hepatitis A. Symptoms include fatigue, nausea, vomiting, abdominal discomfort, dark urine, and jaundice (yellowish discoloration of the eyes and skin). The Food and Drug Administration has approved the vaccine Havrix to protect individuals from contracting hepatitis A. Immunoglobulin is administered for short-term protection and for persons already exposed to hepatitis A.

- *Hepatitis B.* The hepatitis B virus (HBV) lives in the blood and other body fluids and can be transmitted sexually, by sharing contaminated needles, and may be passed by infected mothers to newborns. While some persons are asymptomatic, symptoms of hepatitis B include loss of appetite, nausea, vomiting, fever, fatigue, dark urine, or jaundice. Untreated HBV damages the liver and causes cirrhosis of the liver and liver cancer. Since 1983, a safe and effective vaccine for HBV has made this infection entirely preventable. In the United States, newborns are routinely vaccinated, and HBV is now uncommon.

- *Hepatitis C.* The hepatitis C virus (HCV) lives in the blood. HCV has been dubbed "America's emerging epidemic." Because HCV is a "stealth" virus, symptoms may not appear until 20 or more years after transmission and infection. It is estimated that by the year 2015, there will be more than 19,000 deaths attributed to complications from HCV. It is the most common chronic blood-borne infection in the United States, with an estimated 3.2 million people currently infected. However, the Centers for Disease Control and Prevention (CDC) estimates that 4.1 million persons have infections and that most are chronic. Approximately 10,000 people die annually from cirrhosis, liver cancer, or liver failure due to HCV infection. It is the major reason for liver transplants in the United States. Hepatitis C is most commonly found in persons who have received blood transfusions and those who inject drugs. The virus can be transmitted through pricks by contaminated needles (mainly a risk for health care workers) and sharing razors or toothbrushes with an infected person. It is found more frequently in countries where the blood supply is not screened properly. The rates for sexual transmission are low; however, the virus can be transmitted through high-risk sexual activities (having multiple partners or failing to use condoms). In addition, HCV can be transmitted by snorting cocaine or other drugs using shared paraphernalia and by nonsterile instruments used in tattooing or body piercing. More than half of infected persons experience no symptoms. Symptoms include loss of appetite, fatigue, dark-yellow urine or light-colored stools, and jaundice.

Despite its being the nation's most common blood-borne infection, hepatitis C is not acquired through casual contact (shaking hands, hugging, or sharing eating utensils) with an HCV-infected person. The treatment does not kill the virus; it boosts the infected person's immune system. Currently, the treatment consists of weekly injections (for six months to a year) of the drug interferon alpha in combination with the antiviral drug ribavirin, which is a tablet. Because of the side effects of the medication (depression, fatigue, and GI upset), about 20% of the patients stop the therapy. Pharmaceutical research is ongoing to develop medications (similar to those combination therapies used to treat HIV) that will target areas of the virus and hinder its replication and spread to the liver. There is no vaccine to prevent HCV infection. Persons working in health care settings receive training about exposure risks and are required to take the test for HCV (and other blood-borne pathogens) if exposed to body fluids. Before you decide that you are not at risk for hepatitis C, review the following and make an informed decision.

> **RISKS FOR HCV** *Go to your local public health department, not-for-profit health care facility, or private physician for a blood test for HCV if you have a tattoo (contaminated ink or unsterile needles) and/or body piercing (unsterile equipment), inject drugs or did so (even once and/or "a long time ago when I was experimenting"), received blood-clotting products before 1987 or a blood transfusion or organ/tissue donation before 1993, received (receiving) kidney dialysis, were born to a mother infected with HCV, or have been informed by your health practitioner that your liver enzymes are abnormal.*

- *Hepatitis D.* The hepatitis D virus (HDV) can infect only individuals who are infected with hepatitis B, as it needs the genetic material of that virus to reproduce. It is transmitted in the same ways as hepatitis B. The symptoms for hepatitis D are the same as those for hepatitis B, but typically more severe. Interferon alpha for hepatitis B may have some effect as treatment.

- *Hepatitis E.* The hepatitis E virus (HEV) is found in feces and can be spread by sewage-contaminated water and contaminated undercooked shellfish, fruits, and vegetables. The symptoms include abdominal pain, dark urine, fever, jaundice, nausea, and vomiting. There is no drug treatment or vaccination for hepatitis E. This virus is found rarely in the United States.

## PNEUMONIA

**Pneumonia** can be caused by either bacteria or viruses as well as by environmental chemicals. This infection typically follows a cold or the flu but may be a primary infection.

The four major symptoms are chest pain, abrupt rise in body temperature, coughing, and difficulty breathing. In one type, called walking pneumonia, the only symptom at first may be the cough. Eventual diagnosis by x-ray will reveal the presence of pneumonia. Additional diagnostic measures include analysis of the sputum and listening to the chest with a stethoscope to detect any fluid present in the lungs.

Viral pneumonia generally is treated by bed rest, a high fluid intake, a light diet, and painkillers as necessary. Bacterial pneumonia is treated with antibiotics such as penicillin, plus rest. Conditions that make a person more vulnerable to pneumonia include poor nutrition, chronic bronchitis, emphysema, cancer, alcoholism, sickle cell anemia, and AIDS. People in these risk groups should get a one-time vaccination for pneumococcal pneumonia, which provides protection against most pneumonias. Over-the-counter (OTC) pain relievers, antihistamines, and decongestants can relieve the symptoms. Pneumonia, however, should be treated by a medical professional.

## TUBERCULOSIS

One of the leading causes of death at the turn of the 20th century was **tuberculosis (TB).** During the 1950s TB was virtually put in check by the development of effective antibiotics to treat the infection. Now TB seems to be defying modern medicine and coming back. In 1985 the reported number of cases in the United States was 22,201. By 1992 that number had reached 26,673. Tuberculosis cases began to decline in 1994. There were 16,377 cases reported by the Centers for Disease Control and Prevention in 2000 (latest surveillance data available). It is the leading cause of death by acute infectious diseases other than pneumonia. According to the World Health Organization and the CDC, an estimated 90 million new cases of TB may cause up to 30 million deaths worldwide in the next five years.

One reason for the rising number of TB cases is its association with HIV. HIV-infected individuals are susceptible to other infections including TB because HIV has weakened the immune system. Another reason for the rising rates of TB is that some TB microbes have become strong enough to withstand the drugs that formerly wiped them out. Still, according to Dr. Lee Reichman of the National Tuberculosis Center in Newark, New Jersey, almost all TB is preventable and treatable.

Tuberculosis is caused by the rod-shaped bacterium *Mycobacterium tuberculosis.* The pathogen is spread from person to person through nasal, throat, and lung discharges emitted into the air when an infected person sneezes, coughs, or laughs. Typically, the TB bacteria cause infection in the lungs, but the brain, spine, and other parts of the body may be affected, too.

Anyone can be infected with TB. A person who has been exposed to the TB bacteria may have the TB infection for years but not be aware of it because of the absence of symptoms. If this person is exposed to HIV and becomes infected, the virus weakens the person's immune system and the symptoms of TB appear, first as the prodromal symptoms of fatigue, weight loss, fever, and night sweats. As the condition worsens, symptoms of TB of the lung include a long-term cough, pain in the chest, and coughing blood. These symptoms also apply to several other communicable diseases, so an accurate diagnosis is essential. Also, an early diagnosis is advantageous because TB infection now can be treated by medication before it progresses to TB disease.

The **tuberculin test** is done to diagnose TB infection. Individuals who have a positive reaction are advised to have a follow-up chest x-ray. If the person is found to have TB, he or she is advised and treated appropriately.

Some people with concurrent HIV and TB infections do not react to the TB skin test. Individuals who are HIV-infected and have a negative skin test for TB but have the symptoms of TB infection should have other diagnostic tests to make certain they do not have TB. Untreated TB progressively damages the lungs and can be fatal.

## LYME DISEASE

**Lyme disease** is the best known of the tick-borne diseases. It is carried by a tick (see Figure 6.7) that lives on deer, mice, and other small mammals. The deaths of some people in the late 1980s brought this infectious disease to national prominence. Outbreaks occurred predominantly along the Atlantic coast and in California, Minnesota, Oregon, and Wisconsin.

The disease progresses in stages. The first symptom usually is a rash that erupts two days to five weeks after a tick bite, sometimes accompanied by flulike symptoms. During the second stage, which occurs weeks to months later in 10% to 20% of untreated individuals, the infected person may develop an abnormal heart rhythm, impaired coordination, partial facial paralysis, severe headaches, and memory lapses. These symptoms usually disappear in

### KEY TERMS

**Pneumonia** an inflammation of the bronchial tubes and air sacs of the lungs

**Tuberculosis (TB)** a bacterial infection in the lungs characterized by coughing blood, pain in the chest, fever, and fatigue

**Tuberculin test** a skin test used to diagnose tuberculosis

**Lyme disease** a bacterial infection transmitted by a tick bite

**FIGURE 6.7** ▶ Lyme Disease Is Spread by a Tick That Lives on Mammals

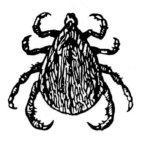

a few weeks. About half of untreated people have chronic or recurring inflammation of the joints, which may be related to a hereditary factor. The disease also can cause miscarriages and birth defects.

Antibiotics are used to treat Lyme disease in its early stages, but preventive measures are best. Two vaccines being tested could halt the disease by killing the Lyme spirochete inside the tick's body as soon as it bites. Precautions include wearing long pants instead of shorts when walking through woods or high grass, using insect repellents containing DEET or a clothing spray containing the insecticide permethrin, and knowing how to identify and remove a tick. A tick may be removed by grasping its mouthparts with tweezers as close to the skin as possible and pulling the entire tick out slowly and steadily. If a tick is on a person less than 24 hours, he or she stands a good chance of not contracting the disease.

Domestic animals can bring the tick indoors with them and can be infected with the disease. Before allowing pets in the house after they have been outdoors, they should be checked for ticks.

## ENCEPHALITIS AND MENINGITIS

West Nile virus encephalitis continues to make news. West Nile virus is an arthropod-borne pathogen that infects birds (crows and exotic birds) and horses. It is spread to humans by mosquito vectors. State surveillance programs are on alert to report infections. Symptoms include fever, headache, muscle weakness and diminished reflexes, and confusion. In extreme cases, the inflammation of the brain can cause permanent neurological damage and death. Precautions against West Nile virus encephalitis infection include using insect repellent containing DEET and wearing long pants and long-sleeved shirts.

## EMERGING AND REEMERGING COMMUNICABLE DISEASES AND THEIR GLOBAL IMPLICATIONS

In the United States, at the beginning of the 20th century, the leading causes of death were communicable diseases (TB, smallpox), not diseases of the heart and

cancers. Advances in science, medicine, and public health helped to make the most deadly communicable diseases an afterthought in this country. However, discoveries and events in the 21st century once again require governmental agencies to predict and plan for communicable conditions as public health threats. This section highlights selected emerging communicable diseases and conditions.

*Anthrax.* The good news is that this condition cannot be transmitted from person to person and that this acute infectious disease is rare in the United States. Anthrax is caused by the bacteria *Bacillus anthracis* that is found in wild animals or cattle, goats, and sheep that ingest anthrax spores from the soil as they graze. The spores can live in the soil for years. Anthrax can infect humans if contaminated animal products are handled, the spores from them are inhaled, or if undercooked meat from a contaminated animal is eaten. Barring exposure to the spores in a bioterrorism attack, the risk of being infected with anthrax is very low. Until recently, the cases of anthrax reported in this country were due to industrial exposure (workers in wool, animal hide/hair industries). The three clinical forms of anthrax infection are: cutaneous or skin, which is the most common form; inhalation; and gastrointestinal. Of the three forms of the disease, inhalation anthrax is the most deadly. After the spores reach the lungs, the bacteria secrete three anthrax-toxin proteins that are lethal to cells. There is a 75% chance that inhalation anthrax will cause death. The symptoms of inhalation anthrax begin with a sore throat, dry cough, fever, muscle aches, chest pain, and fatigue and after several days progress to severe breathing problems and shock. Treatment for anthrax is antibiotics and supportive care.

In February of 2006, anthrax made national news when it was reported that a 44-year-old man (a drum maker from New York) collapsed and was diagnosed and treated for inhalation anthrax at a hospital in Pennsylvania. Investigation by the health departments in both states determined that the source of the man's infection was spores that he inhaled from the hair on the unprocessed animal hides (domestic and imported) that he used to make his drums. Even though the risk of infection is low, if you play drums made of unprocessed hides or have purchased a souvenir drum made from unprocessed hides and experience any unexplained symptoms (fever, skin lesions), report the symptoms and your exposure to your physician.

*Avian Influenza (Bird Flu).* This disease is caused by the virulent avian influenza virus (the variant H5N1 in humans) that usually infects birds (chickens) and water fowl (ducks and swans). Since 1997, 140 million birds (including those destroyed to prevent the spread) have been killed in East Asia. From 1997 to 2005, human cases of bird flu and deaths were reported in Hong Kong (1997),

Thailand, Vietnam, Laos, Cambodia, and Indonesia. In 2005, the virus was discovered in birds in China, Mongolia, Russia, and in countries as far from East Asia as Turkey, Greece, Romania, Macedonia, Croatia, and countries in Africa. For years, this virus rarely produced infection in humans (except for those with occupations related to bird handling). In 2006, 22 deaths from bird flu in humans were reported in Indonesia.

Persons coming in contact with a sick bird's nasal secretions, saliva, or feces are exposed to the virus and are at risk. Unlike other flu viruses that attach to the mucous membranes of the nose and throat, the H5N1 bird-flu virus (or its mutations) "goes for the jugular," attacking the lungs, targeting the alveoli. Symptoms (which usually appear within 48 hours) include high fever, cough and chest pain, difficulty breathing, diarrhea, and bloody nose and gums. Infected persons are isolated and administered the antiviral medications Tamiflu or Relenza. The H5N1 bird flu should be diagnosed and treated immediately to reduce the risk of health complications that include encephalitis; pneumonia; and heart, kidney, and lung failure that can cause death. Presently, there is no vaccine (to confer artificial active acquired immunity—Figure 6.4) to protect against bird flu in humans.

Besides frequent hand washing with soap and water and not eating undercooked eggs and poultry, what can you do to reduce your risk? Public health and medical experts recommend the following: get your annual flu vaccine to protect the respiratory tract against other types of influenza; avoid travel to countries affected by avian influenza (information available on CDC's website); do not visit farms or live animal markets; if you develop a fever or respiratory tract symptoms within 10 days after your travel, alert your physician; practice "social distancing," that is, avoid close contact with people (at large conferences and public events) during the flu season; properly dispose of tissue used when coughing and sneezing. Your state (commonwealth, district, territory) health department's website has valuable information (to include plans in case of an epidemic) about avian influenza. Familiarize yourself and be proactive, not reactive.

The worldwide impact of H5N1 bird flu has the World Health Organization (WHO) and others in the international health community working in concert to control and reduce the spread of this deadly illness. Presently, bird flu has killed more than 110 people; its mortality rate is 50%. Why the lightning response to this communicable disease? It is a rush to prevent a global health disaster, a **pandemic.** First, humans have little or no natural immunity to the bird-flu virus. Second, the virus is just an "international flight away"—the avian influenza virus is carried by migratory waterfowl that contract the virus in contaminated lakes; therefore the virus moves between countries and continents (Asia to Alaska). Third, in the summer of 2006, the first suspected cases of person-to-

person transmission were reported in a village in North Sumatra, Indonesia. A woman and six of her relatives died after exposure to the woman who was sick with H5N1 bird-flu virus. How she was infected is being investigated; neither she nor her family were poultry workers. Has H5N1 bird-flu virus "morphed" into human-to-human transmission? Was the virus spread through coughing, food, or fomites? This has not been determined. If human-to-human transmission is possible, WHO expects that the modes of transmission would be through coughing, sneezing, and kissing. At least 40 countries (including the United States) have developed "sound" pandemic plans for bird flu. Public health measures to slow a pandemic include production of an effective vaccine, the ability to regulate the movement of people, quarantine and isolation, and moving adequate supplies of medications and personnel where needed.

***Bedbugs.*** Yes, they are back. The resurgence of this pest in the urban centers of industrial nations is a 21st-century example of "the revenge of the cooties." The common bedbug, or *Cimex lectularius*, is a blood-sucking insect that grows up to 7 mm in length. Bedbugs have a lifespan from four to 12 months. They hide in cracks and

---

### IS YOUR COLLEGE "ON LOCK" TO STOP H5N1—BIRD FLU?

*Picture an influenza epidemic in your hometown. In ordinary circumstances, the typical flu virus preys on the vulnerable, very young children, seniors, the frail, and those with compromised immune systems. Those are the folks who are given priority when it's time for flu shots. Now picture an epidemic of bird flu in your hometown and on your college campus. These circumstances are not ordinary, and this virus is far from typical. The H5N1 virus has an affinity for the young and able-bodied. The U.S. Department of Health and Human Services estimates that from 209,000 to 1.9 million people in this country could die if H5N1 has the ability to pass from person to person. If someone on your campus is hospitalized for possible bird flu infection, the responsibility of providing medications to those students and staff who might have come in contact with the victim is that of your college health service, not the governmental agencies that are stockpiling Tamiflu. Remember to be proactive. "How has our college prepared for H5N1 bird flu?" is the question that you should be asking your campus health services director.*

crevices of wooden bed frames, baseboards, furniture, and walls by day. They emerge at night to feed on their human hosts. Bedbugs can infest bed linen and mattresses. Unlike other insect parasites discussed in this chapter, bedbugs probably will not be seen. The common symptoms of bedbug bites (the host's reaction to the saliva of the bedbug) are clusters of raised red bumps that itch. Treatment of the symptoms includes the application of topical anti-itch medicines or topical corticosteroids and oral antihistamines.

Nationally, there have been reports of more calls to pest control companies and public health departments about residential infestations. Contrary to what many people believe, bedbugs can infest anyone, not just persons living in shelters. The results of a Canadian study of the problem in urban environments were the following: the majority of the reported bedbug infestations were in single-family dwellings (70%), apartment units (18%), and homeless shelters (8%). There were reports from hotels, community centers, and university dormitories. The study did not determine the reason for the resurgence of bedbug infestations; however, the authors of the study suggested that the increase in world travel and the reluctance to use insecticides (due to toxicity) may be factors.

To reduce your risk of infestation, do not unpack your luggage on your bed, vacuum luggage after traveling, and wash garments after traveling. Infestation occurring in a residence should be handled by a professional pest control service. They will spray approved insecticide in the places where bedbugs hide, vacuum the affected areas, and steam clean and vacuum mattresses.

**Smallpox.** This contagious disease is caused by the variola virus. It is spread by face-to-face contact or direct contact with body fluids from an infected person. Additionally, infection can occur if there is contact with linens or clothing that are contaminated with variola. The incubation period is seven to 17 days. The symptoms progress as follows: high fever, fatigue, headache and body aches; rash that appears in the mouth and on the tongue and skin (face, arms, legs, hands, feet); rash progresses to raised bumps, pustules, crusts, and then to scabs. The scabs fall off, leaving scars. The person is contagious until the last scab falls off (about three weeks after the rash first appeared). About 30% of the cases are fatal. Thanks to the invention of the smallpox vaccination in 1796 and the required vaccinations during the 20th century, the last outbreak of smallpox in the United States was 1949. Routine vaccinations in the United States ended in 1972.

The World Health Organization (WHO) set as its goal to eradicate smallpox from "the earth." Even though the disease was not a public health problem in industrialized countries, it was one of the leading causes of morbidity (permanent disfigurement or blindness) and mortality in Brazil, South Asia, and most parts of the continent of Africa. During the 20th century, smallpox killed 300 million people worldwide. Because of required immunizations in the industrialized countries and the work of Dr. D. A. Henderson and the WHO team to immunize the populations of countries with epidemics, WHO declared smallpox eradicated in 1980. The last human case of naturally occurring smallpox was in 1977 in Somalia. Because smallpox infects only humans and the signs of infection are distinct (visible rash that leaves pockmarks), the disease is easily identified and primary and secondary contacts of the infected person can be vaccinated to prevent its spread. Even though there have been no reported cases in the last 29 years, the threat of bioterrorism has made it necessary to revisit public health strategies to quickly identify smallpox, notify the contacts, and vaccinate those who have been exposed.

***"9/11 Illness" and Hurricane Katrina Fungi.*** The mental and emotional health effects on the survivors of the terrorists' acts on September 11, 2001, and Hurricanes Katrina and Rita on the Gulf Coasts of Louisiana, Mississippi, and Alabama have been documented. The World Trade Center Health Registry is a system that monitors the physical and mental health of 71,437 enrollees for 20 years. The analysis of data from 8,400 adult survivors (excluding rescue/recovery personnel) who were caught in the clouds of dust and debris of the collapsed World Trade Center towers revealed the following reported health problems: new or worsened respiratory problems—56.6%, heartburn/acid reflux—23.9%, and severe headache—21%. Additionally, almost 11% screened positive for serious psychological distress.

The New Orleans Mold Project is a planned scientific investigation of the levels of mold and bacterial endotoxins in posthurricane New Orleans homes. One of the goals of the investigation is to determine which properties of molds impact health. In the fall of 2005, the CDC found that 46% of the inspected homes had visible mold growth and that the residents and workers did not consistently use appropriate respiratory protection equipment. Since the hurricane, residents have reported respiratory symptoms, nose and throat irritation, and coughing ("Katrina cough"). As much of the governmental and academic infrastructure of New Orleans was destroyed or damaged by the hurricanes, continuing investigations by the CDC and other agencies will be challenging.

## SEXUALLY TRANSMITTED INFECTIONS

**Sexually transmitted diseases** are like other communicable diseases in that they are caused and spread by identifiable pathogens, have definite courses of development, and can be treated. Most are curable. These pathogens thrive on warm, moist body surfaces or in body fluids. The pathogens can be exchanged during sexual acts or close physical contact with reproductive structures.

No one has or can develop immunity to any STD. Consequently, having an STD does not protect a person from acquiring it again in the future. Anyone who is sexually active may be exposed to the pathogens causing STDs.

## FYI | MYTHS ABOUT AIDS

These statements are all untrue.

- You can get AIDS by donating blood.
- You can get AIDS through casual contact, such as shaking hands with or hugging an infected person.
- You can catch AIDS if an infected person coughs or sneezes on you.
- You can get AIDS if you play sports with an infected person.
- You can get AIDS from a mosquito.
- You can get AIDS from your doctor or dentist.
- AIDS could spread rapidly through the general population.
- Only gay people get AIDS.
- If you are not gay and do not shoot drugs, you are safe.
- If you do not have symptoms, you are not contagious.
- If you did something risky only once, you cannot get AIDS.
- If you are HIV-positive, you will know it from the symptoms.
- If you test positive for HIV, you have AIDS.
- Abstinence is the only way to protect yourself against AIDS.

**TABLE 6.3 ▶** Classifications of Common Sexually Transmitted Diseases

| TYPE | DISEASE |
| --- | --- |
| Bloodborne | HIV/AIDS<br>Syphilis<br>Hepatitis B |
| Causing vaginitis, cervicitis, or urethritis | Chlamydia<br>Gonorrhea<br>Trichomoniasis<br>Candidiasis |
| Producing lesions | Herpes<br>Genital warts |
| Caused by insect parasites | Pubic lice<br>Scabies |

STDs, race and ethnic risk factors may correlate with other determinants of health status including socioeconomic status, access to quality health care, and reporting biases.

**Risks for STDs.** Various risk factors for STDs have been identified. Upon examining these carefully, two factors emerge as the primary contributors to risk: sex acts without using prophylactics (latex condoms) and unprotected sex acts with multiple partners or with individuals who have multiple partners. Most of the common STDs may be grouped as:

- Being bloodborne (HIV/AIDS, syphilis, hepatitis B); these STDs can damage many body systems after primary invasion of the circulatory system by their causative agents
- Causing vaginitis or urethritis
- Producing lesions
- Being caused by insect parasites

Some of the STDs fall into more than one category because of multiple symptoms that appear during the course of the disease. Table 6.3 gives examples from each category.

## HIV INFECTION AND AIDS

Why is the date June 5, 1981, one that persons who have spent their lives working to reduce the cases of STDs a date to be remembered? This date will always be significant because it officially marked the AIDS epidemic in the United States. Published in the June 5, 1981, issue of the

Statistically, the number of reported cases is highest for 18- to 35-year-olds. More than 25 diseases are spread through sexual contact. About one in four adults in the United States has an STD.

**Incidence of STDs.** The incidence of STDs has surged in recent years. Five of the 10 most common diseases reported to the CDC in 1995 were STDs. The United States has the highest rate of curable STDs of any developed country, according to William Butler of Baylor College of Medicine. More than 12 million people in the United States are newly infected each year, a fourth of whom are teenagers.

Wide discrepancies are found among ethnic groups. For example, the gonorrhea rate for black adolescents is more than 26 times greater than the rate among the corresponding white population. The rate of syphilis in blacks is nearly 60 times that in whites. Syphilis also is about four times as prevalent in Hispanics as in whites. Although no known biologic reasons to explain why racial or ethnic factors alone should influence the risk for contracting

### KEY TERMS

**Sexually transmitted diseases (STDs)** illnesses caused by pathogens that are transmitted during sexual acts

## HIV/AIDS Timeline—Selected Events That Changed the Nation

| | |
|---|---|
| 1981 | CDC reports the first cases of a rare pneumonia (PCP) and a type of skin cancer (KS) in homosexual males. |
| 1982 | The term Acquired Immune Deficiency Syndrome (AIDS) is adopted by CDC (replaced "gay-related immunodeficiency;" GRID). |
| 1984 | Scientists in America and France identify the pathogen that causes AIDS-HIV (HTLV-III and LAV, respectively). |
| 1985 | Rock Hudson, the actor, announces that he has AIDS. |
| 1986 | Surgeon General C. Everett Koop calls for condom use and AIDS education as measures to reduce the spread of AIDS. |
| 1987 | FDA approves AZT for the treatment of AIDS; AIDS Memorial Quilt displayed on the National Mall, Washington, DC<br>*And the Band Played On* by Randy Shilts, the definitive nonfiction book about the AIDS epidemic in America, is published. |
| 1991 | The "Red Ribbon" is adopted as an international symbol for HIV/AIDS advocacy.<br>Ervin "Magic" Johnson announces that he is HIV-positive and retires from the NBA. |
| 1994 | AIDS is the leading cause of death for males ages 25–44 years. |
| 1995 | The first White House Conference on HIV/AIDS.<br>Protease inhibitors, a new class of medications to treat HIV, are marketed. |
| 1996 | FDA approves the first consumer-controlled test kit (home test kit) for HIV. |
| 1998 | CDC announces that African Americans account for 49 percent of all AIDS-related deaths. |
| 1999 | The origins of AIDS (chimps) identified by researchers at the University of Alabama, Birmingham (UAB). |
| 2001 | An estimated 700,000 HIV-positive persons are living in the United States. |
| 2006 | UNAIDS estimates that 40.3 million people worldwide are living with HIV; 25 million have died from AIDS. |

CDC's *Morbidity and Mortality Weekly Report (MMWR)* was an article on five cases of *Pneumocystis carinii* pneumonia (PCP) at the University of California at Los Angeles Medical Center. In July of the same year, a second *MMWR* article described a type of cancer (Kaposi's sarcoma) that is rare in the young diagnosed in 26 men in New York and California and 10 more cases of PCP. The medical community was alerted. At the time, no one would have imagined the report in the *MMWR* would have been the portent of an international health crisis. Slowly the American public began to ask more questions about this disease that appeared to come from nowhere as celebrities became ill and died. The first well-known person revealed to have AIDS was Rock Hudson; he died from AIDS-related complications in 1985. When Earvin "Magic" Johnson announced in November of 1991 that he was retiring from professional basketball because he was infected with HIV, the public was shocked and saddened. When tennis icon Arthur Ashe succumbed to AIDS, people grieved the loss of a fine human being and role model. These incidents, it was hoped, would give credence to the slogan "AIDS does not discriminate."

June 5, 2006, marked 25 years of HIV/AIDS in America. There is no doubt that AIDS changed America (see Timeline). Twenty-five years later, HIV continues to grip America and the world, infecting more than 65 million people; 25 million people have died from AIDS-related conditions. According to the CDC, total deaths in the United States of persons reported with AIDS through December 2004 (latest cumulative data available) numbered 529,113, including 357,712 adults (age 25–44 years), 1,321 adolescents (age 13–19 years), and 5,094 children under age 13.

Although infected individuals are living longer, thanks to new treatments, the essentials have not changed. HIV infection still is incurable and deadly. Scientists know how HIV is and is not transmitted and how people can protect themselves. The American blood supply is protected

**FIGURE 6.8** ▶ Estimated Number of Deaths of Persons with AIDS by Age Category (25–44 years)—Cumulative through 2004

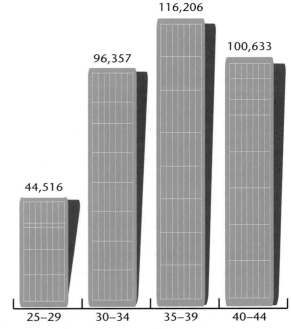

*Source:* Centers for Disease Control and Prevention.

Every year in the United States, about 15 million new cases of sexually transmitted diseases (STDs) are reported. Of that number about one-third (almost five million cases) are among people 25 years and older. According to the National Institute on Aging, approximately 80,000 persons age 50 and older were diagnosed with AIDS in 2001, "almost twice as many as the number of women who will die of breast cancer this year." Is it fair to assume that people 50 years and older are wiser and more experienced about sexual matters? Dr. Mary Jane Minkin cites three reasons that older sexually active people are vulnerable. People 50 years and older are less likely to be exposed to STD/AIDS education than high school and college students, who get the information at school, and have little knowledge about condom use or how HIV is spread. Many older people are returning to dating after the death of a spouse or divorce. People over 50 are less likely to discuss

their sexual behavior with their physician, and they are less likely to get tested and "often mistake symptoms of HIV for the normal aches and pains of aging."

The bottom line is that sexually active people at any age are at risk for STDs. Therefore the risk-reduction measures are the same. Minkin gives the following advice to people who are age 50+.

- Ask your partner about his or her sexual history.
- Use a latex condom every time (because a vagina is a perfect environment for pathogens to grow, a woman is eight times more likely to get HIV from an infected man than a man is to get HIV from an infected woman).
- Limit the number of sexual partners.
- Consider being tested and have an honest conversation with your physician about specific behaviors that increase your risk for STDs.

because of effective screening of donors and donated products and sanitary collection techniques. Reducing the risk of infection with HIV depends on education, behavior changes, and social supports for these changes.

**Acquired immune deficiency syndrome** or **AIDS** was first recognized as a communicable condition in the United States in 1981. Even though much about AIDS remains unknown, enough is known to help people greatly reduce their risk for acquiring the pathogen that causes the condition. The pathogen that causes AIDS, and how it spreads, is no mystery. Anyone who is sexually active can be at risk for acquiring AIDS and other STDs as well. Behavior, not social grouping, is what puts a person at risk for HIV infection and AIDS.

### Incidence of HIV/AIDS and Mortality.
According to the CDC, through December 2004 (most current data available), the cumulative estimated number of the diagnoses of AIDS in the United States was 994,305. Of that number, 934,862 were cases of adults and adolescents (756,399 male and 178,463 female). The number for children under the age of 13 years was 9,443.

During the first half of 1996, 15 years into the epidemic, there was a 13% drop in deaths from AIDS-related illnesses. According to the CDC, for all categories, the estimated number of deaths among persons with AIDS decreased 8% from 2000 through 2004. However, the estimated number of deaths increased in the following categories: *Age group*—13–14, 20–24, 50–54, 55–59, 60–64, 65 and older; *Race/ethnicity*—Hispanics and Indians/Alaska

Natives; *Sex and transmission category*—female and male adults and adolescents exposed through heterosexual contact; *Region*—South and U.S. territories.

### Distribution of Reported Cases.
AIDS is the leading cause of death of American men between ages 25 and 44 and the fourth leading cause of death of women in the same age group. A breakdown of AIDS cases by age at the time of diagnosis is given in Table 6.4.

During the first decade when AIDS was first recognized as a disease in the United States, most of the people identified with symptoms were white gay men. Since 1995, the demographics have changed considerably. Now, black men are almost five times as likely as white men to have AIDS, and black women are nearly 15 times as likely as white women to have the disease. Table 6.5 gives the reported AIDS cases by race or ethnicity. Figure 6.9 gives the percent of persons in the United States living with HIV/AIDS by transmission categories.

- *The Methamphetamine—Public Health Connection.* The methamphetamine crisis in the United States is having an impact on family health, community

### KEY TERMS

**Acquired immune deficiency syndrome (AIDS)** an incurable, sexually transmitted viral disease caused by the human immunodeficiency virus (HIV)

treatment facilities, law enforcement, and reported cases of HIV/AIDS. The connections between the use of alcohol, marijuana, and risky sexual behavior are not new. Under the influence of a psychoactive substance, a person is less likely to make the decision to use a condom. However, data from STD clinics indicate that increased risk for early syphilis is associated with methamphetamine use; methamphetamine use (immediately before or during sexual acts) is consistently associated with MSM and unprotected receptive anal sex (URA). To address public health issues related to methamphetamine use and sexual risk behaviors, in 2005, CDC hosted a national consultation of public health professionals, community leaders, and scientists. The collaboration generated seven research suggestions and six program suggestions that serve as a framework for national, state, and local organizations related to policy, surveillance, and monitoring and intervention strategies. The following is the first two sentences from the "final comment" section of the report: "Methamphetamine use and sexual risk behavior are public health issues in the United States. Methamphetamine use and risk for HIV/STD infection can occur together and are concern for communities of MSM and potentially other populations, although more surveillance and research are needed." (Mansergh, G. et al., p. 131).

■ *The Incarceration and HAART—Public Health Connection.* Research published in *Public Health Reports* revealed an association related to persons incarcerated, released, and reincarcerated. The findings were that while incarcerated and receiving protease inhibitor medications (HAART), the virus was suppressed. Upon reincarceration (nine months after release), five of the eight inmates' viral loads had increased. This is sobering from a personal health and a public health perspective. During confinement, the inmates received their medications as directed; there were no issues hampering their access to treatment. Consequently, the quantity of the virus in their bodies was suppressed. The conclusions of the study were that release from prison has an unexpected harmful effect on viral load; "comprehensive discharge planning" (addressing medical, social, and economic barriers to care) is required so that HIV-positive inmates have access to quality care when they are released; and "follow-up of released inmates may be important in limiting disease progression and transmission in at-risk communities."

**Physiology of HIV/AIDS.** AIDS is caused by a virus known as **human immunodeficiency virus (HIV).** A person does not develop AIDS without being infected with HIV first. HIV is fragile. It does not live on surfaces outside the body for long periods. It cannot survive in extremely cold or hot temperatures, and it can be killed by chlorine bleach. This virus enters the body and survives by invading the chromosomes of white blood cells to duplicate itself. The highest concentrations of HIV are found in blood, semen, vaginal secretions, and breast milk. HIV is not spread through casual contact such as kissing or handshaking. The virus is not spread by vectors such as mosquitoes or by contact with a toilet seat. Trace amounts of HIV found in tears, saliva, and other body fluids have not been found to cause infection. Today, the risk of contracting HIV from blood transfusions is low. Since 1985, the Food and Drug Administration requires that donated blood, blood products, tissue, and organs be screened for HIV.

After 25 years of study, new information continues to be revealed about various aspects of HIV and AIDS. The modes of transmission of the virus that were first reported, however, have not changed. Infection with HIV can occur when blood, semen, vaginal secretions, or breast milk of an affected person comes into contact with the bloodstream or mucous membranes of another person. That is, the virus is spread largely through vaginal, anal, or oral sex; sharing needles to inject drugs or pierce the skin; mother-to-child or fetus transmission; and exposure to infected blood. People who have been exposed to HIV may or may not become infected. Some who have been exposed only once have become infected, while others with multiple exposures remain uninfected.

The incubation period for HIV infection is much shorter than that for AIDS. Antibodies for HIV infection may be detected in a person's blood as early as six weeks after exposure to the virus. Most people, however, convert to seropositive (test positive on a blood test) within three to six months after exposure to HIV. From the moment HIV enters the body, a person is infected for life, can be infectious to others, and is considered **HIV-positive.** Upon being infected, a person may have symptoms similar to flu or mono that go away after a couple of days or weeks (acute HIV infection), or he or she may have no symptoms at all.

**HIV/AIDS in Women and Children.** Thanks to advocacy and medical innovations, there is more information concerning the way HIV/AIDS affects women. Women usually acquire HIV through injectable drug use and unprotected intercourse with an infected partner. Women are more likely than their male partners to become infected with HIV during heterosexual sex, because the concentration of HIV is higher in semen than in vaginal secretions. Additionally, when a male ejaculates, he "injects" semen into the female's vagina, which is lined with mucous membrane.

Women infected with HIV/AIDS reported injection drug use (IDU) and/or sex with men who were infected or had other risk factors for infection (Figure 6.9). To date, there are no confirmed cases of female-to-female transmission of HIV. However, the CDC advises that female-to-female

**TABLE 6.4** ▸ AIDS Cases by Age

| AGE | NUMBER OF AIDS CASES |
|---|---|
| Under 13 | 9,443 |
| Ages 13 to 14 | 959 |
| Ages 15 to 19 | 4,936 |
| Ages 20 to 24 | 34,164 |
| Ages 25 to 29 | 114,642 |
| Ages 30 to 34 | 195,404 |
| Ages 35 to 39 | 208,199 |
| Ages 40 to 44 | 161,964 |
| Ages 45 to 49 | 99,644 |
| Ages 50 to 54 | 54,869 |
| Ages 55 to 59 | 29,553 |
| Ages 60 to 64 | 16,119 |
| Ages 65 or older | 14,410 |

*Source:* Centers for Disease Control and Prevention, cumulative through 2004.

**TABLE 6.5** ▸ AIDS Cases by Race or Ethnicity

| RACE OR ETHNICITY | NUMBER OF AIDS CASES |
|---|---|
| White, not Hispanic | 375,155 |
| Black, not Hispanic | 379,278 |
| Hispanic | 177,164 |
| Asian, Pacific Islander | 7,317 |
| American Indian, Alaska Native | 3,084 |

*Source:* Centers for Disease Control and Prevention, cumulative through 2004.

sexual contact should be considered a means of transmission (HIV transmission through mucous membrane).

Additional kinds of diseases and opportunistic infections are being connected to HIV/AIDS in women. The CDC added invasive cancer of the cervix to the list of opportunistic infections that lead to an AIDS diagnosis. Other female conditions that may signal HIV infection are

- gonorrhea, chlamydia, and pelvic inflammatory disease (PID) that will not go away when treated by a physician
- frequent yeast infections that cannot be explained by other risk factors
- abnormal Pap smear (Class II or III dysplasia)

A woman with any of the above conditions who has engaged in unprotected sex should ask her gynecologist to test for HIV antibodies.

A pregnant woman can pass the virus to the fetus. The virus can be passed before or during birth and through breastfeeding. However, there is good news concerning perinatal transmission of HIV. Because of research and prophylactic treatment for HIV-positive pregnant women with HAART, current rates of perinatal transmission of HIV are less than 2%, compared to 25% to 30% prior to 2003. Also contributing to the decline was the approval (in 2002) by the Food and Drug Administration of a "rapid HIV" test that could be used to identify the HIV status of a woman in labor so that she could receive appropriate therapy to reduce the risk of HIV transmission to her baby. For pregnant women who are identified as HIV-positive, the other interventions that have contributed to this significant decline in the rates of perinatal infection are access to prenatal care and counseling, avoidance of breast-feeding, and the use of elective cesarean section delivery when it is appropriate.

At the beginning of the epidemic, it was assumed that the risk of transmission to the fetus was close to 100%. Groundbreaking research in two areas (trimester of pregnancy for greatest risk or perinatal transmission of the virus and prophylactic treatment of HIV-infected pregnant women) helped to achieve the current successes in the rates of perinatal transmission of HIV. In 1993, a study by Michael St. Louis, reported in the *Journal of the American Medical Association*, found that perinatal infection was more likely if the mother was in the earliest stage of infection (more of the virus present in the circulatory system), when she had AIDS, or if the placental membrane was inflamed. In another study (1996) reported in the *New England Journal of Medicine*, researchers found that risk of transmission of HIV from mother to infant increased significantly when the amniotic sac ruptured more than four hours before delivery. This increased the fetus's risk of HIV infection. The risk to the fetus was reduced when the mother was given **zidovudine (AZT)** during the final trimester of pregnancy. Studies showed that AZT taken according to a strict regimen decreased by nearly 66% the odds of infecting the newborn. In the first 25 years of AIDS in America, the mother-to-fetus transmission rates dropped from an estimated 50% to 30% to 2%—that is great public health news.

**Symptoms.** Most people with HIV infection are completely asymptomatic for years. Some people with HIV have been infected for 10 or more years and remain symptom-free. Unfortunately, HIV attacks special white blood cells (CD4 lymphocytes) of the immune system that are essential in protecting a person from disease. Eventually

## KEY TERMS

**Human immunodeficiency virus (HIV)** a fragile virus spread through the exchange of blood and semen that circulates freely in the bloodstream and always precedes the onset of AIDS

**HIV-positive** determined to have HIV infection by testing

**Zidovudine (AZT)** drug used to treat AIDS and HIV infection

**FIGURE 6.9 ▶** Percentage of HIV/AIDS Cases by Transmission Category in the United States (cumulative through 2004)

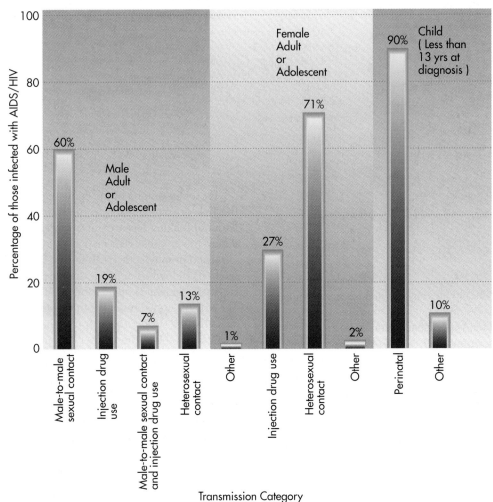

this results in a depressed immune system, which makes a person susceptible to other infections and causes the first noticeable symptoms of HIV disease.

Some HIV-infected persons may enter a middle phase called symptomatic HIV infection. Typical early signs of symptomatic HIV disease include persistent fatigue, dry cough, fever, night sweats, diarrhea, skin rashes, swollen lymph nodes, vaginal yeast infections, and unexplained weight loss. People with HIV can live in this symptomatic phase of HIV disease for months or years and, with treatment, may go through symptom-free periods. Over time, however, the immune system may become so weakened that a person with HIV disease becomes seriously ill, developing **opportunistic infections.** At this point a person is diagnosed with AIDS, the most serious and life-threatening phase of HIV disease.

**Case Definition of AIDS.** The 1993 AIDS Surveillance Case Definition, as defined by the Centers for Disease Control and Prevention, encompasses 26 opportunistic infections that, in an HIV-positive person, lead to an AIDS

diagnosis. According to CDC, a diagnosis of AIDS requires a positive confirmed blood test for HIV antibodies and at least one of these opportunistic infections or conditions. This list includes the following.

- Pneumocystis carinii *pneumonia* (PCP), a deadly lung infection caused by a parasitic protozoan

- *Kaposi's sarcoma* (KS), a rare type of cancer that produces purple-blue skin lesions as well as lesions on the internal organs

- *Candidiasis*, persistent yeast infection of bronchi, trachea, lungs, esophagus, vagina, or skin

- *Cytomegalovirus* (CMV), a viral disease that often infects the retina, leading to blindness

- *Herpes virus infections*, persistant chronic ulcers of the mouth, esophagus, or genitals, and shingles caused by HSV

- *Pulmonary tuberculosis*, a communicable infection caused by bacteria that damage the lungs

- *Invasive cervical cancer*

FYI STATES AND TERRITORIES REPORTING HIGHEST NUMBER OF AIDS CASES

| Geographic Location | Cumulative Number of AIDS Cases |
|---|---|
| *State or territory* | |
| New York | 166,814 |
| California | 135,221 |
| Florida | 96,712 |
| Texas | 64,479 |
| New Jersey | 47,224 |
| Illinois | 31,020 |
| Pennsylvania | 30,526 |
| Georgia | 28,248 |
| Puerto Rico | 28,202 |
| Maryland | 27,550 |

| Geographic Location | Highest Number of AIDS Cases in 2004 |
|---|---|
| New York | 7,641 |
| Florida | 5,822 |
| California | 4,679 |
| Texas | 3,298 |
| New Jersey | 1,848 |
| Illinois | 1,679 |
| Georgia | 1,640 |
| Pennsylvania | 1,629 |
| Maryland | 1,451 |
| North Carolina | 1,137 |

Source: Centers for Disease Control and Prevention, cumulative through 2004.

The case definition of AIDS also includes all people with HIV who have a CD4 lymphocyte count less than $200/mm^3$, whether they do or do not have an opportunistic infection. Some people with AIDS develop **AIDS dementia.** Symptoms range from inability to concentrate and remember, to loss of ability to walk or talk, to incontinence (loss of bladder and bowel control).

The average time from the point of infection with HIV to developing serious enough symptoms for an AIDS diagnosis can be more than 10 years. Although some people progress to AIDS much more quickly than that, it is not yet known if everyone who is infected with HIV will go on to develop AIDS. Some people with AIDS regain their health and live without symptoms for many years; others suffer recurrent bouts of opportunistic infections, often living with more than one at a time; still others die soon after, or even before, an AIDS diagnosis.

Evidence is mounting that some strains of HIV are weaker than others. In an Australian study of 25 people infected by blood transfusions, recipients of blood from donors who developed AIDS 10 or more years after infec-tion were more than twice as likely to be alive 10 years later than recipients of blood from donors who developed AIDS sooner.

**Diagnosis.** In 1985 a reliable blood test was developed to screen blood and blood products for HIV antibodies. HIV infection can be diagnosed by a blood test called **enzyme-linked immunosorbent assay (ELISA or EIA).** This screening test is done to check for antibodies to HIV that a person will develop after being exposed to the virus. ELISA does not test for the presence of the virus in the bloodstream, only antibodies to it.

If a person tests positive on the ELISA, the test is performed a second time. If that test is positive also, another blood test called the **Western blot** is done to confirm the presence of HIV antibodies. AIDS is diagnosed by the presence of HIV antibodies and one or more opportunistic infections or conditions.

Presently, there is one FDA-approved consumer-controlled test kit (home test kit) on the market. The **Home Access HIV-1 Test System®** (better described as a home collection kit) is available in most local pharmacies or retail outlets with pharmacies. This test system is manufactured by Home Access Health Corporation of Hoffman Estates, IL. It is important to note that if the test results are positive, the individual is given referrals for a follow-up test to confirm the Home Access system test as well as information and resources on treatment and support services. The Home Access system testing procedure is as follows:

1. Pricking finger (special device included in the kit) for blood
2. Placing droplets of blood on a specially treated card
3. Mailing card to a licensed laboratory so that the sample can be tested

The individual is given an identification number to use when calling for results, and a counselor is available to

**KEY TERMS**

**Opportunistic infections** illnesses that normally would not be serious but attack a person's body because of a weakened immune system caused by HIV

**AIDS dementia** deteriorated mental and motor capacity caused by HIV-inflicted damage to the central nervous system

**Enzyme-linked immunosorbent assay (ELISA or EIA)** a blood test that diagnoses HIV by exposing the presence of HIV antibodies

**Western blot** a blood test done to confirm results of the ELISA tests

**Home Access HIV-1 Test System** the only Food and Drug Administration approved HIV test for home use

---

**Tips for Action** Should You Take an HIV/AIDS TEST?

The question about whether to get tested for HIV has concerned many individuals. Clouds of fear, suspicion, and misunderstanding still loom large in many communities. Fears of being ostracized by family and friends, being kicked out of school, or losing a job have kept many people who suspect exposure to HIV from being tested. In some cases people simply cannot face the possibility of a positive test and do not want to know. If you are considering having a screening test for HIV:

■ Take your test anonymously in an alternative-site facility where you will be given a number and your name will not be used (some facilities do confidential, not anonymous testing).

■ MAKE SURE THE TESTING SITE DOES COUNSELING BEFORE AND AFTER THE TEST.

---

speak with the person before the test, while waiting for results, and after the results are disclosed to the person. Remember that other home test kits that are marketed are *not* FDA approved; their accuracy cannot be verified.

Fear and embarrassment still keep many people at risk for HIV from testing at their physician's office or an HIV/AIDS clinic. The Home Access HIV-1 Test System® does provide a measure of privacy. Many health care professionals, however, have the following concerns for the individual and for public health when consumer-controlled test kits are used.

1. There is no opportunity for face-to-face counseling. A person receiving the news of a positive test by telephone may hang up before counseling takes place.

2. There is no immediate access to a follow-up test.

3. There is no official partner notification system. The sexual partner of the infected person will have no way of knowing if he or she is infected.

4. Poor people may not be able to afford the test kit, which retails for about $60.00. Testing at the local public health clinic is free.

In May 1996, the Confide® system was the first HIV test intended for home use that was approved by the FDA. Confide® (developed by Direct Access Diagnostics, a subsidiary of Johnson & Johnson) is no longer on the market.

Other diagnostic tests for HIV that are used by health professionals include the following.

■ *Orasure Western blot.* A treated cotton pad is used to collect a tissue sample from between the gum and cheek to test for antibodies. A blood sample is not needed.

■ *Coulter HIV-1 p24 antigen assay.* This is a blood test that screens for HIV antigens, which are detectable earlier than antibodies for HIV. The Coulter test is used in addition to ELISA and reduces the window during which standard testing may show no HIV antibodies even though the person is HIV-positive.

Knowing your serostatus (whether you are HIV-positive or HIV-negative) is important if you are a sexually active person who acts responsibly. At year's end 2003, approximately 1,039,000 to 1,185,000 persons in United States were living with HIV/AIDS. At least 24% to 27% of those are unaware of their infection. A study (on the willingness of patients seeking other services at a public STD clinic to test for HIV) reported in a 2006 issue of *Public Health Reports* validates that there should be no missed opportunities to provide HIV testing and the value of testing for individual and public health. The results showed that 68% (12,176 of 17,875) of the patients accepted being tested for HIV; 68 were HIV-positive for a rate of 5.6 per 1,000. This should be your HIV test "ah-ha" moment. If it is assumed that these 68 people had sexual contact with at least one other person, that means that a minimum of 68 additional individuals should be contacted by the STD clinic and tested. Additionally, 14 of those reporting male-to-male sex were coinfected with syphilis. The majority (85.3%) of the 68 patients who were HIV-positive were located and referred for HIV treatment and support services. In 1995, the National Association of People with AIDS designated June 27 (of each year) as "National HIV Testing Day." Save this date; take the test.

**Treatment.** Effective drug therapies have been developed to prevent or treat specific opportunistic infections. Most of these drugs, however, are toxic and have significant side effects. A class of drugs called reverse transcriptase inhibitors restrains an enzyme crucial to an early stage of HIV duplication. In 1987 the Food and Drug Administration approved the medication Retrovir (commonly known as AZT or zidovudine) to treat HIV and AIDS. Others in this class are Videx (ddl or didanosine), abacavir, Hivid (ddC or balcitabine), and Combivir (AZT and 3TC). They are used to slow the progress of the HIV infection and improve quality of life.

The ability of HIV to adapt and evolve has frustrated efforts to prolong life significantly. A class of anti-AIDS

Phill Wilson is an African-American, HIV-positive, gay man on a mission. His refrain is "Our house is on fire! The fire truck arrives, but we won't come out, because we're afraid the folks from next door will see that we're in that burning house. AIDS is a fire raging in our community, and it's out of control!" Wilson uses this analogy to call attention to the rising rates of HIV infection among African-Americans. Why is there such an urgency in Wilson's message? In 1985 about one-fourth of the reported cases of AIDS were among African-Americans. By 2001, African-Americans accounted for over half of the 40,000 new cases of HIV reported in the United States each year. For women, 60% of all new cases of HIV are among African-American women. As founder of the African American AIDS Policy and Training Institute, which provides unique prevention techniques and training, Wilson's goal is to reduce HIV infection in the African-American community. Through education and community organizing, Wilson wants to prevent AIDS from taking more lives. (Authors' note: As of 2006, among African-Americans, 25% of male infections and 78% of female infections were through heterosexual transmission.)

drugs known as protease inhibitors shows promise. **Protease inhibitors** target a later point in the viral life cycle. Protease inhibitors hinder duplication of the genetic material of HIV (replication) by blocking the action of the HIV protease enzyme. Once inside a healthy cell, HIV needs this enzyme to cut its long chains of viral protein and enzymes into shorter pieces so it can make copies of itself and infect other cells. Physicians prescribe a protease inhibitor with AZT and the other reverse transcriptase inhibitors (a cocktail) because these two types of medications attack HIV during different phases in its replication process. The combination seems to be effective in controlling the amount of virus. The three protease inhibitors that have been approved for use in the United States are Invirase (saquinavir), Norvir (ritonavir), and Crixivan (indinavir).

The use of protease inhibitors in highly active antiretroviral therapy or HAART (the AIDS "cocktail") was approved in 1995 and has caused a dramatic decline in the annual death rate from AIDS. Along with increased access to and specialized medical care and prevention methods, the use of HAART caused the United States AIDS death rate to drop by 47% in 1997. This dramatic decline in AIDS-related deaths was hailed as remarkable. Unfortunately, there were those persons who did not take measures to reduce their risk of infection because they "believed" there was a cure. In the summer of 2006, the FDA approved a medication that combines three antiviral therapies ("cocktail") into a one-dose tablet. The medication, Atripla™, will make it easier for persons on HAART to be in compliance, that is, take the correct dose of the medicine on time, all the time. For personal health and public health, patient compliance is important; it helps slow the evolution of drug-resistant strains of HIV. The medicine is expensive; one month's supply will cost more than $1,100. The medication was approved for use in the United States and 15 countries covered by the President's Emergency Plan for AIDS Relief.

**AIDS Cocktail.** As promising as HAART is, some consider it a two-edged sword. The good news is that deaths from AIDS and mother-to-child transmission of HIV have declined. HIV-infected people are living longer. However, there is some news that is not so good. HAART is not a cure. Even though it lowers the viral load (the measure of new HIV produced by the body), HIV is still present in the body, for example, in the lymph nodes and the brain. Some people on antiretroviral medications believe that they cannot transmit the virus when their viral load is low. This may cause lapses in prevention practices. Some persons on antiretroviral medications experience rapid rebound of the viral load to high levels if the drug therapy is stopped. The drugs' effects are toxic. The most common side effects are depression, diarrhea and nausea, promoting onset or worsening of diabetes mellitus, pain in the hands or feet, and lipodystrophy signaled by the development of a buffalo hump (fat deposits in the back and shoulders) and "Crix belly" or protease paunch (fat deposits in the midsection). Another major concern is that drug-resistant strains of HIV have developed as a result of HAART. Tests now are being done on what are called prototype vaccines.

- *Live virus vaccines*, which stimulate the immune system to attack HIV
- *DNA (deoxyribonucleic acid) vaccines made of synthetic HIV genes* injected directly into a person's

---

**KEY TERMS**

**Protease inhibitors** class of anti-AIDS drugs that target a later point in the viral life cycle and block action of the HIV protease enzyme

## Tips for Action Condom Do's & Don'ts

- **Do** use only latex condoms. Natural membranes have pores through which the virus can travel.

- **Do** use caution when opening a condom. Teeth, fingernails, or other sharp objects could tear the condom.

- **Do** put the condom on as soon as the penis is erect, roll it all the way to the base of the penis, and be sure it stays on until the penis is fully withdrawn. Also make sure there is no air in the tip of the condom.

- **Do** use plenty of water-based lubricant, not oil- or alcohol-based lubricants such as Vaseline or baby oil. These weaken latex and make condoms break more easily.

- **Do not** use a condom past the printed expiration date.

- **Do not** use a condom more than once.

- **Do not** continue using a condom if it breaks during sex. Stop and put on a new condom.

- **Do not** expose condoms to extreme light or temperature. These conditions may cause a condom to dry out and break.

- **Do not** stretch or inflate a condom before use.

- **Do not** use a male condom and the female condom at the same time.

---

muscles, which begin producing HIV proteins, arousing the immune system

- *Recombinant peptide vaccines*, made of synthetic proteins

- *Live attenuated vaccines*, made from HIV that has been weakened so it no longer can cause disease. Experiments in monkeys suggest that these may be the most effective of all the currently available versions, but researchers worry that, after injection, the live virus may revert to its infectious form.

**HIV Drug Resistance.** Many pathogens have the ability to change their genetic structure and become resistant or immune to the medications that once killed them or at least kept them in check. Unfortunately, such is the case with HIV. Researchers at the Fourth International Workshop on HIV Drug Resistance and Treatment Strategies reported that of the 12,000 patients in the United States studied, only 22% had HIV that was sensitive to all three classes of HIV drugs. Twenty-seven percent of the patients had HIV that was resistant to all three classes of HIV drugs, 29% had virus resistance to two classes of drugs, and 22% had HIV resistance to one class of drugs. The implications are that HIV is adapting to HAART, that persons infected with drug-resistant HIV may not respond to traditional HIV therapy, and that HIV has mutated.

**VIEWPOINT** *To stem the tide of HIV infection among drug users who share hypodermic needles, one controversial measure is needle exchange. Do you advocate public funding of needle exchange programs as a preventative measure? Why or why not?*

**Preventing HIV.** Experimentation with sex and drugs, in combination with alcohol use and a sense of indestructibility, makes young people especially vulnerable to HIV infection. Most adolescents know the facts about HIV/AIDS and risk reduction but find it difficult to do what they know. More than 45% of people diagnosed with AIDS were infected with HIV during their teens and twenties. The cumulative data (2004) for age at diagnosis are 13 to 14 years—959 cases and 15 to 19 years—4,936 cases.

Because HIV/AIDS has no cure and currently there is no way to achieve immunity, education and behavior change must slow its progression. U.S. Surgeon General C. Everett Koop announced in 1986 the ways individuals could reduce their risk for HIV infection. He stated that if a person did not choose sexual abstinence, reducing the risk of HIV infection would depend on the following conditions.

- A mutually monogamous sexual relationship with a noninfected partner

- Use of a latex condom with each sexual act that exposes either sex partner to semen, vaginal secretions, or blood

- No sharing of hypodermic needles, syringes, and other paraphernalia by persons using any injectable drug including anabolic steroids

- No sex acts with individuals known to use or suspected of using injectable drugs

The methods for preventing HIV/AIDS espoused by Koop have not changed. Sexually active people must alter their behavior to reduce their risk or thousands more will become infected with HIV before an immunization is discovered. HIV does not discriminate by race, creed, color, occupation, sexual orientation, religious affiliation, or country club membership. Anyone who is engaging in unprotected sex can be exposed to HIV. Therefore, sexually active people must become informed and eliminate risky behavior to reduce their personal risk.

## SYPHILIS

As one of the oldest known STDs, **syphilis** has been researched and documented for centuries. One of the more successful tests for this condition, the Hinton-Davies test for syphilis, was developed by an African-American, William Hinton. Another event linking the African-American community with this disease was an unethical experiment, dubbed the Tuskegee Study, conducted by the U.S. Public Health Service on African-Americans from 1932 to the early 1970s in Macon County, Alabama. African-American men who were exposed to syphilis were supervised medically but were not treated. As the disease ran its course, clinical evidence was gathered at the expense of the health of these unwitting victims. In May 1997, on the behalf of the nation, President Bill Clinton in a White House ceremony issued an official apology to the eight men who were survivors of the study and the families of the other victims. Two years later, the Tuskegee University National Center for Bioethics in Research and Health Care was established.

The syphilis bacterium, a spirochete, has the ability to penetrate the outer layer of skin (the epidermis). The spirochetes can enter the body at virtually any site and invade the circulatory system. Once in the bloodstream, the bacteria move freely through the body systems and leave destruction in their wake. The body systems especially vulnerable to this damage are the cardiovascular system, the central nervous system, and the musculoskeletal system.

The course of syphilis, which takes many years, can be discussed in four separate stages. Each stage has a separate set of symptoms, distinct from the others. If discovered in time, syphilis can be treated and cured so the person will not progress from one stage to the next. In the first stage, primary syphilis, the symptoms appear from 10 to 90 days after the spirochetes invade the body. Usually the symptoms appear within three to five weeks after exposure to the pathogen. A **chancre,** or lesion, appears at the place the bacteria entered the person's body. The chancre is painless and vanishes without treatment. These circumstances may lull the infected person into a false sense that the problem has gone away so diagnosis and treatment are unnecessary. A person who is not familiar with the symptoms of primary syphilis will not connect the appearance of a lesion to a sexual or close physical encounter of several weeks past. Another concern is that the chancre can serve as a portal for HIV to enter the body. Syphilis increases the likelihood of acquiring and transmitting HIV. A person may be infected with more than one STD at a time.

The chancre is the vehicle by which the person passes the syphilis spirochete. Even if not treated, the chancre disappears in a few weeks. The person has no other symptoms and seems to be healthy. Meanwhile the spirochetes continue to circulate through the bloodstream and produce a different set of symptoms later.

The stage of secondary syphilis usually begins weeks to months after the symptoms of primary syphilis leave. In this second stage of syphilis, the symptoms seem totally unrelated to those of primary syphilis. They include low-grade fever, general malaise, swollen glands, and white patches on the mucous membranes of the throat. In addition, a body rash may appear on the torso and even the palms and soles, and the person may lose hair temporarily.

During this stage the person continues to be contagious and, as in primary syphilis, will test positive on a blood test for this condition. Within three to six weeks the symptoms of secondary syphilis disappear as mysteriously as they appeared. If the person is treated during this stage, the pathogens are killed and the progression of this disease ends. If it is not treated, however, the spirochetes continue to circulate freely within the bloodstream and work silently toward the destruction of many body systems.

The stage of latent syphilis disease may begin two to four years after the signs and symptoms of secondary syphilis have disappeared. Unfortunately, latent syphilis has no outward signs. This asymptomatic state presents a two-part problem.

1. The person continues to be contagious during the early part of this phase and is capable of passing the pathogens during intimate contact.

2. The person feels fine and is unaware of the damage to certain systems of the body.

Latent syphilis in people is like termite infestation in a house. The termites begin their silent destruction of the wood structures of the home, and the owner is not aware of the extent of the infestation and the damage until a wooden support gives way.

During the early phases of latent syphilis, the person will test positive on a blood test. As this phase continues, the person no longer is able to infect others during sexual contact, but a woman still can pass along the disease to offspring. If latent syphilis is not treated, damage to the cardiovascular and other body systems continues.

## KEY TERMS

**Syphilis** a sexually transmitted disease caused by the spirochete bacterium *Treponema pallidum*

**Chancre** a painless ulcer that develops at the site where the bacteria enters the body and is the primary symptom of syphilis

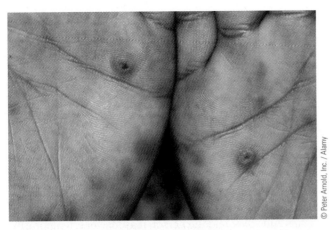

▲ *Rash of secondary syphilis on palms*

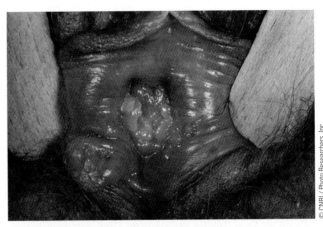

▲ *Chancre on labia of female genitalia*

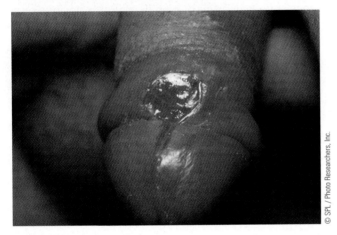

▲ *Chancre on head of penis*

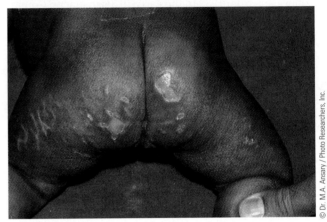

▲ *Congenital syphilis*

Late syphilis, or the tertiary stage, may appear 10 to 20 years after latency. During late syphilis the person's immune system has killed the bacteria, but widespread tissue damage is permanent. Health problems that may arise as a result of untreated syphilis are central nervous system damage (dementia and insanity, blindness, deafness, and partial paralysis), cardiovascular system damage (heart disease and damage to the aorta), and musculo-skeletal system damage (syphilitic arthritis). In late syphilis this damage to the body cannot be reversed by medication, and death usually results from heart failure.

Syphilis is diagnosed through a physical examination and a blood test. Treatment consists of administering penicillin or other antibiotics. Some advanced cases of late syphilis cannot be treated.

Women who are infected with the bacteria of syphilis during pregnancy should seek medical attention immediately. The spirochetes move freely in the mother's bloodstream, so they can and do cross the placenta and invade the circulatory system of the developing fetus. If this situation does occur and is not treated, the fetus will be delivered with **congenital syphilis.** The fetus has gross birth defects or may have no outward signs of infection but may develop neurological and other health problems later in life. To avoid the possibility of genital syphilis, a woman who is receiving prenatal care and who suspects that she has been exposed to syphilis during her pregnancy should report this to her physician or health care provider.

## HEPATITIS B

Hepatitis B (HBV), or serum hepatitis, is caused by a virus that lives in the bloodstream but also is found in semen and vaginal secretions. It causes inflammation of the liver. In the past the risk of acquiring HBV was linked to receiving contaminated blood through transfusions and exposure to contaminated blood in a hospital, and to heroin addicts who inject. Today, many of the reported cases stem from injectable drug use and sexual contact.

The incubation period for HBV ranges from 15 to 180 days. The condition is characterized first by flulike symptoms (low-grade fever, fatigue, joint and muscle pain, nausea, vomiting, and diarrhea). As the liver enlarges, symptoms include jaundice (yellowing of the skin), dark urine, and abdominal pain. If not treated, HBV causes a life-long chronic liver infection. It is the most common cause of liver cancer worldwide, and 5,000 people die each year from hepatitis-related cirrhosis of the liver. The virus damages the liver, causing end-stage liver disease and death.

---

**Tips for Action** How to Reduce Your Chances of Acquiring a Sexually Transmitted Disease

■ Know what you want sexually, and communicate with your partner about choices and strategies for making sex safer.

■ Do not overuse alcohol and drugs as they blur judgment about risks.

■ Limit sexual activity to a relationship in which both partners are not infected with any sexually transmitted disease (STD) and agree to be sexually active with only each other. (Keep in mind that mutual monogamy cannot be verified.)

■ Use latex condoms, water-based lubricants, and spermicides (if allergies are not a problem) every time you have intercourse. Polyurethane condoms are available for men who are allergic to latex condoms.

■ Use latex condoms for oral sex with a male partner (fellatio). For oral sex with a female (cunnilingus) or oral-anal contact, use a latex barrier such as a split condom or dental dam.

■ Urinate before and after intercourse or oral sex to cleanse the urethral opening.

■ Wash hands and genitals before and after sex. Do not douche after sex.

■ Clean sex toys with soap and water. Do not share them without cleaning thoroughly or covering with condoms.

■ Recognize the signs of STDs, and inform your partner if any appear. (The pathogen can be passed before symptoms appear.)

■ Know when self-diagnosis and treatment are appropriate and when they are not.

■ Know where to get medical care if it becomes necessary. Women should get annual Pap tests.

■ If you are sexually active, get tested for STDs if:

— you know or suspect your partner is infected

— you have had unsafe sex with a partner whose health status you do not know

— there are signs of:

■ a vaginal or penile discharge (the drip)

■ rash, warty growths, pimple, itchiness, or sore on genitals

■ persistent lower abdominal pain

■ pain when urinating

■ changes in menstrual flow or unusual bleeding

■ Get tested for HIV if:

— you have had unprotected vaginal, anal, or oral sex with an infected person

— you have shared needles to inject drugs or steroids

— you have had a blood transfusion or received blood products before April 1985

— you have had unprotected sex with an injectable drug user

---

HBV is diagnosed by a blood test and other laboratory analyses. There is no cure for HBV, but it is treatable. Currently, five medications (interferon alpha, three oral antivirals, and a new agent entecavir) are approved for chronic hepatitis B therapy. A nutritional regimen and rest are recommended.

Hepatitis B infection is entirely preventable; a vaccine was developed in the early 1980s. A healthy person at risk should seek the advice of a health professional about being vaccinated for HBV. The virus can be passed from an infected mother to her baby during birth, in which case a shot is recommended 12 hours after birth. Hepatitis B vaccination is recommended as a routine childhood immunization.

## STDS THAT CAUSE VAGINITIS, CERVICITIS, AND URETHRITIS

Symptoms of **vaginitis** and **cervicitis** include pain or discomfort, redness of the tissue, and a vaginal discharge. Both vaginitis and cervicitis sometimes are caused by pathogens that have been transported to the vagina during coitus. Trichomoniasis causes vaginitis. Gonorrhea and chlamydia cause vaginitis and cervicitis.

When men have symptoms of an STD, they generally appear in the urogenital tract. **Urethritis** is the most common condition affecting the male reproductive system. Symptoms of urethritis may include pain or discomfort in the urethra, especially during urination. The STDs associated with urethritis in males are gonorrhea, chlamydia, and trichomoniasis. Women, too, may experience urethritis when they are affected by the STDs that produce vaginal inflammation.

Urethritis is diagnosed by medical examination, sometimes including a bacterial culture. It is treated with antibiotics.

## KEY TERMS

**Congenital syphilis** a condition that is present at birth when the bacteria are transmitted by the mother during pregnancy

**Vaginitis** inflammation of the vagina

**Cervicitis** inflammation of the cervix

**Urethritis** inflammation of the urethra

## CHLAMYDIA

**Chlamydia** has been called the "silent epidemic." This STD is caused by the bacteria *Chlamydia trachomatis* (not to be confused with *Chlamydia pneumoniae*). Approximately 75% of women and 50% of men are asymptomatic or have very mild symptoms and have no idea that they should seek treatment and notify their partners. Chlamydia is now the most common STD in the United States. Approximately 3 million new cases of chlamydia are reported each year, and actual cases will exceed these reported. In females the signs and symptoms may not appear until several months after exposure. However, they usually appear within one to three months of exposure. In some cases they are so mild that the woman does not notice them or may even ignore them. Symptoms include inflammation of the cervix and whitish discharge from the vagina, bleeding between menstrual periods, and abdominal pain. Some women have discomfort during urination. The discharge, whether it comes from the cervix or the urethra, contains the chlamydia organism. It can be passed during coitus and other sex acts.

Chlamydia infection may go undetected in women for months or even years as the organism moves to the upper reproductive tract. If untreated, the woman may develop **pelvic inflammatory disease.** Complications of PID include lower back pain, scarring of the fallopian tubes (which increases the risk of ectopic pregnancy), and tubal factor infertility. In addition, the results of a longitudinal study published in the January 3, 2001, *Journal of the American Medical Association* indicate a link between past *Chlamydia trachomatis* infection and the development of squamous cell cervical cancer.

If a woman has a chlamydia infection, the organisms may be passed to the fetus during vaginal delivery, causing complications such as eye infection (conjunctivitis) and pneumonia in the baby. More than 30,000 infants are born with chlamydia each year. The risk for spontaneous abortion and stillbirth is high.

The signs and symptoms of chlamydia are more likely to appear sooner in men than women. Still, they may not become apparent until several weeks after exposure. Symptoms usually include urethritis, with a characteristic fluid and mucous discharge from the penis and discomfort during urination. Swelling in the testicles may occur.

*Chlamydia trachomatis* can infect the urethra of men, causing a seemingly innocuous infection called **nongonococcal urethritis (NGU).** Symptoms include discharge from the penis and burning during urination. For the purpose of effective treatment, NGU should be considered an STD infection and not a simple urinary tract infection. Untreated NGU can become serious. The organisms can move to the prostate gland, vas deferens, and epididymis, causing complications in the urogenital tract such as epididymitis. In women and men, infection with chlamydia also has been associated with a twofold to fourfold increased risk of acquiring HIV infection.

Screening for chlamydia can be done with a recently introduced specific urine test. Diagnosis of chlamydia also can be done within half an hour by taking a sample of secretions from the cervix or the urethra. Treatment for chlamydia is with an antibiotic such as tetracycline. Neither penicillin nor any OTC medication is effective in treating chlamydia. Treatment options may consist of a seven-day regimen of antibiotic treatment or the preferred single dose treatment of oral azithromycin (Zithromax) that was approved by the FDA in 1997. Individuals being treated for chlamydia who choose to have intercourse should use a latex condom to prevent spread of the pathogens to the other sex partner.

## GONORRHEA

**Gonorrhea** is one of the most common STDs in the United States. The highest incidence is among 20–24-year olds according to the Centers for Disease Control and Prevention. One of the fortunate aspects of gonorrhea infection is that, at least in men, it is not easily ignored. Sometimes called the clap, the bacteria thrive on warm, dark, and moist body surfaces. It can survive in the reproductive tract for years. The gonococcus is passed during coitus and produces urethritis in men and cervicitis in women. If individuals engage in oral or anal sex, the bacteria living in the pus discharge can invade the mucous lining of the throat or anus and cause infection at those sites.

In men the incubation period usually is about two to 10 days after exposure. Symptoms in men include pus discharge from the urethra in the penis and burning during urination. This discomfort usually is enough to send men to a physician for prompt treatment. Because the incubation period is so brief, men generally are aware of their infection within a week. As with any STD, the advantage of a short incubation period is that the infected person will notice the symptoms and seek treatment promptly. Again, any partner should be advised to seek treatment.

Untreated gonorrhea infection in men can have serious consequences. The gonococcus can spread, infecting the urinary tract, vas deferens, and testes. Scar tissue that forms in the urogenital tract as a result of the infection can cause problems with urination and possibly lead to sterility.

The signs of early gonorrheal infection in women are not detected easily. Generally, women are asymptomatic. Some have a pus discharge from the vagina and burning during urination. In any case, the bacteria continue to live in the reproductive tract, infecting the uterus, fallopian tubes, and ovaries. Untreated gonorrhea in women may lead to pelvic inflammatory disease and infertility.

Gonorrheal infection of the female poses a threat to the newborn in vaginal delivery. The gonococcus may invade the eyes of the fetus while passing through the vagina during delivery. This may cause inflammation of the eyes, which can produce blindness. Today this complication is averted by routinely placing silver nitrate or penicillin drops in the eyes of newborns immediately after delivery to prevent infection.

The most reliable test to diagnose gonorrhea is analysis of bacteria cultured from discharges of the urethra, vagina, throat, or anus of the person seeking treatment. Penicillin (or some other antibiotic if a person is allergic to penicillin or has a case of penicillin-resistant gonorrhea) is the most effective treatment. Gonorrhea cannot be cured using over-the-counter preparations. People who have been exposed and are with or without symptoms should seek treatment by appropriate health care professionals.

---

**VIEWPOINT** *The risk of acquiring any sexually transmitted disease (STD) increases if a person engages in the risk behaviors of unprotected sex, with multiple or anonymous partners. Meeting these partners in bars, clubs, parks, and bathhouses is not unusual. An Internet chat room is becoming the newest risk environment for sexually transmitted diseases according to two investigations reported in the July 26, 2000,* Journal of the American Medical Association. *One study compared Internet sex seekers with those who do not use the Internet to seek sex partners. The study subjects were clients of a public health department HIV testing and counseling site. The conclusions of this study were that Internet chat room sex seekers appear to be at greater risk for STDs than those who did not seek a sex partner via the Internet. Cyberspace facilitates meeting people with common interests and offers more opportunities for people's paths to cross. If you do not seek sex partners using the Internet, does this impact your risk for acquiring an STD? How will meeting sex partners using the Internet impact the functions of public health departments to control the spread of STDs through diagnosis and treatment, partner notification, and education?*

*Source:* May McFarlane, Sheana S. Bull, and Cornelis A. Rietmeiger, "The Internet as a Newly Emerging Risk Environment for Sexually Transmitted Diseases," *Journal of the American Medical Association,* 248:4 (July 26, 2000), pp. 443, 447.

## TRICHOMONIASIS

One form of vaginitis is known as **trichomoniasis (trich or TV).** As with other pathogens that cause STDs, the trichomonad of TV thrives in warm, dark, and moist environments. The reproductive structures of men and women alike are ideal environments for these protozoa to survive. They emerge when the body's defense mechanisms are weakened.

Men usually are asymptomatic while the TV organisms are living in the urogenital tract. During coitus a man can transmit the protozoa to the female's vagina, where they multiply. Signs and symptoms of trichomoniasis in women are itching of the vagina, labia, and perineal area, as well as a translucent discharge from the vagina that is bubbly or foamy, green-yellow in color, and malodorous.

This discharge contains the trichomonad and therefore is contagious. If exchanged during sexual intercourse, the male partner could become infected and have symptoms of urethritis. In some cases men may remain asymptomatic and simply pass on the trichomonads to another sexual partner.

The TV organism does not limit its invasion to the vagina or the urethra of men. It moves to the upper regions of the reproductive tract of both women and men, where topical medications cannot reach it. To reduce the risk of continuous or recurring infections, TV should be treated as soon as symptoms appear. Trichomoniasis is diagnosed easily by a gynecologist or urologist, who can identify the trichomonad in the discharge from the vagina or the urethra. TV cannot be treated with OTC medications. The most effective treatment is an oral prescription medicine called Flagyl, which should be taken as directed.

To reduce the risk of ping-pong infection, both partners should be treated simultaneously even if one is asymptomatic. If the couple is to engage in coitus during treatment, the man should wear a latex condom to protect both partners from exchange of body secretions that may contain the trichomonads that have yet to be killed by the medication.

The first national data on trichomoniasis and bacterial vaginosis were presented at the 2006 National STD Prevention Conference. A health survey of a nationally representative sample of about 2,000 women (ages 14–49 years) in the United States was conducted in 2001 and 2002. The analysis of the data by the CDC indicated that the prevalence of TV in women in the United States was 3%. The prevalence among African-American women was 13.5%, 1.2% among white women, and 1.5% among Mexican-American women. The lead author of the study (Emilia Koumans, M.D., M.P.H.) said that the disproportionate impact of TV on African-American women is likely related to socioeconomic factors (income,

---

### KEY TERMS

**Chlamydia** a common STD caused by the bacteria *Chlamydia trachomatis*

**Pelvic inflammatory disease (PID)** inflammation of the uterus, fallopian tubes, and ovaries

**Nongonococcal urethritis (NGU)** infection in the urethra of men, usually caused by the *Chlamydia* bacteria

**Gonorrhea** STD caused by the bacteria *Neisseria gonorrhoeae*

**Trichomoniasis (trich or TV)** STD caused by the protozoan *Trichomonas vaginalis*

limited access to health care). This condition has long-term health consequences and must be diagnosed and treated when the symptoms appear. Untreated trichomoniasis increases a women's risk for premature or low-birthweight babies and acquiring HIV.

## BACTERIAL VAGINOSIS

When the normal balance of bacteria in the vagina is disrupted and a proliferation of other bacteria causes inflammation of the vagina, the condition is known as **bacterial vaginosis** or BV. The symptoms of BV include vaginal discomfort (pain, itching, irritation), a "fishy" odor, and a discharge. Bacterial vaginosis should not be treated with over-the-counter preparations; they do not kill the bacteria, even though the symptoms may be temporarily relieved. Bacterial vaginosis is effectively treated with a prescribed, single-dose oral medication or a course of intravaginal antibiotics.

The information that follows comes from the first nationl data gathered and reported on BV (2006 National STD Prevention Conference—see Trichomoniasis). Bacterial vaginosis is a common infection (27.4% prevalence) in women of childbearing age in the United States. However, as noted by Dr. Koumans and her colleagues at the CDC, African-American women are disproportionately affected by BV. White women had a prevalence of 22%, Mexican-American women had a prevalence of 28%, and African-American women had a prevalence of 50.3%. Analysis of the data showed that the factors associated with bacterial vaginosis were douching, annual family income below $20,000, having been pregnant, a new sex partner, and for white women, increasing numbers of sex partners.

## CANDIDA

As a result of advertisements on television and in women's magazines, **candida** has received better coverage in recent years. This common condition, affecting at least half a million American women a year, also is known as candidiasis, moniliasis, and yeast infection. It is caused by one of four varieties of the *Candida* fungus, of which *Candida albicans* is the most common. These fungi inhabit the vagina normally but will multiply and cause problems if certain agents and conditions are present. Diabetes, lowered immunity, birth control pills, pregnancy, and antibiotics all can decrease the acidity of the vagina and render it a fertile arena for excessive growth of the fungi.

Symptoms of yeast infection include itching or burning of the vagina and labia, redness of the vagina and labia, and lumpy or curdlike discharge from the vagina that clings to the vaginal walls and labia.

The white discharge contains the fungi and can be passed during sex acts. A woman usually avoids coitus during the time of infection because the vagina is irritated and intercourse is uncomfortable. Men usually are asymptomatic for candida even though they may be carriers of the fungi.

Until 1990 the most effective treatments for candida were the prescription fungicides clotrimazole and miconazole nitrate. Now these medications are available to women in over-the-counter medications as preparations to be inserted into the vagina and rubbed on the labia.

Any woman with a first-time vaginal yeast infection should consult a gynecologist for a diagnosis before using an OTC medication. If her self-diagnosis is not correct, the medication will not kill the pathogens causing the symptoms, the condition will worsen, and the woman can expose her sex partner. If she is advised to use an OTC medication, the woman should follow the manufacturer's instructions and use the medicine as directed to be sure that all of the fungi present will be killed.

Most recently an oral, prescription medication (fluconazole) is available for the treatment of vaginal yeast infections. Unlike the traditional treatments, this medication

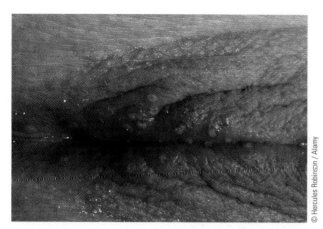
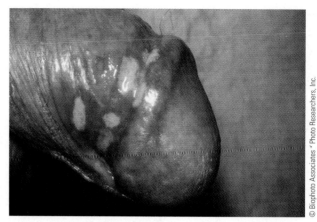

▲ *Genital herpes appears as blisters on the labia of a woman and on the male penis*

is in the form of a one-dose tablet. Side effects include headache, nausea, and stomach pain. If the woman chooses to have vaginal intercourse during the course of treatment, her partner should wear a condom. This will reduce the risk of ping-pong infection.

No matter if the fungi of candidiasis were transmitted sexually or multiplied for some other reason, the condition can recur if it is not treated properly. Because no one develops immunity to candida, a person can be reinfected.

## HERPES

**Herpes** is a viral STD that produces distinctive lesions. Approximately a half million new cases are reported to the CDC each year, and CDC estimates the total prevalence at 20 million Americans. Other herpes viruses are *herpes zoster* or varicella, which causes chickenpox and shingles, and the Epstein-Barr virus, which causes mononucleosis. The herpes virus is capable of producing lesions in the form of blisters on the epidermis (skin) as well as on mucous tissue. Herpes simplex virus (HSV) Type 1 produces oral lesions, called fever blisters or cold sores, on the lips, in the mouth, and sometimes in the nose. HSV Type 2 is transmitted sexually and is referred to as genital herpes. It produces lesions or blisters on the genitalia. Oral-genital contact can introduce HSV Type 1 to the genital area and HSV Type 2 to the mouth and face.

The signs and symptoms of genital and oral herpes are similar for both sexes. Usually within two weeks after exposure, painful clusters of blisters appear on the genitals (penis, scrotum, vagina, cervix), thighs, buttocks, anal area, lips, or mouth of the infected person. These fluid-filled lesions contain the virus and make the person contagious. The blisters remain for several days, then disappear without treatment. Generally the first outbreak (primary outbreak) of herpes is the most painful and lasts 10–14 days. The secondary outbreak (if there is one) may last about seven days and, usually, is not as severe as the first.

Infection with HSV Types 1 and 2 are permanent. The virus never leaves the person; it lies dormant in nerve endings in the cheek and lower back, respectively. During times of physiological or psychological stress, or any condition that suppresses the immune system, the virus can activate outbreaks weeks, months, or even years after the first one. Before the outbreak (prodromal period) some people have vague signs such as irritability, fever, and a tingling or burning sensation in the area where the blisters will appear. Some people learn to recognize the prodromal signs and prepare for subsequent outbreaks.

Women who are infected with herpes have a higher risk for cervical cancer. If a woman with active herpes lesions delivers a baby vaginally, the baby has a one in four chance of becoming infected. If infected, the baby can become blind, incur damage to internal organs, have mental retardation, or die. A cesarean section delivery or antiviral medications given in the last month of pregnancy lower the risk of infecting the baby.

Herpes is diagnosed by a visual inspection of the lesions by a clinician and microscopic examination and culture of the fluid contained in the blisters. It has no cure, although it can be treated with topical over-the-counter preparations that ease the pain and dry the blisters. A more effective treatment is with one of three prescription medicines. Zovirax® (acyclovir) is a cream that can be applied directly to the lesion or taken orally in capsule form. Acyclovir is available as an intravenous medication. Other treatments include Valtrex® (valacyclovir), which is used to treat genital herpes and herpes zoster (shingles) in adults, and Famvir (famciclovir). The oral medication, taken daily, tends to reduce the number of recurring outbreaks but should be taken only under medical supervision. A person who has more than six attacks a year is a candidate for antiviral suppressive therapy.

## KEY TERMS

**Candida** common STD caused by the fungus *Candida albicans*

**Herpes** an STD caused by the herpes simplex virus (HSV)

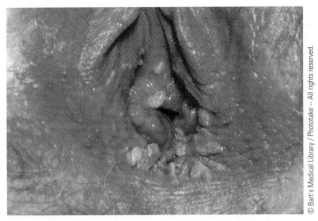
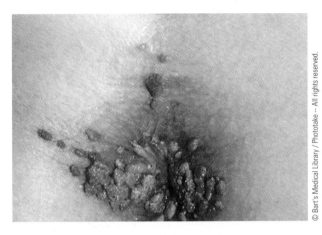

▲ *Genital warts*

Individuals applying ointment or otherwise handling the lesions should wash their hands thoroughly before touching other parts of the body so they will not introduce the herpes simplex virus to other body sites, called **autoinoculation.** Because a person may be contagious prior to the appearance of active lesions, honesty with sex partners about this condition is important so the partner can make an informed decision about sexual activity.

There is no cure for herpes. Research continues for a way to block HSV's ability to enter the bloodstream and prevent infection. In animal research reported in the journal *Nature,* Palliser and colleagues used genetically altered materials, anti-HSV-2 siRNAs (small interfering RNA) and cationic lipids to create a vaginal microbicide. The agent prevented viral infection and protected the mice against HSV-2 by preventing the expression of the HSV-2 gene, thus blocking the replication and spread of the virus. This research is significant because an effective microbiocide is a less expensive prophylaxis than the current medication.

## GENITAL WARTS

Genital HPV infection is estimated at 6.2 million new cases annually in the United States; many of these infections do not persist and the infected person has no symptoms. **Genital** or **venereal warts** are one of the most prevalent STDs in the United States, infecting up to a million Americans each year. It is the most common STD for which students seek medical attention at college clinics, and it is most prevalent in ages 16–25. Over 100 types of human papillomavirus (HPV) have been identified. About 35 of these are associated with infections of the anal-genital area and are considered STDs.

About 60% of those exposed to the HPV develop genital warts (those with a weak immune system are more susceptible), some people never develop symptoms, and some women reveal symptoms only under internal medical examination by **colposcopy** or a new photographic procedure using a cerviscope or a DNA probe.

When symptomatic, the first and only sign of HPV infection in women is the appearance of painless cauliflowerlike warts on the labia, in the vagina, on the cervix, or near the anus. These areas are warm and moist and thus are ideal environments for the warts to thrive. The warts are unsightly in appearance and occasionally can block the entrance to the vagina or cervix or obstruct the urethra. They may grow faster during pregnancy and shrink after the baby is born. The virus can be transmitted from mother to child during birth, sometimes causing the baby to develop warts in the throat, which obstruct breathing.

A persistent infection with oncogenic (a virus that produces tumors) HPV types causes long-term health problems for women and men. Of the sexually transmitted HPVs, the high-risk types HPV type 16 and HPV type 18 (oncogenic HPV types) are responsible for approximately 70% of cases of cancers of the cervix, genitals (to include the penis), and anus; HPV types 6 and 11 cause an estimated 90% of the cases of genital warts. Reducing the risk of being infected with HPV is important for long-term health. Because anogenital HPV causes cervical cancer, it is imperative that a woman with HPV infection have a Pap smear annually.

Research reported in the *Journal of the National Cancer Institute* found that women are five to 11 times more likely to develop cancer of the cervix if their male sexual partners have sex with prostitutes or have multiple sexual partners. The study linked cervical cancer with HPV, which is passed during intercourse.

In men, genital warts may form on the glans or shaft of the penis, on or near the anal opening, or in the rectum. Genital warts are found more often in uncircumcised than circumcised males.

Because the warts are so distinctive, they usually can be diagnosed by a simple physical exam. As with the other STDs caused by viruses, HPV has no cure. The warts (not the virus) may be removed by surgery (including laser surgery), cauterization, freezing (cryosurgery), or applying chemicals to the affected areas.

In the summer of 2006, the Centers for Disease Control and Prevention (CDC) recommended the use of a quadrivalent (prepared with four types of viruses) vaccine to protect against HPV types 16 and 18 and HPV types 6 and 11. The Food and Drug Administration approved vaccine, Gardasil® (Merck & Company, Inc.), is administered in a three-dose series (zero, three, and six months at $120 per dose) and is licensed for girls and women ages nine to 26 years. The immune response is stronger in younger people, and, after the third dose, the vaccine is effective for 2.5 to 3.5 years. The Advisory Committee on Immunization Practices (advises CDC on vaccine policy) recommended that all 11- and 12-year-old girls be immunized. The committee's recommendation is not a state health department requirement, but it is controversial, especially for "abstinence until marriage" advocates. However, since at least 35% of youth are sexually active before entering high school, some parents may consider the vaccine for their daughter.

It is important to note that the HPV vaccine does not confer immunity for other STDs. Therefore, recommended methods to reduce the risk of STDs must continue to be used.

## PUBIC LICE

Often called crab lice or crabs, **pubic lice** infest the pubic hair of their host. These lice are transmitted when the pubic hair of the partners rubs together during sexual activity. Further, crabs can be contracted from contaminated clothing, towels, or linen that has had contact with the carrier's pubic area. Even though crab lice are associated with pubic hair, they may infest the facial hair (beards, mustaches, eyebrows) of partners if oral-genital contact has occurred. The incubation period is brief, 24 to 48 hours.

To ensure continuous infestation, the female lice lay eggs, called nits, that attach to the hair shaft. After several days these eggs hatch and another generation of crabs emerges. Signs and symptoms of **pediculosis** are intense itching of the pubic and perineal areas, skin irritation (even sores, from scratching), and visual identification of lice in hair and nits on hair shafts.

The advantage of the short incubation period is that an infested person is likely to seek treatment promptly and can identify the source of the infection. To prevent reinfestation, the treatment for lice (pubic, head, or body) must include a method for both killing the lice and removing the nits. Several OTC preparations come in the form of special shampoos. Lindane and Ovide are available by prescription. The instructions should be followed, and the treatment should be repeated in seven days to kill any lice that hatched from eggs that were not removed during the initial treatment. Contaminated clothing and linens need not be destroyed, but these items should be washed and dried or dry-cleaned.

## SCABIES

Like pubic lice, **scabies** is caused by a multicellular parasite (the mite *Sarcoptes scabiei hominis*) that completes its life cycle on humans. Usually, the mite is too small to see without magnification. The worldwide prevalence is estimated at 300 million cases yearly. Scabies occurs in males and females, all ages, and all ethnicities and socioeconomic levels. In "classic" scabies (skin eruptions), about five to 15 female mites infest the host. They burrow into the skin and lay eggs. The incubation period is usually three to six weeks for the first infestation; it may be days for reinfestation.

The mode of transmission of scabies is direct skin-to-skin contact. The mites usually can crawl one inch per minute on warm skin; at room temperature, they can survive up to 36 hours and are able to infest and burrow. Signs and symptoms of scabies are intense itching of infected areas (usually not the face); the itching is worse at night. The skin lesions appear in the pubic area—on the genitals, buttocks, legs, and abdomen.

The recommended diagnosis and treatment guidelines by CDC for scabies are confirmed diagnosis of skin scrapings and application of the topical medication Permethrin (with topical crotamiton or oral ivermectin as alternative therapies). Unlike crab lice, classic scabies is usually not transmitted by fomites (towels, linens, clothing). This infestation does not have dire consequences, though it certainly is not pleasant.

## LYMPHOGRANULOMA VENEREUM

**Lymphogranuloma venereum (LGV)** is a system-wide STD that is caused by a particular form of *Chlamydia* bacteria. In a person engaging in anal sex, the symptoms (bleeding, inflammation of the rectum, abdominal pain) may be mistaken for other anorectal conditions. After a short incubation period, the first symptom is a small, painless, pimplelike lesion that usually appears on or near the genital region. In the secondary stage of LGV, symptoms include fever, chills, and headaches stemming from the systemic involvement. The lymph nodes in the groin enlarge (forming buboes), become firm, and then soften

---

### KEY TERMS

**Autoinoculation** spreading a pathogen from one part of one's body to another part

**Genital or venereal warts** an STD caused by the human papillomavirus (HPV)

**Colposcopy** an internal medical examination performed to detect the presence of genital warts in women who are asymptomatic

**Pubic lice** small insects (metazoa) that infest the host's pubic hair; *Phthirius pubis*

**Pediculosis** infestation with lice

**Scabies** condition caused by the *Sarcoptes scabiei* parasite, which burrows under the skin and lays eggs

**Lymphogranuloma venereum (LGV)** an STD that affects the lymph nodes and is caused by a type of chlamydia

and rupture. Late complications, because of blockage of the vessels of the lymphatic system, are swollen limbs and genitals (elephantiasis).

Findings from research conducted in New York City and presented at the 2006 National STD Prevention Conference identified links between LGV, HIV, and syphilis among men who have repeated, unprotected anal sex with men. Additionally, 84% of the men with LGV were "coinfected" with HIV. Until recently, sophisticated labs were need to diagnose LGV. Scientists at CDC have developed a new genetic test that is easy to use, offers faster results, and detects *Chlamydia* DNA specific for LGV. Both of these reports are good news, especially before LGV has a chance to become a public health threat in the United States. LGV is treated with antibiotics, but the course of treatment is longer than for other chlamydia infections. Typically, LGV is more common in tropical cli-

mates; however, outbreaks in the United States have been reported since 2004.

**Chancroid. Chancroid** sometimes is known as soft chancre. The incubation period ranges from two to 14 days and averages about two to five days. Symptoms of chancroid are small bumps or papules appearing on the genitals or in the perineal area. These lesions erode and become soft, painful ulcers that produce a discharge. Lymph nodes in the groin also may be affected. Treatment for chancroid includes keeping the affected areas clean of discharge so surrounding tissue will not be infected, plus the use of antibiotics.

**Granuloma Inguinale.** Sometimes called donovanosis, **granuloma inguinale** is most common in tropical and subtropical areas of the world. Few cases are reported in the United States. The incubation period is eight to 80 days.

**FIGURE 6.10 ▶** Rates for Contracting Various Sexually Transmitted Diseases after One Heterosexual Unprotected Act of Intercourse

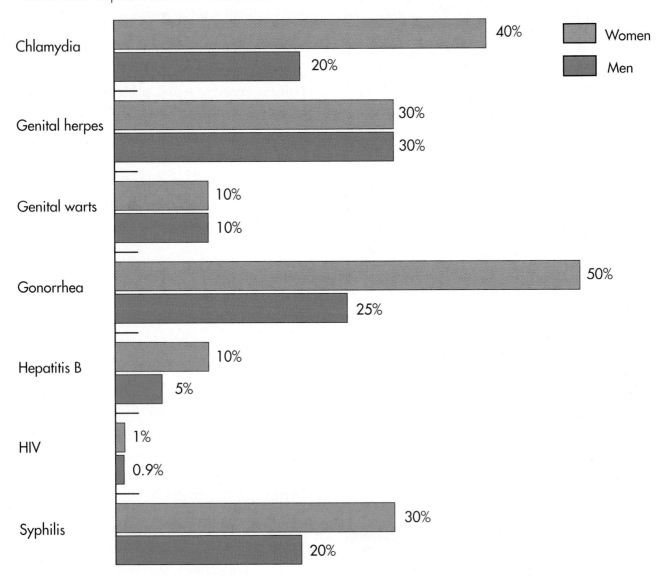

**TABLE 6.6 ▶** Summary of Common Sexually Transmitted Diseases

| DISEASE | PATHOGEN TYPE | DISTINGUISHING SIGN OR SYMPTOM | DIAGNOSIS | TREATMENT |
|---|---|---|---|---|
| Bacterial vaginosis (BV) | Bacterium | itching/burning; discharge; fishy odor | Identification of symptoms | Oral prescription or intravaginal antibiotics |
| Candidiasis (yeast infection) | Fungus | *Female:* cottage cheese-like discharge, strawberry-red color of vagina and labia, pain in genital area <br> *Male:* usually asymptomatic | Identification of discharge | Prescription or over-the-counter (OTC) fungicide (miconazole) (cure) |
| Chlamydia | Bacterium | *Male:* watery discharge from urethra; pains when urinating; can cause prostatitis <br> *Female:* usually asymptomatic; sometimes a similar discharge; leading cause of pelvic inflammatory disease (PID) | Culture of discharge | Antibiotics other than penicillin (cure) |
| Genital herpes | Virus | Blisters in genital and rectal areas | Presence of blisters and laboratory identification of virus in fluid of blister | Zovirax (acyclovir) (not a cure) |
| Genital warts (venereal warts) | Virus (human papilloma virus) | Cauliflowerlike growths in genital and rectal areas; itching and irritation; sometimes no symptoms | Presence of lesions; Pap smear | Removal of lesions by laser surgery, freezing, or chemicals (not a cure) |
| Gonorrhea (clap) | Bacterium | *Male:* pus discharge from urethra, burning during urination <br> *Female:* usually asymptomatic; can lead to PID; sterility (in both) | Culture of discharge | Antibiotics (ceftriaxone), sodium (cure) |
| HIV/AIDS | Virus | Asymptomatic at first; opportunistic infections | Blood test; usually none in initial stages | AZT, ddI protease inhibitors, ddC, HAART (not a cure) |
| Pubic lice (crabs) | Metazoan | Intense itching of areas covered with pubic hair | Presence of lice and nits (eggs) on pubic hair | Prescription or OTC pediculocide shampoo (cure) |
| Syphilis | Bacterium (spirochete) | *Primary:* chancre <br> *Secondary:* rash <br> Latent: asymptomatic <br> *Late:* irreversible damage to central nervous system, cardiovascular system | Specific blood test | Penicillin or other antibiotic (cure) |
| Trichomoniasis | Protozoan | *Female:* frothy, foul odor, vaginal discharge, itching of genital area <br> *Male:* usually asymptomatic | Identification of trichomonad in discharge | Flagyl (metronidazole) (cure) |

Granuloma inguinale is recognized by the appearance of hard, painless nodules (bumps) on the genitals. These lesions erode and create larger beefy-red lesions on adjacent areas, including the area near the anus. This condition is treated with antibiotics.

## REDUCING THE RISK FOR STDS

Abstaining from sexual acts that include a partner will eliminate the chances of acquiring an STD. Some people have chosen abstinence and masturbation as a means of reducing their risk. If abstinence is not a viable alternative, other measures can be taken to sharply reduce the risk of acquiring STDs, although they do not eliminate the

### KEY TERMS

**Chancroid** STD named for the genital lesions it produces; caused by bacterium *Haemophilus ducreyi*

**Granuloma inguinale** STD caused by bacterium *Calymmatobacterium granulomatis*

risk completely. Each person must take responsibility for reducing his or her own risks. Figure 6.10 presents the risks for contracting various STDs by gender.

## Diagnosis, Treatment, and Other Concerns

Prompt, effective treatment and education about safer sex are necessary to reduce the spread of STDs. If a private practitioner is not available or affordable, a person can be diagnosed and treated for STDs at the city or county public health department STD clinic. Because this service is supported by taxes, individuals are treated regardless of their ability to pay. The telephone number of the clinic usually can be found in the government listings section (Blue Pages in some cities) of the local telephone directory under a heading of Department of Health, Infectious Disease, or Specialty Clinics.

Diagnosis and treatment are the first steps in controlling STDs. People reporting to the clinic are examined, and any tests necessary are performed to diagnose or discover which STD is the cause of the problem. Administration of appropriate medication should follow the diagnosis. Patients will be instructed on proper use of the medication and any necessary follow-up. Medications must be used as directed so the symptoms do not come back. Even during treatment individuals may be contagious and should take precautions not to infect partners if sexual activities continue during treatment.

Because they have been exposed to the pathogen, sexual partners of infected individuals also should be contacted so they can be treated. Assistance in notifying partners and in investigating cases are important functions of public health departments in controlling the spread of STDs in the community. Individual rights and privacy are protected by confidentiality and anonymity.

Before leaving a public STD clinic, those reporting for treatment should be counseled about their health, the risk of infecting others, and ways to reduce the risk of exposure and new infection. There is no immunity to any STD. Educating the client about the risk reduction is a vital function of the public health department. Table 6.6 lists relevant information pertaining to selected sexually transmitted diseases.

## Summary

- Pathogens have been classified here as viruses, bacteria, fungi, protozoa, and metazoa.
- The course of infectious disease begins with exposure and infection, followed by an incubation period, then a prodromal period, the clinical stage, recovery (or relapse to an earlier stage), and, finally, termination.

- A person can become infected through the skin or other body surface, by inhaling an airborne pathogen, by eating contaminated food or drinking contaminated water, or through fomites such as contaminated hypodermic needles or bed linens.
- The first defenders against disease are the skin and the mucous membranes.
- Immunity may be either natural (inherited) or acquired (conferred by antibodies in the immune response).
- Immunodeficiencies result from failure of the immune system to react to pathogens. In autoimmune diseases the immune system attacks the body's own cells and tissues.
- Infectious childhood diseases for which immunizations are recommended include polio, diphtheria, pertussis (whooping cough), tetanus (lockjaw), rubeola (red measles), rubella (German measles), mumps, hepatitis B, *Hib* disease or H-flu, and chickenpox.
- Of all human diseases the cold is the most common. It is medically elusive because types of cold viruses number in the hundreds.
- Tuberculosis, once one of the leading causes of death, is on the rise again, often in connection with HIV/AIDS.
- Of the sexually transmissible diseases, HIV/AIDS is the most devastating because a vaccine has not been found and the disease leaves the body vulnerable to attack by opportunistic diseases.
- Two blood-borne STDs are syphilis and hepatitis B.
- STDs that cause vaginitis or urethritis are candida, trichomoniasis, chlamydia, and gonorrhea.
- Genital herpes (HSV Type 2) and genital warts (human papillomavirus) are lesion-producing STDs. Infection with either of these has been linked to the development of cervical cancer.
- Parasites produce pubic lice and scabies.
- Prompt diagnosis and treatment can reduce the spread of most STDs. Risk reduction through abstinence or use of latex condoms is imperative.

## Personal Health Resources

Thomson**NOW** Visit the ThomsonNOW website at http://thomsonedu.com/thomsonnow for valuable resources that will:

- Help you evaluate your knowledge of the material.
- Guide you through tutorials to help you understand and apply the material.
- Allow you to take an exam-prep quiz to better prepare for class tests.

AIDS Education Global Information System (AEGIS). This site has over 300,000 documents on HIV/AIDS. 949-248-5843

**www.aegis.com**

Centers for Disease Control and Prevention (CDC). Available are health-related databases and documents by the CDC; full text of the *Morbidity and Mortality Weekly Report;* access to CDC WONDER, an online public health information system; and the *HIV/AIDS Surveillance Report,* and publications from the National Center for Health Statistics.

**www.cdc.gov**

Centers for Disease Control and Prevention (CDC) Travel Information provides information on current disease outbreaks around the world, summaries from inspections of international cruise ships, the book *Health Information for International Travel* with CDC recommendations about vaccination requirements and health hints for travelers and precautions for HIV-infected travelers, and schedules for recommended childhood immunizations and boosters.

**www.cdc.gov/travel**

Healthy People 2010: Understanding and Improving Health lists objectives related to communicable diseases (including sexually transmitted diseases) and discusses responsible sexual behavior.
1-800-367-4725

**www.health.gov/healthy people/**

HIV InSite has information on prevention and social issues, statistics about AIDS in each state, lists of clinical trial sites, and *The AIDS Knowledge Base* textbook.

**www.hivinsite.ucsf.edu**

Journal of the American Medical Association (JAMA) Sexually Transmitted Disease Information Center. This site contains a collection of fact sheets about STDs, daily news articles, articles from *JAMA* and other medical journals, statistics on STDs, and contact information on patient support groups.

**www.ama-assn.org/special/std**

National Institute of Allergy and Infectious Diseases (NIAID). Information is available on HIV/AIDS, other STDs, and other diseases and medical conditions. The site also includes a glossary of AIDS-related terms, vaccine study news, and the *AIDS Daily Summary* from CDC.

**www.niaid.nih.gov**

Office of Disease Prevention and Health Promotion Lists federal health clearinghouses, calendar of national health observances, and the report *Nutrition and Your Health: Dietary Guidelines for Americans.*

**www.odphp.osophs.dhhs.gov**

Office of Minority Health Resource Center (OMHRC). Available are *Minority Health Resource Pocket Guide* (source of health information and materials for minority populations), the newsletter *Closing the Gap*, the *Funding Guide*, and lists of health professionals who volunteer to provide technical assistance to community-based organizations.

**www.omhrc.gov**

## It's Your Turn for Study and Review

1. Differentiate between a communicable disease and a noncommunicable disease or condition using the concepts related to pathogens, vectors, chain of infection, and immunity.

2. Explain the concept of disease immunity by responding to the following situation: You had rubella in the third grade. Your best buddy, Kendall, was immunized for rubella. Both of you have acquired immunity to rubella. Differentiate between your active immunity and Kendall's active immunity. Include in your response the terms *antigen* and *antibody*.

3. The MMR immunization confers lifetime immunity; the immunization for influenza does not. Explain why a person getting a flu shot must get one yearly.

4. Differentiate among syphilis, chlamydia, genital warts, and pubic lice by the following: pathogen, signs and symptoms, diagnosis and treatment, long-term health consequences.

5. You, Sydney, and Aidan (members of your personal health class) are discussing HIV infection and AIDS. Sydney says that if a person has HIV, he or she has AIDS. Aidan says that is wrong. Because you scored 96 on the last test, they ask you about the matter. Which of your classmates is correct? Respond to their statements by using the following: definition of HIV, transmission modes of HIV, CDC's definition of AIDS.

6. Related to STDs, one of the objectives of *Healthy People 2010* is to eliminate sustained domestic transmission of primary and secondary syphilis. Explain why the elimination of syphilis would "reduce the likelihood of human immunodeficiency virus (HIV) transmission."

7. Name the STDs that can be acquired by transmission from mother to fetus. For each, give the classification and the specific name of each pathogen. Explain how the pathogen is transmitted from mother to fetus.

8. Differentiate the treatments for the following STDs by name, prescription or OTC medication, and treatment only or no cure: HIV and AIDS, genital herpes, HPV, gonorrhea, syphilis, trich, and yeast infection.

9. Identify the functions of a public health department in the control of communicable diseases, especially the STDs.

## Thinking about Health Issues

Is chronic fatigue syndrome a real illness?
David L. Stevens, "Chronic Fatigue: Straight to the Point," *Western Journal of Medicine,* 175:5 (November 2001); p. 315.

1. What are the major symptoms of chronic fatigue syndrome (CFS)?

2. What are some of the psychological manifestations that are frequently found in patients with chronic fatigue syndrome? What is the relationship between these symptoms and the onset of fatigue?

3. Why is it difficult for many doctors to make the diagnosis of CFS? When does simple fatigue become disabling enough to be considered part of CFS?

4. What are some therapeutic measures that have shown promise in helping patients with CFS?

## Selected Bibliography

Adler, J. "The Fight Against the Flu." *Newsweek,* 146:18, October 31, 2005, pp. 38–45.

Anttila, T., et al. "Serotypes of *Chlamydia trachomatis* and Risk for Development of Cervical Squamous Cell Carcinoma." *Journal of the American Medical Association,* 285, 2001, pp. 47–51.

Ashe, A. *Days of Grace: A Memoir.* New York: Alfred A. Knopf, 1993.

Begley, S. "AIDS at Twenty." *Newsweek,* June 11, 2001, pp. 34–51.

Bosch, F., et al. "Male Sexual Behavior and Human Papillomavirus DNA: Key Risk Factors for Cervical Cancer in Spain." *Journal of the National Cancer Institute,* 88:15, August 7, 1996, pp. 1060–1067.

Boyce, N. "AIDS Is Far from Over." *U.S. News and World Report,* February 19, 2001, p. 56.

Brink, S. "Improved AIDS Treatments Bring Life and Hope—At a Cost." *U.S. News and World Report,* January 29, 2001, pp. 44–46.

Burroughs Wellcome Co. *What You Need to Know about Sexually Transmitted Diseases, HIV Disease, and AIDS.* Distributed at American Medical Association Conference on Sexually Transmitted Diseases: Risk Assessment, Diagnosis, and Treatment, February 1996.

Campos-Outcalt, et al. "Integrating Routine HIV Testing into a Public Health STD Clinic." *Public Health Reports,* 121:2, March–April 2006, pp. 175–180.

Center for Biologics Evaluation and Research—U.S. Food and Drug Administration. "Donor Screening Assays for Infectious Agents and HIV Diagnostic Assays." Available at www.fda.gov/cber/products/testkits.htm. Accessed June 25, 2006.

Centers for Disease Control and Prevention. "CDC Health Update: Inhalation Anthrax Case in Pennsylvania." February 22, 2006. Available at www.bt.cdc.gov/agent/anthrax/han022206.asp. Accessed July 25, 2006.

Centers for Disease Control and Prevention. "Cluster of HIV-Infected Adolescents and Young Adults—Mississippi 1999." *Morbidity and Mortality Weekly Report,* 49:38 (September 29, 2000), pp. 861–864.

Centers for Disease Control and Prevention. "HIV/AIDS among Men Who Have Sex with Men and Inject Drugs—United States, 1985–1998." *Morbidity and Mortality Weekly Report,* 49:21, June 2, 2000, pp. 465–470.

Centers for Disease Control and Prevention. "HIV/AIDS among Women Who Have Sex with Women." June 2006. Available at www.cdc.gov/hiv/pubs/brochure/atrisk.htm. Accessed July 15, 2006.

Centers for Disease Control and Prevention. *Surveillance Report: HIV Infection and AIDS in the United States, 2004.* 2006. Available at www.cdc.gov/hiv/topics/surveillance/reports/2004report/print/commentary. Accessed June 25, 2006.

Chosidow, O. "Scabies." *New England Journal of Medicine,* 354:16, April 20, 2006, pp. 1718–1726.

Cohen, J. "HIV/AIDS: Latin America & Caribbean" (Special Section). *Science,* 313:5786, July 28, 2006, pp. 467–490.

Cose, E. "A Cause That Crosses the Color Line." *Newsweek,* January 17, 2000, p. 49.

Cowley G. "Cannibals to Cows: The Path of a Deadly Disease." *Newsweek,* March 12, 2001, pp. 53–61.

Crowley, L. V. *Introduction to Human Diseases,* 4th ed. Sudbury: Jones and Bartlett Publishers, 1997.

Fauci, A. "Twenty-Five Years of HIV/AIDS" (Editorial). *Science,* 313:5786, July 28, 2006, p. 409.

Forsman, K. E. "Pediculosis and Scabies: What to Look for in Patients Who Are Crawling with Clues." *Postgraduate Medicine,* 98, 1995, pp. 89–100.

Gershman, K., et al. "Update: Multistate Outbreak of Mumps—United States, January 1–May 2, 2006." *Journal of the American Medical Association,* 295:23, June 21, 2006, pp. 2712–2714.

Goetz, T. "The Battle to Stop Bird Flu." *Wired,* 114:1, January 2006, pp. 111–115.

Guglielmo, W. "Had All Your Shots?" *Newsweek,* May 21, 2001, pp. 60–61.

Hader, S. L., Smith, D. K., Moore, J. S., and Scott, S. H. "HIV Infection in Women in the United States: Status at the Millennium. *Journal of the American Association,* 285, 2001, pp. 1186–1192.

Hampton, T. "High Prevalence of Lesser-Known STDs." *Journal of the American Medical Association,* 295:21, June 7, 2006, p. 2467.

Hampton, T. "Lymphogranuloma Venereum Targeted—Those at Risk Identified; Diagnostic Test Developed." *Journal of the American Medical Association*, 295:22, June 14, 2006, p. 2592.

Hampton, T. "Scientist Plan New Orleans Mold Project." *Journal of the American Medical Association*, 295:23, June 21, 2006, p. 2710.

Harder, B. "Flora Horror." *Science News*, 169:7, February 18, 2006, p. 104.

Hayden, T. "Bugs, Bared." *U.S. News and World Report*, November 12, 2001, p. 68.

Healy, D. "The Young People's Plague." *U.S. News & World Report*, 140:16, May 1, 2006, p. 63.

"Health Effects from 9/11." *Journal of the American Medical Association*, 295:20, May 24/31, 2006, p. 2347.

Henkel, J. "Attacking AIDS with a 'Cocktail' Therapy." *FDA Consumer*, July/August 1999, pp. 12–17.

Henkel, J. "Hepatitis C—New Treatment Helps Some, but Cure Remains Elusive." *FDA Consumer*, 33, March/April 1999, pp. 23–29.

"Hepatitis C Prevalence." *Journal of the American Medical Association*, 295: 24, June 28, 2006, p. 2839.

Hillemanns, P., et al. "Screening for Cervical Neoplasia by Self-Assessment for Human Papillomavirus DNA." *Lancet*, 354, 1999, p. 1970.

Hinig, R. "D. A. Henderson—Eradicating One of History's Deadliest Diseases Was Just the Beginning." *Smithsonian*, 36:8, November, 2005, pp. 70–71.

Hoofnagle, J. H. "Hepatitis B—Preventable and Now Treatable." *New England Journal of Medicine*, 354, March 9, 2006, pp. 1074–1076.

Hwang, S., et. al. "Bed Bug Infestations in an Urban Environment." *Emerging Infectious Diseases*, 11:4, April 2005, pp. 533–538.

Jefferson, D. "How AIDS Changed America." *Newsweek*, 147:20, May 15, 2006, pp. 36–41.

Johnson, D. "Silencing Herpes Simplex Virus with a Vaginal Microbicide." *New England Journal of Medicine*, 354, March 2, 2006, pp. 970–971.

Jaret, P. "The Health Breakthroughs That Matter to You." *Health*, 20:1, January/February 2006, pp. 128–133, 199–200.

Johnson, E. "Magic." *What You Can Do to Avoid AIDS*. New York: Random House, 1991.

Jones, J. H. *Bad Blood: The Tuskegee Syphilis Experiment*. New York: Free Press, 1981.

Kalb, C. and Andrew Murr. "Battling a Black Epidemic." *Newsweek* 147:20, May 15, 2006, pp. 42–48.

Kennedy, A., Brown, C. and Gust, D. "Vaccine Beliefs of Parents Who Oppose Compulsory Vaccination." *Public Health Reports*, 120:3, May–June 2005, pp. 252–258.

Klausner, J. D., et al. "Tracing a Syphilis Outbreak through Cyberspace." *Journal of the American Medical Association*, 284, 2000, pp. 447–449.

Kotloff, K. L., et al. "Detection of Genital Human Papillomavirus and Associated Cytological Abnormalities among College Women." *Sexually Transmitted Diseases*, 25, 1998, p. 243.

Landseman, S. H., et al. "Obstetrical Factors and the Transmission of Human Immunodeficiency Virus Type 1 from Mother to Child." *New England Journal of Medicine*, 334, June 20, 1996, pp. 1617–1623.

Letvin, N. L., Bloom, B. R., and Hoffman, S. L. "Prospects for Vaccines to Protect against AIDS, Tuberculosis, and Malaria." *Journal of the American Medical Association*, 285, February 7, 2001, pp. 606–611.

Levine, S. "No Safety in the Numbers—AIDS Rises among Young." *U.S. News and World Report*, June 11, 2001, p. 31.

Lloyd, J. "The Bird Flu–Are We Ready for a Pandemic?" *UN Chronicle*, 42:4, December 2005-February 2006, pp. 64–66, 68–69.

Mandelbrot, L., et al. "Lamivudine-Zidovudine Combination for Prevention of Maternal-Infant Transmission of HIV-1." *Journal of the American Medical Association*, 285, April 25, 2001, pp. 2083–2093.

Mansergh, G., et al. "CDC Consultation on Methamphetamine Use and Sexual Risk Behavior for HIV/STD Infection: Summary and Suggestions." *Public Health Reports*, 121:2, March–April 2006, pp. 127–133.

Marcus, M. "Peace of Mind after a Pap Test?" *U.S. News and World Report*, March 5, 2001, p. 63.

Markowitz, L., et al. "Quadrivalent Human Papillomavirus Vaccine Recommendations of the Advisory Committee on Immunization Practices (ACIP)." *Morbidity and Mortality Weekly Reports*, 56 (RR02); March 23, 2007, pp. 1–24.

McFarlane, M., Bull, S. S., and Rietmeijer, C. A. "The Internet as a Newly Emerging Risk Environment for Sexually Transmitted Diseases." *Journal of the American Medical Association*, 284, 2000, pp. 443–446.

Meisler, J. G. "Toward Optimal Health: The Experts Discuss Herpes." *Journal of Women's Health and Gender-Based Medicine*, 9, 2000, pp. 825–830.

Minkin, M. "STDs: A Risk in Your 50s?" *Prevention*, April 2002, pp. 107–108.

Mofenson, L., et al. "Achievements in Public Health: Reduction in Perinatal Transmission of HIV Infection—United States, 1985–2005." *Morbidity and Mortality Weekly Reports*, 55:21, June 2, 2006, pp. 592–597.

"Outbreak of Syphilis among Men Who Have Sex with Men—Southern California, 2000." *Journal of the American Medical Association*, 285, 2001, pp. 1285–1287.

Pagan, C. N. "The -itis Epidemic." *Health*, 20:4, May 2006, pp. 98–102.

Palliser, D., Chowdhury, D., Wang, Q-Y, et al. An siRNA-based Microbicide Protects Mice from Lethal Herpes Simplex Virus 2 Infection. *Nature*, 439, 2006, pp. 89–94.

"Primary and Secondary Syphilis—United States, 1999." *Journal of the American Medical Association*, 285, 2001, pp. 1284–1285.

Purvis, A. "The Global Epidemic." *Time*, December 30, 1996–January 6, 1997, pp. 76–78.

Querna, B. "Emerging Epidemic." *U.S. News & World Report*, 140:9, March 13, 2006, pp. 60–62.

Reinhardt, E. "Public Health Tools—Vaccines, Antivirals and Other Interventions." *UN Chronicle*, 42:4, December 2005–February 2006, p. 67.

St. Louis, M., et al. "Risk for Perinatal HIV-I Transmission According to Maternal, Immunologic, Virologic, and Placental Factors." *Journal of the American Medical Association*, June 9, 1993, pp. 2853–2859.

Sawaya, G. F., et al. "Current Approaches to Cervical Cancer Screening." *New England Journal of Medicine*, 344, 2001, pp. 1603–1607.

Sepkowitz, K. A. "AIDS—The First 20 Years." *New England Journal of Medicine*, 344, 2001, pp. 1764–1772.

Seppa, N. "Small Wonder—Taking the Bite Out of Anthrax Toxin." *Science News*, 169:17, April 29, 2006, p. 262.

Shilts, R. *And the Band Played On: Politics, People, and the AIDS Epidemic.* New York: Penguin Books, 1988.

Shute, N. "A World of Worry." *U.S. News & World Report*, 140:21, June 5, 2006, pp. 52–54.

Sobel, R. "Herpes Tests Give Answers You Might Need to Know." *U.S. News and World Report*, June 18, 2001, p. 53.

Steinbrook, R. and Drazen, J. M. "AIDS—Will the Next 20 Years Be Different?" *New England Journal of Medicine*, 344, June 7, 2001, pp. 1781–1782.

Steinbrook, R. "The Potential of Human Papillomavirus Vaccines." *New England Journal of Medicine*, 354, March 16, 2006, pp. 1109–1112.

Stephenson, B., et al. "Effects of Release from Prison and Re-Incarceration on the Viral Loads of HIV-Infected Individuals." *Public Health Reports*, 120:1, January/February 2005, pp. 84–88.

Tyler, K. L. "West Nile Virus Encephalitis in America." *New England Journal of Medicine*, 344, June 14, 2001, pp. 1858–1859.

Walsh, C., Anderson, L. A., and Irwin, K. "The Silent Epidemic of *Chlamydia trachomatis:* The Urgent Need for Detection and Treatment in Women." *Journal of Women's Health and Gender-Based Medicine*, 9, 2000, pp. 339–343.

Voelker, R. "HIV Drug Resistance." *Journal of the American Medical Association*, 284, 2000, p. 169.

Zakaria, F. "A Threat Worse than Terror." *Newsweek*, October 31, 2005, 146:18, p. 46.

Zamula, E. "Shingles: An Unwelcome Encore." *FDA Consumer*, 35, May/June, 2001, pp. 21–25.

Name _____    Course _____

Date _____    Section _____

Place a checkmark (✔) in the box for each immunization you have received.

| VACCINE | MONTHS | | | | | YEARS | |
|---|---|---|---|---|---|---|---|
| | 2 | 4 | 6 | 12–15 | 15 | 4–6 | 14–16 |
| Diphtheria, tetanus, pertussis (DTP) | | | | | | | |
| Oral polio vaccine (OPV) | | | | | | | |
| Measles, mumps, rubella (MMR) | | | | | | | |
| *Haemophilus influenzae* type b *(Hib)* | | | | | | | |
| Chicken pox | | | | | | | |
| Td—contains tetanus and diphtheria vaccines (for children seven years and older) | | | | | | | |
| | Birth | 1–2 Mos. | 4 Mos. | 6–18 Mos | | (or other) | |
| Hepatitis B (Hep B) | | | | | | | |

Name _____     Course _____

Date _____     Section _____

| | Yes | No |
|---|---|---|
| **1.** AIDS is the end stage of infection caused by HIV. | _____ | _____ |
| **2.** HIV is a chronic infectious disease that spreads among individuals who engage in risky behaviors such as unprotected sex or the sharing of hypodermic needles. | _____ | _____ |
| **3.** AIDS now has a cure. | _____ | _____ |
| **4.** Abstaining from sex is the only 100% sure way to protect yourself from HIV infection. | _____ | _____ |
| **5.** Condoms are 100% effective in protecting you against HIV infection. | _____ | _____ |
| **6.** If you are sexually active, latex condoms provide the best protection against HIV infection. | _____ | _____ |
| **7.** The number of HIV infections in teens has increased year by year. | _____ | _____ |
| **8.** A person can become HIV-infected by donating blood. | _____ | _____ |
| **9.** You can tell by looking at someone if he or she is HIV-infected. | _____ | _____ |
| **10.** The only means to determine whether someone has HIV is through an HIV antibody test. | _____ | _____ |
| **11.** HIV can completely destroy the immune system. | _____ | _____ |
| **12.** The HIV virus may live in the body 10 years or longer before AIDS symptoms develop. | _____ | _____ |
| **13.** People infected with HIV have AIDS. | _____ | _____ |
| **14.** Once infected with HIV, a person never becomes uninfected. | _____ | _____ |
| **15.** HIV infection is preventable. | _____ | _____ |

*Source:* Adapted from *Test Your Survival Smarts: Self-Quiz on Drugs and AIDS*, Washington, DC: U.S. Department of Health and Human Services, National Institute on Drug Abuse, 1995.

## Answers

1. Yes. AIDS is the term used to define the manifestation of opportunistic diseases and cancers that occur as a result of HIV infection.

2. Yes. People do not get HIV because of who they are but, rather, because of what they do. Almost all of the people who get HIV do so because they choose to engage in risky behaviors.

3. No. AIDS has no cure.

4. No. Abstinence does protect a person from getting HIV infection from sex, but it can still be contracted by sharing hypodermic needles.

5. No. Only abstaining from sex gives you 100% protection. If they are used correctly, however, condoms are effective in protecting against HIV infection.

6. Yes. Proper use, however, is necessary to minimize the risk of infection.

7. Yes. In the early 1990s the number of infected teens increased by 96% over a short span of two years. Probably about 20% of the AIDS patients today were infected as teenagers.

8. No. A myth regarding HIV is that it can be transmitted by donating blood. People cannot get HIV from giving blood. Health professionals use a new needle every time they draw blood. These needles are used only once and are destroyed and thrown away immediately after each individual has donated blood.

9. No. The symptoms of AIDS often are not noticeable until several years after a person has been infected with HIV.

10. Yes. Nobody can tell if an HIV infection exists unless an HIV antibody test is done. Upon HIV infection, the immune system's line of defense against the virus is to form antibodies that bind to the virus. On the average the body takes three months to manufacture enough antibodies to show up positive in an HIV antibody test. Sometimes it may take six months or longer.

11. Yes. The virus multiplies, attacks, and destroys white blood cells. These cells are part of the immune system, and their function is to fight off infections and diseases in the body. As the number of white blood cells killed increases, the body's immune system gradually breaks down and may be destroyed.

12. Yes. Up to 10 years may go by before the person develops AIDS.

13. No. Being HIV-positive does not necessarily mean the person has AIDS. On the average, it takes seven to eight years following infection before the individual develops the symptoms that fit the case definition of AIDS. In essence, from the point of infection, the individual may have the chronic disease 10 years or longer.

14. Yes. There is no second chance.

15. Yes. The best prevention technique is to abstain from sex until the time comes for a mutually monogamous sexual relationship. In the absence of sharing needles, that one behavior, according to Dr. James Mason, former director of the Centers for Disease Control and Prevention in Atlanta, will almost completely remove the risk of contracting HIV or developing any other sexually transmitted disease.

Name _____     Course _____

Date _____     Section _____

To assess your risk of being HIV-infected, answer the following questions.

|  |  | Yes | No |
|---|---|---|---|
| 1. | Have you had unprotected sex with someone other than one faithful partner? | _____ | _____ |
| 2. | Have you had sex with a prostitute? | _____ | _____ |
| 3. | Have you had a sexually transmitted disease, such as syphilis or genital herpes? | _____ | _____ |
| 4. | Have you ever shared needles or syringes to inject drugs? | _____ | _____ |
| 5. | If you are male have you had sex with other males? | _____ | _____ |
| 6. | Did you receive a blood transfusion before 1985? | _____ | _____ |
| 7. | Have you been sexually assaulted? | _____ | _____ |
| 8. | Have you had sex with anyone who would answer "yes" to any of these questions? | _____ | _____ |

If you answered "yes" to any of these questions, seriously consider being tested for HIV for your own sake as well as the health of your sexual partners.

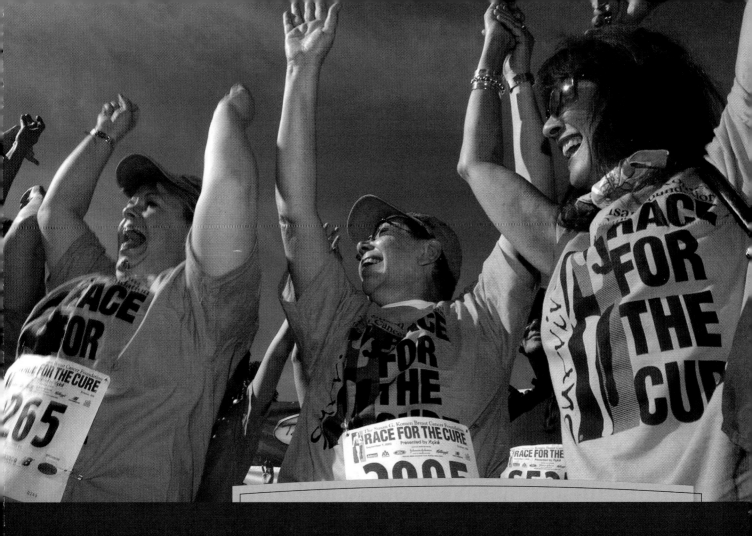

# Chapter Seven Noncommunicable Diseases

**OBJECTIVES** ■ Explain the mechanism by which cancers develop. ■ List the personal health choices that reduce an individual's risk of developing cancer. ■ Define chronic obstructive lung disease (COLD) and describe its manifestations. ■ Identify and differentiate the types of anemia. ■ Differentiate type 1 and type 2 diabetes. ■ Define rheumatic diseases and give examples. ■ Identify three skin conditions related to ethnicity. ■ Give examples of diseases of the digestive tract.

ThomsonNOW™ Log on to ThomsonNOW at http://thomsonedu.com/ thomsonnow to access and explore self-assessments, interactive tutorials, and practice quizzes.

The top killers in the United States at the beginning of the 20th century were communicable diseases—tuberculosis, diphtheria, scarlet fever, polio, and other highly infectious diseases—that ravaged communities and sometimes wiped out entire families. Today, the leading causes of death in the United States are all noncommunicable diseases, those that cannot be transmitted from one person to another. The top three killers in the United States are cardiovascular conditions, cancers, and stroke. The No. 1 killer, cardiovascular disease, is covered in Chapter 8.

# Cancer

Just the mention of cancer arouses fear in people. Although it still is the second leading cause of death of adults in the United States (23.5%), following heart disease, many cancers now are preventable and curable. In 2006 there were approximately 564,830 deaths from cancer, or 205 per 100,000. One goal of *Healthy People 2010* is to reduce the annual death rate for cancer to 159.9 per 100,000. From 1998 to 2002, the mortality rates (death rates) from cancer were as follows:

| Population | Cancer Deaths per 100,000 (All Sites) | |
|---|---|---|
| | Male | Female |
| American Indian and Alaska Native | 159.7 | 113.8 |
| Asian American and Pacific Islander | 148.0 | 99.4 |
| Black or African American | 339.4 | 194.3 |
| White | 242.5 | 164.5 |
| Hispanic or Latino | 171.4 | 111.0 |

For the first time since cancer statistics began to be kept in the 1930s, overall mortality from cancer was level from 1991 to 1994 and declined 1.4% per year from 1994 to 1998 (latest figures available), reversing a 6.4% rise from 1971 to 1990, according to the National Cancer Institute (NCI). Some of the success may be attributable to the decline in smoking as well as improved treatment methods and preventive measures. More specifically, the NCI *Annual Report to the Nation on the Status of Cancer, 1973–1998: Featuring Cancers with Recent Increasing Trends* shows that deaths from:

- Lung cancer—decreased 1.9% per year from 1992 to 1998 in men but increased 0.8% per year from 1992 to 1998 in women

- Breast cancer fell 3.4% per year between 1995 and 1998

- Colorectal cancer dropped 7% in men and 4.8% in women

- Prostate cancer declined by 6.3%

- Ovarian cancer decreased 4.8%

## THE MECHANISM OF CANCER

Normally, as cells become worn out, they reproduce themselves in an orderly way. With the exception of gametes and red blood cells, each of the body's approximately 100 trillion cells has a nucleus that contains 23 pairs of chromosomes. On these chromosomes are located genes, the basic units of heredity, which contain an ordered sequence of the body's **genetic code.**

During cell division the genetic material in each cell is supposed to duplicate in an orderly pattern to produce normal cells. Scientists at Princeton University and the Johns Hopkins University Oncology Center have discovered a gene that suppresses disorderly cell growth. The gene, called p53, is located on the short arm of chromosome 17. A healthy p53 gene makes p53 protein, which keeps tumors from forming by incorporating itself into the cells' DNA. The p53 acts as a tumor killer by stopping a cancerous cell from making copies of itself or by killing the cancer cell to prevent other tumors from forming.

In some cases, a **mutation** in p53 occurs. If this happens, the gene cannot suppress tumor growth because the cell lacks its natural tumor killer protecting gene. A defective gene p53 has been implicated in at least 52 types of cancers including lung, breast, cervix, colon, and skin.

An enzyme called **telomerase** allows the cells to reproduce indefinitely, forming a **tumor.** If it remains self-contained and does not spread, it is termed benign. Although most **benign tumors** have little effect on body functioning and are harmless, they may cause discomfort or damage if they press against adjacent tissues or organs.

The disease called **cancer** is a group of diseases characterized by uncontrolled growth and the spread of abnormal cells. The normal cells are overcome and eventually die. A cancer, a **malignant tumor,** begins as a localized tumor, confined to one area. If, however, the tumor continues to grow and begins to invade surrounding tissues and organs, it is called an **invasive tumor.** Cancer can be found in any body tissue. When cells break off from a malignant tumor, migrate to other parts of the body through the circulatory or lymphatic system, and form new cancers, **metastasis** has occurred.

Most adults have precancerous or cancerous cells in their bodies. If the immune system is healthy, it can keep these cells in check. Just one errant cell, however, can produce cancer, of which some types take years to develop and others mobilize rapidly.

Research has uncovered a variety of agents, both internal and external, that can instigate cancer. These cancer-causing agents, known as **carcinogens,** include:

- Occupational hazards and pollutants (such as nickel and asbestos)

- Chemicals in food and water

- Certain viruses (human papillomavirus, hepatitis B, and hepatitis C, for example)
- Radiation (including the natural radiation from the sun)

Other factors that contribute to the development of cancer include a genetic predisposition and psychological factors that compromise the immune system.

Some misconceptions regarding cancer have been passed from one generation to the next. Some people have resigned themselves to the mistaken idea that cancer just happens and a person can do little to avoid it. One of the most disturbing consequences is that some people are paralyzed into inaction when they notice a symptom or sign that a health professional should investigate.

The news about cancer is much better than one might think. Many forms of cancer that account for the highest incidence (number of cases in the population) and mortality (death) rates are related to lifestyle factors that a person can alter or even eliminate to reduce the risk of cancer. Further, the most successful treatment of cancer comes in the early stage. If people would be proactive against cancer, much of it could be halted. Attitude also plays a role in cancer. Many people underestimate their ability to reduce their risk and turn the prognosis in their favor. Figure 7.1 shows the estimated role of major cancer-causing agents.

## ETHNICITY AND CANCER

Even though anyone can develop cancer, incidence and death rates from cancer are generally higher in African Americans than Caucasians. The cancer incidence rates for all sites (1998–2002) for African Americans were 682.6 per 100,000 for males and 398.5 per 100,000 for females compared to 556.4 per 100,000 and 429.3 per 100,000 for Caucasian males and females, respectively. For those same years the death rates (per 100,000) for African-American males and females were 339.4 and 194.3, respectively, compared to 242.5 and 164.5 for Caucasian males and females, respectively. African Americans have a higher incidence of death rates for cancers of the esophagus, stomach, liver, larynx, prostate, and cervix. African-American women are more than twice as likely to die of breast cancer within five years of diagnosis than Caucasian women are.

The use of recommended screening tests for the early diagnosis and treatment of cancer varies between racial and ethnic groups. Dr. William Eley of the Emory University School of Public Health asserts that the disease in African Americans tends to be diagnosed in later stages. According to the American Cancer Society, more than 90% of women whose breast cancer is diagnosed before it spreads survive at least five years, whereas survival drops to as low as 18% in women whose cancer has spread before it is diagnosed.

**FIGURE 7.1 ▶** Estimate of the Relative Role of the Major Cancer-Causing Agents

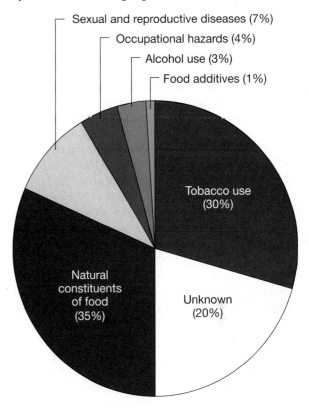

- Sexual and reproductive diseases (7%)
- Occupational hazards (4%)
- Alcohol use (3%)
- Food additives (1%)

Tobacco use (30%)

Unknown (20%)

Natural constituents of food (35%)

### KEY TERMS

**Genetic code** chemicals in genes designated in combinations of the letters A, T, C, and G

**Mutation** a disruption in the order of chemicals in the genetic code that produces an anomaly or, in the case of cancer, growth and spread of tumors

**Telomerase** enzyme that allows the cells to reproduce indefinitely, forming a tumor

**Tumor** an abnormal mass of tissue that grows independently of surrounding tissue and serves no useful function; neoplasm

**Benign tumor** tumor that remains self-contained; noncancerous

**Cancer** group of diseases characterized by uncontrolled growth and spread of abnormal cells that kill normal cells

**Malignant tumor** a tumor that is cancerous

**Invasive tumor** tumor that continues to grow and encroaches upon surrounding tissues and organs

**Metastasis** the process of new cancers forming when cells from a malignant tumor break off and travel to other parts of the body

**Carcinogen** cancer-causing agent or substance

Table 7.1 summarizes diagnosed cancers by site of the cancer, sex, and ethnic group. These numbers give incidence and mortality rates within each group.

Florence Bonner, a sociology professor at Howard University and principal investigator for the National Black Leadership Initiative on Cancer, commented that the African-American community historically has viewed good health as a privilege and remains reactive instead of proactive toward health care. In regard to cancer, Bonner commented that people of lower economic status within the African-American community are more fatalistic about being diagnosed ("once you're diagnosed, you're dead").

Linda Burhansstipanov of the Native American Research Consortium in Denver reported that language barriers and different communication patterns in the Native American community may be a barrier when non-Native health care professionals are serving Native Americans. Most indigenous languages have no word for cancer. In the Hispanic-Latino community, too, language differences may present problems.

In addition to the socioeconomic (lack of health insurance or transportation) and cultural (attitudes about screening tests) differences that may erect barriers to patient care, misunderstanding of medical jargon or directions on how to take medications may present problems.

## DIAGNOSIS AND TREATMENT OF CANCER

Because cancer is not a single condition but instead encompasses a group of conditions, no one diagnostic test can be used to determine if cancer is present. Some of the general procedures are

- **Biopsy.** A small piece of tissue is removed through a special hollow needle and examined microscopically to determine if a tumor is benign or malignant.

- **Magnetic resonance imagery (MRI).** Magnetic fields and radio waves produce a computer image of body tissue that may reveal abnormalities. The newer models can scan the full body in 18 seconds instead of the usual 45 minutes. They also are starting to be used instead of biopsies to detect breast lumps.

**TABLE 7.1 ▶** Incidence and Mortality Rates by Site, Race, and Ethnicity, United States, 1998–2002

| | WHITE | AFRICAN AMERICAN | ASIAN AND PACIFIC ISLANDER | AMERICAN INDIAN AND ALASKA NATIVE | HISPANIC LATINO |
|---|---|---|---|---|---|
| **Incidence** | | | | | |
| All sites | | | | | |
|   Males | 556.4 | 682.6 | 383.5 | 255.4 | 420.7 |
|   Females | 429.3 | 398.5 | 303.6 | 220.5 | 310.9 |
| Breast (female) | 141.1 | 119.4 | 96.6 | 54.8 | 89.9 |
| Colon and rectum | | | | | |
|   Males | 61.7 | 72.5 | 56.0 | 36.7 | 48.3 |
|   Females | 45.3 | 56.0 | 39.7 | 32.2 | 32.3 |
| Lung and bronchus | | | | | |
|   Males | 76.7 | 113.9 | 59.4 | 42.6 | 44.6 |
|   Females | 51.1 | 55.2 | 28.3 | 23.6 | 23.3 |
| Prostate | 169.0 | 272.0 | 101.4 | 50.3 | 141.9 |
| Uterine cervix | 8.7 | 11.1 | 8.9 | 4.9 | 15.8 |
| **Mortality** | | | | | |
| All sites | | | | | |
|   Males | 242.5 | 339.4 | 148.0 | 159.7 | 171.4 |
|   Females | 164.5 | 194.3 | 99.4 | 113.8 | 111.0 |
| Breast (female) | 25.9 | 34.7 | 12.7 | 13.8 | 16.7 |
| Colon and rectum | | | | | |
|   Males | 24.3 | 34.0 | 15.8 | 16.2 | 17.7 |
|   Females | 16.8 | 24.1 | 10.6 | 11.8 | 11.6 |
| Lung and bronchus | | | | | |
|   Males | 75.2 | 101.3 | 39.4 | 47.0 | 38.7 |
|   Females | 41.8 | 39.9 | 18.8 | 27.1 | 14.8 |
| Prostate | 27.7 | 68.1 | 12.1 | 18.3 | 23.0 |
| Uterine cervix | 2.5 | 5.3 | 2.7 | 2.6 | 3.5 |

*Note:* Rates are per 100,000, age-adjusted to the 2000 U.S. standard population. Hispanic/Latinos are not mutually exclusive from whites, African Americans, Asian Americans and Pacific Islanders, and American Indians and Alaska Natives.
*Source:* National Cancer Institute, Division of Cancer Control and Population Science, Surveillance, Epidemiology, and End Results Program, 2000. Mortality derived from data originating from the Centers for Disease Control and Prevention, National Center for Health Statistics, 2000.

## FYI | FIGHTING CANCER WITH WHAT YOU EAT

To protect yourself from cancer:

- Cut dietary fats to no more than 30% of your total calories by
  —trimming all fat from meat and removing skin from poultry before cooking
  —cutting down on the amount of fat and oil used in cooking
  —substituting low-fat for high-fat dairy products
  —limiting intake of meat to no more than three to six ounces a day
  —using less fat and oil in cooking
- Eat more fruits and vegetables—at least two or three a day. Include cabbage, yellow vegetables, onions, garlic, potatoes, peas, green leafy vegetables, and citrus fruits.
- Eat vegetables raw or cook them by steaming or stir-frying. Eat fruits raw, as canned and preserved fruits lose nutrients.
- Eat plenty of fiber—in whole-grain cereals and breads—and use whole-wheat flour in baking.
- Substitute fruit and vegetable juices for coffee, tea, and soda.
- Drink two to four glasses of low-fat milk each day.
- Eat fish two or three times a week.
- Cook by baking, broiling, steaming, poaching, and roasting instead of frying or barbecuing.
- Drink alcohol only in moderation.

- **Computerized axial tomography (CAT scan).** Radiation allows the viewing of internal organs that usually are not visible by x-ray.

Early detection and treatment of any cancer are important. Survival rates are linked to the stage at which the cancer is first diagnosed. Cancers are easier to treat when the tumor is localized. The American Cancer Society recommends regular screening tests for early detection in people who do not have symptoms. Table 7.2 lists some of the screening measures for various cancer sites and how often they should be done.

The treatment plan for cancer must be tailored to the individual. The form of treatment depends on variables such as the type of cancer, site of the malignancy, how early it was diagnosed, and the patient's general health. In many cases, more than one method is used. The physician who specializes in treating cancer is called an **oncologist.**

The most widely utilized methods of treatment are

- **Surgery.** The tumor and its surrounding tissue are removed by excising them.

- **Radiation.** Often combined with surgery, x-rays are aimed at the site of the tumor to destroy or stop the growth of cancerous cells. A **radiologist** determines how much radiation is necessary. A drawback of radiation therapy is that it destroys some healthy cells at the same time.
- **Chemotherapy.** Any or a combination of more than 50 drugs is administered intravenously to kill cancerous cells. Chemotherapy is a **systemic** treatment used when cancer cells have spread throughout the body.
- **Hormone therapy.** Tamoxifen or aromatase inhibitors are used.

## REPRESENTATIVE CANCERS: AN OVERVIEW

The most common cancers are of the lung, colon and rectum, breast, prostate, testicles, uterus (cervix and endometrium), ovaries, skin, and oral cavity. The American Cancer Society estimates of cancer incidence and deaths by site and sex are shown in Figure 7.2. The highest incidence for men is prostate cancer, and for women, breast cancer. The highest number of deaths from cancer for both men and women is due to lung cancer.

**Lung and Bronchus.** Lung cancer is the leading cause of death in men and women alike. Lung cancer accounts for approximately 12% of cancer diagnoses. Since 1987, more women have died from lung cancer than breast cancer. What is most disturbing is that lung cancer is one of the most preventable forms of cancer because the greatest risk factor for this condition is cigarette smoking.

### KEY TERMS

**Biopsy** microscopic examination of a small piece of tissue that has been removed with a special needle; one of the cancer diagnostic tests

**Magnetic resonance imagery (MRI)** use of radio waves and magnetic fields that produce a computer image of the body to locate abnormalities

**Computerized axial tomography (CAT scan)** use of radiation to view internal organs that do not show up on an x-ray

**Oncologist** physician who specializes in treating cancer (tumors)

**Surgery** removal of a tumor and surrounding tissue

**Radiation** emission of rays of energy from a common center that can destroy cancerous cells

**Radiologist** a physician who specializes in the use of radiation to diagnose and treat disease

**Chemotherapy** drugs taken intravenously to kill cancer cells

**Systemic** pertaining to the whole body

**TABLE 7.2 ▶** Summary of American Cancer Society Recommendations for the Early Detection of Cancer in Asymptomatic People

| TYPE OF CANCER | CHECKUP |
| --- | --- |
| **Breast** | Women 40 and older should have an annual mammogram checkup, an annual clinical breast examination (CBE) by a health care professional, and should perform monthly breast self-examination (BSE). The CBE should be conducted close to and preferably before the scheduled mammogram. Women aged 20–39 should have a clinical breast examination by a health care professional every three years and should perform monthly BSE. |
| **Colon and rectum** | Beginning at age 50, men and women at average risk should follow one of the following examination schedules: 1) fecal occult blood test (FOBT) every year, 2) flexible sigmoidoscopy every five years, 3) FOBT every year and flexible sigmoidoscopy every five years, 4) double-contrast barium enema every five years, or 5) colonoscopy every 10 years. (The American Cancer Society prefers option 3 of the first three options.) A digital rectal exam should be done at the same time as sigmoidoscopy, colonoscopy, or double-contrast barium enema. People who are at increased or high risk for colorectal cancer should talk with a doctor about a different testing schedule. |
| **Prostate** | Beginning at age 50, the prostate-specific antigen (PSA) test and the digital rectal exam should be offered annually to men who have a life expectancy of at least 10 years. Men at high risk (African-American men and men who have a first-degree relative who was diagnosed with prostate cancer at a young age) should begin testing at age 45. Patients should be given information about the benefits and limitations of tests so they can make an informed decision. |
| **Uterus** | Cervix: All women who are or have been sexually active or who are 18 and older should have an annual Pap test and pelvic examination. After three or more consecutive satisfactory examinations with normal findings, the Pap test may be performed less frequently. Discuss the matter with your physician.<br>Endometrium: Beginning at age 35, women with or at risk for hereditary nonpolyposis colon cancer should be offered endometrial biopsy annually to screen for endometrial cancer. |

*Note:* A cancer-related check is recommended every three years for people aged 20–40 and every year for people age 40 and older. This exam should include health counseling and, depending on a person's age, might include examinations for cancers of the thyroid, oral cavity, skin, lymph nodes, testes, and ovaries, as well as for some nonmalignant diseases.

The death rate for lung cancer could be cut in half if people did not smoke cigarettes. Because black males tend to smoke cigarettes with a higher tar and nicotine content, they are at greater risk for developing lung cancer than other groups. Black females do not smoke as much as other groups. Other risk factors for lung cancer include exposure to asbestos, radiation and certain chemicals, and secondhand smoke (discussed in Chapter 13).

Signals that should be reported to a physician as soon as they appear are a nagging or persistent cough, blood in the sputum (phlegm coming from the lungs), pain in the chest, shortness of breath, hoarseness or voice change, weight loss, loss of appetite, anemia, and recurring lung infections such as bronchitis. Early detection of lung cancer is difficult, though, because some of the symptoms that people are taught to look for do not appear until the lung cancer is advanced. Clinicians are hopeful that a newer test, low-dose spiral computed tomography (spiral CT), which is used to screen persons at high risk for lung cancer, will reduce the mortality rate.

If lung cancer is diagnosed early, the person has a 43% chance of surviving 12 months. If the tumor is localized, the person has a 48% chance of surviving five years.

Unfortunately, only 15% of lung cancers are discovered early. Treatments other than or in addition to surgery include radiation, chemotherapy, and targeted biological therapies.

*Lung Cancer and Women.* In 2006, 73,000 women in the United States are expected to die from lung cancer. The death of Dana Reeves (widow of Christopher "Superman" Reeves) from lung cancer renewed interest in how this condition affects women. Research published in the *Journal of the American Medical Association (JAMA)* confirms that women are more susceptible to the carcinogens in tobacco than men. However, women who develop lung cancer have better survival rates from the disease after diagnosis. Additionally, the research results suggest that antismoking campaigns for girls and women need to be more aggressive than those for boys and men. Screening for lung cancer in women smokers should be used with women who report lower levels of smoking history than men.

**Colon and Rectum.** The colon and rectum is the third leading cancer site both in women and in men. The 2006 estimates for new cases of cancer of the colon are 106,680 and about 42,000 for rectal cancer. A major risk factor for colorectal cancer is a family history of colorectal cancer or **polyps.** During 1998 to 2002, the incidence rates decreased by 1.8% per year. Health promotion campaigns that encourage persons to have a colonoscopy, to include the removal of polyps (if present), are partially responsible for the decline. Diets high in fat and low in fiber have been linked to increased risk. Death rates (for men and women) from colon and rectum cancer have declined over the last 20 years; the estimated number of deaths for 2006 was slightly more than 55,000.

Signals of colorectal cancer include bleeding from the rectum, blood in the stool (the bowel movement), and

**FIGURE 7.2 ▶** Leading Sites of New Cancer Cases and Deaths, 2006 Estimates

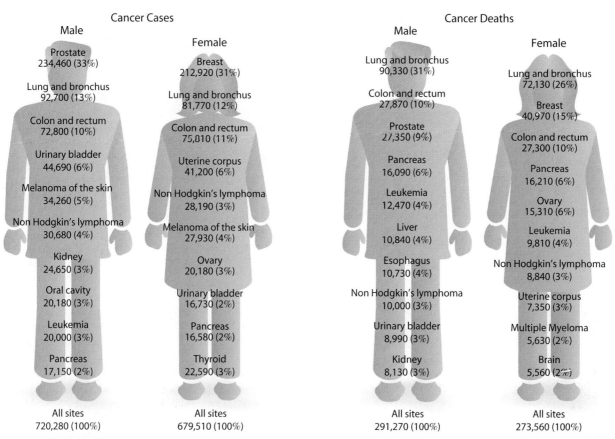

*Note:* Cancer cases exclude basal and squamous cell skin cancers and in situ carcinomas except urinary bladder.
*Source:* American Cancer Society.

changes in bowel habits, cramping pain in the lower abdomen, or characteristics such as recurring constipation or diarrhea.

A physician can detect colorectal cancer in its early stages (even if the person reports no symptoms) by performing a digital rectal examination, a stool blood test (to detect hidden blood or occult blood in the feces), and a proctoscopic examination in some combination. Also, consumer-controlled test kits now are available to use at home.

If problems are indicated, more extensive diagnostic tests should be done. The most common treatment is surgery, sometimes followed by radiation. Chemotherapy also is used in some cases. The target therapies approved by the FDA to treat metastatic colorectal cancer are bevacizumab and cetuximab.

**Breast.** The American Cancer Society has estimated that 212,920 new cases of invasive breast cancer in women and 1,720 new cases of breast cancer in men would be diagnosed in the United States in 2006. One in every eight women develops cancer of the breast. It is the second leading cause of cancer death in women. A woman's age (over 40) is "the most important factor affecting breast cancer risk." The incidence of breast cancer increases with age. Women with a family history or personal history

of breast cancer, early onset of menstruation, and late age at menopause are at risk. Other risk factors include never having a child and having a first birth after age 30. Figure 7.3 shows the risk factors for breast cancer.

*Genes and Breast Cancer.* A woman who has inherited mutations in the *BRAC1* and *BRAC2* cancer susceptibility genes has a 45% to 65% lifetime risk of developing breast cancer. For these women, the risk reduction methods recommended have been prophylactic mastectomy and annual mammography beginning at age 25. A study published in *JAMA* (May 24/31, 2006) reported that using contrast-enhanced breast magnetic resonance imaging (MRI) is cost-effective in screening women (ages 35–54) with inherited mutations in the *BRCA1* gene. In this population of high-risk women, MRI ($1,000 and up vs. $50–$150 for mammographic screening) detects breast

## KEY TERMS

**Polyps** small growths on the wall of the colon or rectum

## FIGURE 7.3 ▶ Risk Factors for Breast Cancer

| Risk factor | Lower risk | | High risk |
|---|---|---|---|
| Country of birth | ASIA AFRICA | | NORTH AMERICA, NORTHERN EUROPE |
| History of premenopausal bilateral breast cancer in family | NO | | YES |
| History of cancer in one breast | NO | | YES |
| Socioeconomic class | LOWER | | UPPER |
| Age at first full-term pregnancy | < 20 | | 30 + |
| Removal of ovaries | YES | | NO |
| Body build after menopause | THIN | | OBESE |
| History of fibrocystic disease | NO | | YES |
| Any first-degree relatives with breast cancer | NO | | YES |
| History of primary cancer in ovary or endometrium | NO | | YES |
| Radiation to chest | SMALL DOSES | | LARGE DOSES |
| Marital status | HAVE BEEN MARRIED | | NEVER MARRIED |
| Place of residence | RURAL | | URBAN |
| Race | BLACK | | WHITE |
| Age at menarche (onset of menstruation) | LATE | | EARLY |
| Age at menopause | EARLY | | LATE |

*Note:* Although mortality rate among blacks is higher than that of whites, their incidence rate is lower.
*Source:* National Center for Health Statistics.

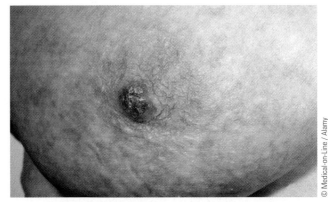

▲ *Dimpling around the nipple is one of the signs of breast cancer.*

**Mammography** is another diagnostic method. It does not seem to reduce breast cancer mortality for premenopausal women. For postmenopausal women, however, this screening may reduce deaths from breast cancer as a result of early detection.

If breast cancer is diagnosed early and the tumor is localized, the woman has a 97% chance of surviving five years. Chemotherapy and radiation are used in any combination and sometimes in conjunction with surgery. In a mastectomy, the entire breast is surgically removed. In a lumpectomy only the lump is removed.

Since breast cancer is now recognized as a "collection" of more than one specific disease, drug treatments have advanced to target the specific type of tumor. A hormonal therapy, such as a selective estrogen receptor modulator (SERM) tamoxifen or raloxifene, is used to reduce the risk of invasive and noninvasive breast cancer if the tumor is stimulated by estrogen or progesterone. Herceptin® is a drug treatment that blocks the HER 2 protein that causes aggressive cell growth.

cancer earlier than mammography and should be added to mammography screening. Women with *BRCA1* gene mutations are at greater risk for developing breast cancer, and their cancer is more aggressive than cancer that develops in women with *BRCA2* gene mutations. Other risk factors for breast cancer include family history, high breast tissue density, and being overweight (BMI of 25–29) or obese (BMI ≥ 30) after menopause (see Figure 7.3). Presently, the best way to reduce the number of deaths from breast cancer is through early detection. The American Cancer Society recommends that women 20 years of age and older should do a breast self-examination (BSE) once a month, after the menstrual period, to spot any irregularity or unusual lump. Signs and symptoms that should be reported to a physician immediately include a persistent lump, swelling, thickening, or distortion of the breast, persistent pain, tenderness of the nipple, and discharge of blood or other fluid from the nipple. Figure 7.4 illustrates different sizes of lumps in the breast and mode of detection.

**Prostate.** The prostate gland is about the size of a walnut and is located in front of the rectum, behind the base of the penis, and under the bladder. Like breast cancer, prostate cancer has a higher incidence rate in older individuals. An estimated 234,460 new cases occurred in 2006. Prostate cancer is the second leading cause of death in men. Risk factors include age, race, diet (diet high in saturated fat), and family history (5% to 10% of prostate cancer). The greatest risk factors, unfortunately, are two that cannot be controlled: being over age 65 and being African American or Jamaican of African descent. One in nine African-American males will develop prostate cancer. This rate, the highest in the world, is 37% higher than for Caucasian men.

Symptoms of prostate cancer are similar to those of other problems of the prostate and urogenital tract. Therefore, a man with any of these symptoms should report to a physician for an examination and diagnostic tests. Signs of a problem include weak or interrupted

**FIGURE 7.4 ►** Size of Tumors Found by Mammography and Breast Self-Exam

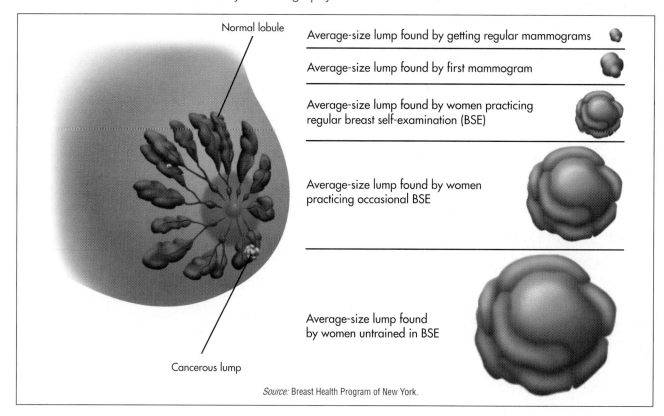

Normal lobule

Average-size lump found by getting regular mammograms

Average-size lump found by first mammogram

Average-size lump found by women practicing regular breast self-examination (BSE)

Average-size lump found by women practicing occasional BSE

Average-size lump found by women untrained in BSE

Cancerous lump

*Source:* Breast Health Program of New York.

urine stream; inability to urinate or difficulty starting or stopping urination; frequent urination, especially at night; blood in the urine; pain or burning during urination; continuing lower back pain, pelvic pain, pain in upper thighs; fatigue; and anemia.

The American Cancer Society recommends an annual digital (finger) rectal examination (DRE) and the prostate-specific antigen (PSA) blood test for men of average risk beginning at age 50. African American, Jamaican, and men with a strong family history should begin annual screening at age 45.

If prostate cancer is diagnosed early, the man has a high chance of recovery, as this is a slow-growing cancer. More than half of all prostate cancers are diagnosed when the tumor is localized. The five-year survival rate for early detection is 99%. Treatment options depend on age, stage of the cancer, and other factors.

Treatments include the following.

1. *Surgery.* The two most common surgical operations are radical prostatectomy (total removal of the prostate and some surrounding tissue) and transurethral resection of the prostate or TURP (removal of only part of the gland).

2. *Radiation.* This is sometimes used to treat prostate cancer that is still confined to the prostate. External beam radiation or brachytherapy (radioactive seed implants) may eliminate the need for surgery.

3. *Hormone therapy.* This often is used with patients whose prostate cancer has metastasized or recurred after treatment. This treatment does not cure the cancer, but it does lower the level of male testosterone, which causes prostate cancer cells to grow.

4. *Chemotherapy (anticancer drugs).* This treatment is used with patients whose prostate cancer has spread outside of the prostate and for whom hormone therapy has failed. It has limited success in treating advanced cases, although it may slow tumor growth and reduce pain. It also is not effective against early prostate cancer.

5. *Careful observation/expectant therapy* ("watchful waiting"). This can be appropriate for older men with prostate cancer that is slow-growing (less aggressive tumor).

The first test to detect if prostate cancer has spread to other tissues was recommended for approval by the Food and Drug Administration (FDA) in 1997. The test, Prostascint, can detect whether cancer has spread 65% of the time, says Dr. Michael Manyak, who led studies at the George Washington University Medical Center. The

## KEY TERMS

**Mammography** an x-ray used to detect breast cancer

**Tips for Action** Breast Self-Exam

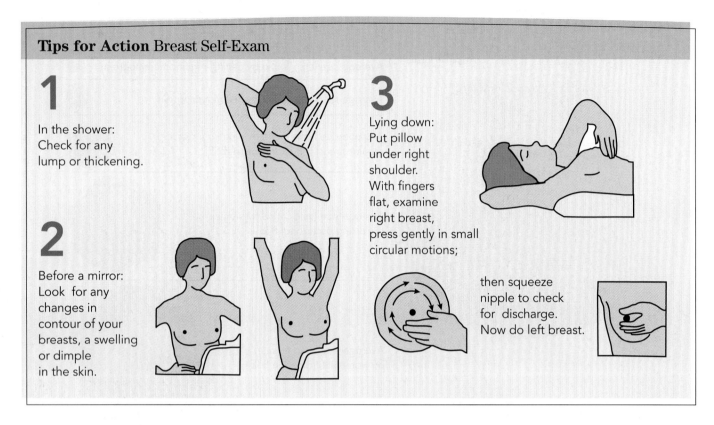

**1**

In the shower:
Check for any
lump or thickening.

**2**

Before a mirror:
Look for any
changes in
contour of your
breasts, a swelling
or dimple
in the skin.

**3**

Lying down:
Put pillow
under right
shoulder.
With fingers
flat, examine
right breast,
press gently in small
circular motions;

then squeeze
nipple to check
for discharge.
Now do left breast.

test uses a radioactive particle that emits a beacon showing the location of traveling cancer cells. The test results will enable the patient to avoid unnecessary surgery and radiation.

**Testicles.** Testicular cancer is one of the most common cancers in males at early adulthood, with the highest risk between ages 15 and 34. The rates for Caucasian males are four times greater than among African Americans. Probable causes have not been identified, except that males who had undescended testicles during childhood seem to have the greatest risk. Testicular cancer may run in families. Also, men who have had mumps have a higher rate of testicular cancer.

In early stages this cancer is painless. Because the first symptom is an enlargement or thickening of the testis, a regular testicular self-examination is advised. The procedure takes only three minutes and is best done after a warm bath or shower. Cure rates are close to 80% as a result of advances in managing the disease.

**Uterus: Cervix and Endometrium.** Cancer of the cervix, at the neck of the uterus, is the more common of the two forms of uterine cancer. Mortality rates have dropped due to aggressive awareness campaigns and screenings. In 2006, 3,700 deaths were estimated compared to 6,600 in 2001 who would die from the disease. When it is found in its early or precancerous stage (**carcinoma *in situ***), it is highly curable. Warning signs of cervical cancer are abnormal uterine bleeding or spotting,

abnormal discharge or bleeding from the vagina, or bleeding after sexual intercourse.

The primary cause of cervical cancer is infection of the cervix by certain "high-risk" types of the human papillomavirus (HPVs 16, 18, 31). Detailed information on HPV and the FDA-approved vaccine to prevent cervical cancer is in Chapter 6 of the text. Other risk factors for cervical cancer are early age at first intercourse, multiple sex partners, and infection with the sexually transmitted disease herpes simplex virus (HSV2). Because the risk factors for cervical cancer are related to sexual behaviors, teens and young women should know them so they can reduce their risk. The five-year survival rate is 91% for localized cancers of the cervix.

Females should have regular pelvic examinations and **Pap tests** for early detection of cervical cancer. The annual screening should begin three years after first intercourse and no later than age 21 (every two years with the liquid-based test). Women age 30 and older should discuss the frequency of the screening with their health care provider. Screening after a hysterectomy (to include removal of the cervix) is necessary if the surgery was done as a treatment for cancer of the cervix. In the regular Pap test (named for the Greek physician George Papanicolaou) a sample of cells is taken from the cervix for microscopic examination.

When diagnosed and treated early, invasive cervical cancer (localized) has a five-year survival rate of 92%. However, Caucasian women are more likely to have invasive cervical cancer diagnosed at the localized stage (56%) than African-American women (48%). It is

## Tips for Action Testicular Self-Exam

1. Roll each testicle gently between the thumb and fingers of both hands.
2. If you find any hard lumps or changes in the normal configuration, see your doctor. Although you can spot the symptoms, only a physician can make a definite diagnosis.

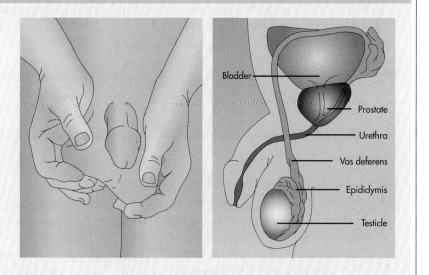

imperative that all women (especially African-American women) have an annual Pap test. Again, early detection is the key to recovery. Treatments include cryotherapy, electrocoagulation, or local surgery for preinvasive lesions. Invasive cancer is treated with surgery, radiation, and sometimes chemotherapy.

Cancer of the endometrium or the lining of the uterus occurs more frequently in women over age 50. Any woman who is experiencing abnormal bleeding should see a physician. This is important for women who have gone through menopause. Risk factors include estrogen exposure (estrogen replacement therapy without progestin), early menarche, late menopause, and polycystic ovary syndrome.

Early detection of endometrial cancer is through an annual pelvic examination. Treatment consists of surgery in the early stages and radiation in later stages. The five-year survival rate is 96% if endometrial cancer is discovered early.

**Ovaries.** Ovarian cancer is difficult to detect. As a result, by the time the most noticeable symptoms appear, the cancer is in its advanced stage. When a woman reports to her physician with symptoms such as bloating (enlargement of the abdomen), abdominal pain, and gas, these may be considered as indicative of a gastrointestinal problem such as an ulcer. Ovarian cancer accounts for about 3% of cancer cases (20,180 new cases in 2006) in women. An estimated 15,310 women died of cancer of the ovary in 2006.

The risk for ovarian cancer is related directly to a woman's lifetime number of ovulations. A high number of ovulations can increase by nine times the chances of producing cells with a genetic flaw that often leads to ovarian cancer, says Andrew Berchuck, professor of gynecologic

oncology at the Duke University Medical Center. Anything that lowers the number of lifetime ovulation cycles reduces the risk. If you have one baby, it decreases the risk by about 13%, he says. If you have three babies your risk is about half that of women who had no babies. Other risks for ovarian cancer include inherited mutations in the *BRCA1* or *BRCA2* cancer susceptibility genes and women who have had breast cancer or have a family history of breast or ovarian cancer.

Birth control pills, which control ovulation, reduce the risk of ovarian cancer. Women should have thorough pelvic examinations regularly to detect ovarian problems. Tests used to diagnosis ovarian cancer (transvaginal ultrasound and a blood test for the tumor marker *CA125*) are offered to women who have high risk or have symptoms. These are not routine screening tests. A biopsy of the ovary is used to confirm a diagnosis. The Pap test cannot be used to detect cancer of the ovaries. Treatments include surgery (removal of the ovaries, uterus, and fallopian tubes) and chemotherapy. The five-year survival rate is 57% for women younger than 65 and 28% for those 65 years and older.

**Skin.** Almost anyone can develop skin cancers. They are more common, however, in males, in light-skinned people

### KEY TERMS

**Carcinoma *in situ*** an early cancer that does not extend beyond the surface layer

**Pap test** diagnostic test for cancers of the cervix, uterus, and vagina, performed by taking a sample of cells from the cervix for examination under a microscope

HEALTHY PEOPLE 2010 Objectives for Cancer

- Reduce the lung cancer, breast cancer, cancer of the cervix, and colon cancer death rates.
- Increase the proportion of women who receive a Pap test.
- Increase the proportion of women aged 40 years and older who have received a mammogram within the preceding two years.

- Increase the proportion of cancer survivors who are living five years or longer after diagnosis.

## FYI | PAP TEST RESCREENING

The Food and Drug Administration has approved two new systems for detecting abnormal cells in a Pap test that might be missed by the cytotechnologist during manual screenings.

1. PAPNET uses computer technology that reads the Pap slides (containing sample cells from the cervix) and creates enlarged color images of cells that are likely to be abnormal based on computer-developed guidelines that were created by feeding a series of digitized images of Pap slides into the computer.
2. AutoPap 300 QC is a computerized system that uses image processing and pattern recognition techniques (size, shape, texture of cells) to classify cells as abnormal.

Women should ask if the laboratory where their Pap smears are sent uses either of these rescreening technologies.

Even with these new technologies, some women will be told that their Pap test is normal because of too few cells on the slide or cell samples were not taken from both the inside and the surface of the cervix. Douching or using vaginal spermicides one or two days before a Pap test can wash away abnormal cells and reduce the tests' accuracy.

Another form of skin cancer that is not as prevalent but is much more serious is **malignant melanoma.** This form of skin cancer affected approximately 62,000 people in 2006 in the United States, killing an estimated 10,710. A person's risk of malignant melanoma can be calculated from the number, size, and appearance of moles on the skin. Diagnosis hinges on the presence of abnormal moles, called **dysplastic nevi.** Research at the National Cancer Institute identified risk factors for melanoma: the number of abnormal moles (10 or more) or unusual moles or large moles (a tumor nine inches long). The increased risk is roughly equivalent to the risk conferred by multiple sunburns. Other risk factors for all skin cancers include the use of tanning beds/booths, immunosuppression conditions, and occupational exposure to chemicals such as coal tar and creosote.

Changes in moles and other skin lesions should be brought to a physician's attention as soon as they are found. To reduce the risk of skin cancers in the first place, people should avoid unnecessary exposure to the sun or ultraviolet rays for long periods (especially 10 a.m. to 4:00 p.m.). Individuals with light skin pigmentation are more at risk. When outdoors, people should wear protective clothing, such as a hat with a brim, wear sunglasses, and use waterproof sunscreen. The American Academy of Dermatology recommends a sunscreen product with a **sun protection factor (SPF)** of 15 or higher. The SPF number can be found on the label of the product. Since severe sunburn in early childhood may increase the risk of skin cancer, children should be protected.

**Oral Cavity.** The major risk factors for cancer of the oral cavity are combustible and smokeless tobacco products and excessive use of alcohol (see also Chapter 13). If one form of cancer is related directly to a person's behavior, this is it. Anyone who smokes (cigarettes, cigars, pipe) or uses chewing tobacco or snuff should examine the mouth regularly, including the lips and tongue, for lesions.

Signs to be alerted to are sores that bleed or will not heal and a red or white lesion (patch) that will not go away. These may appear on the area of the lip where the cigarette or cigar rests or inside the lip where the chewing tobacco or snuff is placed. Other symptoms, such a persistent sore throat, should be reported to a physician

(easily sunburned; naturally blond or red hair), and people who live at a high altitude (the states of AZ, CA, CO, ID, MT, NV, NM, OR, UT, WA, WY). Other than having light skin pigmentation or being male, the main risk factor is too much exposure to the **ultraviolet (UV) rays** of the sun. Of all skin cancers, 90% occur on parts of the body not usually covered with clothing—the face, hands, forearms, and ears.

The two types of skin cancers that have the highest incidence are **basal cell carcinoma** and **squamous cell carcinoma.** Most of these skin cancers are curable, especially if they are treated early. More than 1 million cases occur annually.

A type of skin cancer called malignant melanoma is not the most common form, but it is the most deadly. Approximately 40,300 new cases are diagnosed each year; about 8,000 people die of the condition annually. Many African Americans have a lower risk for malignant melanoma because they have more skin pigment, melanin, which protects against skin cancer. Malignant melanoma occurs 10 times more often among whites than African Americans and four times more often among whites than Latinos.

African Americans with lighter skin can develop malignant melanoma. Dark-skinned African Americans may develop malignant lesions on the lighter areas of the body, such as the palms, soles, or inside the mouth. Even though the risk is lower, African Americans and Latinos (especially those with lighter skin) should take the same precautions as whites to reduce the risk of skin cancer. Avoid unnecessary exposure to the sun, and use a sunscreen with a sun protection factor (SPF) of 15 or higher.

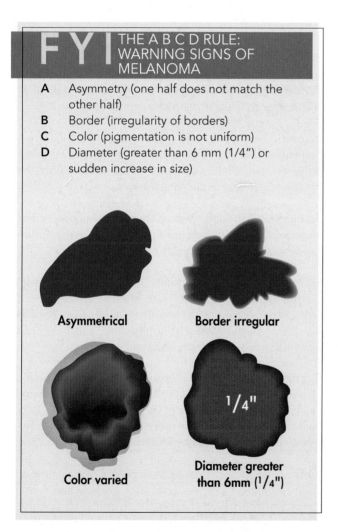

## FYI THE A B C D RULE: WARNING SIGNS OF MELANOMA

**A** Asymmetry (one half does not match the other half)
**B** Border (irregularity of borders)
**C** Color (pigmentation is not uniform)
**D** Diameter (greater than 6 mm (1/4″) or sudden increase in size)

**Asymmetrical**

**Border irregular**

**Color varied**

**Diameter greater than 6mm (¹/₄″)**

1/4″

has pointed out health choices that might reduce an individual's risk of cancer.

**Smoking.** Cigarette smoking is responsible for 90% of lung cancers among men and 79% among women—about 87% overall. Smoking accounts for about 30% of all cancer deaths. Those who smoke two or more packs of cigarettes a day have lung cancer mortality rates 12 to 25 times greater than those who don't smoke.

**Nutrition and Diet.** According to a 1997 report from the Harvard University School of Public Health, 3 to 4 million people need not have developed cancer if they had adhered to a healthy diet.

Some guidelines are as follows.

1. *Maintain recommended weight.* For people who are obese, weight reduction is a good way to lower cancer risk. Weight maintenance can be accomplished by

### KEY TERMS

**Ultraviolet (UV) rays** beams of radiation from the sun that contribute to the development of skin cancer when a person is exposed to them

**Basal cell carcinoma** common type of skin cancer that usually does not metastasize

**Squamous cell carcinoma** common type of skin cancer that affects the squamous layer of the epidermis

**Malignant melanoma** a more serious type of cancer in the form of a pigmented mole or tumor

**Dysplastic nevi** flat, irregularly shaped moles, mottled in color with indistinct borders; a warning sign of malignant melanoma

**Sun protection factor (SPF)** the numerical rating given to a product that informs the consumer how effectively the product protects from the sun's ultraviolet rays

or dentist. Oral cancer is easy to detect and cure in its early stages.

## CANCER PREVENTION

If everything known about the prevention of cancer were applied, up to two-thirds of cancers would not occur. The following are areas in which the American Cancer Society

---

**Tips for Action** How to Help Prevent Skin Cancer

■ Avoid the sun. Try to stay out of the sun from 10 a.m. to 3 p.m., when sun rays are strongest.

■ Cover up. When you are out in the sun, wear wide-brimmed hats, long-sleeved shirts, and pants. Keep your neck covered.

■ Use a sunscreen with a sun protection factor (SPF) of 15. Sunscreen keeps out the ultraviolet rays. Apply it at least 15–30 minutes before going in the sun. Put on more after swimming or sweating.

■ Beware of cloudy days. You still can get burned then.

■ The sun's rays can reach through three feet of water, so even though you may feel cool in the water, the sun can still burn you.

■ Watch out for the sun in wintertime. Snow reflects sunlight, which can burn you.

■ Do not use sunlamps, tanning parlors, or tanning pills. They can be just as harmful to your body as the sun.

■ Look at your skin. Check moles, spots, and birthmarks monthly. If they change in appearance or grow, consult a doctor.

---

reducing intake of total calories and by maintaining a physically active lifestyle.

2. *Eat a varied diet.* Variety in the diet and moderation offer the best hope for lowering the risk of cancer.

3. *Include a variety of vegetables and fruits in the daily diet.* Daily consumption of vegetables and fresh fruits is associated with decreased risk of lung, prostate, bladder, esophagus, colorectal, and stomach cancers.

4. *Eat more high-fiber foods such as whole-grain cereals, breads, and pasta, and vegetables and fruits.* High-fiber diets are a healthy substitute for fatty foods and may reduce the risk of colon cancer.

5. *Cut down on total fat intake.* A diet high in fat may be a factor in the development of certain cancers, particularly breast, colon, and prostate. The American Cancer Society recommends reducing total fat intake to 30% or less of total calorie intake.

6. *Limit consumption of alcohol, if you drink at all.* Heavy drinking, especially when accompanied by cigarette smoking or smokeless tobacco use, increases risk of cancers of the mouth, larynx, throat, esophagus, and liver.

7. *Limit consumption of salt-cured, smoked, and nitrite-cured foods.* Areas of the world where salt-cured and smoked foods are eaten frequently have a higher incidence of cancer of the esophagus and stomach. Modern methods of food processing and preserving seem to avoid the cancer-causing by-products associated with older methods of food treatment.

**Sunlight.** Almost all of the more than 1 million cases of basal and squamous cell skin cancer diagnosed each year in the United States are sun-related (ultraviolet radiation). Sun exposure is a major factor in the development of melanoma, and the incidence increases for those living near the equator.

**Physical Activity.** Recently the importance of physical activity in preventing cancer has received attention. The Harvard report recommends a brisk hour-long walk daily and at least an hour of vigorous exercise each week.

**Alcohol.** Oral cancer and cancers of the larynx, throat, esophagus, and liver occur more frequently among heavy drinkers of alcohol, especially when accompanied by smoking cigarettes or chewing tobacco.

**Smokeless Tobacco.** Use of chewing tobacco or snuff increases the risk of cancer of the mouth, larynx, throat, and esophagus, and it is highly addictive.

**Estrogen.** Estrogen treatment to manage menopausal symptoms can increase the risk of endometrial cancer. Using progesterone with the estrogen, however, lessens this risk. Consultation with a physician will help each woman assess her personal risks and benefits.

**Occupational Hazards.** Exposure to certain industrial agents (such as nickel, chromate, asbestos, and vinyl chloride) increases the risk of various cancers. The risk of lung cancer from asbestos increases greatly when exposure to asbestos is combined with cigarette smoking.

**Ionizing Radiation.** Excessive exposure to ionizing radiation can increase cancer risk. Most medical and dental x-rays are adjusted to deliver the lowest dose possible without sacrificing image quality.

## Diseases of the Respiratory System

Following cardiovascular diseases and cancer on the list of leading causes of death in the United States is the category of **chronic obstructive lung disease (COLD),** also called chronic obstructive pulmonary disease (COPD).

## Tips for Action Some Symptoms of Common Cancers

See your physician promptly if you notice these symptoms of common cancers.

■ **Lung:** chronic cough or hoarseness; coughing up blood; chest pain or shortness of breath; regular pneumonia or bronchitis

■ **Breast:** a new lump; thickening or pain in the breast or armpit that persists; nipple tenderness or discharge; retraction or distortion of the breast

■ **Colon and Rectum:** blood in stool; major change in bowel habits; regular constipation or diarrhea; unusual abdominal pain or cramping.

■ **Prostate:** blood in urine; painful or difficult urination; inability to urinate or difficulty starting; persistent pain in lower back, pelvis, or upper thigh

■ **Uterus and Cervix:** abnormal vaginal bleeding; unusual abdominal pain or swelling that persists; pain during intercourse

■ **Skin:** a sore that will not heal; change in shape, size, or color of a mole; sudden appearance of a mole or lump

■ **Oral:** a sore on lips or mouth that will not heal; swelling or lumps in mouth, neck, lips, or tongue; chronic hoarseness or coughing; trouble swallowing

*Source:* American Medical Security.

The major lung diseases, aside from cancer, are chronic bronchitis, emphysema, and chronic asthma. Most are caused by cigarette smoking (discussed in Chapter 13). Environmental pollution (discussed in Chapter 15) is a contributing factor.

The respiratory system consists of the nose, throat, larynx, trachea, bronchi, and lungs (see Figure 7.5). Its function is to supply the blood with oxygen and relieve it of carbon dioxide. This exchange of oxygen and carbon dioxide takes place in the lungs. Air enters the lungs through the nose, where it is warmed, moistened, and filtered before it goes into the throat and **trachea** (windpipe). The trachea divides into two main **bronchi,** which connect to each of the two lungs.

In the lung the bronchi divide and subdivide, forming smaller passageways called bronchioles, and ending in air sacs called **alveoli.** The exchange of gases takes place in the alveoli, through tiny capillaries. During inhalation and exhalation the lungs expand and contract by movements of the rib cage and the diaphragm. The **pleurae,** membranes that line the chest cavity, allow the surfaces of the lungs and chest cavity to move past each other smoothly.

## BRONCHITIS

Chronic **bronchitis** is more than a bad case of the common cold. It can be a serious, even life-threatening respiratory disorder. It is characterized by inflammation and

**FIGURE 7.5** ▶ Respiratory System

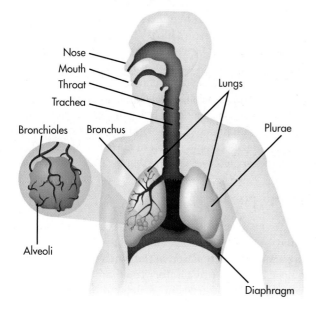

Nose
Mouth
Throat
Trachea
Lungs
Bronchioles
Bronchus
Plurae
Alveoli
Diaphragm

### KEY TERMS

**Chronic obstructive lung disease (COLD)** lung diseases characterized by decreased breathing functions; includes chronic bronchitis, emphysema, and chronic asthma; COPD or COBD

**Trachea** tube that connects the larynx to the lungs; windpipe

**Bronchi** two main passageways that connect to each lung from the trachea

**Alveoli** air sacs in the lungs where the exchange of gases takes place

**Pleurae** membranes that line the chest cavity and reduce friction during respiration

**Bronchitis** inflammation of the bronchial tubes in the lungs

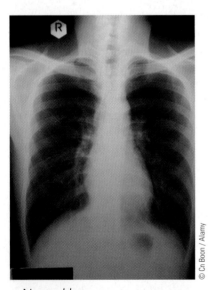

▲ *Normal lung*

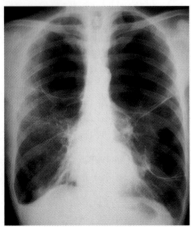

▲ *Lung with emphysema*

swelling of the bronchi, which impair normal respiratory function. The increased mucous secretion further clogs the bronchi and has to be coughed up to keep the breathing tubes free. Symptoms of bronchitis include a cough, wheezing, and shortness of breath, persisting for several weeks.

Over time, chronic bronchitis may cause the bronchial tubes to become severely obstructed. The heart enlarges because it has to pump harder than usual to deliver oxygen to the rest of the body.

Diagnosis is by chest x-ray and special machines that measure the amount of air flowing in and out of the lungs. Medical treatment consists of drinking plenty of water, being in humid surroundings, and taking bronchodilator medications that expand the cavity of the bronchial tubes.

## EMPHYSEMA

**Emphysema** is a progressive lung disease that eventually destroys the alveoli so that people who are affected have more and more difficulty breathing. The alveoli become nonfunctional and stiff instead of elastic. As the disease progresses, the oxygen supply in the blood is diminished, which overburdens the cardiovascular system and damages the heart. Tobacco smoke and air pollutants are the most common causes of emphysema.

The main symptom is shortness of breath, accompanied by a cough and difficulty breathing. Advanced-stage patients tire easily because of the large effort involved in merely breathing. Overinflation of the lungs produces the barrel-shaped chest often identified with people who have emphysema. The lack of oxygen may cause the lips, ear lobes, skin, and fingernails to be tinged blue.

Except for the few cases caused by a genetic disorder, no one test can be used to diagnose emphysema. Blood tests and chest x-rays do not uncover emphysema in its early stages. Only through a series of tests can it be diagnosed. Unfortunately, effects of the disease cannot be reversed, and the person's life is shortened.

The disease can be slowed, however, by removing the irritants that led to it, and those affected can be made more comfortable by drinking large amounts of fluids, getting adequate rest, eating a balanced diet, and, upon the advice of a physician, exercising moderately. Vaporizers and humidifiers may be helpful. In addition, several prescription drugs act to loosen mucus (an indication of chronic bronchitis) and expand the air passages. Oxygen therapy may be necessary.

## HAY FEVER

**Hay fever** is considered a mild respiratory ailment related most often to agents in the environment that induce an allergic reaction in the mucous membranes of the nose and upper respiratory tract. It often is seasonal, evoked by buds on trees in spring and the pollens from

## FYI THE POSSIBLE ROLE OF ALLERGY IN ASTHMA

| Symptoms | Probable Cause |
|---|---|
| Is your asthma worse in certain months? If so, are these symptoms at the same time of allergic rhinitis—sneezing, itching, runny and obstructed nose? | Pollens and outdoor molds |
| Do symptoms appear when visiting a house that has indoor pets? | Animal dander |
| Do eyes itch and become red after handling a pet? If the pet licks you, does a red, itchy welt develop? | Animal dander |
| Do symptoms appear in a room where carpets are being vacuumed? | Animal dander, mites, dust |
| Does making a bed cause symptoms? | Mites |
| Do symptoms develop when you go into a damp basement or a vacation cottage that has been closed up for some time? | Molds |
| Do symptoms develop related to certain job activities, either at work or after leaving work? | Environmental agents, indoor pollution |
| If symptoms develop at work, do they improve when away from work for a few days? | Indoor pollution |

*Source:* U.S. Department of Health and Human Services, National Institutes of Health, Public Health Service, 1994.

various plants in autumn. Characterized by sneezing and itchy, watery eyes and nose, hay fever seems to run in families. An overly active immune system is what precipitates the allergic reaction. Medical relief usually is found in the form of antihistamines. Hay fever, though not considered serious in itself (although the discomfort is not denied), sometimes leads to asthma.

## ASTHMA

**Asthma** is a respiratory disease characterized by acute attacks of wheezing and difficulty breathing, caused by obstruction (or narrowing) of the bronchioles. It is most common in children and often disappears with the passing of time. Three distinctly different causes are allergens; nonallergen, stress-related causes (discussed in Chapter

3); and exercise-induced asthma. The latter type is most common in athletes. It is brought on by overexertion, particularly in cold weather, which dries out the bronchi. It is easily treated and usually can be prevented by warming up 10 minutes before vigorous exercise.

In the first type, agents such as pollen, dust, animal fur, bee venom, or specific foods bring on the asthma attack. It can be prevented or treated by **immunotherapy,** in which the person is desensitized through injections of weakened allergens. Antihistamines and corticosteroid drugs also are successful in reducing inflammation. Once an attack has begun, bronchodilator drugs are taken through an inhaler. This usually restores breathing to normal.

The number of people who have asthma has risen markedly since 1982, especially in women and minorities. Death rates from asthma are highest among people who are at least 55 years old. Even though overall death rates still are relatively low (about five per million), the death rate for urban African Americans in the age range 15–44 years is five times higher than that for Caucasians. Hispanics also have higher asthma-related death rates.

A study conducted by researchers at Hahnemann University Hospital in Philadelphia concluded that metropolitan air pollution apparently is not the cause, as outdoor pollution declined during the period when the death rates from asthma went up. Other suspected reasons are indoor air pollution and secondhand smoke.

A long-term study of nearly 2,500 asthma patients in Rochester, Minnesota, concluded that the life expectancy of asthmatics is no different from people who do not have asthma. The exception is the patients who were at least 35 years old when their asthma was diagnosed and people who had additional lung diseases.

## Blood Disorders

The blood disorders that most often come to mind are the anemias—iron-deficiency anemia and pernicious anemia. An inherited form of anemia, sickle cell anemia, is associated largely with African Americans.

### KEY TERMS

**Emphysema** progressive lung disease that eventually destroys the alveoli and greatly reduces lung functioning

**Hay fever** mild respiratory ailment caused by environmental agents that provoke the body to produce histamines

**Asthma** chronic respiratory disease characterized by attacks of wheezing and difficulty breathing caused by narrowing of the bronchi that may be triggered by allergens

**Immunotherapy** desensitization to allergens through periodic injections of weakened allergens

## ANEMIA

**Anemia** is a condition in which a person has an insufficient quantity or quality of red blood cells. The function of these cells is to carry oxygen to the tissues and organs so the bodily systems can function normally. Oxygen is carried on the red blood cells by the chemical **hemoglobin,** which also is responsible for the cell's red color. Individuals with anemia have reduced hemoglobin (and oxygen in circulation) and may experience fatigue and other symptoms. If the anemia becomes too severe, the person is susceptible to infection and may have trouble healing.

In many cases anemia is the result of inadequate amounts of iron in the diet. Called **iron-deficiency anemia,** it can be corrected by an iron supplement. Chapter 9 contains additional information on iron in the diet. Sometimes health conditions such as cancer or heavy menstrual flow may cause a person to be anemic. The cause has to be diagnosed so the proper treatment can follow.

Another type of anemia, which stems from a nutritional deficiency, is called **pernicious anemia** or **vitamin $B_{12}$ deficiency anemia.** In this condition the person has a deficiency in vitamin $B_{12}$ because the body is not able to absorb it, or it may develop in vegans who do not take vitamin supplements. Pernicious anemia is treated by vitamin $B_{12}$ injections.

## SICKLE CELL DISEASE

Some forms of anemia are attributable to an inherited trait. One type of genetic-based anemia, or **hemoglobinopathy,** is called **sickle cell disease (SCD).** Approximately 72,000 African Americans have sickle cell disease. The sickle cell gene also is carried by people whose ancestors come from countries around the Mediterranean Sea, the Arabian Peninsula, and portions of India. According to the March of Dimes, one in every 1,000 to 1,500 Latinos living in the United States has sickle cell disease. In addition, many people carry one sickle gene or have the sickle cell trait. This means that, although they do not have the disease itself, they can pass the gene to their children.

Generations of Africans living in the malaria belts of the African continent were protected genetically from malaria when, over time, they developed a sickle gene that altered the composition of their red blood cells. Those who carried one sickle gene were more resistant to the blood-borne parasite that causes malaria. This inherited protection, the sickle cell gene, was passed to successive generations and was brought to the Americas with the slave trade. This is why one in 10 or 12 African Americans carries the sickle gene and has sickle cell trait. Sickle cell anemia is just one of several sickle cell diseases. Other common sickle cell diseases are sickle hemoglobin C disease (SC disease) and sickle cell thalassemia disease (S/Thal).

Normally, red blood cells are soft, round, doughnut-shaped cells that are able to pass through even the tiniest blood vessels. Sickle cells, in contrast, take on the sickle shape for which the disease is named (see Figure 7.6). Instead of passing through the blood vessels, these cells clump together and clog tiny vessels (impeding the flow of oxygen-carrying blood), which is painful. Most people with sickle cell disease have at least one or two crises, called painful episodes, each year, and 15% to 20% endure these crises more frequently.

**Inheritance.** Because sickle cell anemia is a recessive trait-inherited condition, two recessive genes (sickle genes) have to be present to produce sickle cell anemia in a child. One sickle cell gene has to come from the mother and the other from the father. Figure 7.7 illustrates the way the sickle cell gene is inherited. *A* designates the gene for normal hemoglobin, and *s* denotes the sickle cell gene. Because the child gets half of his or her genetic material from each parent, *AA* designates two inherited genes for normal hemoglobin. The child who inherits one gene for normal hemoglobin and one for sickle cell hemoglobin is designated *As* and has the sickle cell trait. The letters *ss* indicate that the child inherited two sickle genes, one from each parent, and has sickle cell anemia.

If both parents have normal hemoglobin (*AA*), any children they conceive will have normal hemoglobin as well. Conversely, if both parents have sickle cell anemia (*ss*), any children they conceive will have the disease like their parents. If, however, both parents have sickle trait (*As*), the probability or odds for each child to have the genes *AA*, *As*, or *ss* are as follows.

- 25% risk of inheriting two sickle genes and thus sickle cell anemia (*ss*)

**FIGURE 7.6** ▶ Normal Red Blood Cell and Sickle Cell

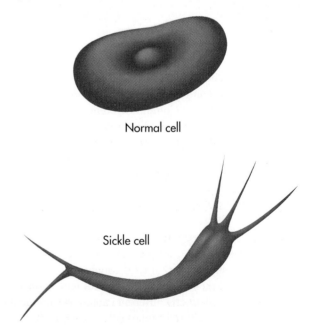

Normal cell

Sickle cell

**FIGURE 7.7** ▶ How Sickle Cell Anemia Is Inherited

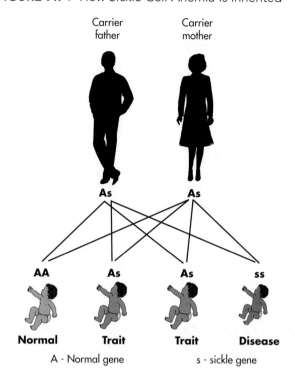

Carrier father          Carrier mother

As          As

AA          As          As          ss

Normal          Trait          Trait          Disease

A - Normal gene          s - sickle gene

- 25% chance of inheriting two normal genes and thus normal hemoglobin (*AA*)

- 50% chance of inheriting one normal and one sickle gene and thus sickle cell trait (*As*)

**Symptoms, Diagnosis, and Treatment.** Individuals with sickle cell trait usually have no apparent symptoms. Though healthy, the person carries an inherited sickle cell gene that can be passed on to any children conceived. Sometimes individuals with sickle cell trait become short of breath temporarily or have some pain if they are in an environment in which the oxygen levels are lower than normal, such as at high altitudes while traveling in the mountains, when deep-sea diving, or after receiving general, inhalation-type anesthesia for surgery.

People with sickle cell anemia may develop symptoms as early as six months of age. One sign is pain and swelling in the hands or feet. Babies with sickle cell disease may stop making red blood cells for a short time, called an **aplastic crisis.** Symptoms include inactivity, pallor, and rapid breathing and heartbeat. As its name implies, aplastic crisis requires immediate medical attention.

In the summer of 2006, a national campaign, "Be Sickle Smart," was initiated to educate persons with SCD and their families about SCD and iron overload, which is a consequence of repeated blood transfusions that may be used as treatment. The NFL player Tiki Barber partnered with Novartis Pharmaceuticals to launch AskTiki.com.

A person with sickle cell anemia has a weakened immune system and thus is susceptible to infection. A fever over 100°F may indicate an infection. In the past, many people with sickle cell anemia died by age 20, and few survived past 40. Now infants and young children (under six years) are prescribed **prophylactic penicillin therapy** as a preventive measure against infections such as meningitis, hepatitis B, and pneumonia, which are major causes of complications and death. Penicillin, however, does not cure sickle cell anemia.

In early 1995 the National Institutes of Health (NIH) announced a new treatment for severe cases of sickle cell anemia for adults over 18 years. The cancer drug hydroxyurea proved to be so effective in alleviating the pain of sickle cell episodes that the NIH ended drug trials four months early and made the drug available to physicians. It seems to work by stimulating the body to increase the production of fetal hemoglobin that resists sickle cell clumping. Although this drug is not a cure, it is a welcome advance in the treatment of sickle cell disease. More research is needed to investigate the long-term effects. However, hydroxyurea is considered to be safe for children between the ages of five and 15 years.

The emphasis is shifting to prevention through education and genetic counseling. The basic screening test used to determine if a person carries the sickle gene is a blood test called hemoglobin electrophoresis. With the aid of this test, couples who are considering conceiving a child are able to weigh their risk of having a child with sickle cell anemia.

**KEY TERMS**

**Anemia** condition characterized by an insufficient quantity or quality of red blood cells (RBCs)

**Hemoglobin** a chemical in red blood cells that carries oxygen and is responsible for the RBCs' color

**Iron-deficiency anemia** anemia caused by an iron deficiency. It can be cured with an iron supplement

**Pernicious anemia** or **vitamin B$_{12}$ deficiency anemia** a condition in which the stomach does not produce intrinsic factor to combine with and transport vitamin B$_{12}$ to the bloodstream

**Hemoglobinopathy** abnormal hemoglobin in the blood

**Sickle cell disease** an inherited form of anemia that produces sickle-shaped cells that clump together and clog tiny blood vessels

**Aplastic crisis** interruption in the body's production of RBCs; may occur in persons with sickle cell disease

**Prophylactic penicillin therapy** use of penicillin to prevent infections from occurring in infants and young children with sickle cell anemia

# A Disease of the Metabolism: Diabetes

The glands of the **endocrine system** manufacture the body's hormones and secrete them directly into the bloodstream. The ductless glands include the pituitary, thyroid, parathyroid, adrenal, ovary, testis, and part of the pancreas. The hormones are responsible for regulating body functions.

**Diabetes mellitus,** usually called diabetes or "sugar diabetes," is a chronic condition in which a person has excessive amounts of glucose or blood sugar in the circulatory system because of insufficient production of the hormone **insulin** or insensitivity of the body's cells to insulin. Normal blood sugar ranges from 70 to 110 mg/dL. (Factors such as time of day, meals, illness, stress, and medications can cause a person's blood sugar to increase.) It affects 20.8 million Americans and is one of the leading (in the top 10) causes of death in the United States. Approximately 800,000 new cases are diagnosed annually, making diabetes mellitus a growing public health concern. In 2005, 1.5 million new cases were diagnosed. Insulin is produced by the beta cells of the pancreas in the **islets of Langerhans** and is secreted into the bloodstream. Insulin has two major functions.

1. To move glucose from the blood to the cells of the body where it is used as energy.

2. To convert excess glucose to glycogen, stored as an energy reserve in the liver and muscles.

## TYPES OF DIABETES

People with diabetes are unable to process glucose properly and, as a result, the glucose accumulates in the blood. The form of diabetes in which the pancreas is not producing insulin is called **type 1 diabetes** or **insulin-dependent diabetes.** This form, the more serious of the two, requires regular insulin injections. Although it accounts for only about 5% to 10% or less of all diabetes in the United States, that figure represents as many as a half million cases.

Type 1 diabetes is unknown or rare in some ethnic groups, including the Japanese, Chinese, Polynesians, and South African blacks. Meanwhile, Scandinavians (specifically Swedish and Finnish peoples) have much higher rates than the U.S. population overall.

Evidence indicates that type 1 diabetes may be triggered by a virus that infects only people whose genes make them vulnerable to the disease. According to Dr. Massimo Trucco of the University of Pittsburgh, if the virus can be identified, a vaccine might be devised to administer to newborns and thereby prevent them from contracting diabetes.

In the more common form, **type 2 diabetes** or **non-insulin-dependent diabetes,** the pancreas produces some insulin, but the cells of the body are not able to use it effectively. As many as 90% of diabetics over age 20 are

**FYI** RISK FACTORS FOR DIABETES

- A family history of diabetes
- Overweight (BMI 25–29) or obese (BMI ≥ 30)
- Over age 45 (although Hispanics over age 30 are at high risk)
- Lack of exercise
- Ethnic background, including African Americans, Hispanics, American Indians, and Pacific Islanders, who are more likely to develop diabetes and run a greater risk of complications
- Women who have had a baby weighing more than nine pounds at birth or developed diabetes while pregnant

of this type. Type 2 diabetes (formerly called adult-onset diabetes) usually occurs after age 40. Scientific evidence indicates that the inherited SHIP2 gene may double the odds of developing type 2 diabetes. However, those persons represent only about 20% of the cases of type 2 diabetes. The majority of the cases are due to overweight and obesity, dietary patterns, and lack of regular exercise.

Type 2 diabetes is about twice as prevalent in minority groups (except Asians) as in Caucasians. In African Americans it is the fourth leading cause of death from disease. African-American women are more than twice as likely as Caucasian women to develop diabetes. About one in 10 African Americans between ages 45 and 65 has diabetes, and the incidence increases with advancing age. One in four African-American women over age 55 has diabetes. The rate for Hispanics is even higher. Diabetes is the third leading cause of death in Hispanic women. The typical high-fat diet of this as well as African-American cultures makes them more prone to the disease. Figure 7.8 shows the proportional prevalence of type 2 diabetes by various ethnic minorities in the United States. Other risk factors for type 2 diabetes include having a family history of the condition and being overweight. American Indians have the highest rate of type 2 diabetes in the world. The overall prevalence of type 2 diabetes is over 12.8% in American Indians compared with 7% in the general population. Some experts believe that American Indians carry a gene that slows the body's use of calories, causing the body to store fat instead of burning it.

In both type 1 and type 2 diabetes, when the diabetic person eats a meal, the glucose accumulates in the blood and produces a condition called **hyperglycemia,** or high blood sugar. Because the cells of the body cannot get glucose for energy from the blood and the body has no glycogen reserve, the cells burn protein and fat as their source of fuel. The burning of fat in the absence of glucose causes the formation of acid substances called ketones.

**FIGURE 7.8** ▶ Prevalence of Diabetes and Pre-diabetes in U.S. Subpopulations, 2005

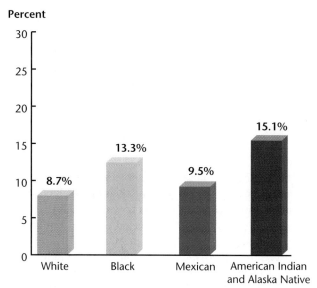

Percent

Source: American Diabetes Association, 2007.

The accumulation of these ketones leads to **ketoacidosis** or **ketosis,** which can result in coma and death.

## SIGNS AND SYMPTOMS OF DIABETES

The symptoms of type 1 diabetes appear suddenly and dramatically. In some cases people develop ketoacidosis before they even think about seeing a physician. Symptoms of type 1 diabetes include fatigue and irritability, abnormal hunger and thirst, frequent urination, and weight loss. Some of the same symptoms occur in type 2 diabetes. The signals seem to be more subtle for type 2 diabetes, and the person may not notice them until a blood test is done during a routine health examination. Other signs that may signal type 2 diabetes are drowsiness, blurred vision, itching, slow-healing cuts, skin infections, and numbness of fingers or toes.

If you have the following risk factors, you should be tested at least every other year beginning at age 20: waist circumference greater than 35 inches (women) or 40 inches (men) or a BMI ≥ 25; a first-degree relative with the disease; diabetes during pregnancy; African American, Hispanic/Latino American or Asian American; rarely exercise. There is a link between diabetes and the CVDs (heart disease, stroke, atherosclerosis). You can reduce your risk by lowering your **A**1C (a test that measures blood sugar) to less than 7, and keeping your Blood pressure below 130/80 and your LDL "bad" Cholesterol below 100—the A-B-Cs of diabetes.

Syndrome X (metabolic syndrome) also is a risk factor for diabetes mellitus and CHD. It is characterized by excess abdominal fat (apple shape) causing at least two of the following: insulin resistence, elevated blood lipids, and high blood pressure.

In type 1 diabetes two life-threatening complications can arise if the person's blood sugar level becomes too high or too low because of an imbalance of insulin: diabetic coma and insulin reaction. In **diabetic coma** the amount of insulin the person has injected is not enough to process the glucose in the bloodstream. This causes hyperglycemia and leads to ketoacidosis. If this problem is not corrected, it can lead to coma and death.

The person experiences the same symptoms as those when type 1 diabetes was first diagnosed. Additional symptoms include dry skin and mouth, labored breathing, nausea and vomiting, a sweet or fruity breath odor, large amounts of ketones in the urine, and a blood sugar level of more than 300 mg/dL. Because diabetic coma develops slowly, the person usually can be transported to a hospital in time to receive insulin treatment.

If a person has injected too much insulin, skipped a meal, or engaged in excessive physical activity, the blood sugar level may drop below normal levels. The result is called **insulin shock,** a form of **hypoglycemia** or low blood sugar (<40 to 50 mg/dL of blood). Unlike diabetic coma, the onset of insulin reaction is sudden. Some of the symptoms are a weak or faint feeling, hunger, trembling, moist skin, headache, confused or irritable behavior that may escalate to rapid heartbeat, shallow breathing, and

### KEY TERMS

**Endocrine system** body system composed of glands that manufacture and secrete hormones directly into the blood; ductless glands

**Diabetes mellitus** chronic condition characterized by excessive amounts of glucose in the blood due to abnormal metabolism of glucose

**Insulin** hormone essential for processing glucose in the body

**Islets of Langerhans** cells in the pancreas that produce insulin

**Type 1 diabetes** or **insulin-dependent diabetes (IDDM)** form of diabetes in which the pancreas does not produce insulin

**Type 2 diabetes** or **noninsulin-dependent diabetes (NIDDM)** form of diabetes in which the pancreas produces some insulin but the body's cells are insensitive to it

**Hyperglycemia** high blood sugar caused by the body's inability to process glucose in the blood

**Ketoacidosis** or **ketosis** accumulation of acid substances (ketones) caused by incomplete burning of fat for energy

**Diabetic coma** unconsciousness induced by ketoacidosis

**Insulin reaction** low blood sugar caused by too much insulin; insulin shock

**Hypoglycemia** low blood sugar

■ Reduce diabetes-related deaths in general.

■ Reduce diabetes-related deaths among American Indians and Alaska Natives.

■ Reduce the most severe complications of diabetes:

—End-stage renal disease

—Blindness

—Lower extremity amputation

—Perinatal mortality

—Major congenital malformation

---

loss of consciousness. An insulin reaction can be stopped by giving the person candy, orange juice, or anything sweet. Sometimes proper first aid is delayed or no aid is given because insulin reaction is mistaken for diabetic coma or alcohol intoxication.

Individuals with both types of diabetes should receive long-term medical care from a physician so the condition can be controlled and serious health complications will not develop. Over time diabetes affects the cardiovascular system and the central nervous system severely. If diabetes is not controlled, the following chronic conditions can develop.

■ *Diabetic retinopathy*, a disease of the retina, which can lead to blindness

■ *Cardiovascular complications (macrovascular disease)* such as atherosclerosis, heart attack (diabetics are twice as likely as nondiabetics to have a heart attack), hypertension, stroke, poor circulation to the legs and feet, and gangrene and subsequent amputation

■ *Kidney (renal) diseases* such as kidney infections and kidney failure

■ *Diabetic neuropathy*, a disease of the nerves, which can lead to numbness of the hands and feet, muscle weakness, skin disorders, impaired bladder functioning, and sexual impotence

■ *Infections (bacterial and fungal)* due to impaired T-cell function

In addition, the infant of a mother with type 1 diabetes has a higher-than-average risk of birth defects, stillbirth, respiratory distress, and other problems at birth.

## CONTROL OF DIABETES

Normal blood glucose levels range from 70 to 110 milligrams/deciliter (mg/dL) of blood. Factors such as time of day, meals, illness, medicines, and stress can cause a person's glucose level to rise or fall. Regardless of the time the last meal was consumed, a blood sugar level of more than 200 mg/dL suggests a problem. A physician uses a blood test called the glucose tolerance test to diagnose diabetes.

For both types of diabetes, the diabetic person has to be able to balance blood sugar, food intake, and

activities. Type 1 diabetics are able to achieve this balance in most cases by monitoring their blood glucose and adjusting the amounts of insulin they inject daily (or continuously infuse by a pump) based on food intake and daily activities meal by meal. In March 2001, the FDA approved the GlucoWatch, which is a glucose monitoring device (worn like a watch) that detects blood glucose through the skin. Type 1 diabetes, then, is controlled by proper diet, exercise, and daily injections of the hormone insulin. There are four basic types of insulin, each with a different duration of action. A physician decides the type for the patient based on the individual's lifestyle and blood glucose level.

In January 2006, the FDA approved an inhaled form of insulin. Exubera® (an inhaled powder form of recombinant human insulin) was approved for treatment of adults with type 1 and type 2 diabetes. Clinical trials demonstrated that the inhaled insulin reached peak levels in the bloodstream in about 50 minutes compared to 105 minutes with injectible insulin. This medication is not recommended for diabetics who smoke, have asthma, bronchitis, or emphysema. Patients who are prescribed Exubera® must monitor blood sugar as with injectible insulin.

Type 2 diabetes can be controlled through diet and exercise. Oral medication (antidiabetic agents that stimulate the pancreas to release more insulin) might be required in some cases, but daily insulin injections are not. Individuals with type 2 diabetes should be under the care of a physician who has expertise in treating the disease. Often the condition can be controlled without medication if regular physical activity is combined with a weight-loss diet.

In October 2006, the FDA approved Januvia® (a DPP-IV inhibitor) to treat type 2 diabetes. It is an oral medication that can be used alone or in combination with two other commonly prescribed oral medications when these medications (along with diet and exercise) do not provide "adequate blood sugar control." This new class of drug prolongs the activity of proteins that increase the release of insulin after a meal by blocking the enzyme DPP-IV (dipeptidyl peptidase IV).

Public health epidemiologist Susan Helmrich suggests that an increase in physical activity can be effective in preventing type 2 diabetes in the first place.

**FIGURE 7.9 ▶** Normal and Arthritic Joints

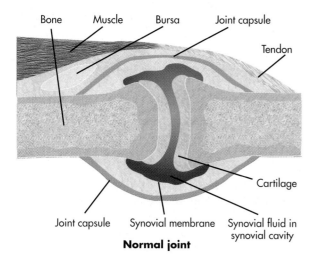

**Normal joint**

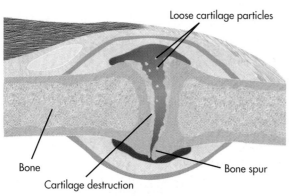

**Arthritic joint**

## Arthritis and Rheumatic Diseases

**Arthritis** refers to a group of more than 100 **rheumatic diseases** that affect (inflame) the joints. Arthritis includes the conditions osteoarthritis, rheumatoid arthritis, fibromyalgia, gout, carpal tunnel syndrome, bursitis, scleroderma, and lupus. The Arthritis Foundation estimates that in 2006, 46 million people (1 in 5 adults) had arthritis or chronic joint symptoms; 42.7 million of that number had the disease diagnosed by a physician. It is the second leading cause of work-related disability in the United States. Arthritis affects people of all ages; however, more than half are under age 65. It is more common in women, 25.9 million (men—16.8 million and children—300,000). It is estimated by the year 2030, about 67 million people 18 years and older living is the United States will have some form of doctor-diagnosed arthritis. The prevalence of rheumatic conditions is higher in African Americans (53% of total cases) than Caucasians (46%). The rheumatic disease lupus, which is also an autoimmune disorder, and three types of arthritis are highlighted in this chapter. Osteoporosis, the most common form, is discussed in Chapter 14.

Any place in the body where two bones meet is a joint. The ends of the bones are covered by **cartilage.** The entire joint is enclosed in a capsule lined by the inner skin called the **synovial membrane,** which releases a lubricating synovial fluid between the bones and facilitates movement. Surrounding the joint are muscles, **tendons,** and **ligaments. Bursae** keep all these structures moving smoothly against each other when everything is functioning normally. Figure 7.9 contrasts a normal joint with an arthritic joint.

When the joints are traumatized or invaded by a foreign object, **inflammation** is the body's reaction. In arthritis the joint (arthro) is what becomes inflamed (itis). Onset can be slow or sudden. Once a person has arthritis, it usually is for life.

### LUPUS

Lupus erythematosus, more commonly called **lupus,** is an immune system disorder that causes inflammation of tissues and vital organs of the body. The joints can be affected, complicating the disease. The normal function of the immune system is to protect healthy tissue and organs. People with lupus instead produce antibodies that attack normal cells, producing inflammation, cell injury, and cell destruction. Although the cause of lupus is unknown, individuals may be genetically predisposed to lupus, and certain environmental factors, such as sunlight, may trigger it.

Lupus is an insidious condition in that it develops gradually and subtly. The symptoms come and go and mimic

### KEY TERMS

**Arthritis** general classification of numerous diseases that cause swelling and pain in the joints, muscles, and bones

**Rheumatic diseases** disorders that involve inflammation and swelling of the joints and that restrict range of motion

**Cartilage** elastic tissue at ends of bones that acts as a shock absorber and buffer between bones

**Synovial membranes** lining of joints that releases a lubricating fluid

**Tendons** cordlike structures that connect bones to each other

**Ligaments** structures that attach muscles to bones

**Bursae** fluid-filled sacs that keep muscles, bones, ligaments, and tendons moving smoothly against each other

**Inflammation** body's reaction to pathogens or trauma characterized by redness, pain, and swelling

**Lupus** an arthritic, chronic disorder of the immune system accompanied by inflammation of various parts of the body

---

**Tips for Action** 12 Joint Savers

1. Respect pain.
2. Avoid extra stress on involved joints.
3. Control your weight.
4. Relax and stretch to avoid stiffness.
5. Use your strongest joints and muscles.
6. Spread the weight of an object over many joints.
7. Balance rest and activity.

8. Plan ahead and set priorities.
9. Organize work and storage areas.
10. Sit to work.
11. Use labor-saving devices.
12. Ask for help.

*Source:* Arthritis Foundation.

---

other illnesses, which makes diagnosis difficult. Lupus may be mild in some people, affecting just a few body organs. In others it may cause serious, even life-threatening, health problems.

Approximately 1.5 million people in the United States have lupus, with about 6,000 new cases each year. Lupus is most common in women and develops most often between the ages of 15 and 44. According to the Arthritis Foundation, lupus is more common in African American, Hispanic, American Indian, and Asian American women than in other groups.

One of the two main types of lupus, discoid (cutaneous) lupus, is confined to the skin. It is characterized by persistent flushing of the cheeks in disklike lesions (a rash) that appear in the butterfly area of the face, on the neck, scalp, ears, arms, and other areas exposed to ultraviolet light. Discoid lupus is not life-threatening.

About 10% of these cases develop into systemic lupus erythematosus (SLE), which affects a number of body systems. In some people it may involve only the skin and joints. In others it may affect the joints, kidneys, blood, and central nervous system, causing arthritis and nephritis (inflammation of the kidney). SLE is characterized by periods of remission when the person has less severe symptoms and by flare periods during which the condition becomes highly active again.

A third, and rare, type of lupus is drug-induced. Certain prescribed medications create a lupus-like syndrome similar to SLE, but the nervous system is rarely affected. Two medications associated with drug-induced lupus are hydralazine (to treat hypertension) and procainamide hydrochloride (to treat irregular heart rhythm). This form of lupus is more common in men. Only 4% of those who take these drugs will develop lupus, and when the medication is discontinued, the symptoms of lupus fade in those who do.

The onset of lupus is gradual, with only vague signs of the disease. Until specific symptoms develop, the following symptoms are found commonly in people in the early stages of lupus.

- Fever and fatigue
- Loss of appetite, weight loss
- Aches and pains, swollen glands
- Nausea and vomiting
- Headache
- Depression
- Easy bruising
- Hair loss
- Edema and swelling

In addition to these generalized symptoms, the following are more suggestive of lupus.

- Rash over the cheeks and bridge of the nose (hence, the moniker "wolf disease")
- Discoid lupus lesions
- Development of rash after exposure to sun and fluorescent light
- Bald spots
- Ulcers inside the mouth
- Swelling and pain of two or more joints
- Pleuritis (inflammation of membranes that cover the lungs)
- Seizure
- Raynaud's phenomenon (fingers or toes turning white or blue in the cold)

Several tests have been developed to diagnose lupus. Including a thorough physical examination and health history, the test used to make the initial diagnosis is the immunofluorescent antinuclear antibody (ANA or FANA) test. In conjunction with lab tests, the American College of Rheumatology developed a set of 11 diagnostic criteria to help differentiate lupus from other diseases. A person would have to meet at least four of the criteria to be diagnosed with lupus.

Nonsteroidal anti-inflammatory drugs (NSAIDs) such as ibuprofen and naproxen and corticosteriod drug therapy often are prescribed to those diagnosed with lupus, along with adequate rest. No cure has been found. As reported in February 2001, researchers at the University of California, San Diego, School of Medicine found that mice with a genetic mutation in the enzyme alpha-mannosidase II developed lupus-type symptoms, including high levels of antibodies and kidney inflammation. Additional research will lead to better understanding of the genetic links among other autoimmune disorders such as multiple sclerosis and rheumatoid arthritis as well as more accurate diagnostic tests for systemic lupus. Most cases can be managed through proper treatment, although about 5,000 people die from this disease each year in the United States. Of those diagnosed, 80% to 90% live more than 10 years after diagnosis, and most people with lupus can expect a normal lifespan.

In 2006, the FDA approved a large-scale clinical trial to compare the effectiveness of a new stem cell treatment to that of medications currently available.

## OTHER RHEUMATIC CONDITIONS

**Osteoarthritis** affects almost 16 million people in the United States, but rarely in people under age 45. This disease occurs primarily in the hands and the weight-bearing joints—the knee and hip. It has been called the wear-and-tear disease. People who are born with slight defects that make their joints fit together incorrectly or move incorrectly may be more likely to develop osteoarthritis. In some families osteoarthritis possibly is the result of a hereditary defect in one of the genes responsible for a major protein component of cartilage called collagen.

African-American women have higher rates of osteoarthritis than Caucasian women do. This may be related in some part to a genetic predisposition and also to the greater propensity of African-American women to be overweight (discussed in Chapter 10).

Studies have shown that people who carry extra weight in their twenties greatly increase their risk of developing arthritis of the knees and hips later in life. This is true for moderately overweight as well as obese individuals. Dr. Allan Gelber, a Johns Hopkins University School of Medicine rheumatologist, said that each 20-pound increment of extra weight raises a person's chances of developing osteoarthritis by 50%. Research has indicated that vitamin E can be effective in reducing the pain somewhat.

**Rheumatoid arthritis** is one of the more severe arthritis conditions because it can affect all joints of the body. It is an autoimmune disorder characterized by pain and joint inflammation that results in crippling deformities. It strikes most commonly between

**TABLE 7.3 ▶** Comparison of Osteoarthritis and Rheumatoid Arthritis

| OSTEOARTHRITIS | RHEUMATOID ARTHRITIS |
|---|---|
| Usually begins after age 40 | Usually begins between ages 25 and 50 |
| To age 45, more common in men; after age 54, more common in women | Women outnumber men 3 to 1 |
| Usually develops slowly, over many years | Often develops suddenly, within weeks or months |
| Often affects joints on only one side of the body | Usually affects same joint on both sides of the body (for example, knees) |
| Usually does not cause joint inflammation | Causes inflammation of the joint |
| Affects only certain joints; rarely affects elbows or shoulders | Affects many joints, including elbows and shoulders |
| Does not cause a general feeling of sickness | Often causes a general feeling of sickness, fatigue, weight loss, fever |

*Source:* Arthritis Foundation, Atlanta, GA.

ages 20 and 45. Of the estimated 2 million people afflicted in the United States, an estimated 80% are women in their childbearing years. Table 7.3 compares rheumatoid arthritis with osteoarthritis.

**Treatment.** The most successful original treatment for arthritis, still used, is aspirin. Other available remedies encompass the following.

- Various medications (nonsteroidal anti-inflammatory agents and cortisones)
- Exercise
- Rest or relaxation

## KEY TERMS

**Osteoarthritis** most common form of arthritis (affects primarily the hands and weight-bearing joints), caused by erosion of cartilage resulting in joint deformation, stiffness, and pain

**Rheumatoid arthritis** more severe form of arthritis that causes inflammation and swelling of tissues lining the joints; affects all joints of the body

**Tips for Action** How to Prevent Razor Bumps

■ Before shaving, lather the beard area thoroughly.

■ Use only disposable razors, and throw them away after one use to prevent reintroducing bacteria to the affected area.

■ Avoid electric razors; they produce a sharper hair tip.

■ Do not stretch the skin. Once tension is released, the hairs retract and penetrate the follicle.

■ Keep the skin scrupulously clean.

■ Use a baby shampoo to prevent irritation to sensitive skin.

■ Shave only every other day.

■ If you spot an embedded hair, release it with a clean needle.

■ Massage the beard area daily with a washcloth or coarse sponge.

If the condition does not clear up in a few weeks, an antibiotic ointment or oral antibiotics may be prescribed.

*Source:* Colonel Madison Patrick, M.D., U.S. Army Health Clinic, Oahu, HI.

■ Application of heat or cold

■ Joint protection (by brace or other device)

■ Surgery

■ Weight control (long term)

A growing body of evidence confirms the importance of a sensible exercise program in relieving the pain and disability of arthritis sufferers. Regular exercise is vital to maintaining maximum range of motion around the joints, according to the Arthritis Foundation. Walking, swimming, stretching, and aerobics can help reduce joint pain and stiffness, build stronger muscles and bones, and improve overall health. Walking may be one of the best all-around exercises. Best of all, however, may be water exercise, as the water cushions the impact of exercise on the joints.

**Fibromyalgia. Fibromyalgia,** or fibromyositis, is the second most common rheumatic disease. The onset occurs most often in women between the ages of 20 and 55. This disease does not involve inflammation of tissues but, rather, unexplained muscle pain (myalgia). People with fibromyalgia may feel deep muscular aching, throbbing, burning, or stabbing pain, along with total fatigue. Related symptoms include disturbances in deep-level sleep, headaches, chest pain, dizziness, and abdominal pain.

However painful, fibromyalgia does not seem to damage connective tissues or organs permanently, and it does not lead to deformity. The lack of objective physical evidence and absence of overt signs make diagnosis difficult. Because x-rays and typical blood tests are normal, this disease has been largely unrecognized and underreported until recently.

The cause remains elusive. Proposed theories include trauma to the central nervous system, an infectious agent such as the flu virus, and changes in muscle metabolism, among others.

## Skin Conditions

Skin conditions cover a wide range from psoriasis to eczema to ringworm. Some conditions are particularly applicable to African Americans because of their unique skin characteristics. Some African Americans' hair texture is like that of people of European ancestry. Typically, however, African-Americans' hair is coarser and curlier than that of other ethnic groups.

### PSEUDOFOLLICULITIS

The curlier hair texture can cause a skin problem for African-American men known as **pseudofolliculitis barbae,** a condition that occurs when curved beard hairs are cut during shaving. Shaving gives the tips of the curled hair sharp points that penetrate the skin, causing a painful and irritating rash (razor bumps). The affected follicles may become inflamed, requiring antibiotics to treat the infection. Permanent scarring may result.

A logical solution is to stop shaving, and this may be a reason many African-American men wear beards. Some men use a chemical depilatory (a shaving powder) to remove facial hair. Several studies have indicated that nearly 45% of African Americans in the military who shave develop razor bumps sooner or later.

### VITILIGO

**Vitiligo** is an autoimmune skin disorder characterized by a gradual destruction of the **melanocytes.** As a result, the person with vitiligo begins to lose pigment in the skin and hair. Even though it can affect individuals of any race, it is particularly disfiguring and unsettling to people who have dark pigmentation. The cause of vitiligo is unknown, but a family history of the condition has been reported in at

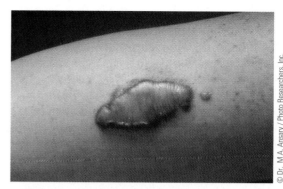

▲ *Keloid with hyperpigmented overlying skin*

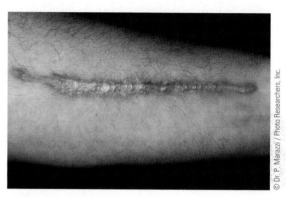

▲ *Keloid on the arm*

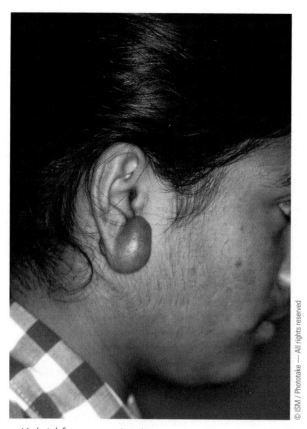

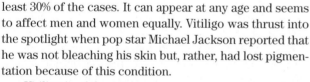

▲ *Keloid from ear piercing*

least 30% of the cases. It can appear at any age and seems to affect men and women equally. Vitiligo was thrust into the spotlight when pop star Michael Jackson reported that he was not bleaching his skin but, rather, had lost pigmentation because of this condition.

Vitiligo is of three types.

1. In *localized* or *patterned vitiligo*, the person may have one or several patches of white spots, areas of depigmentation (macules), on one or two areas of the body.

2. *Generalized vitiligo* is characterized by large or small macules scattered on the body in no special pattern. These macules often are symmetrical. In one form of generalized vitiligo, the macules are confined to the tips of fingers and toes and the lips. In some cases the person loses all skin pigmentation (turns white).

3. In *mixed vitiligo*, the loss of pigmentation can be widespread and localized.

Vitiligo is treated using PUVA photochemotherapy (psoralens and ultraviolet light) and corticosteroids. Even after treatment some areas of the body will not repigment. Some people with vitiligo use special cosmetic preparations to cover the white areas.

## KELOIDS OR CICATRICES

A **keloid,** or cicatrix, may look like a blister filled with fluid, but it is not. The irregularly shaped scar becomes progressively larger because of excessive amounts of **collagen** that forms during the healing process. The scar that forms does not stop growing as it is supposed to and extends beyond the original area of the injury or trauma.

### KEY TERMS

**Fibromyalgia** arthritis-related disease marked by widespread pain, fatigue, stiffness, but no evidence of inflammation, or joint or muscle degeneration

**Pseudofolliculitis barbae** a skin condition of black males in which the sharp points of shaved hair penetrate the skin of the face causing a painful rash (razor bumps)

**Vitiligo** an autoimmune skin disorder characterized by gradual destruction of the pigment-producing cells

**Melanocytes** pigment-producing cells of the skin

**Keloid** raised scar that results from overgrowth of fibrous tissue following a cut, piercing, or burn to the skin

**Collagen** fibrous protein found in connective tissue

A keloid can form on many surfaces of the body. The face, neck, and upper chest are the most common sites. The configuration or pattern of the keloid can be unusual, depending on the site and the type of trauma. You may have seen the Greek letter Ω in the form of a dark, raised scar on the upper arm or chest of a fraternity member. This scar is the result of trauma to the skin by a hot branding iron.

Although keloids can form on individuals of any ethnic group, they are more common in African Americans and people with a family history of keloid formation. People with a propensity for keloid skin should be careful when considering ear piercing, body piercing, cosmetic surgery, or other forms of adornment that cause trauma to the skin.

Removing a keloid by cutting it away may seem like a simple proposition. Surgically removing the keloid, however, would result in another scar that would heal as a keloid. Keloids should be treated by a dermatologist or a plastic surgeon with experience in skin disorders of African Americans. In treating a keloid, the physician has to consider the size and location of the keloid, as well as how long the person has had it. Nonsurgical treatments include massage, ultrasound, and corticosteroid creams and ointments that soften and shrink the scar. In some cases steroids are injected directly into the keloid. Some physicians use laser surgery to remove the keloid because it leaves a smaller scar. Silastic gel sheeting, or SGS, used to reduce scar tissue formation after burns, has been approved to treat keloids. This treatment makes the keloid flatter and reduces the symptoms of burning and itching.

## Disorders of the Digestive Tract

As with the other body systems, the digestive tract can function abnormally from a number of different causes. Figure 7.10 illustrates the digestive tract and the organs that may be affected.

**Peptic ulcers** can form in the lining of the stomach (gastric ulcers) or the small intestine (duodenal ulcers) as the result of the corrosive effect of digestive juices. The juices irritate the lining, reduce the protective mucus, and begin to digest the tissue itself. About 20 million Americans develop at least one ulcer during their lifetime, according to the *PIA Medical Sciences Bulletin.*

For nearly a century, peptic ulcers were blamed solely on lifestyle factors such as stress and diet. Although these still have a role in some cases, research at the University of Washington and other institutions shows that as much as 90% of peptic ulcers develop as a result of infection caused by the *Helicobacter pylori* bacterium. The propensity for ulcers also seems to run in families, and they do tend to develop in people who are under chronic stress, those whose diet is high in fat, and those who consume large amounts of alcohol. The most prominent symptom of peptic ulcer is pain that appears in the same area and that

is related to the digestive cycle. Among the diagnostic tools are endoscopic and x-ray examinations, as well as lab testing for the *H. pylori* bacteria.

The former standard recommendation to alleviate ulcers by drinking milk was found to be faulty because it causes the stomach to secrete more acid to digest the lactose and fat in milk. Currently, drugs that reduce stomach secretions or soothe irritated linings are prescribed. In addition, people with ulcers should avoid high-fat foods, alcohol, and other substances that irritate the stomach lining.

**Colitis** is a recurring inflammation of the large intestine. Because the cause is basically unknown, treatment focuses on relieving the symptoms, which include abdominal pain and frequent diarrhea. Anti-inflammatory drugs and steroids are the main treatments, along with increasing dietary fiber intake.

**Diverticulosis** is a painful condition resulting when the intestinal wall, usually of the large intestine, becomes weakened. Small pouches develop and fill with fecal matter passing through the intestine, which causes them to become irritated. This disease is most prevalent at middle age or after, though it can develop at any age. If it persists, bleeding and chronic obstruction may occur, which can be life-threatening. In some cases a person may have an attack that seems like it could be appendicitis, but the discomfort of diverticulosis occurs on the left side of the body instead of the right because of the configuration of the intestine.

**Gastroesophageal reflux disease (GERD)** is a condition of the digestive tract in which the stomach acid flows backward from the stomach into the esophagus. It has no single cause; however, the lower esophageal sphincter (LES) is supposed to act with the diaphragm to keep stomach acid from back flowing. For many persons, triggers for GERD may include lying down after a meal, wearing tight fitting clothing, or even bending over. Symptoms include heartburn more than once a week, which is more severe at night (may keep the person from sleeping), and esophagitis (inflammation of the esophagus). GERD is a chronic disease that usually has to be controlled on a long-term basis, even if the symptoms are under control, and should be diagnosed by a physician. Complications include inflammation of the vocal chords or throat, breaks in the lining of the esophagus, laryngitis and esophageal ulcers, and narrowing of the esophagus.

Another complication that is far less common is Barrett's esophagus in which the normal lining of the esophagus is replaced with abnormal epithelium. Barrett's esophagus has been linked to cancer. In addition, there is a link between asthma and reflux of stomach acid up in the throat and down into the lungs. According to the International Foundation for Functional Gastrointestinal Disorders, 5% to 7% of the global population experience gastric problems, and heartburn or acid regurgitation experienced weekly has been found to occur in 19.8% of individuals.

**FIGURE 7.10 ▶** Digestive Tract

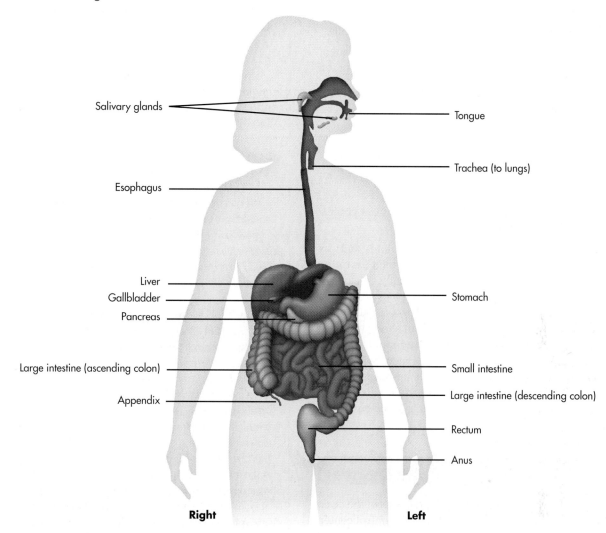

Salivary glands

Tongue

Trachea (to lungs)

Esophagus

Liver

Gallbladder

Pancreas

Stomach

Large intestine (ascending colon)

Appendix

Small intestine

Large intestine (descending colon)

Rectum

Anus

**Right**                                    **Left**

Representative of the stones that form in kidneys and other organs are **gallstones,** which form in the gallbladder. The process begins in the liver, which manufactures bile. Although some of the bile empties directly into the upper intestine, most is diverted to the gallbladder. The bile is stored in the gallbladder until it is required by the small intestine for digestion.

About 80% of gallstones develop when the amount of cholesterol in the body is disproportionately larger than the other components of bile. In these cases, cholesterol precipitates out of the bile, forming many small crystals within the gallbladder. Over a number of years these develop into stones, which may range in size from that of a pea to that of a marble. Most gallstones are not harmful and cause no symptoms. If a stone is squeezed from the gallbladder into the bile duct, however, it can produce recurrent abdominal pain to severe infection and extreme pain.

**KEY TERMS**

**Peptic ulcers** irritations in the lining of the stomach or the small intestine caused by an infection and the corrosive effect of digestive juices

**Colitis** recurring inflammation of the large intestine

**Diverticulosis** a painful condition caused by weakened places on the large intestine that bulge, fill with fecal matter, and become irritated

**Gastroesophageal reflux disease (GERD)** a condition of the digestive tract characterized by persistent heartburn, esophagitis, and other serious symptoms due to back flow of acid from the stomach up into the esophagus

**Gallstones** structures composed of mineral salts and cholesterol that form in the gallbladder

The greatest risk factors for gallstones are

- *Ethnic origin.* American Indians have a genetic predisposition to secrete high levels of cholesterol into bile.

- *Estrogen.* At puberty and as hormone replacement therapy, estrogen increases cholesterol concentration in the bile.

- *Hypertriglyceridemia.* People experience high levels of triglycerides, including those with diabetes.

- *Certain cholesterol-lowering drugs.* These include clofibrate and gemfibrozil.

- *Obesity.* This increases the risk for women but not for men.

- *Rapid weight loss.* This introduces excess cholesterol into bile as body fat is metabolized.

Gallstones are detected by ultrasound and by cholescintigraphy, a scanning procedure using a radioactive injection. Treatment nowadays usually consists of removal by laparoscopic surgery. Another, less permanent treatment is ursodeoxycholic acid to dissolve gallstones. A third treatment is lithotripsy, the use of shock waves to pulverize the stones. This has been used more successfully with kidney stones, as gallstones recur within five years in about 50% of patients who have lithotripsy.

**Lactose intolerance,** resulting from a deficiency of the lactase enzyme in the stomach, is discussed in Chapter 9.

## Neurological Disorders

The **central nervous system (CNS)** consists of the brain and the spinal cord. The brain is the body's control center. It sends messages to and receives stimulation from all parts of the body via the nervous system. The brain, not surprisingly, is the most complex organ in the body. It is the receptacle of thoughts, feelings, behaviors, physical sensations, movements, and senses. The brain also controls involuntary functions such as breathing and swallowing. It houses an intricate network of nerve cells called **neurons,** which form the foundation of this complex electrochemical communications system.

Unlike most other cells in the body, neurons cannot be replaced if they die. Therefore, death of neurons has a severe impact on memory, cognition, and behavior. This is the case with Alzheimer's disease, discussed in Chapter 14. Representative brain disorders discussed here are headaches and epilepsy.

### HEADACHES

The headache is the most common assault on the brain. More than 45 million Americans suffer from chronic, recurring headaches, a statistic that continues to grow every year, according to the National Headache Foundation. The

**VIEWPOINT** *The promise of the great benefits from stem cell research to medicine has been in the news. The possibilities for medical uses include treatment for neurological disorders (Alzheimer's disease and Parkinson's disease), management of autoimmune diseases such as systemic lupus and type 1 diabetes, treatment of spinal-cord injury, and development of treatments for cancer. The controversy does not derive from the benefits of the research, but from bioethical issues. Should tax dollars fund scientific investigation conducted on human embryos? Any national policy would probably follow the recommendations of the National Bioethics Advisory Commission, which were to "use only fertilized human ova left over from in vitro fertilization (IVF) procedures." The pro-life argument is that "human life . . . has dignity and merits protection." Supporters, including media celebrities Michael J. Fox and Mary Tyler Moore, who suffer from Parkinson's and type 1 diabetes, respectively, recognize the potential of the therapeutic benefits and think that tax-funded research should be approved. An alternative view is that stem cell research should be limited to the use of adult stem cells (from blood or bone marrow). As the technology develops, several bioethical questions must be addressed. Should the National Institutes of Health fund embryonic stem cell research? Should privately funded stem cell research be banned? Should a frozen embryo left over from IVF be compared with a lab-created embryo for the purpose of research or an embryo in a uterus?* **What is your opinion?**

four categories of headache covered here are 1) tension (ache in the area where the muscles of the head and neck meet), 2) vascular (migraine and cluster), 3) organically caused (tumors and disease), and 4) rebound (medication-induced).

**Tension Headaches.** About 90% of headaches are classified as tension headaches. Those occurring one to 15 days per month are classified as frequent tension headaches; chronic tension headaches occur 15 or more days per month. The pain typically is generalized all over the head. Some people have headaches almost daily. They usually awaken in the morning with the headache and frequently have an accompanying sleep disorder. This type of headache often is caused by depression or other emotional problems.

Others have episodic headaches (fewer than one a month). As the name indicates, these headaches occur spasmodically and seem to have no pattern. Symptom relief may include relaxation techniques and the use of over-the-counter medications. If they continue over time, a physician should be consulted.

### Vascular Headaches—Migraines, Cluster, and Toxic Headaches.

**Migraine headaches** usually have a hereditary component. If both parents have them, their children have a 75% chance of having them also. If one parent has migraines, each child has a 50% chance of getting them. African Americans seem to have a lower prevalence of migraines than Caucasians. A comparison of migraine headaches in blacks and whites is shown in Figure 7.11. About 29.5 million people have migraine headaches.

Migraines can be brought on by stress, poor sleeping habits, and changes in altitude and temperature. In addition, foods and beverages including chocolate, red wine, and aged cheese can provoke a migraine, as can noise, certain odors, bright lights, and watching TV. Hormone headaches, such as a menstrual migraine, are triggered by the hormone serotonin's interaction with estrogen. In addition, women taking hormonal contraceptives may experience more menstrual migraines.

Some migraines are preceded by a warning signal known as an **aura,** tingling or numbness of limbs, speech impairment, or visual disturbances such as flashing spots in front of the eyes. This is followed by severe pain on one side of the head. The pain may be so extreme that it causes nausea and vomiting, cold hands, shaking, and sensitivity to light and sound. Attacks last several minutes to several days.

Drug treatments include ergotamine and preventive medications including beta blockers, NSAIDs (nonsteroidal anti-inflammatory drugs), and antidepressants. Nondrug therapies include diet control, relaxation tapes, and biofeedback to manage the muscle contractions and swelling of blood vessels.

As their names implies, **cluster headaches** come in groups, up to four headaches per day during a cluster period. A headache can last 15 minutes to several hours, and a cycle can last days, weeks, or months, eventually retreating into long periods of remission. The pain is intense. Excess smoking and alcohol consumption can trigger these headaches. Prescription medications that have proven successful include special nose drops, ergotamine, and oxygen therapy (inhaling pure oxygen through a facial mask).

An allergic reaction or inflammation of the sinuses can produce a constant, gnawing pain in the sinuses. A fever may accompany the headache. Despite what most people believe, sinus headaches are rare. Many people who think they have a sinus headache actually have a tension or migraine headache.

### Organically Caused Headaches.

An organic headache is one caused by an abnormality of the brain or the skull. Organic headaches account for less than 5% of all headaches. These, however, often are symptomatic of more serious disorders such as tumors, brain infection, or cerebral hemorrhage. If left untreated, organic headaches can have serious health consequences. Signs such as sudden sharp, intense, severe pain; lack of balance; confusion; or difficulty speaking during the headache episode should be reported to the doctor immediately.

### Other Types of Headaches.

**Rebound headache** is medication-induced and occurs when a person is using prescription or over-the-counter medications and exceeds the

---

**FIGURE 7.11** ▶ Prevalence of Migraine, by Sex and Race

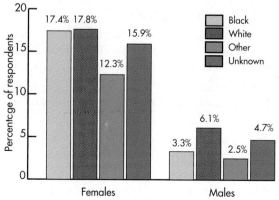

*Source:* National Headache Foundation Newsletter, Summer 1992.

---

### KEY TERMS

**Lactose intolerance** a digestive disorder caused by a deficiency of the enzyme lactase that is characterized by stomach pains and gas when a person consumes dairy products

**Central nervous system (CNS)** the portion of the nervous system composed of the brain and the spinal cord

**Neuron** a nerve cell that is the foundation for the electrochemical communication system in the brain

**Migraine headache** a vascular form of headache characterized by severe pain

**Aura** sensory warning signals that may precede migraine headache

**Cluster headaches** headaches that occur in groups and cycles, characterized by intense pain

**Rebound headache** a headache induced by pain medication that is not used according to the manufacturer's dosing instructions

recommended dose. This is common if the OTC medication contains caffeine (which is added to speed the action of the main ingredients of the headache medicine). Be aware that even though caffeine is a beneficial additive, use of caffeine while taking headache medications makes a person vulnerable to a rebound headache.

A dull ache in and around the ear that gets worse when a person chews, talks, or yawns may be a result of dysfunction of the temporomandibular joint (TMJ) of the jaw. A health care provider should be consulted to diagnose TMJ. Treatments may consist of heat, massage, painkillers, and a bite plate. Relaxation techniques also may be effective.

In general, behavioral management techniques have proven helpful in managing chronic headaches. These methods include

- *Biofeedback and relaxation training.* Biofeedback techniques (introduced in Chapter 3) are used to measure physical activity that may be contributing to the headaches. The activity measured may be muscle tension, blood flow, skin resistance, or skin temperature. The patient learns to use this feedback to exert voluntary control over a physical function. Between a third and a half of individuals with vascular and tension headaches seem to benefit from these treatments.

- *Cognitive-behavioral psychotherapy.* The patient learns problem-solving and coping skills that can be used to manage stress and situations thought to increase the frequency and intensity of headaches. Cognitive therapies focus on the relationships among thoughts, feelings, and behaviors and how to replace dysfunctional patterns with functional ones.

- *Operant behavioral treatment.* Treatment consists of withdrawal from all medications with addictive potential, increasing physical activity, and developing positive reinforcements (rewards) for positive behaviors. Candidates for this technique are those who experience chronic headaches over at least a three-month period, have not responded to medical treatment, and are functionally disabled by the headaches. These techniques usually are reserved for the most difficult and disabled patients.

In addition, headache sufferers are advised to avoid caffeine altogether. Headaches that are persistent or recurring should be diagnosed by a physician.

## SEIZURE DISORDERS

The more common term for seizure disorder is **epilepsy.** Approximately 1% of all Americans have some form of seizure-related disorder. Caused by abnormal electrical activity in the brain, they are characterized by muscular malfunctioning that ranges from minor twitching in the mildest form to convulsions and loss of consciousness in the extreme form. The most common forms of seizures are

1. *Grand mal.* Major convulsions throughout the body, often preceded by an aura, culminate in a loss of consciousness from 30 seconds to several minutes or longer.

2. *Petit mal.* Minor twitching of muscles occurs, with no convulsions. A minor loss of consciousness may not even be noticed.

3. *Psychomotor.* Characteristics are mental confusion and listlessness, accompanied by unusual repetitive movements and behaviors such as lip smacking.

4. *Jacksonian seizure.* This begins in one part of the body and moves into the hand, arm, or other parts, usually on only one side of the body.

In about half of the cases of epilepsy, the cause is identified as head injury, congenital abnormality related to inflammation of the brain or spinal column, drug poisoning, tumors, nutritional deficiency, or hereditary factors. In the other half of cases, the cause is unknown.

Because of effective medications, most people with epilepsy can lead a normal life. The disease does not get progressively worse, nor is it fatal.

## Summary

- Cancer is a number of diseases resulting from a mutation of genetic material, followed by uncontrolled growth of abnormal cells. It is the second leading cause of death in the United States.

- Chronic obstructive lung disease (COLD) consists primarily of chronic bronchitis and emphysema.

- Sickle cell disease is an inherited blood disease.

- Diabetes mellitus has two forms—type 1, the more serious of the two, and type 2, or adult-onset—both involving deficient insulin production in the body.

- Rheumatic diseases, commonly termed arthritis, consist of about 100 conditions involving inflammation of the joints and supporting tissues.

- Skin conditions that are almost exclusively a problem of African Americans are pseudofolliculitis barbae, vitiligo, and keloids.

- Representative digestive disorders are peptic (stomach and small intestine) ulcers, colitis, diverticulosis, gallstones, and gastroesophageal reflux disease.

- The major types of headache are tension, vascular (migraine and cluster), organic, and rebound.

- The most common forms of epileptic seizure are grand mal, petit mal, psychomotor, and Jacksonian.

## Personal Health Resources

**ThomsonNOW**  Visit the ThomsonNOW website at http://thomsonedu.com/thomsonnow for valuable resources that will:

- Help you evaluate your knowledge of the material.
- Guide you through tutorials to help you understand and apply the material.
- Allow you to take an exam-prep quiz to better prepare for class tests.

American Cancer Society (ACS). Sponsored by the nation's premier voluntary health organization dedicated to fighting cancer, this site offers current and consumer-friendly educational and statistical information on cancer to patients, families, survivors, the general public, and health professionals. Information is available in Spanish. "In My Community" connects users to activities, events, and resources in their local areas.
1-800-ACS-2345

**www.cancer.org/**

National Cancer Institute (NCI). This federal agency is part of the National Institutes of Health (NIH) and is the nation's primary agency for cancer research. Information (including morbidity and mortality data) is available on various types of cancers, treatments, screenings, and health disparities. This site provides information to consumers and professionals.
1-800-4-CANCER (Cancer Information Service)

**www.nci.nih.gov/**

National Heart, Lung, and Blood Institute (NHLBI). This federal agency is part of NIH and provides information on lung diseases and disorders. The site provides health information, scientific resources, news and press releases, links to Healthy People 2010, and the consumer-friendly "HLBI Express."

**www.nhlbi.gov/index.htm**

The Sickle Cell Information Center (sponsored by the Georgia Comprehensive Sickle Cell Center at Grady Health System, Sickle Cell Foundation of GA Inc., Emery University School of Medicine, and Morehouse School of Medicine). This site provides up-to-date information on sickle cell disease and other hemoglobinopathies to patients, professionals, and consumers. It includes news, research updates, and access to worldwide sickle cell resources.

**www.emory.edu/PEDS/SICKLE/**

National Institutes of Health (NIH). This federal agency is the gate to hundreds of information and statistical resources on chronic and infectious diseases. Links to the more than 20 institutes that are part of NIH can be accessed here.

**www.nih.gov/**

American Diabetes Association. This association is a recognized not-for-profit organization dedicated to fighting diabetes through education and research. The site offers current information to diabetics and others interested in the disease and its management.
1-800-DIABETES (342-2383)

**www.diabetes.org**

## It's Your Turn For Study and Review

1. Differentiate between an invasive malignant tumor and metastasis.

2. List the top four leading cancer sites for females and males. List the leading cancer deaths for females and males. Compare the two lists.

3. Indicate four behaviors that you can adopt that will reduce your risk of developing the cancers you listed in review item #2.

4. Differentiate between biopsy and surgery (treatment) related to certain cancers. Indicate two physicians that specialize in the treatment of cancers.

5. Mrs. Jones is AA and pregnant with her first baby. Her husband is As. Determine the following for Baby Jones: percent chance of normal hemoglobin, percent chance of sickle cell trait, and percent chance of sickle cell disease.

6. Regarding diabetes mellitus, describe hyperglycemia and its relationship to ketosis.

7. Differentiate among vascular headache, tension headache, and rebound headache.

8. Identify and describe the skin condition that may result from body piercing.

## Thinking about Health Issues

What are the scientific, political, and ethical issues associated with embryonic stem cell research?
James Trefil, "Brave New World: Everything You Wanted to Know about Stem Cells, Cloning and Genetic Engineering but Were Afraid to Ask." *Smithsonian*, December 2001, p. 38.

### KEY TERMS

**Epilepsy** a seizure disorder caused by abnormal electrical activity in the brain

1. According to the article, what were some of the controversial medical discoveries over the past century? Why were they considered controversial at the time?

2. What are some of the benefits and potential risks of stem cell research, genetic engineering, and human cloning?

3. What are the major ethical versus the scientific positions concerning stem cell research?

## Selected Bibliography

Adler, J. and Rogers, A. "The War against Migraines." *Newsweek*, January 11, 1999, pp. 46–52.

Altshul, S. "The Diabetes-Parkinson's Connection." *Prevention*, 58:11, November 2006, p. 41.

American Cancer Society. *Cancer Facts and Figure 2006*. Atlanta: American Cancer Society, 2006.

American Cancer Society. *Cancer Facts and Figures for African Americans*. Atlanta: ACS, 1996.

Andrews, M. "A Guiding Hand." *U.S. News & World Report*, 141:4, July 31, 2006, pp. 59–62.

Arthritis Foundation. "The Facts about Arthritis." Available at www.arthritis.org/. Accessed September 1, 2006.

Beers, M. and Porter, R. (Eds.). (2006). *The Merck Manual of Diagnosis and Therapy*. Merck Research Laboratories, Whitehouse Station, NJ.

Begley, S. "The Race to Decode the Human Body." *Newsweek*, April 10, 2000, pp. 50–57.

Begley, S. "The War over Stem Cells." *Newsweek*, July 9, 2001, pp. 22–27.

Brand-Miller, J., et al. *The Glucose Revolution*. New York: Marlowe and Company, 1999.

Brinks, S. "Prostate Dilemmas." *U.S. News and World Report*, May 22, 2000, pp. 66–81.

Campos, G. M., et al. "The Pattern of Esophageal Acid Exposure in Gastroesophageal Reflux Disease Influences the Severity of the Disease." *Archives of Surgery*, 134, 1999, pp. 882–887.

Carper, J. *Food: Your Miracle Medicine*. New York: Harper-Collins, 1994.

Carson, M. and Lo, D. "The Push-Me Pull-You of T Cell Activation." *Science*, July 27, 2001, pp. 618–619.

Caruana, C. "Scar Wars." *Essence*, October 1993, p. 24.

Centers for Disease Control and Prevention/Association of Public Health Laboratories. *Newborn Screening Quality Assurance Program Report*, 16:3, Quarter 3, August 2006.

Charache, S., et al. "Effect of Hydroxyurea on the Frequency of Painful Crisis in Sickle Cell Anemia." *New England Journal of Medicine*, 332:20, May 18, 1995, pp. 1317–1322.

Coltrera, F. "Breast Cancer: The News That Has Doctors Cheering." *The Oprah Magazine*, 7:10, October 2006, pp. 232, 234.

Cowley, G. "The Real 'Hot Zone.'" *Newsweek*, November 27, 2000, pp. 66–67.

Crute, S. "New Hope for Babies with Sickle-Cell Anemia." *Heart and Soul Magazine*, December/January 2002, p. 52.

DeCross, A. J. and Peura, D. A. "Role of *H. pylori* in Peptic Ulcer Disease." *Contemporary Gastroenterology*, 5:4, 1992, pp. 18–28.

Department of Health and Human Services. *Healthy People 2010: Understanding and Improving Health*. Washington, DC: U.S. Government Printing Office, 2000.

Dixon, B. M. *Good Health for African Americans*. New York: Crown Publishing, 1994.

Dunkin, M. A. "Fibromyalgia." *Arthritis Today*, September/October 1993.

*Facts about Lupus*. Rockville, MD: Lupus Foundation of America.

Finch, A., et al. "Salpingo-oophorectomy and the Risk of Ovarian, Fallopian Tube, and Peritoneal Cancers in Women with a *BRCA1* or *BRCA2* Mutation. *Journal of the American Medical Association*, 296:2, July 12, 2006, pp. 185–192.

"First Inhaled Insulin Product Approved." *FDA Consumer*, 40:2, March–April 2006, pp. 28–29.

Fischer, J. "The Cell Wars Begin." *U.S. News and World Report*, December 20, 2001, pp. 56–57.

Fischman, J. "Delaying Diabetes: Lifestyle Changes Help More than Drugs." *U.S. News and World Report*, August 20–27, 2001, p. 19.

Fischman, J. "Facing Down a Killer Disease." *U.S. News and World Report*, June 25, 2001, pp. 58–68.

"Five Ways to Outsmart Diabetes." *Redbook*, 207:1, July 2006, p. 56.

Gaston, M., et al. "Oral Prophylaxis with Penicillin in Children with Sickle Cell Anemia." *New England Journal of Medicine*, 314:25, June 19, 1986, pp. 1593–1599.

Graham, J. "You Can Prevent Breast Cancer." *Redbook*, 207: 4, October 2006, pp. 96, 100.

Griffin, K. "Baffled by Choices." *AARP The Magazine*, 49:5A, September/October 2006, pp. 40, 42–44, 128–129.

Harrar, S. "Don't Forget the Follow-up." *Prevention*, 58:4, April 2006, p. 48.

Harrar, S. "Beat Diabetes before It Starts." *Prevention*, November 2001, pp. 140–149.

Henry, W. L., Jr., Johnson, K. A., and Villarosa, L. *Black Health Library Guide to Diabetes*. New York: Henry Holt and Co., 1993.

Herman, W., et al. "Diabetes Mellitus and Its Complications in an African American Community: Project DIRECT." *Journal of the National Medical Association*, 90, 1998, pp. 147–156.

International Early Lung Cancer Action Program (I-ELCAP) Investigators. "Women's Susceptibility to Tobacco Carcinogens and Survival after Diagnosis of Lung Cancer." *Journal of the American Medical Association*, 296:2, July 12, 2006, pp. 180–184.

Jaret, P. "Seven Must-Have Medical Tests." *Health*, December 2001, pp. 52–58.

Lewis, C. "Diabetes a Growing Public Health Concern," *FDA Consumer*, 36:1, January/February 2002, pp. 26–33.

Loman, N., et al. "Family History of Breast and Ovarian Cancers and BRCA1 and BRCA2 Mutations in a Population-Based Series of Early-Onset Breast Cancer." *Journal of the National Cancer Institute*, 93, 2001, pp. 1215–1223.

Lupus Foundation of America. "Lupus Facts and Overview: Criteria for Diagnosing Lupus." Available at www.lupus.org/. Accessed August 15, 2006.

MacNeil, J. "Don't Drink and Smoke: Two Vices' Bad Synergy." *U.S. News and World Report*, June 26, 2000, p. 63.

Marwick, C. "Embryonic Stem Cell Debate Brings Politics, Ethics, to the Bench." *Journal of the National Cancer Institute*, 93, 2001, pp. 1192–1193.

Mayfield, E. "New Hope for People with Sickle Cell Anemia." *FDA Consumer*, May 1996, pp. 16–21.

Meadows, M. "Encouraging Women to Take Charge of Diabetes." *FDA Consumer*, 35:6, November/December 2001, pp. 7–8.

Mone, G. and Svoboda, E. "The 6 Biggest Ideas in Medicine (and One Cautionary Tale)." *Popular Science*, 269:2, August 2006, pp. 55–57.

Moran, M. "Autoimmune Diseases Could Share Common Genetic Etiology." *American Medical News*, October 8, 2001, www.amednews.com.

Needham, C. "Cultural Differences Shape Cancer Care." *Journal of the National Cancer Institute*, 86:4, February 16, 1994, pp. 261–262.

"New Vaccine Prevents Cervical Cancer." *FDA Consumer*, 40:5, September/October 2006, p. 37.

*Newborn Screening for Sickle Cell Disease and Other Hemoglobinopathies*, 6:9, April 6–8, 1987.

Pagan, C. N. "The –itis Epidemic." *Health*, 20:4, May 2006, pp. 98–102.

Patlak, M. "New Devices Aim at Improving Pap Test Accuracy." *FDA Consumer*, October 1996, pp. 9–13.

Plevritis, S., et al. "Cost-effectiveness of Screening *BRAC1/2* Mutation Carriers with Breast Magnetic Resonance Imaging." *Journal of the American Medical Association*, 295:20, May 24/31, 2006, pp. 2374–2384.

Ries, L. A. G., et al., eds. *SEER Cancer Statistics Review, 1973–1997*. Bethesda, MD. National Cancer Institute, 2000.

Rosenbloom A., et al. "Emerging Epidemic of Type 2 Diabetes in Youth." *Diabetes Care*, 22, 1999, pp. 345–354.

Sauer, G. C. *Manual of Skin Diseases*, 6th ed. Philadelphia: J. B. Lippincott Co., 1991.

Seppa, N. "Stem Cell Treatment for Lupus." *Science News*, 169:5, February 4, 2006, pp. 67–68.

Seppa, N. "Enzyme Shortage May Lead to Lupus." *Science News*, June 10, 2000, p. 372.

Shon, E. "Therapy by the Pound: Human Fat Is a Source of Coveted Stem Cells." *U.S. News and World Report*, April 23, 2001, p. 54.

"Vitiligo." *Update: Dermatology in General Medicine*. New York: McGraw-Hill Book Co., 1983.

Vogel, V., et al. "Effects of Tamoxifen vs Raloxifene on the Risk of Developing Invasive Breast Cancer and Other Disease Outcomes." *Journal of the American Medical Association*, 295:23, June 21, 2006, pp. 2727–2751.

Woodward, K. L. "The Debate on Embryonic Research." *Newsweek*, July 9, 2001, p. 31.

Name _____    Course _____

Date _____    Section _____

## Introduction

You can reduce your risk of developing some types of cancers, such as lung cancer, by changing your lifestyle behaviors. For other types of cancers, such as breast and colorectal cancers, your chance for cure is greatly increased if the cancer is found at an early stage through periodic screening examinations.

This questionnaire has been designed by the American Cancer Society to help you learn about your risk factors for certain types of cancers and the chances that cancer would be found at an early stage when a cure is possible.

## Testing Scoring Directions

Read each question concerning each site and its specific risk factors. Be honest in your responses. Circle the number in parenthesis next to your response.

For example, question #2 on lung cancer, below: If you are 53 years old (50–59) then circle 5 as your score. Total your scores in each section.

Men: Complete the first three sections only. Women: Complete all sections unless otherwise noted.

## About Your Answers

You may check your own risks with the answers contained in this assessment. You are advised to discuss this assessment with your physician if you are at higher risk.

## Important: React to Each Statement

Individual numbers for specific questions are not to be interpreted as a precise measure of relative risk, but the totals for a given site should give a general indication of your risk.

## LUNG CANCER

1.  **SEX:**       a. Male (2)       b. Female (1)

2.  **AGE:**       a. 39 or less (1)     b. 40–49 (2)      c. 50–59 (5)      d. 60+ (7)

3.  **EXPOSURE TO ANY OF THESE:**

    a. Mining (3)       b. Asbestos (7)    c. Uranium and radioactive products (5)    d. None (0)

4.  **HABITS:**   a. Smoker (10)*     b. Nonsmoker (0)*

5.  **TYPE OF SMOKING:**

    a. Cigarettes or little cigars (10)    b. Pipe or cigar, but not cigarettes (3)    c. Nonsmoker (0)

6.  **NUMBER OF CIGARETTES SMOKED PER DAY:**

    a. 0 (1)    b. Less than ½ pack per day (5)      c. ½–1 pack (9)      d. 1–2 packs (15)     e. 2+ packs (20)

7.  **TYPE OF CIGARETTE:**

    a. High tar/nicotine (10)**    b. Medium tar/nicotine (9)**    c. Low tar/nicotine (7)**    d. Nonsmoker (1)

8.  **LENGTH OF TIME SMOKING:**

    a. Nonsmoker (1)    b. Up to 15 years (5)    c. 15–25 years (10)    d. 25+ years (20)

Subtotal _____

*If you stopped smoking more than 10 years ago, count yourself as a nonsmoker. If you have stopped smoking in the past 10 years, you are an ex-smoker. Ex-smokers should answer questions 4 through 8 according to how they previously smoked. Then ex-smokers may reduce their point total on questions 5 through 8 by 10% for each year they have not smoked. Current smokers also answer questions 5 through 8.

**High tar/nicotine: 20 mg. or more tar/1.3 mg. or more nicotine; medium tar/nicotine: 16–19 mg. tar/1.1–1.2 mg. nicotine; low tar/nicotine: 15 mg. or less tar/1.0 mg. or less nicotine.

9.    I am stopping smoking today. (If yes, subtract 2 points)          Yes          No

                                                                                TOTAL _____

## COLORECTAL CANCER

### Risk Factors

1.    **AGE:**      a. 40 or less (2)      b. 40–49 (7)      c. 50 and over (12)

2.    **HAS ANYONE IN YOUR FAMILY EVER HAD:**
      a. Colon cancer (18)      b. Colon polyps (18)      c. Neither (1)

3.    **HAVE YOU EVER HAD:**
      a. Colon cancer (25)      b. Colon polyps (25)          c. Ulcerative colitis for more than seven years (18)
      d. Cancer of the breast, ovary, uterus, or stomach (13)      e. None of the above (1)

                                                                                TOTAL _____

### Symptoms

1.    Do you have bleeding from the rectum?                              Yes          No

2.    Have you had a change in bowel habits (such as altered frequency, size, consistency, or color of stool)?          Yes          No

### Reducing Your Risks and Detecting Cancer Early

1.    I have altered my diet to include less fat and more fruits, fiber, and cruciferous vegetables (broccoli, cabbage, cauliflower, brussels sprouts).          Yes          No

2.    I have had a negative test for blood in my stool within the past year.          Yes          No

3.    I have had a negative examination for colon cancer and polyps within the past year (proctosigmoidoscopy, colonoscopy, barium enema, x-rays).          Yes          No

## SKIN CANCER

1.    I live in the southern part of the United States.                  Yes          No

2.    I frequently work or play in the sun.                              Yes          No

3.    I have a fair complexion or freckles (natural hair color of blonde, red, or light brown, or eye color of grey, green, blue, or hazel).          Yes          No

4.    I work in mines, around coal tars or radioactivity.               Yes          No

5.    I experienced a severe, blistering sunburn before age 18.         Yes          No

6.    I have family members with skin cancer or a history of melanoma.  Yes          No

7.    I had skin cancer or melanoma in the past.                        Yes          No

8.    I use or have used tanning beds or sun lamps.                      Yes          No

9.    I have large, many, or changing moles.                            Yes          No

## Reducing Your Risks and Detecting Cancer Early

10. I cover up with a wide-brimmed hat and wear long-sleeved shirts and pants.      Yes      No

11. I use sunscreens with a sun protection factor (SPF) rating of 15 or higher when going out in the sun.      Yes      No

12. I examine my skin once a month for changes in warts or moles.      Yes      No

## BREAST CANCER

1. **AGE GROUP:**      a. Under 35 (10)    b. 35–39 (20)    c. 40–49 (50)    d. 50 and over (90)

2. **RACE:**    a. Mongoloid (10)   b. Hispanic (10)   c. Black (20)   d. White (25)

3. **FAMILY HISTORY:**    a. None (10)    b. Mother, sister, daughter with breast cancer (30)

4. **YOUR HISTORY:**
   a. No breast disease (10)    b. Previous lumps or cysts (15)    c. Previous breast cancer (100)

5. **MATERNITY**
   a. First pregnancy before 30 (10)    b. First pregnancy at 30 or older (15)    c. No pregnancies (20)

## Detecting Cancer Early

6. I practice self-examination monthly. (If yes, subtract 10 points.)      Yes      No

7. I have had a negative mammogram and examination by a physician in accordance with American Cancer Society Breast Health Guidelines. (If yes, subtract 25 points.)      Yes      No

**TOTAL** _____

## CERVICAL CANCER
(Lower portion of uterus)

These questions do not apply to a woman who has had a total hysterectomy.

1. **AGE GROUP:**
   a. Less than 25 (10)    b. 25–39 (20)    c. 40–54 (30)    d. 55 and over (30)

2. **RACE:**    a. Mongoloid or white (10)    b. Black (20)    c. Hispanic (20)

3. **NUMBER OF PREGNANCIES:**    a. 0 (10)    b. 1 to 3 (20)    c. 4 and over (30)

4. **VIRAL INFECTIONS:**
   a. Viral infections of the vagina such as genital warts, herpes, or ulcer formations (10)
   b. Never (1)

5. **AGE AT FIRST INTERCOURSE:**
   a. Before 15 (40)    b. 15–19 (30)    c. 20–24 (20)    d. 25 and over (10)
   e. Never had intercourse (5)

6. **BLEEDING BETWEEN PERIODS OR AFTER INTERCOURSE:**    a. Yes (40)    b. No (1)

7. **SMOKER:**    a. Nonsmoker (2)    b. Smoker (3)

**Subtotal** _____

## Detecting Cancer Early

8. I have had a negative Pap smear and pelvic examination within the past year. (If yes, subtract 50 points.)

Yes      No

**TOTAL** _____

## ENDOMETRIAL CANCER
(Body of uterus)

These questions do not apply to a woman who has had a total hysterectomy.

1. **AGE GROUP:**    a. 39 or less (5)      b. 40–49 (20)      c. 50 and over (60)

2. **RACE:**      a. Mongoloid (10)      b. Black (20)      c. Hispanic (20)      d. White (20)

3. **BIRTHS:**      a. None (15)      b. 1 to 4 (7)      c. 5 or more (5)

4. **WEIGHT:**    a. 50 or more pounds overweight (50)      b. 20–49 pounds overweight (15)
   c. Normal or underweight for height (10)

5. **DIABETES** (elevated blood sugar):    a. Yes (3)      b. No (1)

6. **ESTROGEN HORMONE INTAKE:**\*\*\*    a. Yes, regularly (15)    b. Yes, occasionally (12)    c. None (10)

7. **ABNORMAL UTERINE BLEEDING:**    a. Yes (40)      b. No (1)

8. **HYPERTENSION (HIGH BLOOD PRESSURE):**    a. Yes (40)    b. No (1)

**Subtotal** _____

## Detecting Cancer Early

9. I have had a negative pelvic examination and Pap smear or endometrial tissue sampling (endometrial biopsy) performed within the past year. (If yes, subtract 50 points.)    Yes      No

**TOTAL** _____

\*\*\*Excludes birth control pills.

## Answers and Test Analysis

### LUNG

1. Men have a higher risk of lung cancer than women. Because women are smoking more, their incidence of lung and upper respiratory tract (mouth, tongue, and voice box) cancer is increasing.

2. The occurrence of lung and upper respiratory tract cancer increases with age.

3. Cigarette smokers may have 20 times or even greater risk than nonsmokers. However, the rates of ex-smokers who have not smoked for 10 years approach those of nonsmokers.

4. Pipe and cigar smokers are at a higher risk for lung cancer than nonsmokers. Cigarette smokers are also at a much higher risk for lung cancer than nonsmokers or pipe and cigar smokers. All forms of tobacco, including chewing or dipping, markedly increase the user's risk of developing cancer of the mouth.

5. Male smokers of less than 1/2 pack per day have a five times higher lung cancer rate than nonsmokers. Male smokers of 1–2 packs per day have a 15 times higher lung cancer rate than nonsmokers. Smokers of more than 2 packs per day are 20 times more likely to develop lung cancer than nonsmokers.

6. Smokers of low tar/nicotine cigarettes have slightly lower lung cancer rates. Smokers of low tar/nicotine cigarettes may unconsciously smoke in a manner that increases their exposure to these chemicals, however.

7. The frequency of lung and upper respiratory tract cancer increases with the duration of smoking.

8. Exposures to materials used in these and other industries have been shown to be associated with lung cancer, especially in smokers.

If your total is:

24 or less. . . . . . You have a low risk for lung cancer.
25–49. . . . . . . . You may be a light smoker and would have a good chance of kicking the habit.

50–74. . . . . . . . As a moderate smoker, your risks for lung and upper respiratory tract cancer are increased. The time to stop is now.

75 or more. . . . . As a heavy cigarette smoker, your chances of getting lung cancer and cancer of the upper respiratory or digestive tract are greatly increased.

**REDUCING YOUR RISK**—Make a decision to quit today. Join a smoking cessation program. If you are a heavy drinker of alcohol, your risks for cancer of the head, neck, and esophagus are further increased. Use of spitting tobacco increases your risks of cancer of the mouth. Your best bet is not to use tobacco in any form. See your doctor if you have a nagging cough, hoarseness, persistent pain, soreness in the mouth or throat, or lumps in the neck.

## COLORECTAL

1. Colon cancer occurs more often after the age of 50.
2. Colon cancer is more common in families with a previous history of this disease.
3. Polyps and bowel diseases are associated with colon cancer. Cancer of the breast, ovaries, or stomach may also be associated with an increased risk of colon cancer.
4. Rectal bleeding may be a sign of colon or rectum cancer.

### I. RISK FACTORS*
If your total is:

5 or less. . . . . . You are currently at low risk for colon and rectum cancer. Eat a diet high in fiber and low in fat and follow cancer checkup guidelines.

6–15. . . . . . . . You are currently at moderate risk for colon and rectum cancer. Follow the American Cancer Society guidelines for early detection of colorectal cancer. These are: a digital rectal exam every year after 40 and a fecal occult blood test every year and sigmoidoscopic, preferably flexible, exam every three to five years after age 50.**

16 or more. . . . You are in the high-risk group for colon and rectum cancer. This rating requires a lifetime, ongoing screening program that includes periodic evaluation of your entire colon. See your doctor for more information.

### II. SYMPTOMS—The presence of rectal bleeding or a change in bowel habits may indicate colon or rectum cancer. See your physician right away if you have either of these symptoms.

### III. REDUCING YOUR RISKS AND DETECTING CANCER EARLY—Regular tests for hidden blood in the stool and appropriate examinations of the colon will increase the likelihood that colon polyps are discovered and removed early and that cancers are found in an early, curable state. Modifying your diet to include more fiber, cruciferous vegetables, and foods rich in vitamin A and less fat and salt-cured foods may result in a reduction of cancer risk.

## SKIN

1. The sun's rays are more intense the closer one lives to the equator.
2. Excessive ultraviolet light from the sun causes cancer of the skin.
3. These materials can cause cancer of the skin.
4. Persons with light complexions are at greater risk for skin cancer.
5. A severe sunburn while growing up may increase one's risk for melanoma.
6. A tendency to have precancerous moles or melanomas may occur in certain families.
7. Persons with a previous skin cancer or melanoma are at increased risk for developing a skin cancer or melanoma.
8. Tanning beds use a type of ultraviolet ray that adds to skin damage by the sun, contributing to skin cancer formation.
9. Any change in a mole may be a sign of melanoma.

If you answered "yes" to any of the first nine questions, you need to use protective clothing and use a sunscreen with an SPF rating of 15 or greater whenever you are out in the sun and check yourself monthly for any changes in warts or moles. An answer of "yes" to question 10, 11, and 12 can help reduce your risk of skin cancer or possibly detect skin cancer early.

**REDUCING YOUR RISKS AND DETECTING CANCER EARLY**—Numerical risks for skin cancer are difficult to state. For instance, a person with dark complexion can work longer in the sun and be less likely to develop cancer than a person with a light complexion. Furthermore, a person wearing a long-sleeved shirt and wide-brimmed hat may work in the sun and be at less risk than a person who wears a bathing suit for only a short time. The risk for skin cancer goes up greatly with age.

Melanoma, the most serious type of skin cancer, can be cured when it is detected and treated at a very early stage. Changes in warts or moles are important and should be checked by your doctor.

## BREAST

If your total is:

Under 100 . . . . . Low risk. You should practice monthly breast self-examination (BSF), have your breasts examined by a doctor as part of a regular cancer-related checkup, and have mammography in accordance with American Cancer Society guidelines.

100–199 . . . . . . Moderate risk. You should practice monthly BSE, have your breasts examined by a doctor as part of a cancer-related checkup, have periodic mammography in accordance with American Cancer Society guidelines or more frequently as your physician advises.

200 or higher. . . High risk. You should practice monthly BSE, have your breasts examined by a doctor, and have mammography more often. See your doctor for the recommended frequency of breast physical examinations and mammography.

**DETECTING CANCER EARLY**—One in 9 American women will get breast cancer in her lifetime. Being a woman is a risk factor. Most women (75%) who get breast cancer do not have other risk factors. BSE and mammography may diagnose a breast cancer in its earliest stage with a greatly increased chance of cure. When detected at this stage, cure is more likely and breast-saving surgery may be an option.

## CERVICAL

1. The numbers represent the relative risks for invasive cancer in different age groups. The highest incidence of invasive cancer is among women over 40 years of age. However, abnormal changes and early noninvasive cancers occur more commonly in the 20s and 30s age groups. These early changes can be found with the Pap test.

2. Puerto Ricans, blacks, and Mexican Americans have higher rates for cervical cancer.

3. Women who have delivered more children have a higher occurrence.

4. Viral infections of the cervix and vagina are associated with cervical cancer.

5. Women with earlier age at first intercourse and with more sexual partners are at a higher risk.

6. Irregular bleeding may be a sign of uterine cancer.

If your total is:

40–69 . . . . . . . . This is a low-risk group. Ask your doctor for a Pap test and advice about frequency of subsequent testing.

70–99 . . . . . . . In this moderate-risk group, more frequent Pap tests may be required.

100 or more. . . You are in the high-risk group and should have a Pap test (and pelvic exam) as advised by your doctor.

**DETECTING CANCER EARLY**—Early detection of this cancer by the Pap test has markedly improved the chance of cure. When this cancer is found at an early stage, the cure rate is extremely high and uterus-saving surgery and childbearing potential may be preserved.

## ENDOMETRIAL

1. Endometrial cancer is seen among women in older age groups. Numbers in parentheses by the age groups represent approximate relative rates of endometrial cancer at different ages.

2. Caucasians have a high occurrence.

3. The fewer children one has delivered the greater the risk of endometrial cancer.

4. Women who are overweight are at greater risk.

5. Cancer of the endometrium is associated with diabetes.

6. Cancer of the endometrium may be associated with prolonged continuous estrogen hormone intake, which occurs in only a small number of women. You should consult your physician before starting or stopping any estrogen medication. The medical use of estrogen in combination with progesterone does not appear to increase risk and may have other health benefits in this case.

7. Women who do not have cyclic regular menstrual periods are at greater risk. Any bleeding after menopause may be a sign of this cancer.

8. Cancer of the endometrium is associated with high blood pressure.

If your total is:

45–59. . . . . . .   You are at very low risk for developing endometrial cancer.

60–99. . . . . . .   Your risks are slightly higher. Report any abnormal bleeding immediately to your doctor. Tissue sampling at menopause is recommended.

100 and over. . .   Your risks are much greater. See your doctor for tests as appropriate.

**DETECTING CANCER EARLY**—Once again, early detection is a key to your chance of a cure for this cancer. Regular pelvic examinations may find other female cancers such as cancer of the ovary.

\* If your answers to any of these questions change, you should reassess your risk.

\*\* The digital rectal exam has an additional advantage in that it is also an early detection method for cancer of the prostate in men.

Name _____    Course _____

Date _____    Section _____

Write in the points next to each statement that is true for you. Before each statement that is not true for you place a zero. Then add up your total score.

1. I have been experiencing one or more of the following symptoms regularly.

   ■ Excessive thirst                                         Yes 3  _____

   ■ Frequent urination                                       Yes 3  _____

   ■ Extreme fatigue                                          Yes 1  _____

   ■ Unexplained weight loss                                  Yes 3  _____

   ■ Blurry vision from time to time                          Yes 2  _____

2. I am over 30 years old.                                    Yes 1  _____

3. I am more than 20% overweight.                             Yes 2  _____

4. I am a woman who has had more than one baby weighing over nine pounds at birth.    Yes 2  _____

5. I am of Native American descent.                           Yes 1  _____

6. I am of Hispanic or African-American descent.             Yes 1  _____

7. I have a parent with diabetes.                             Yes 1  _____

8. I have a brother or sister with diabetes.                 Yes 2  _____

                                                             **Total**  _____

Scoring 3–5 points
You probably are at low risk for diabetes. Do not just forget about it, though, especially if you are 30, overweight, or of African American, Hispanic, or Native American descent.

Scoring over 5 points
You may be at high risk for diabetes. You may even have diabetes already.

What to do about it
See your doctor promptly. Find out if you have diabetes. Even if you do not have diabetes, know the symptoms. If you experience any of them in the future, you should see your doctor immediately.

*Note:* This test is meant to educate and make you aware of the serious risks of diabetes. Only a medical doctor can determine if you do have diabetes.
*Source:* American Diabetes Association.

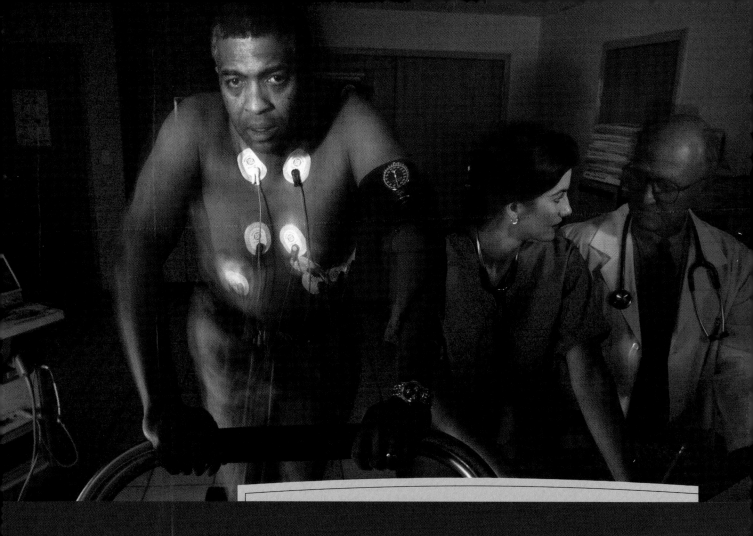

# Chapter Eight Cardiovascular Disease

**OBJECTIVES** ■ Describe the circulatory system and identify the parts of the heart. ■ Identify the causes and major risk factors for cardiovascular diseases. ■ Explain how blood pressure is measured and the significance of the measurements. ■ Describe the role and types of blood lipids in the body. ■ Describe how atherosclerosis occurs. ■ Identify the four conditions that precipitate stroke. ■ Identify selected new treatments for heart conditions.

ThomsonNOW™ Log on to ThomsonNOW at http://thomsonedu.com/ thomsonnow to access and explore self-assessments, interactive tutorials, and practice quizzes.

Diseases affecting the heart and the cardiovascular system are foremost among the noncommunicable diseases. More than 900,000 people in the United States die of cardiovascular diseases each year, representing 43.8% of all deaths in the country. The leading cardiovascular diseases are atherosclerosis, heart attack, angina, and stroke. Of these, coronary heart disease (heart attacks and angina) is most common, and the cerebrovascular condition stroke is singled out as the third leading cause of death of adults in the United States. Although some of the risk factors for cardiovascular disease cannot be avoided, many more are related to diet, exercise, and other lifestyle habits and thus are preventable.

Figure 8.1 shows the death rates for coronary heart disease and stroke. Although people over age 40 are most at risk for heart disease, many deaths occur before that time. According to the National Center for Health Statistics, the death rate from heart disease for African-Americans exceeded the rate for Caucasians by 38%, and deaths from strokes were 82% higher for African-Americans

than Caucasians. Table 8.1 compares the death rate from cardiovascular disease among race and ethnicity and gender.

# The Cardiovascular System

The cardiovascular system consists of the heart and two main types of blood vessels—the arteries and the veins (see Figure 8.2). This system is responsible for transporting blood throughout the body. Blood, which amounts to about five or six quarts in the average human body, has many functions. It carries nutrients, waste products, hormones, and enzymes; regulates body temperature, water levels in the cells, and acidity levels; and helps the body defend against invading pathogens.

As the **arteries** that carry oxygen-rich blood leave the heart, they divide into smaller blood vessels called **arterioles** and then into even smaller vessels called **capillaries.** The capillary walls are so thin that they allow nutrients, oxygen, waste products, hormones, and enzymes to pass through. The **veins** and the smaller **venules** return to the heart the blood that carries waste products and carbon dioxide. This deoxygenated blood is pumped to the lungs, where it dispenses the impurities, picks up oxygen, and is returned to the heart. The entire cycle is repeated about once a minute.

The organ that makes blood circulation possible is the heart, illustrated in Figure 8.3. The heart is a muscular pumping organ situated slightly left of center of the chest and just behind the ribs. Even though the heart is only slightly larger than a fist, it is strong enough to pump five to six quarts per minute, 75 gallons per hour, and 2,000 gallons of blood per day. The heart beats (contracts and expands) approximately 100,000 times a day throughout a person's life. The contraction is called **systole,** and the relaxation between contractions is termed **diastole.**

The heart is bisected lengthwise by a wall called the **septum,** which separates the right side from the left so blood that has returned to the heart to be pumped to the lungs for oxygen (pulmonary circulation) will not mix with blood on the left side, which has received oxygen and is on its way back to nourish the body systems. The heart has four compartments or chambers. The two upper chambers, or receivers, are called **atria,** and the two lower chambers, or pumpers, are the **ventricles.** The right atrium receives blood through the largest veins in the body, the superior **vena cava** and the inferior vena cava. The left atrium receives blood returning from the lungs with oxygen that soon will be on its way back to the body. The right ventricle pumps blood in need of oxygen to the lungs, and the left ventricle pumps blood rich in oxygen through the **aorta** to arteries that nourish the body systems.

On the exterior of the heart are located blood vessels that encircle the heart and supply the heart muscle with blood. These blood vessels are called **coronary arteries.**

**FIGURE 8.1** ▶ Coronary Heart Disease and Stroke Deaths, United States, 1979–1998

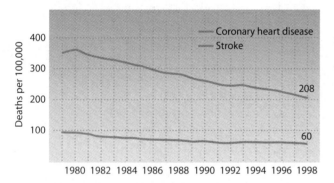

*Note:* Age adjusted to the year 2000 standard population.
*Source:* Centers for Disease Control and Prevention, National Center for Health Statistics, National Vital Statistics System.

**TABLE 8.1** ▶ Coronary Heart Disease Deaths, 2003

| POPULATION CATEGORY | CORONARY HEART DISEASE DEATHS (RATE PER 100,000) |
| --- | --- |
| Overall | 162.6 |
| **Race and ethnicity** | |
| American Indian or Alaska Native | 114.0 |
| Asian or Pacific Islander | 98.6 |
| Hispanic or Latino | 138.3 |
| **Race and Gender** | |
| White male | 209.2 |
| African-American male | 241.1 |
| White female | 125.1 |
| African-American female | 160.3 |

*Source:* Centers for Disease Control and Prevention, National Center for Health Statistics.

**FIGURE 8.2** ▶ Circulatory System

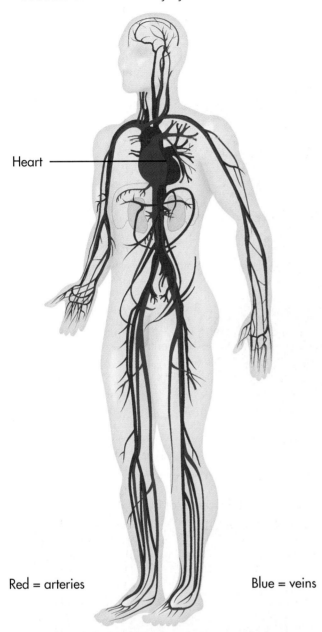

Heart

Red = arteries                    Blue = veins

## Major Risk Factors for Cardiovascular Disease

Over the years certain conditions or **risk factors** for cardiovascular disease (CVD) have been identified. The major predisposing or unchangeable risk factors are

- *Heredity.* Tendencies toward various CVDs, particularly atherosclerosis and hypertension, run in families.
- *Age and sex.* Heart attacks occur across the age spectrum. About half of those who die from heart attacks are men in the 40–65 age group. Recent statistics are showing that nearly as many women as men die from heart attacks. A woman's risk for heart attack increases

after menopause. Heart disease is the No. 1 killer of men and women alike.

African-Americans and Hispanics are at greater risk for CVDs than Caucasians. African-Americans have severe hypertension three times as often as Caucasians.

The major modifiable, behaviorally related risk factors—the risk factors that you can change—are hypertension, high levels of blood lipids, overweight or obesity, cigarette smoking, and lack of exercise. Contributing risk factors also include diabetes and stress. Figure 8.4 shows the interrelationships of various risk factors.

## HYPERTENSION (HIGH BLOOD PRESSURE)

Blood pressure is the force of the blood against the walls of the arteries caused by the heart pumping. The pressure, greatest during the heart's contraction, is known as **systolic blood pressure.** The lower pressure during the heart's relaxation phase is termed the **diastolic blood pressure.**

### KEY TERMS

**Arteries** blood vessels leaving the heart with blood full of oxygen

**Arterioles** very small arteries

**Capillaries** extremely small blood vessels with thin walls that allow nutrients and oxygen to pass through

**Veins** blood vessels that return the blood with carbon dioxide to the heart

**Venules** very small veins

**Systole** contraction segment of heartbeat

**Diastole** relaxation of the heart between beats

**Septum** wall that bisects the heart lengthwise

**Atria** the two upper chambers of the heart which receive blood (atrium is singular)

**Ventricles** the two lower chambers of the heart which pump blood

**Vena cava** either of the two largest veins in the body that return blood to the right atrium—inferior vena cava brings blood from the lower limbs and abdomen; superior vena cava brings blood from the head, neck, and upper limbs

**Aorta** artery through which oxygen-rich blood is transported from the heart to arteries that nourish the body systems

**Coronary arteries** blood vessels that surround the exterior of the heart and supply heart muscle with blood

**Risk factors** conditions or situations that predispose a person to develop a disease

**Systolic blood pressure** force in the blood vessel during the heart's contraction

**Diastolic blood pressure** force in the blood vessel during the heart's relaxation phase

**FIGURE 8.3** ▶ Circulation in the Heart

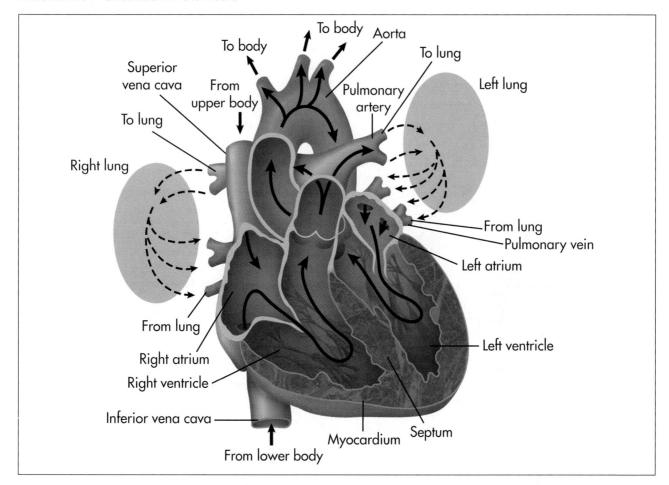

Blood pressure is measured by an instrument called a **sphygmomanometer,** which displays a column of mercury that rises and falls with the blood pressure. Blood pressure readings are given as two numbers, the top one of which is the systolic pressure and the bottom of which is the diastolic pressure. Because normal blood pressure depends on a variety of factors, it is given in ranges. A blood pressure slightly lower or higher than the "textbook" or average of 120/80 mm Hg is no cause for alarm. A systolic pressure consistently above 140 and a diastolic pressure consistently above 90 are considered abnormal. Individuals with these readings should see a physician. Table 8.2 gives the classification of blood pressure.

High blood pressure, **hypertension,** is a risk factor for several conditions, including heart attack and stroke. When the blood pressure is constantly above normal ranges, it increases the workload of the heart, eventually enlarging it. High blood pressure strains the blood vessels, which can become scarred, hardened, and narrower, restricting the needed blood flow. Occasionally clots may form, obstructing the arteries. The American Heart Association estimates that one in four American adults has high blood pressure. African-Americans, Puerto Ricans, Cubans, and Hispanics are more likely to have high blood pressure than Caucasians.

**TABLE 8.2** ▶ Classification of Blood Pressure

| CATEGORY OF ADULTS AGED 18 YEARS AND OLDER | SYSTOLIC (mm Hg) | DIASTOLIC (mm Hg) |
|---|---|---|
| Normal | <130 | <85 |
| High normal | 130–139 | 85–89 |
| Hypertension |  |  |
| Stage 1 (mild) | 140–159 | 90–99 |
| Stage 2 (moderate) | 160–179 | 100–109 |
| Stage 3 (severe) | 180–209 | 110–119 |
| Stage 4 (very severe) | ≥210 | ≥120 |

*Source:* American Medical Association.

Unfortunately, hypertension usually has no symptoms or warning signs. The American Heart Association has estimated that about 28% of the people with high blood pressure are not aware of it. This is why hypertension sometimes is called "the silent killer."

In 2004 (latest cumulative data available), hypertension killed 54,186 people in the United States. It contributes to thousands of deaths from stroke, heart disease, and kidney failure annually. Among persons with hypertension, about 72% know they have it, 61% are being treated,

**FIGURE 8.4 ▶** Interrelationship of Risk Factors and Cardiovascular Disease

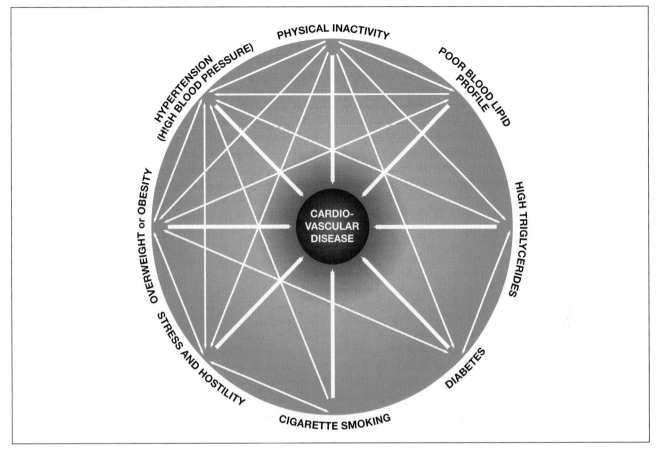

**TABLE 8.3 ▶** Medications for Hypertension

| CATEGORY | ACTION |
|---|---|
| Diurectics | Rid the body of excess water and salt |
| Beta blockers | Reduce heart rate and heart's output of blood |
| Sympathetic nerve inhibitors | Discourage nerves from constricting blood vessels |
| Vasodilators | Cause muscles in artery walls to relax and allow artery to widen |
| ACE inhibitors | Interfere with body's production of angiotensin, which causes arteries to constrict |
| Calcium channel blockers | Reduce heart rate and relax blood vessels |
| ACE inhibitor and calcium channel blocker (combination) | Interferes with body's production of angiotensin, which causes arteries to constrict, reducing heart rate |

and only 35% have it under control. Even though scientists have identified factors that contribute to hypertension, in most cases (90%–95%) of hypertension, the cause is unknown. This type of hypertension is called essential hypertension. In cases in which kidney disease or tumor of the adrenal glands may cause high blood pressure, the problem can be corrected and the blood pressure usually returns to a normal range. This type of hypertension is called secondary hypertension.

Essential hypertension can be treated and controlled. Home remedies should not be used to treat hypertension. Drinking vinegar, vinegar water, or lemon juice will not lower blood pressure. A physician will develop a treatment plan that consists of some combination of diet, exercise, and medication. Medications used to lower blood pressure, listed in Table 8.3, are called **antihypertensives.** These are available only by prescription. Reacting to stress in unhealthy ways (hot reactors) may be changed through behavior modification methods, discussed in Chapter 3. Avoidable risk factors that have been identified for hypertension are being overweight, consuming too much salt in the diet, using oral contraceptives, and, possibly, being exposed to lead through flaking lead-based paint and lead water pipes.

## KEY TERMS

**Sphygmomanometer** instrument used to measure blood pressure

**Hypertension** also known as high blood pressure; a chronic increase in blood pressure above the normal range

**Antihypertensives** medications used to lower blood pressure

## Atherosclerosis

At birth the interior lining of the blood vessels is smooth, with no obstruction. Year by year matter that floats through the blood vessels (blood containing fats, calcium, fibrin, debris from cells) begins to adhere to the lining of the blood vessels, forming **plaque.** The resulting condition is **atherosclerosis.** Figure 8.5 shows how plaque builds up in the arteries over time, obstructing the flow of blood. In some instances individuals speed this process as a result of their lifestyle. Three causes of damage to the arterial wall are

- Elevated cholesterol and triglyceride levels in the blood
- High blood pressure
- Cigarette smoke

Diets high in saturated fat and lack of regular exercise hasten plaque formation and contribute to premature atherosclerosis. Even children are not immune.

## BLOOD LIPIDS

The American Heart Association has named elevated levels of **blood lipids** or **lipoproteins** as one of the main causes of damage to the blood vessels that can lead to cardiovascular diseases. The culprits are cholesterol and triglycerides. Cholesterol is a soft, fatlike substance manufactured by the liver and needed in small amounts by the body to form cell membranes and hormones. Unfortunately, most people consume too much additional cholesterol in animal foods such as meat and dairy products. Foods from plants do not contain cholesterol.

Just as oil cannot dissolve in water, cholesterol cannot dissolve in blood. It is transported throughout the circulatory system by the cholesterol carrier **low density lipoprotein (LDL).** Some of the circulating cholesterol is used by body tissues to build cells, and some of the cholesterol is returned to the liver. A problem arises if the bloodstream is carrying excess cholesterol. The excess is deposited on the lining of the arteries and contributes to plaque formation and atherosclerosis. For this reason

**FIGURE 8.5 ▶** The Atherosclerotic Process

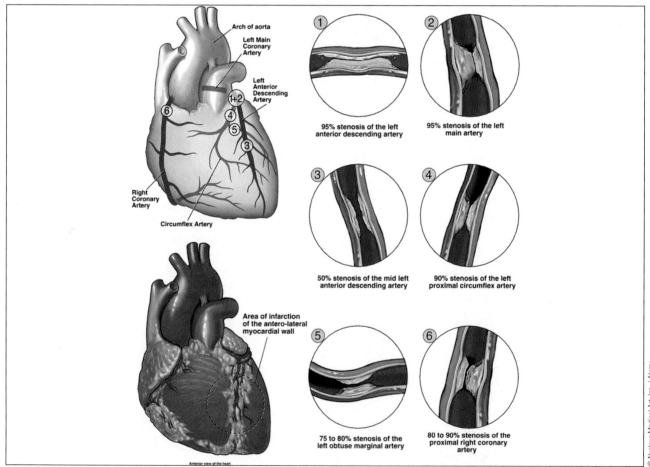

© Nucleus Medical Art, Inc. / Alamy

*Source:* Werner W. K. Hoeger and Sharon A. Hoeger, *Lifetime Physical Fitness and Wellness,* 5th edition (Belmont, CA: Wadsworth, 1998).

LDL cholesterol is called the "bad" cholesterol. People with high levels of LDL cholesterol have a greater risk for cardiovascular disease.

Another type of lipoprotein, **high density lipoprotein (HDL)** cholesterol, picks up other cholesterol circulating in the bloodstream and returns it to the liver for reprocessing or excretion. Because HDL cholesterol clears cholesterol out of the system, it is known as the "good" cholesterol.

Individuals with a higher ratio of HDL cholesterol to LDL cholesterol have a lower risk for CVDs. African-American men and women have lower HDL levels than Caucasian men and women. This may be related to cultural dietary factors, as the African-American diet tends to be higher in saturated fat than the average Caucasian diet.

A third type of lipoprotein, **very low density lipoprotein (VLDL),** carries a form of fatty substance called **triglycerides,** also manufactured by the liver. Triglycerides are broken down in the capillaries and either used for energy or stored by muscle or fat cells. Excess triglycerides in the arteries contribute, along with LDL cholesterol, to fatty deposits and atherosclerosis.

Generally speaking, women have higher HDL levels than men do, because the female sex hormone estrogen tends to raise HDL levels. This may explain partially why women are better protected against heart disease until estrogen production ends during menopause and, coincidentally, their rate of heart disease increases. As people get older or fatter or both, their triglyceride and cholesterol levels tend to rise. Children are not immune. Plaque formation has been documented in children under the age of two years.

Blood lipid levels can be assessed through a blood test. The guidelines for serum cholesterol levels, published by the National Cholesterol Education Program, are given in Table 8.4, and the triglyceride levels in Table 8.5. Chapter 9 contains a discussion of blood lipids in relation to nutrition and dietary fat.

In the longest running study of heart disease, the Framingham study, not one person in its 48-year duration with a cholesterol level of 150 or lower died of heart disease. In Japan the typical rural resident has a cholesterol level of 120 and the average city dweller has a level of 140. In contrast, Japanese Americans who have lived in the United States a number of years have readings in the 200s. Denver cardiologist Dr. Richard J. Flanigan says, "We have taught them how to die."

Obese people (BMI ≥30) are more likely to develop heart disease or a stroke. Approximately 45% of Americans are overweight (BMI 25–29). This problem, too, is more prevalent in certain ethnic minority populations (especially among the women) than Caucasians (see Figure 8.6). Chapters 9, 10, and 11 provide more information on regulating cholesterol levels through nutrition, weight management, and physical fitness, respectively.

**TABLE 8.4 ▶** Serum Cholesterol Guidelines

|  | AMOUNT | RATING |
|---|---|---|
| **Total cholesterol** | ≤200 mg/dL | Desirable |
|  | 200–239 mg/dL | Borderline high |
|  | ≥240 mg/dL | High risk |
| **LDL cholesterol** | <130 mg/dL | Desirable |
|  | 130–159 mg/dL | Borderline high |
|  | ≥160 mg/dL | High risk |
| **HDL cholesterol** | ≥50 mg/dL | Desirable |
|  | 36–49 mg/dL | Moderate risk |
|  | ≤35 mg/dL | High risk |

**TABLE 8.5 ▶** Triglyceride Guidelines

| AMOUNT | RATING |
|---|---|
| <125 mg/dL | Desirable |
| 126–400 mg/dL | Borderline high |
| >400 mg/dL | High risk |

## CIGARETTE SMOKING

The risk of heart attack for smokers is twice that of people who do not smoke. The nicotine in tobacco smoke constricts blood vessels, and the gases displace oxygen in the bloodstream. Chapter 13 provides more

### KEY TERMS

**Plaque** material composed of fat and cholesterol that adheres to the walls of the blood vessels

**Atherosclerosis** condition that results when the blood vessel walls become coated with plaque, obstructing blood flow

**Blood lipids** or **lipoproteins** fatty substances carried through the blood

**Low density lipoprotein (LDL)** fatty substances produced by the liver that carry cholesterol to arterial walls; "bad" cholesterol

**High density lipoprotein (HDL)** fatty substance that picks up cholesterol in the bloodstream and returns it to the liver; "good" cholesterol

**Very low density lipoproteins (VLDL)** largest of the lipoproteins; allows cholesterol to circulate in bloodstream

**Triglycerides** fatty substances used for energy or stored by muscle or fat cells

**FIGURE 8.6** ▶ Trends in Being Overweight (BMI 25–29) and Obese (BMI ≥ 30) by Sex and Race, Adults Age 20–74

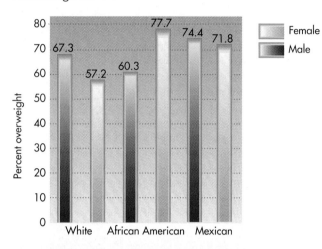

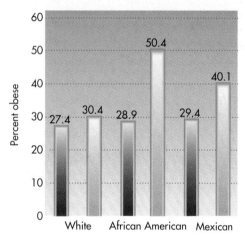

information on the detrimental effects of cigarette smoking on health.

## LACK OF EXERCISE

Physical inactivity unquestionably contributes to cardiovascular disease. Regular aerobic exercise strengthens the heart muscle and lowers serum cholesterol levels. Chapter 11 contains more information on the benefits of aerobic exercise.

## CONTRIBUTING RISK FACTORS

Diabetes increases the risk for problems of the circulatory system, such as heart attack, stroke, and kidney disease. Diabetes is discussed in Chapter 7.

The effects of stress in daily life cannot be ignored. Psychological stress may be related to the job, environment, or socioeconomic status. Stress has been linked to high blood pressure and, hence, CVD. Stress is the topic of Chapter 3.

Researchers also have found a link between hostility and heart disease. The toxic core of the Type A personality (discussed in Chapter 2), which includes cynicism, anger, and aggression, can translate to higher blood pressure and coronary heart disease. Finally, using cocaine or crystal methamphetamine (illicit stimulant psychoactive drugs) can produce heart attacks and sudden death.

## Disorders of the Heart

Coronary heart disease (CHD) is the general term covering heart attacks and angina pectoris. Both of these conditions involve an insufficient supply of blood to the coronary arteries and the consequent lack of oxygen to the heart muscle. Even though CHD is the leading cause of death (for men and women) in the United States, more than 7 million living Americans have survived a heart attack. The lifetime risk of developing CHD after age 40 is 49% for men and 32% for women.

The term for any condition in which a body tissue is not receiving enough oxygen is **ischemia.** As many as 3 to 4 million Americans may have ischemic episodes without knowing it, called silent ischemia. Other heart conditions are abnormal heart rhythm (bradycardia and tachycardia), sudden cardiac death, congestive heart failure, rheumatic heart disease, and congenital heart defects.

### HEART ATTACK (ACUTE MYOCARDIAL INFARCTION)

A heart attack, or **acute myocardial infarction (MI),** occurs when the blood supply from the coronary arteries to the heart muscle, the **myocardium,** is reduced (ischemia) substantially. This is caused by blockage from a blood clot (thrombus) or plaque. The area of heart muscle that is deprived of oxygen and dies is called an **infarct.** Depending

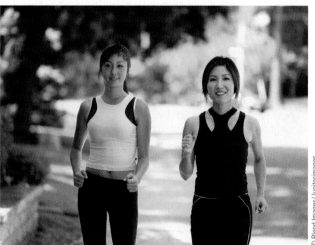

▲ *Walking maintains a healthy heart*

on how much heart muscle is damaged, the person can incur permanent disability or die. Heart attack is the leading heart disease. In 2006, approximately 565,000 Americans experienced their first heart attack and 300,000 a recurrent heart attack. The average age for the first MI is 65.8 for men and 70.4 for women.

Symptoms of heart attack are

- A crushing or heavy discomfort or pain in the chest that lasts more than a few minutes or goes away and returns (described by some as feeling like a blow by a fist to the chest)
- Pain that begins in the chest and may spread to the shoulders, neck, jaw, or arms
- Symptoms similar to heartburn accompanied by nausea or vomiting
- Sweating
- Lightheadedness, dizziness, or fainting

Anyone experiencing all or a combination of these symptoms should receive medical assistance immediately. Delay of treatment because of denial is a mistake.

## HEART ATTACK—IT'S DIFFERENT FOR WOMEN

Studies indicate that a woman's heart is not just a smaller model of a man's. Heart attack is the leading cause of death of women in the United States. Women under 50 years of age are twice as likely to die from a heart attack than men under 50. Additionally, 38% of women who survive a heart attack die within the first year compared to 21% of men. However, for many women, symptoms of heart attack are different from the "classic" signs that men often experience and sometimes are more difficult to detect. A woman might tell her physician that she experiences breathlessness ("I get winded") doing routine activities. Other symptoms of a heart attack that a woman may experience include upper back, shoulder, and/or abdominal pain (similar to indigestion), dizziness, and unusual fatigue. These symptoms might even occur (at a lower intensity) four to six weeks before the heart attack.

According to a National Institutes of Health (NIH) study of heart disease in 1,000 women over a 10-year period, the "gold-standard" x-ray procedure, the angiogram, is less effective in detecting heart disease. This is because microvascular disease, which is more common in women than in men, is more difficult to identify. Microvascular disease, in which plaque is deposited uniformly on the lining of the coronary arteries, decreases the diameter of the blood vessel's interior and thus the blood flow to the heart muscle. The plaque buildup does not appear as a blockage on an angiogram, and a woman having a heart attack may be misdiagnosed by her physician and sent home.

Even when women seek medical assistance when experiencing the symptoms of a heart attack, at least 33% of women with these symptoms do not get a diagnosis or are misdiagnosed. It is imperative that women recognize the symptoms, seek immediate medical assistance, and insist that the cardiologist not immediately rule out heart disease if the angiogram shows no blockage.

## ANGINA PECTORIS

Another result of coronary artery disease is **angina pectoris.** This is a symptom of myocardial ischemia. The chest pain is usually described by the victim as the sensation of squeezing or gas. The usual blood supply to the heart may be enough for normal needs but not enough for increased exertion, such as running to catch the bus or shoveling snow. Angina can be a sign that a person is at risk for heart attack. It also can occur during periods of great emotional stress. Angina is more often reported by women. The female-to-male ratio is 1.7:1.

More than 6 million people suffer from angina pectoris, and about 1.2 million people in the United States are hospitalized with angina each year. This makes it the leading cause of admission to coronary care facilities. An estimated 350,000 new cases occur every year.

Angina is treated with medications such as nitroglycerin, which relaxes the blood vessels and increases blood flow to the myocardium. The condition can be treated with a class of medications (beta blockers and calcium antagonists) that affect the heart's demand for oxygen. Medications to lower blood pressure are prescribed in some cases, and in still others surgery may be required.

A class of medications known as glycoprotein IIb/IIIa receptor antagonists (anticoagulant drugs) block the process that leads to formation of blood clots. One of the pioneer medications, Aggrastat®, was approved in 1998 for use in the United States. Anticoagulants are used to treat angina and are prescribed after angioplasty or other procedures to open clogged blood vessels because they block platelet formation.

---

## KEY TERMS

**Ischemia** lack of oxygen to body tissue

**Acute myocardial infarction** a condition that occurs when blood supply to heart muscle is cut off and the tissue dies; heart attack

**Myocardium** heart muscle

**Infarct** area of tissue deprived of oxygen that dies

**Angina pectoris** chest pain that occurs when the heart muscle does not get enough blood

---

## Tips for Action How to Lower Your Risk for Heart Disease

■ **Get 7 to 8 hours of sleep every night.** Your body and your brain need that time to rest, repair, and regroup.

■ **Get your blood pressure and cholesterol levels checked.** If you do not know your blood pressure, total cholesterol, and HDL (good) cholesterol levels, get them measured soon. You may be at risk without knowing it.

■ **Eat a low-fat, low-salt diet; eat fish three times a week.** Cutting back on fatty foods will lower your total cholesterol. That, in turn, may help you lower your blood pressure and raise your HDL cholesterol. Restrict salt in your diet, as high salt intake is linked to high blood pressure in some cases. The omega-3 fatty acids in the fish promote the health of your CVS.

■ **Exercise.** Walking (or some form of moderate exercise) at least 30 minutes **every** day can reduce your risk for heart attack. People who do more vigorous activities have an even lower heart attack risk. The exercise will help you reach or maintain a healthy body mass index—BMI of 19 to 24.

■ **If you smoke, quit. If you don't smoke, avoid being in "smoke-filled rooms."** Smoking increases your risk for heart attack. The more you smoke, the higher are your risks for heart attack and stroke. Your risk for heart disease drops dramatically soon after you quit smoking. Passive smoking (see Chapter 13) puts you at risk for heart and lung disease.

■ **Take medications.** If lifestyle changes are not enough to lower your risk, your doctor may prescribe cholesterol and blood pressure-lowering drugs.

■ **Follow the oral health "2-2-2 Rule": brush and floss twice daily—see your dentist twice a year.** Inflamed gums (gingivitis) and other oral infections increase your risk for heart problems.

■ **Reduce stress.** Stress and anxiety are risk factors for CVDs. Use a relaxation technique to take the edge off stressors, especially those at work or school. Decrease anxiety using time management strategies and by following a budget.

*Source: "How to Save Your Own Heart." The Oprah Magazine,* October 2006.

---

## ARRHYTHMIAS

In a normal heart, electrical impulses spread in a systematic way throughout the heart, causing the heart to beat in a regular rhythm. **Arrhythmia,** which means irregular heartbeat, refers to any change in this pattern. Some arrhythmias are so brief that they do not affect the overall heart rate. If they last for some time, though, they may cause the heart to beat too slowly or too rapidly. **Bradycardia** describes a heart rate of fewer than 60 beats a minute. **Tachycardia** means a heart rate of more than 100 beats per minute.

Most arrhythmias are acquired as the result of atherosclerosis, hypertension, or an imbalance of minerals such as potassium, magnesium, and calcium, which play a vital role in starting and maintaining normal heart impulses. Alcohol, tobacco, cocaine, and other substances also can provoke arrhythmias.

Symptoms of arrhythmias are wide-ranging, from barely perceptible to cardiovascular collapse and death. Slower rates may produce fatigue, lightheadedness, loss of consciousness, or even death, depending upon the amount of oxygen deprivation in the heart muscle. Arrhythmias also can lead to damage to other organs such as the brain, kidneys, lungs, or liver during prolonged cardiac arrest. Blood clots can form and break free, causing a stroke or damaging other organs.

The standard diagnostic tool is an **electrocardiogram (ECG or EKG),** which shows the timing of the electrical events in the heart. Treadmill testing sometimes is done to provoke exercise-related arrhythmias. Electrophysiologic testing has become valuable for inducing otherwise infrequent arrhythmias so they can be studied. Performed under local anesthesia, it involves placing temporary electrode catheters strategically within the heart. With fluoroscopic guidance, the heart's electrical signals are mapped.

Potentially life-threatening bradycardia may be treated with medication to increase and improve the heart rate. Temporary or permanent **pacemakers** sometimes are implanted surgically. Tachycardia is treated with a variety of drugs, administered intravenously or orally. Increasingly, ablative techniques such as cauterization via a catheter are used to destroy the malfunctioning heart tissue. Many tachycardias can be stopped by delivering electric shocks to the heart through a device called a **defibrillator.**

American Airlines was one of the first U.S. airlines to equip planes with portable defibrillators and train at least one attendant per plane to use them. These devices are to be added to longer flights over water, where emergency landings are not possible. About 60 people die each year on planes from a variety of medical causes. Cardiologist James Atkins, of the University of Texas Southwestern

Medical Center, has estimated that about 20 of them could be saved with the use of defibrillators on domestic flights.

## SUDDEN CARDIAC DEATH

About half of all adult deaths from heart disease in the United States, or 330,000 each year, are sudden and unexpected. **Sudden cardiac death (SCD)** is the result of an unresuscitated cardiac arrest stemming from rapid activity of the heart, which may be caused by all known heart diseases.

Sudden cardiac arrest is reversible in most victims if it is treated with **cardiopulmonary resuscitation (CPR)** and electric shock within seven to 10 minutes after the event. Few resuscitation attempts are successful after 10 minutes have elapsed. Survival rates improved dramatically after the defibrillator and bedside monitoring were developed in the 1960s, and later through cardiopulmonary resuscitation. Underlying heart disease (atherosclerotic heart disease) often is found in victims of SCD.

Anxiety is proving to be one of the strongest risk factors—even more so than smoking, says Dr. Ichiro Kawachi of the Harvard University School of Public Health. In studies he led, the risk of SCD was four and a half times higher in anxious participants in one study, and six times higher among the most anxious than among those who had no symptoms of phobic anxiety. For reasons yet unknown, intense psychological stress may trigger irregular heart rhythms.

Treatment is as varied as the underlying conditions causing the SCD or the damage done to the heart muscle scarred by the attack. Reducing deaths from SCD depends on a "chain of survival" to rescue victims. This includes early notification of the emergency, early CPR, early defibrillation, and early advanced medical care.

## CONGESTIVE HEART FAILURE

**Congestive heart failure** comes about because the heart muscle is damaged or overworked. This can stem from high blood pressure, a heart attack, atherosclerosis, and other conditions that place a strain on the heart. The damaged heart is not strong enough to keep blood circulating normally throughout the body. As the blood flow from the heart slows, blood returning to the heart through the veins backs up, causing congestion in the tissues.

Symptoms usually include swelling (edema) in the legs and ankles and possibly in other parts of the body as well. The person may be short of breath as fluid collects in the lungs. Congestive heart failure affects the kidneys' ability to remove water from the body. Weight gain is a common effect as well.

Treatment for congestive heart failure usually involves rest, proper diet, prescribed daily exercises, and medication. If a specific cause of congestive heart failure is

---

### KEY TERMS

**Arrhythmia** irregular heartbeat

**Bradycardia** heart rate of fewer than 60 beats per minute

**Tachycardia** heart rate of more than 100 beats per minute

**Electrocardiogram (ECG)** measurement of electrical activity in the heart

**Pacemaker** device implanted near the heart to regulate heartbeat

**Defibrillator** a device that delivers electrical shocks to the heart in an attempt to restore normal rhythm

**Sudden cardiac death (SCD)** result of an electrical malfunction that throws the heart off rhythm and ends with the abrupt loss of heart function

**Cardiopulmonary resuscitation (CPR)** manual method of providing oxygen to the brain, heart, and other vital organs, reversing sudden cardiac death

**Congestive heart failure** condition caused when blood flow from the heart slows and blood returning to the heart backs up in the veins, causing blood to collect in the tissues

- Reduce deaths from coronary heart disease and strokes.

- Increase the proportion of people with high blood pressure whose blood pressure is under control.

- Increase the proportion of adults with high blood pressure who are taking action (for example, losing weight, increasing physical activity, or reducing sodium intake) to help control their blood pressure.

- Increase the proportion of adults aged 20 years and older who are aware of the early warning symptoms and signs of a heart attack and the importance of accessing rapid emergency care by calling 9-1-1.

- Increase the proportion of adults with high blood cholesterol who are aware of their condition and are taking action to reduce their blood cholesterol to recommended levels.

- Increase the proportion of adults who have had their blood pressure measured within the preceding two years and can state whether their blood pressure was normal or high.

- Increase the proportion of adults who have had their blood cholesterol checked within the preceding five years.

discovered, it should be treated or corrected. Most cases are treatable.

## RHEUMATIC HEART DISEASE

If strep throat is not treated early, it can develop into rheumatic fever, which can cause inflammation of heart muscle and valves and culminate in damage to the heart known as **rheumatic heart disease.** Rheumatic fever appears most often in children ages five to 15.

A culture taken in response to a suspect sore throat can reveal the strep infection, but no lab test is available to identify rheumatic fever. The first symptoms are a high fever and sore joints. Chest pains or shortness of breath indicates that the heart is affected, which can be verified by chest x-ray and electrocardiogram.

A heart valve that does not close completely lets blood leak into the chamber from which it was pumped, mixing with the blood that flows normally. The added volume puts extra strain on the heart muscle. When a valve does not open enough, the heart has to pump harder than normal to force blood through the narrower opening. In their most advanced state, these conditions may turn into congestive heart failure.

A technique called echocardiography is used to detect the condition. Sound waves sent into the chest rebound from the heart's walls and valves, showing the shape, texture, and movement of the valves and size and functioning of the heart chambers.

To decrease the risk of rheumatic heart disease related to strep throat, the best cure is prevention. Strep throat is treated successfully with antibiotics, such as penicillin, that prevent rheumatic fever from ever developing. If a person has had one attack, the goal is to prevent another (to which he or she is susceptible). If the heart valves are damaged, valve replacement surgery may be performed.

## CONGENITAL HEART DEFECTS

**Congenital heart defects** are present in almost 1% of live births, the most frequent congenital malformation in newborns. Sometimes they are the product of the mother's having had German measles (or some other viral disease) during the first trimester of pregnancy or of her drinking alcohol or using drugs such as cocaine. In most cases, however, the cause is unknown.

One class of defects is called **stenoses,** or constrictions in a heart valve, artery, or vein. A second class consists of **septal defects,** which allow the blood to flow abnormally between the right and left chambers. Another defect, **patent ductus arteriosus**—more common in premature babies—allows blood to mix between the pulmonary artery and the aorta because a duct that normally closes after birth fails to do so.

In still another classification, **cyanotic defects,** blood pumped to the body carries too little oxygen. This results in cyanosis, a blue discoloration of the skin of newborns (often called blue babies). A rare defect occurs when the heart is formed incompletely.

Congenital heart defects usually are diagnosed at birth or during infancy, when a doctor detects a heart murmur or cyanosis. Tests may include a chest x-ray, an electrocardiogram, an echocardiogram, and a cardiac catheterization. Some heart defects are treated with medication and others with surgery to repair the defect.

## OTHER HEART CONDITIONS

**Bacterial endocarditis** is a serious infectious disease involving the heart valves or tissues. It is rare, but when it does occur, it poses a serious threat to people who already have structural damage to or dysfunctions of the heart. As a prophylactic measure, the American Heart Association recommends antibiotics when people undergo

## Tips for Action Nutritional Aids to a Healthy Heart

- **Eat more fiber.** Eating fruits, vegetables, cereals, or grains can reduce the risk for heart attack by up to 20%.

- **Drink tea.** Tea drinkers historically have had less heart disease. It may neutralize the ability of bad LDL cholesterol to clog arteries. Two or three cups a day of green or black tea, with or without caffeine, hot or iced, will do the trick. Herbal tea does not offer these benefits.

- **Eat beans.** Legumes contain much soluble fiber and other cholesterol-lowering components. All kinds of beans work.

- **Eat garlic.** Taking garlic supplements daily (equivalent to eating 1/2 to 11/2 garlic cloves) lowers cholesterol 9%–12%.

- **Take vitamin E.** In one study at Cambridge University in England, taking 400 IUs of vitamin E for 18 months slashed nonfatal heart attacks in cardiovascular patients by 77%.

- **Get enough vitamin C.** This means 2,000 mg of vitamin C daily. Orange juice is a good source.

- **Get B vitamins.** These include folic acid, B6, and B12. Good sources include green leafy vegetables and orange juice.

- **Eat fish.** The omega-3 oils in fish thin the blood, ward off clot formation, boost good HDL cholesterol, and help stave off irregular heartbeat. Two or three servings a week should be enough.

- **Eat flavonoids.** These denote foods rich in antioxidants and include grapes, red wine, onions, apples, and tea. Restrict wine to no more than one or two glasses a day, though.

- **Cut back on saturated (animal) fats.** These are contained in meat, cheese, butter, and milk (except nonfat or skim milk). Also restrict margarine. The safest fat is the type in olives and olive oil, almonds, walnuts, avocados, and canola oil.

*Source: Jean Carper, Stop Aging Now!* (Farmington Hills, MI: Macmillan Library Reference, 1999).

---

dental procedures that may cause the gum or mouth to bleed, as well as certain other surgeries.

A childhood heart condition that appears more often among those of Asian ancestry is **Kawasaki disease,** striking most often boys under age eight. (Girls are half as likely to get it.) The heart (coronary arteries or heart muscle) is involved in about 20% of those affected. Kawasaki disease and acute rheumatic fever are the two leading causes of acquired heart disease in American children. Symptoms are fever, rash, swollen hands and feet, red eyes, swollen lymph glands in the neck, and inflammation of the mouth, lips, and throat. The cause is unknown. Treatment is aspirin and intravenous gamma globulin.

## DIAGNOSIS

As a result of advances in technology, several means have been developed to diagnose the severity of damage to the heart after a heart attack occurs and to detect potential heart anomalies before a problem arises. The **cardiologist** is the physician who has been trained to diagnose these problems and to treat the problems that do not require surgery.

1. *Electrocardiogram.* The ECG or "EKG" is one of the most widely used diagnostic tests. The electrical activity of the heart is measured while the person is resting or while the person is walking or running on a treadmill (exercise ECG or stress test). The latter is a better measure of which parts of the heart are deprived of oxygen.

2. *Coronary angiography.* A catheter (a thin, hollow tube) is threaded through the heart's blood vessels and a radioactive dye is released through the tube. The dye, which is visible on x-ray, shows the precise areas of blockage in the coronary arteries. If a cardiologist

---

### KEY TERMS

**Rheumatic heart disease** damage to the heart caused by strep throat

**Congenital heart defects** heart malformations present at birth

**Stenoses** heart defects characterized by obstructions to a valve, artery, or vein

**Septal defect** heart defect characterized by abnormal blood flow between the left and right heart chambers

**Patent ductus arteriosus** heart defect caused by a duct remaining open between the pulmonary artery and the aorta allowing the blood to mix

**Cyanotic defect** heart defect characterized by too little oxygen in the blood

**Bacterial endocarditis** infectious disease involving the heart valves or tissues

**Kawasaki disease** childhood disease most common to Asian children; affects the heart in about 20% of the cases

**Cardiologist** physician trained in the diagnosis and treatment of heart conditions

recommends this diagnostic procedure, he or she should discuss with the patient the health risks.

3. *Magnetic resonance imaging (MRI).* Powerful magnets and computer-generated images of heart muscle identify damage caused by a heart attack.

4. *Radionuclide imaging* (includes thallium test, multiple gated acquisition (MUGA) scan, and acute infarct scintiphotography). Substances called radionuclides are injected into the bloodstream so computer-generated pictures can find them in the heart. These tests show how well the heart muscle is supplied with blood and how well the heart's chambers are functioning. They also identify the part of the heart damaged by heart attack.

## TREATMENTS

In 1893 the African-American physician Daniel Hale Williams performed the first successful open-heart surgery and so became a pioneer among cardiac surgeons, who now perform a variety of procedures that have been perfected during the last 30 years.

- *Pacemaker.* In heart problems related to rhythm, the pacemaker often has truly been a lifesaver. This device contains a battery that stimulates the heart through electrical charges. The pacemaker may be permanent or may be removed surgically.

- *Coronary artery bypass graft surgery.* Blood supplying the heart muscle is rerouted around the blockage in the coronary artery that is causing the problem. A vein from the patient's thigh is removed, spliced into sections, and attached or grafted above and below the blocked blood vessel. If the surgery is successful, circulation is restored to the damaged heart muscle because blood is able to bypass the blockage.

- *Balloon angioplasty.* Percutaneous transluminal coronary angioplasty (PTCA) is the medical term for the procedure commonly known as balloon angioplasty. A catheter is threaded to the blocked coronary artery. Then a smaller, balloon-tipped tube is pushed through the catheter to the blockage. As the balloon is inflated, the blockage is pushed to the side, allowing more blood to circulate to the heart muscle. Because the coronary artery is much smaller near the tip of the ventricle portion of the heart, balloon angioplasty works best when the blockage is closer to the upper portion of the artery.

- *Atherectomy.* In this procedure, the plaque-blocked coronary artery is opened by grinding away the plaque with a rotating disk (rotating at about 200,000 rpm) that is located on the end of a catheter that has been threaded through a blood vessel in the leg to the coronary artery. This procedure may be followed by PTCA.

- *Intracoronary stenting.* A collapsed metal framework is inserted into a narrowed coronary artery on a balloon catheter that is inflated to expand the framework, which stays in place and keeps the artery from narrowing.

- *Heart transplant.* If the heart muscle or other structures are so damaged that neither drug therapy nor surgery can solve the problem, the heart may have to be replaced. The healthy heart of a donor is transplanted surgically into the patient. In 2005, 2125 heart transplants were done in the United States. Because of the shortage of available hearts for transplant, many people in need of a new heart will not survive if suitable organ donors are not found.

- *Mechanical heart.* If a mechanical heart could be perfected, it would solve the current problems of heart transplant, including finding a compatible donor and the body's rejecting the transplanted organ. In the summer of 2001, Robert Tools, age 59, became the first recipient of a self-contained, artificial heart. The titanium and plastic AbioCor® "heart" is battery powered and attached to a coil implanted under the skin. Blood flow is regulated by an implanted, "microchip-packed controller." Using the coil recharger, the mechanical heart is recharged by an external battery pack or by plugging the coil recharger directly into a wall outlet. Technology has improved the size of the controller; previous controllers were large and cumbersome to the patient. However, mechanical or artificial hearts have drawbacks. They still depend on an external power source and have caused serious health complications such as stroke, infection, and seizures. As the medical technology improves, the mechanical heart will move closer to being an acceptable alternative to the heart transplant. Tools lived for 151 days. In September 2006, the FDA approved the first totally implanted artificial heart for patients with advanced heart failure involving both pumping chambers of the heart. The AbioCor® Implantable Replacement Heart is intended for patients who are not eligible for a heart transplant, for whom no alternative treatments are available, and who are unlikely to live more than a month without intervention. This system consists of the two-pound mechanical heart (diseased heart removed during the implantation process) and a power transfer coil. A controller and an internal battery are implanted in the patient's abdomen. The system's two external batteries allow free movement for up to two hours. This replacement heart was approved under the Humanitarian Use Device (HUD) provisions of the Food, Drug, and Cosmetic Act.

- *Drug therapy.* The best known nonsurgical treatment for heart disease is the simple medication aspirin, which thins the blood. The value of aspirin in preventing unstable angina and myocardial infarction has been demonstrated. The American Heart Association, however, strongly cautions people not to begin taking aspirin on a long-term basis without first consulting their doctor. Physicians have to evaluate each candidate individually. In particular, they have to weigh a person's risk of myocardial infarction and coronary heart disease and death against the potential for adverse reactions to prolonged aspirin therapy.

A class of medications called statins, which were usually prescribed for people with dangerously high cholesterol, is being used to treat people with marginally high cholesterol. Statins (brand names such as Baycol, Lipitor, Zocor) control blood cholesterol by lowering LDLs and raising HDLs. Research is ongoing to determine the safety of statins. The risk that is most often cited is liver damage.

---

**VIEWPOINT** *In addition to the great expense of heart transplants, compatible donors are difficult to secure. This means that the list of people awaiting a heart transplant is lengthy. What, if any, restrictions should be placed on those allowed to receive a heart transplant? Should eligible candidates be prioritized? For example, should younger patients receive priority over older ones?* **What is your opinion?**

---

## STROKE

**Stroke,** also known as brain attack, or **cerebrovascular accident (CVA),** is the second leading cause of death worldwide and the third leading cause of adult death in the United States. It is the most common cause of adult disability, including paralysis, loss of speech, and memory lapses. During the 1970s and 1980s Americans cut the death rate for stroke nearly in half, but that trend has leveled off. Each year approximately 700,000 Americans have a first (500,000) or recurrent stroke (200,000); every 45 seconds someone has a stroke.

A stroke occurs when blood circulation to the brain is blocked or disrupted. Brain cells, robbed of vital supplies of oxygen and nutrients, can die quickly (cerebral infarct). Among the many risk factors for stroke are heart disease, hypertension, cigarette smoking, high red blood cell count (increasing the risk for blood clots), diabetes mellitus, and the use of oral contraceptives (the pill) after age 35.

Data from the CDC indicate that African-Americans and Hispanics are at greater risk than whites of dying from a stroke at an early age. African-Americans between ages 45 and 59 were found to be at least three times more likely to die of a stroke than whites in the same age range. The risk was also higher, though not by

---

**FYI | FACTS ABOUT STROKE**

- Stroke killed 150,147 people (58,660 males and 91,487 females) in the United States in 2004 (latest cumulative data) and continues to be the third largest cause of death, ranking behind diseases of the heart and cancer.

- Approximately 5.7 million U.S. stroke survivors are alive today (3,300,000 women and 2,400,000 men), many with permanent stroke-related disabilities.

- 28% of the people who have a stroke in a given year are under age 65.

- The incidence of stroke more than doubles in each successive decade over age 55.

- Women account for more than six in 10 (61.4%) stroke deaths.

- Because of hypertension, African-Americans have 1.8 times greater rate of fatal stroke and 4.2 times greater rate of kidney failure than whites.

- From 1988 to 1998 the death rate from stroke declined 15.1% overall.

*Source:* American Heart Association, *Heart Disease and Stroke Statistics: 2007. Update At-a-Glance* (Dallas: AHA, 2007).

---

as much, for Hispanics. Between ages 60 and 74 the risk margin for African-Americans was double that for whites and Hispanics.

The two major causes of stroke involve blockages (ischemic strokes), which comprise 80% of all strokes, and bleeding, the remaining 20%. As shown in Figure 8.7, these causes of stroke take four forms.

1. **Cerebral thrombus.** A blood clot forms on plaque lining the blood vessel in the brain and completely occludes (blocks) the blood vessel.

2. **Cerebral embolism.** A moving blood clot (embolus) partially or totally blocks a blood vessel in the brain.

---

### KEY TERMS

**Stroke (cerebrovascular accident** or **CVA)** disruption of blood flow to the brain, causing destruction of brain cells; also known as brain attack

**Cerebral thrombus** blood clot that gets caught on plaque in a blood vessel in the brain, causing complete blockage of the blood vessel

**Cerebral embolism** moving blood clot that partially blocks a blood vessel in the brain

**FIGURE 8.7 ►** Causes of Stroke

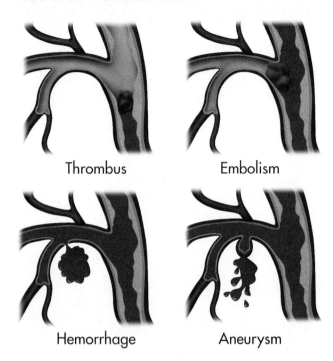

Thrombus          Embolism

Hemorrhage          Aneurysm

3. **Cerebral hemorrhage (bleeding).** A blood vessel in the brain ruptures and saturates surrounding brain tissue. (In a subarachnoid hemorrhage a blood vessel on the surface of the brain breaks and bleeds into the space between the skull and the brain.)

4. Ruptured **aneurysm.** A sac formed by distention or dilation of the artery wall breaks open.

A stroke resulting from cerebral embolism or thrombosis usually is related to atherosclerosis and hypertension. A stroke also can occur if an aneurysm bursts as a result of a blow or injury to the head.

Warning signs and symptoms of a stroke are

- Sudden weakness or loss of feeling in the face, arm, or leg on one side of the body
- Sudden severe headache with no known cause
- Dizziness, unsteadiness, or sudden falls, especially with any of the other signs
- Twisting of the mouth to one side or dropping of the bottom lip
- Temporary blurred, double, or loss of vision (especially in one eye)
- Temporary loss of speech; difficulty speaking or understanding speech

A person with one or more of these signs should call or have someone call 9-1-1 immediately. Stroke is a medical emergency. The Joint Commission on the Accreditation of Health Care Organizations (JCAHO) approves hospitals as certified primary stroke centers. Your local hospital may be able to treat stroke even if it is not a primary stroke center.

Sometimes warning signs last only a few moments and then disappear. These brief episodes, known as **transient ischemic attacks** or **TIAs,** sometimes are called ministrokes. They reveal an underlying serious condition that is progressive; half of them predate a major stroke by a year or less. Unfortunately, because TIAs do go away temporarily, many people ignore them. As with stroke, symptoms of TIAs should be reported to a physician immediately.

The most common form of TIA is called **transient monocular blindness,** in which a person experiences blurred vision in one eye. A second form is **transient hemispheral attack,** in which the person may have difficulty thinking and communicating and, in addition, experience numbness or weakness in one arm, one leg, or the face because of diminished blood flow to one side of the brain.

In June 1996, the Food and Drug Administration (FDA) approved the clot-dissolving agent tissue plasminogen activator (TPA) as the first treatment for acute ischemic stroke. The FDA first approved TPA to treat heart attacks in progress. Because this new therapy must be administered within three hours of the beginning of symptoms of stroke, the signs of stroke must not be ignored and medical help delayed. The American Heart Association has developed medical guidelines for the use of TPA in appropriate patients.

Other treatments show promise, too. In one study, funded by the National Institute of Neurological Disorders and Stroke, two drugs that reduce the tendency of the blood to clot—aspirin and warfarin—lowered the risk of stroke 50% to 80% in patients with atrial fibrillation, a type of irregular heartbeat. People with this condition have five times the normal risk for stroke. It is associated with some 70,000 strokes each year in the United States, and about 15% of all patients who have had a stroke have atrial fibrillation.

For people who have already had one stroke or its warning signs and who have severe stenosis (narrowed arteries), a surgical procedure called **carotid endarterectomy** has proved beneficial in preventing future strokes. In this procedure fatty deposits are removed from one of the two main arteries in the neck that supply blood to the brain.

## Summary

- The cardiovascular system consists of the heart and blood vessels, responsible for pumping oxygen throughout the body.
- The major risk factors for cardiovascular disease are the predisposing factors of heredity, age, sex, and more important variables that can be changed, including high blood pressure, physical inactivity, poor

- Higher than normal stroke risk has been identified in ten states: Alabama, Arkansas, Georgia, Louisiana, Mississippi, North Carolina, South Carolina, Tennessee, Florida, and Virginia.
- For people ages 35 to 54, the stroke death rate was 2.1 times higher than the U.S. average in a 153-county region along the southeastern coast.
- Among people ages 55 to 74, the rate was 1.7 times higher in the same area.

- For people in both age groups, the death rate from stroke in the eight-state stroke belt was 1.3 times the national average.

The reasons for this concentration in the Southeast remain a mystery. Theories range from genetic anomalies to trace metals and other micronutrients in the drinking water.

*Source:* George Howard, Bowman Gray School of Medicine, Winston-Salem, NC.

blood lipid profile, high triglyceride level, cigarette smoking, diabetes, obesity, and stress and hostility.

- Coronary heart disease (heart attack and angina) results from an insufficient supply of blood to the arteries of the heart and subsequent lack of oxygen to the heart muscle.

- Arrhythmias, which result from atherosclerosis, hypertension, or a mineral imbalance in the body, range from imperceptible to life-threatening.

- Congenital heart defects, the most frequent congenital condition in newborns, are classified as stenoses, septal defects, and cyanotic defects.

- The four conditions leading to stroke are cerebral embolism, cerebral thrombus, cerebral hemorrhage, and cerebral aneurysm.

## Personal Health Resources

ThomsonNOW Visit the ThomsonNOW website at http://thomsonedu.com/thomsonnow for valuable resources that will:

- Help you evaluate your knowledge of the material.
- Guide you through tutorials to help you understand and apply the material.
- Allow you to take an exam-prep quiz to better prepare for class tests.

American Heart Association. Provides information for the consumer and the health professional about cardiovascular diseases, risk factors, and measures that can be used to reduce risks for America's leading cause of death. Information is available on family health, nutrition, risk awareness, advocacy, and the Reference Guide to Heart and Stroke. Biostatistical Fact Sheets, which include risk factors, are available for a variety of populations. Links have been set up to the American Stroke Association, government agencies, and Reuters Professional Health News. 1-800-AHA-USA1 (1-800-242-8721)

**www.americanheart.org**

American Stroke Association. This division of the American Heart Association provides detailed health information on cerebrovascular accidents, including risk assessment. The site also includes the "Heart and Stroke A–Z Guide," guides to professionals about research grants and conferences, access to *Stroke Connection Magazine*, and much more. 1-888-4-STROKE (1-888-478-7653)

**www.strokeassociation.org**

Canadian Cardiovascular Society. Information is available for the consumer and health professional about coronary heart diseases (CHDs). The site provides access to the *Canadian Journal of Cardiology*, the society's newsletter, updated wire service medical and health news about CHDs, and links to other Canadian and American sites devoted to CHDs.

**www.ccs.ca/**

### KEY TERMS

**Cerebral hemorrhage** bleeding from a ruptured blood vessel in the brain

**Aneurysm** sac formed by distention or dilation of an artery wall

**Transient ischemic attack (TIA)** brief or temporary interference with blood supply to the brain; a mini stroke

**Transient monocular blindness** form of TIA characterized by blurred vision in one eye

**Transient hemispheral attack** form of TIA in which difficulty in thinking and communicating occurs along with numbness in one arm, leg, or the face because of less blood flow to one side of the brain

**Carotid endarterectomy** removal of fatty deposits from one of the two main arteries in the neck that supply blood to the brain

## Tips for Action For a Heart-Healthy Attitude

Positive coping strategies can reinforce cardiac treatments and help stop the progression of heart disease. Some of the most effective steps you can take are the following.

■ Exercise to increase your energy and stimulate physical changes that minimize anxiety and depression.

■ Maintain a healthy diet to increase your energy and promote a sense of well-being.

■ Schedule yearly drug reviews to identify medications and interactions that may influence your mood or temperament.

■ Manage your time effectively so you will have an opportunity to cultivate rewarding relationships, participate in enjoyable activities, and practice a relaxation technique such as meditation, biofeedback, or guided meditation.

■ Create comfortable surroundings that minimize anxiety-producing distractions such as noise and overcrowding.

■ Whenever possible, plan major life changes so they occur only one at a time.

*Source:* Johns Hopkins Medical Letter, July 1997.

---

Centers for Disease Control and Prevention (CDC). The CDC site offers a great variety of information on public health and communicable and noncommunicable diseases. It contains databases, books, documents, and links to the National Center for Health Statistics and the Office of the U.S. Surgeon General.

**www.cdc.gov**

Heart and Stroke Foundation of Canada. This organization has up-to-date information on CHDs and healthy living. Information is in English and French.

**www.heartandstroke.ca**

## It's Your Turn For Study and Review

1. Identify the coronary arteries, and describe their function. In your response, use the terms *myocardium*, *ischemia*, and *infarct*.

2. Describe the sequence of events that leads to the development of atherosclerosis.

3. Alvin's total serum cholesterol level is 225 mg/dL (HDL cholesterol 33 mg/dL; LDL cholesterol 165 mg/dL). Describe his risk for cardiovascular disease and coronary heart disease.

4. Identify the risk factors for heart attack and stroke.

5. Differentiate the signs of heart attack between women and men.

6. Stroke or brain attack is caused by a blockage or bleeding. Differentiate the four forms that these causes of stroke may take.

7. Describe the development of hypertension and its role in cardiovascular disease and coronary heart disease.

8. As a special assignment for your health class, you have been asked to create a poster that identifies behaviors that should be used to lower risk for cardiovascular disease and coronary heart disease. Identify at least five actions that a person could take to reduce the risk of developing CVD and CHD.

9. Identify at least two diagnostic tools and the physician that is involved in the diagnosis and treatment of cardiovascular disease and coronary heart disease.

## Thinking about Health Issues

When is a person considered dead?
Raymond Hoffenberg, "Christiaan Barnard: His First Transplants and Their Impact on Concepts of Death," *British Medical Journal*, 323:7327, December 22, 2001, p. 1478.

1. What are the ethical parameters to consider before contemplating heart transplantation on a patient with irreversible heart disease?

2. What are the controversies concerning the definition of "brain death"?

3. What spiritual and ethical controversies were prevalent at the time of the first cardiac transplant?

## Selected Bibliography

American Heart Association. "Emergency Stroke Treatment Enters New Era." *Heart Style*. Dallas: AHA, Fall 1996.

American Heart Association. *Heart and Stroke Facts*. Dallas: AHA, 2006.

Batchelor, S. "The Beat of a Different Heart." *Ms. Magazine*, 16:1, Winter 2006, pp. 61–62.

"Body Wise—Your Vital Signs." *The Oprah Magazine*, 7:10, October 2006, pp. 189–220.

Comarow, A. "Heart Trouble Could Come Straight from Your Parents." *U.S. News and World Report*, February 12, 2001, p. 60.

Comarow, A. "Statins Are Magic When You Gotta Have Heart." *U.S. News and World Report*, April 16, 2001, pp. 54–55.

Comarow, A. "Your Cholesterol Might Have to Come Down—Way Down." *U.S. News and World Report*, May 28, 2001, pp. 46–48.

"Consensus Panel Statement on Prevention of Heart Disease." *Urban Cardiology*, 2:5, September/October 1995.

Cool, L. "Stopping a Stroke." *Reader's Digest*, March 2007, pp. 136–143.

Cowley, G. "The Real 'Hot Zone.'" *Newsweek*, November 27, 2000, pp. 66–67.

Dixon, B. M. *Good Health for African Americans.* New York: Crown Publishing, 1994.

Dworetzky, T. "A Walking Miracle." *Discover*, January 2002, p. 47.

FDA Updates. "Totally Implanted Artificial Heart." *FDA Consumer*, 40:6, November/December 2006, p. 7.

Gatehouse, J. "The Cure for Everything." *Maclean's*, 120:3, January 29, 2007, pp. 32–38.

Harrar, S. "Stroke's Sneaky Symptoms." *Prevention*, 57:12, December 2005, p. 38.

Hobson, K. "Back on the Right Beat." *U.S. News & World Report*, 140:9, March 13, 2006, p. 63.

Hoeger, W. W. K. and Hoeger, S. A. *Lifetime Physical Fitness and Wellness*, 5th ed. Englewood, CO: Morton Publishing, 1998.

"How to Save Your Own Heart." *The Oprah Magazine*, 7:10, October 2006, p. 220.

Huddleston, J. In *The Wellness Book*, Benson, H., and Stuart, E., eds. New York: Birch Lane Press, 1992.

Kahn, J. "Mending Broken Hearts." *National Geographic*, 221:2, February 2007, pp. 40–65.

MacMillan, A. "New Test for Stroke Risk." *Prevention*, 57:12, December 2005, p. 32.

McVeigh, G. "A Diet Your Heart Loves." *Prevention*, 58:11, November 2006, p. 78.

Meadows, M. "Brain Attack—A Look at Stroke Prevention and Treatment." *FDA Consumer*, 39:2, March–April 2005, pp. 20–27.

Perry, M. "Health Secrets from the Morgue." *Men's Health*, April 2006, pp. 151–155, 160.

*Physicians' Desk Reference*, 61st ed. Montvale, NJ: Thomson PDR, 2007.

Shepelavy, R. "Fatigue . . . Do You Know What Heart Disease Feels Like?" *Redbook*, 207:5, November 2006, pp. 188–192, 194.

Wilson, T. W. and Grimes, C. E. "Biohistory of Slavery and Blood Pressure Differences in Blacks Today: A Hypothesis." *Hypertension*, 17:1, January 1991 (supplement).

Woodman, S. "Death by Couch Potato." *My Generation*, November/December 2001, p. 12.

U.S. Department of Health and Human Services. *Healthy People 2010: Understanding and Improving Health.* Washington, DC: U.S. Government Printing Office, 2000.

Name _____

Course _____

Date _____

Section _____

*Directions:* Student will access the following website to complete, print, and return the printout to the instructor.

**http://hp2010.nhlbihin.net/atpiii/calculator.asp?usertype=pub**

*Source:* National Institutes of Health/National Heart, Lung, and Blood Institute.

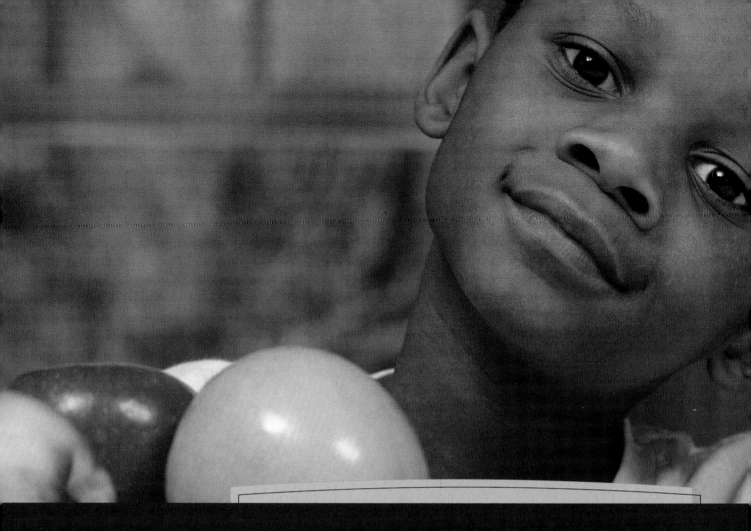

© trbfoto/Brand X Pictures/Jupiterimages

# Chapter Nine The Basics of Nutrition

**OBJECTIVES** ■ Define nutrition, nutrients, and calories. ■ **List and define the three energy or fuel nutrients.** ■ Explain the role of dietary fiber in the body. ■ **Define antioxidants and free radicals.** ■ Describe the requirements of the food label. ■ **List five nutrition guidelines of the MyPyramid system.** ■ Describe the key themes of the USDA MyPyramid System. ■ **Explain the Mediterranean Diet Pyramid.** ■ Define the different types of vegetarians and the vegetarian diet. ■ Explain the problems of fast food and junk food and how to avoid them. ■ Discuss dietary supplements and food additives. ■ List the food safety hazards and describe prevention measures.

ThomsonNOW™ Log on to ThomsonNOW at http://thomsonedu.com/ thomsonnow to access and explore self-assessments, interactive tutorials, and practice quizzes.

People's bodies are examples not only of what they eat but also of what they do not eat. Proper nutrition helps people to feel good and to live well. Recent advances in nutrition—the science that shows a connection between the body and food—have revealed that daily diet affects both how healthy people are and how many years they will live. During the typical lifetime a person will spend approximately six years eating about 60 tons of food prepared in 70,000 meals. Only 100 foods will account for 75% of the total amount of food consumed.

While millions of people are dying each year of starvation throughout the world, many people in the United States are dying as an indirect result of an overabundance of food. In addition to overeating, Americans are not eating a balanced diet. Their diet is too high in calories, sugar, sodium, fats, cholesterol, and alcohol. The *Healthy People 2010* report highlights some of the most important dietary changes that can safeguard health and well-being. They include reducing the consumption of fat and sodium, increasing the consumption of complex carbohydrates (starch) and dietary fiber, and consuming adequate amounts of iron, calcium, and other vitamins and minerals.

Among the many diseases related to poor **nutrition** are coronary heart disease, stroke, cancers, atherosclerosis, and adult-onset diabetes. Consuming the proper **nutrients** over time is essential to prevent disease and improve health and well-being. Healthy eating provides people with energy and increases productivity.

## Nutrition and Nutrients

Foods contain approximately 50 nutrients that the body is unable to manufacture for itself. These are used for three essential purposes.

1. They provide energy.
2. They form body structures (growth and repair of body tissues).
3. They help to regulate the body's biochemical reactions, collectively called metabolism.

The six classes of essential nutrients, discussed in this section, are carbohydrates, fats, proteins, vitamins/minerals, and water. The first three are sources the body uses to supply energy, and the last three regulate body processes (see Figure 9.1). Energy is measured in **kilocalories (kcal),** commonly referred to simply as **calories.** Calorie consumption depends on a person's height, gender, weight, and activity level. A dietitian can offer specific goals for individuals. According to federal standards, adults should consume 45% to 65% of calories from carbohydrates, 20% to 35% from fat, and 10% to 35% from protein. Children's fat intake should be higher with 25% to 40% of their caloric intake.

The **energy value** of a food is computed by multiplying the number of grams of each energy nutrient in a serving of food by the caloric values per gram of carbohydrate,

**FIGURE 9.1** ▶ Approximate Proportions of Nutrients in the Human Body

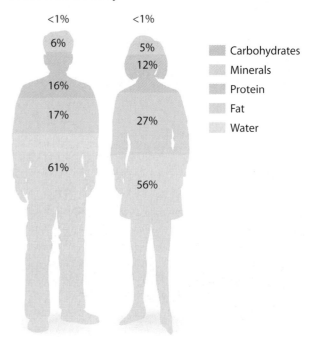

*Source*: W. W. K. Hoeger and S. A. Hoeger, *Principles and Labs for Physical Fitness*, 3rd ed. (Belmont, CA: Wadsworth, 2002), p. 55.

protein, and fat. For example, if a food has 10 grams of carbohydrates, 5 grams of protein, and 4 grams of fat, the caloric value is calculated as shown in Figure 9.2.

Figure 9.3 graphically depicts the caloric value of major energy foods. Alcohol does contribute energy (7 calories per gram), but it is not considered a nutrient.

The process of converting nutrients so the body can use them is known as **metabolism.** The number of calories needed per day is the body's **metabolic rate (MR).** Metabolic rate depends upon the person's age, sex, body-frame size, weight, percentage of body fat, emotional state, glandular function, and exercise level as well as the climate (hot or cold weather, altitude) and the **basal metabolic rate (BMR)**—the number of calories used while resting. MR is a combination of BMR and calories expended in normal daily activities. Regardless if you consume carbohydrates, protein, or fat, if you consume more calories than required to maintain your size and don't

**FIGURE 9.2** ▶ Energy Values

|  | Total grams | × | Calories (kcal per gram) |  |
|---|---|---|---|---|
| Carbohydrate | 10 | × | 4 | = 40 |
| Protein | 5 | × | 4 | = 20 |
| Fat | 4 | × | 9 | = 36 |
|  |  |  | Total | = 96 calories |

**FIGURE 9.3 ▶** Caloric Value Per Gram of Major Energy Nutrient

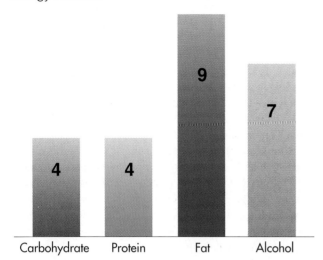

expend these calories in some way with physical activity, your body will convert the excess to fat. These concepts are expanded in Chapter 11.

## CALORIE GOALS

Calorie consumption depends on a person's height, weight, sex, and physical activity level. A dietitian can be helpful with specific goals for individuals. The National Diabetes Education Program offers this guide:

| Weight (Pounds) | Fat Goal (Grams) | Calorie Goal |
|---|---|---|
| 120–174 | 33 | 1,200 |
| 175–219 | 42 | 1,500 |
| 220–249 | 50 | 1,800 |
| 250+ | 55 | 2,000 |

## The Process of Digestion

In **digestion,** the body breaks down food and drink into substances that can be absorbed. As shown in Figure 9.4, nutrients reach the body's structures through the process of digestion. Food not broken down is passed as waste out of the body. Several body organs contribute to the digestive process by breaking down food substances chemically or mechanically into small molecules that can be absorbed into body cells.

## The Energy Nutrients

**Carbohydrates** are organic compounds that provide bodies and brains with **glucose,** their basic fuel. The body receives approximately 90% of its energy from metabolism of carbohydrates. Approximately 45%–65% of the diet should be composed of carbohydrates—45%–55%

**FIGURE 9.4 ▶** Food Is Broken Down by the Organs of the Digestive System

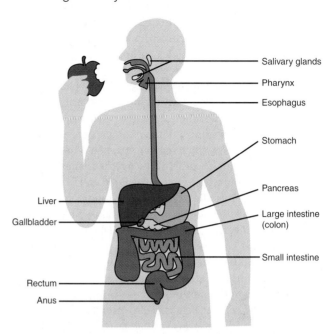

*Source:* Diane Hales, *An Invitation to Health*, 12th ed. (Belmont, CA: Wadsworth, 2007), p. 147.

### KEY TERMS

**Nutrition** the study of nutrients in foods and in the body

**Nutrients** chemical substances or nourishing elements found in food

**Kilocalorie (kcal)** the amount of energy required to raise the temperature of 1 gram of water 1°C

**Calorie** a term meaning the same as kilocalorie; measurement of energy

**Energy value** the result of multiplying the number of grams of each energy nutrient in a serving of food by the caloric values per gram of carbohydrate, protein, and fat

**Metabolism** process of converting nutrients into body tissue and functions

**Metabolic rate (MR)** total amount of energy the body expends in a given amount of time

**Basal metabolic rate (BMR)** amount of energy (calories) a person uses when totally inactive

**Digestion** process of breaking down food and drink into substances the body can absorb

**Carbohydrates** compounds composed of carbon, hydrogen, and oxygen used by the body to create 90% of its energy

**Glucose** a simple sugar; body's basic fuel

complex carbohydrates and 10% or less simple carbohydrates (see Figure 9.5). Both complex and simple carbohydrates have 4 calories per gram. The two major types of carbohydrates are **complex carbohydrates** (starches and fiber) and **simple carbohydrates** (sugars).

Foods containing complex carbohydrates, or starches and fiber, are not rich in protein (although they may have some, and a few such as dried peas and beans have a considerable amount). Also, they are not necessarily lower in fat and calories (for example, biscuits, pancakes, and croissants). Americans get most of their complex carbohydrates from refined grains, which may be stripped of many nutrients and fiber. Only 1% of what the average American consumes comes from whole grains. The Food and Drug Administration (FDA) has allowed claims by food companies to promote the health benefits of whole grains, such as those in Wheaties, Cheerios, and other breakfast cereals, that can protect against cardiovascular disease and are associated with a reduced risk for rectal, colon, gastric, endometrial, tongue, oral, pharyngeal, and esophageal cancer. The best sources of complex carbohydrates are plants, including grains, breads, cereals, pastas, yellow fruits and vegetables (carrots, yams), cruciferons vegetables (broccoli, cabbage, and cauliflower), certain root vegetables, such as potatoes, and dark green leafy vegetables. Whole grains are made up of all of the components of the grain: the bran (or fiber-rich outer layer), the endosperm (middle layer), and the germ (the nutrient-packed inner layer). The 2005 Dietary Guidelines recommend that Americans increase their consumption of whole-grain foods. The American Heart Association, the American Cancer Society, the National Institutes of Health, and the American Society for Clinical Nutrition recommend that Americans increase their whole-grain consumption to at least three servings every day. Research evidence shows that those who eat whole-grain products each day have about a 15% to 25% reduction in death from all causes, including heart disease and cancer. When checking the food label, notice the ingredient list; the first ingredient on the list should be whole grain, such as "whole-grain wheat," "whole wheat," or "whole-grain oats."

Simple carbohydrates are sugars found naturally in foods such as fruit, vegetables (peas and beets), and milk. Words that end in "ose" (glucose, fructose, galactose, sucrose, maltose, dextrose) designate simple carbohydrates. Refined and processed sugars, including corn syrup and sorghum, are also simple carbohydrates. Foods high in simple sugars are "empty calorie" foods if they lack other nutrients. Examples of "empty calorie" foods include cakes, candy, jellies, rolls, fruit drinks, fruit punch, and regular soft drinks. Sugars comprise 16% of the average American's calories and 20% of the average teenager's calories. A diet in which too many simple carbohydrates are consumed can contribute to dental cavities, obesity, and health conditions such as diabetes, hyperglycemia, hypoglycemia, and heart disease. Suggestions to increase your fruits and vegetables intake include:

Start the day with a glass of juice and strawberries or other fruit on cereal.

**FIGURE 9.5 ▶** The American Diet: Current and Recommended Carbohydrate, Fat, and Protein Intake

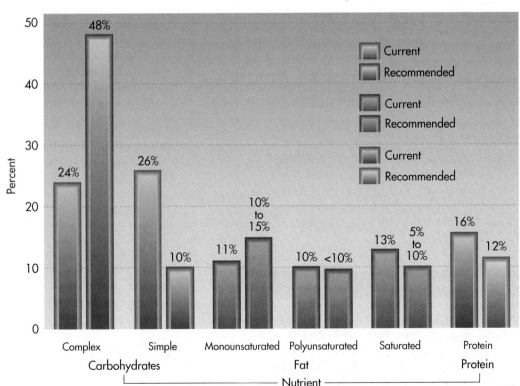

*Source:* W. W. K. Hoeger and S. A. Hoeger, *Principles and Labs for Physical Fitness*, 3rd ed. (Belmont, CA: Wadsworth, 2002), p. 56.

Toss fruit into a green salad for variety, crunch, color, and flavor.

Buy precut vegetables for snacking or dipping instead of using chips.

Make or order sandwiches with extra tomatoes or other vegetable toppings.

Suggestions to increase your intake of grains include:

Add brown rice or barley to soups.

Choose whole-grain, ready-to-eat cereals.

Check labels of rolls and bread, and choose those with at least 2 to 3 grams of fiber per slice.

## FIBER

Often referred to as "bulk" or "roughage," **fiber** is the indigestible portion of plant foods (leaves, stems, skins, and seeds) found in the walls of plant cells and in the tough structural part of plants. High-fiber foods, including whole-grain and enriched breads and cereals, are high in B vitamins and iron. These foods keep the digestive system in good working order by delaying absorption of cholesterol and other nutrients, and soften stools by absorbing water. Fiber helps to control weight by creating a feeling of fullness without adding extra calories. Fiber may be **soluble** or **insoluble.**

Insoluble fibers—cellulose, lignin, and some hemicellulose—increase the bulk in feces, preventing constipation, hemorrhoids, obesity, and diverticulosis (a painful inflammation of the bowel), and they may lower the risk of heart disease and stroke. Colon and rectal cancer is rarer in countries having diets high in fiber and low in animal fat. Several research studies contribute to the theory that fiber-rich diets, those including insoluble fiber, prevent the development of precancerous growths. Is it that more fiber helps to move foods through the colon faster (reducing the colon's contact time with cancer-causing substances) or because insoluble fiber reduces bile acids and certain bacterial enzymes that may promote cancer? There is still controversy over the mechanics and potential health benefits of fiber. Many research studies have shown that insoluble fiber provides protection against breast cancer, constipation, diverticulosis (painful inflammation of the bowel), heart disease, diabetes, and obesity. Research does support the many benefits of fiber and is still exploring the link between fiber and the protection against cancer. However, a large-scale study of almost 90,000 women found no such correlation between fiber and colon cancer. Most experts do agree that Americans should double their current consumption of dietary fiber to 20–35 grams per day and perhaps to 40–50 grams for others.

The National Cancer Institute recommends about 20 to 35 grams and the American Dietetic Association recommends 25 to 35 grams of fiber per day, the equivalent of five or six servings of high-fiber foods such as whole-grain cereals and fruits. However, the average intake is about 11 to 13 grams (see Table 9.1 for good fiber sources).

**TABLE 9.1 ▶** Good Fiber Sources

| High-fiber options for breakfast | | |
|---|---|---|
| Whole-grain toast | 1 slice | 2 g |
| Bran cereal | | |
| Bran flakes | 1 cup | 7 g |
| All Bran | ⅓ cup | 10 g |
| Raisin bran | ¾ cup | 5 g |
| Oat bran | ⅓ cup | 5 g |
| Bran muffin, with fruit | 1 small | 3 g |
| Strawberries | 10 | 2 g |
| Raspberries | ½ cup | 3 g |
| Bananas | 1 medium | 2 g |
| **Lunches that include fiber** | | |
| Whole-grain bread | 1 slice | 2 g |
| Baked beans | ½ cup | 10 g |
| Carrot | 1 medium | 2 g |
| Raisins | ¼ cup | 2 g |
| Peas | ½ cup | 6 g |
| Peanut butter | 2 tablespoons | 2 g |
| **Fiber on the menu for supper** | | |
| Brown rice | ½ cup | 2 g |
| Potato | 1 medium | 3 g |
| Dried cooked beans | ½ cup | 8 g |
| Broccoli | ½ cup | 3 g |
| Corn | ½ cup | 5 g |
| Tomato | 1 medium | 2 g |
| Green beans | ½ cup | 3 g |
| **Fiber-filled snacks** | | |
| Peanuts | ¼ cup | 3 g |
| Apple | 1 medium | 2 g |
| Pear | 1 medium | 4 g |
| Orange | 1 medium | 3 g |
| Prunes | 3 | 2 g |
| Sunflower seeds | ¼ cup | 2 g |
| Popcorn | 2 cups | 2 g |

*Source:* From Judith E. Brown, *Nutrition Now,* 3rd ed. (Belmont, CA: Wadsworth, 2002).
*Note:* Prunes contain fiber, but their laxative effect is primarily due to a naturally occurring chemical substance that causes an uptake of fluid into the intestines and the contraction of muscles that line the intestines.

Fiber intake should be increased gradually in the diet through fiber foods, not supplements, to avoid intestinal gas, cramps, diarrhea, and bloating (from fermentation of

## KEY TERMS

**Complex carbohydrates** important source of energy for the body found in fruits, vegetables, legumes, and grains

**Simple carbohydrates** sugars found naturally or added in the processing of foods

**Fiber** or **roughage** nondigestible complex carbohydrate needed to keep the digestive system in good working order

**Soluble** dissolvable in water

**Insoluble** not dissolvable in water

**Tips for Action** Boosting the Fiber Content in Your Diet

- Substitute brown rice for white rice.
- Eat the skins of baked potatoes.
- Add brown rice, millet, bulgur, or barley to soups, stews, and casseroles.
- Snack on dried fruits.
- Cook with recipes that include bran and other good sources of fiber, and bake with whole-wheat flour.
- Do not overcook vegetables. Steaming and stir-frying are two methods that prevent the breakdown of fiber.
- Eat legumes at least three times a week.
- Sprinkle wheat germ or bran on applesauce, pudding, yogurt, cottage cheese, custard, and ice cream.
- Whenever you can, eat unpeeled fresh fruits (scrubbed well). Among the fruits with the highest fiber content are apples, oranges, strawberries, and pears.

- Choose high-fiber snacks (such as popcorn, fruits, and raw vegetables).
- Read labels and look for whole-grain breads, macaroni, egg noodles, and cereals.
- Choose high-fiber breakfast cereals.
- When buying bread, look for "stone-ground wheat" or "whole wheat" as the first ingredient. Other breads usually are made from refined flour (with the bran removed) that has been colored brown.
- Use spinach or romaine lettuce instead of iceberg lettuce in salads.
- As you increase your fiber intake, drink more water, too.

fiber and sugars in the colon). When increasing fiber in the diet, water intake should be increased as well. Excellent sources of insoluble fiber are leafy greens, wheat, rice, corn bran (outer layer), seeds of fruits (such as strawberries), skins of fruits, and root vegetables.

Soluble fibers are digested in the large intestine. These fibers (pectin, some hemicellulose, and gums) help lower the blood cholesterol level. They stay in the stomach longer (give a sense of fullness), slow the absorption of sugars from the small intestine, and thus may assist in controlling blood sugar levels. Soluble fiber is present in dried beans, barley, oats, oat bran, corn bran, many vegetables, and fruits such as citrus, apples, prunes, and pears. Whole-grain breads are excellent sources of fiber, as opposed to breads made with white or refined wheat flour in which the fiber-rich bran may have been removed mechanically. Food labels list the fiber content in breads.

From the abundance of cereals on the market, selecting the healthier ones is difficult. Cereals made from oats, corn, or rice are low in fat and calories. Granola and muesli often are packed with nuts, coconut, and dried fruits, and sweetened with honey—a combination that can add up to more than 10 grams of fat and 200 calories in 1/2 cup. Low-fat cereals are made with puffed rice and more dried fruits than nuts.

When choosing a cereal, look for the following on the label: no more than 6 grams of sugar, 2 grams of fat, and at least 3 grams of fiber per serving. Beware of the claims of cereal sweetened with honey or fruit juice, not sugar. They are all equally damaging to the teeth, and the body breaks them down into plain old sugar.

## DIETARY FAT

The average person in the United States eats more fat than is considered healthy. Fats should compose 20% to 35% of daily calories. The diet of African-Americans is more fat-laden than Caucasians since it consists primarily of fatty meat, bacon, sausage, poultry skin, and fat. Fat packs more than twice the number of calories (250 per ounce) as pure proteins and carbohydrates do (115 calories per ounce). Diets that are high in fat can lead to Type 2 diabetes, heart disease, high blood pressure, stroke, and cancers of the colon, uterus, breast, and prostate. Fats, or **lipids,** however, do serve significant purposes in the body and are needed in reasonable amounts. Fats provide insulation against the cold, regulate body temperature, suppress hunger pangs, protect vital organs against injury, transport four fat-soluble vitamins (A, D, E, K) in the body, contribute to growth, regulate hormones, are essential for healthy skin, and provide fuel for energy. In addition, fat supplies 9 calories of energy per gram, and it is a concentrated source of energy when carbohydrate supplies are insufficient, such as during prolonged exercise. High- and low-fat diets can be unhealthy. With very low levels of fat and very high levels of carbohydrates, the levels of **high-density lipoprotein (HDL),** the so-called good cholesterol, declines. High-fat diets, on the other hand, can lead to obesity and its related health dangers.

Dietary fats are either saturated (solid at room temperature) or unsaturated (liquid at room temperature) and are distinguished by the types of fatty acids in their chemical structures. All dietary fats are a mix of saturated and

## TABLE 9.2 ▶ Types of Fats and Examples

| SATURATED FATS | | MONOUNSATURATED FATS | POLYUNSATURATED FATS | TRANS FATS |
|---|---|---|---|---|
| Bacon | Meat | Canola oil | Corn oil | Cakes, Cookies |
| Butter | Milk, whole | Cashews | Cottonseed oil | Crackers, |
| Cheese | Palm kernel oil | Olive oil | Fish | Pies, Bread |
| Chocolate | Palm oil | Peanut oil | Margarine, tub | Animal products |
| Coconut oil | Poultry | | Mayonnaise | Fried potatoes |
| Cream cheese | Shortening | | Nuts (most varieties) | Potato/Corn chips |
| Egg yolk | Sour cream | | Safflower oil | Popcorn |
| Hydrogenated (hard) fats | | | Soybean oil | |
| Lard | | | Sunflower oil | |
| | | | Unhydrogenated peanut butter | |

unsaturated fats but are predominantly one or the other. Unsaturated fats, such as oils, are likely to be liquid at room temperature and saturated fats, such as butter, are likely to be solid. Vegetable and fish oils are generally unsaturated and animal fats are saturated. See Table 9.2 for the types of fats with examples of each.

**Saturated fats** usually are found in animal products including lard, butter, cheese, milk, pork, beef, bacon, veal, lamb, poultry skin, hot dogs, luncheon meats, nondairy cream substitutes, chocolate, and cocoa. Exceptions to the solid rule are coconut oil, palm oil, and palm kernel oil (tropical oils), which are almost solid at room temperature. Although they are referred to as oils, they are highly saturated fats and will raise blood cholesterol levels. They are the major culprits in colorectal cancer.

Unsaturated fats include monounsaturated fats and polyunsaturated fats. **Monounsaturated fats (MUFA)** are found in foods such as olives, peanuts, and cashews, as well as canola oil, peanut oil, and olive oil. **Polyunsaturated fats (PUFA)** are found in mayonnaise, margarine, pecans, almonds, walnuts, sunflower oil, soybean oil, sesame oil, safflower oil, and corn oil, among others. Table 9.2 lists examples of each of the types of fats, and Table 9.3 gives the percentage of fat calories in selected foods.

**Hydrogenated trans-fatty acids (TFAs)** are unsaturated fatty acids formed when vegetable oils are processed and made more solid or into a stable liquid. This processing is called hydrogenation. Hydrogen is added to increase shelf life, improve the texture of the product, and make it more spreadable. This process also increases the saturation, and the resulting trans-fatty acids may increase the risk of heart disease and cancer. Therefore, hydrogenated fat may be as dangerous as saturated fat. Processed foods and oils provide approximately 80% of trans fats in the diet, compared with 20% that occur naturally in food from animal sources. The trans fats content in processed foods has changed and is likely to continue to change as the industry reformulates products. Trans fats are found in most foods made with partially hydrogenated oils, such as coconut and palm oil, baked goods, and fried foods and some margarine products.

Stick margarine is more hydrogenated and contains more trans-fatty acids than tub margarine. Spray oils are the best. To cut down on both saturated and trans fats, choose soybean, corn, olive, canola, safflower, and sunflower oils, and look for reduced-fat, fat-free, and trans fat-free versions of snacks, baked goods, and other processed foods. Suggestions to limit your fats include:

Restrict animal fats such as milk, butter, ice cream, cheese, and other full-fat dairy products, fatty meat, bacon, sausage, poultry skin, and fat.

Reduce the number of foods made with partially hydrogenated vegetable oils.

Reduce your intake of organ meats and eggs.

Substitute fat-free sour cream or nonfat plain yogurt for sour cream.

Add low-fat milk instead of water to oatmeal and other hot cereals.

Eat cereals with added calcium and with low-fat milk.

Top salads or soups with low-fat shredded cheese.

## KEY TERMS

**Lipids** blood fats

**High-Density Lipoprotein (HDL)** "good cholesterol" molecule containing high concentration of protein

**Saturated fats** fats mainly found in animal products; increase levels of blood fat cholesterol

**Monounsaturated fats** fats with only one double bond of unsaturated carbons in carbon atom chain

**Polyunsaturated fats** fats that contain two or more double bonds between unsaturated fats along the carbon atom chain

**Hydrogenated trans-fatty acids (TFAs)** fats or oils that have been treated by a process that adds hydrogen to some of the unfilled bonds in the fat molecule, thereby hardening the fat or oil

**TABLE 9.3 ▶** Percentage of Fat Calories in Selected Foods

| TYPE OF FOOD | LESS THAN 15% OF CALORIES FROM FAT | 15%–30% OF CALORIES FROM FAT | 30%–50% OF CALORIES FROM FAT | MORE THAN 50% OF CALORIES FROM FAT |
|---|---|---|---|---|
| Fruits and vegetables | Fruits, plain vegetables, juices, pickles, sauerkraut | | French fries | Avocados, coconuts, olives |
| Bread and cereals | Grains and flours, most breads, most cereals, corn tortillas, pita, matzo, bagels, pasta | Cornbread, flour tortillas, oatmeal, soft rolls and buns, wheat germ | Breakfast bars, biscuits and muffins, granola, pancakes and waffles, doughnuts, taco shells, pastries, croissants | |
| Dairy products | Nonfat milk, cottage cheese, nonfat cottage cheese, nonfat yogurt | Buttermilk, low-fat yogurt, 1% milk, low-fat cottage cheese | Whole milk, 2% milk, creamed cottage cheese | Butter, cream, sour cream, half & half, most cheeses (including part-skim and lite cheeses) |
| Meats | | Beef round; veal loin, round, and shoulder; pork tenderloin | Beef and veal, lamb, fresh and picnic hams | All ground beef, spareribs, cold cuts, bacon, sausages, corned beef, hot dogs, pastrami |
| Poultry | Egg whites | Chicken and turkey (light meat without skin) | Chicken and turkey (light meat with skin, dark meat without skin), duck and goose (without skin) | Chicken and turkey (dark meat with skin), chicken and turkey hot dogs and bologna, egg yolks, whole eggs |
| Seafood | Clams, cod, crab, crawfish, flounder, haddock, lobster, perch, sole, scallops, shrimp, tuna (in water) | Bass and sea bass, halibut, mussels, oyster, tuna (fresh) | Anchovies, catfish, salmon, sturgeon, trout, tuna (in oil, drained) | Herring, mackerel, sardines |
| Beans and nuts | Dried beans and peas, chestnuts, water chestnuts | | Soybeans | Tofu, most nuts and seeds, peanut butter |
| Fats and oils | Oil-free and some lite salad dressings | | | Butter, margarine, all mayonnaise (including reduced calorie), most salad dressings, all oils |
| Soups | Bouillons, broths, consomme | Most soups | Cream soups, bean soups, "just add water" noodle soups | Cheddar cheese soup, New England clam chowder |
| Desserts | Angel food cake, jello, some fat-free cakes | Pudding, tapioca | Most cakes, most pies | |
| Frozen desserts | Sherbet, low-fat frozen yogurt, sorbet, fruit ices | Ice milk | Frozen yogurt | All ice creams |
| Snack foods | Popcorn (air-popped), pretzels, rye crackers, rice cakes, fig bars, raisins, marshmallows, most hard candy, fruit rolls | Lite microwave popcorn, plain crackers, caramels, fudge, gingersnaps, graham crackers | Snack crackers, popcorn (popped in oil), cookies, candy bars, granola bars | Most microwave popcorn, corn and potato chips, buttery crackers, chocolate |

*Source:* American Heart Association and U.S. Department of Agriculture.

# LECITHIN

**Lecithin** is a complex fatlike substance in foods such as liver, eggs, peanuts, and soybeans. It is composed of polyunsaturated (phospholipids) fatty acids and, as an emulsifier, helps disperse fat particles in water. Lecithin is added to many processed foods such as ice cream, chocolate, and margarine.

One component of lecithin is choline, an essential nutrient for some animals. Humans need choline, but human cells manufacture it. Human bodies use choline and

- Promote health and reduce chronic disease risk, disease progression, debilitation, and premature death associated with dietary factors and nutritional status among all people in the United States.

- Reduce the consumption of fat and sodium.

- Increase the consumption of complex carbohydrates (starch) and dietary fiber.

- Increase the proportion of persons age two and older who consume at least three daily servings of vegetables, with at least one-third being dark-green or deep-yellow vegetables.

- Consume adequate amounts of iron and calcium.

other lecithin components in making membranes around nerve fibers and helping to transmit nerve impulses.

Although lecithin supplements have been promoted as curing liver disease, cancer, and AIDS; lowering blood cholesterol; and preventing memory loss and Alzheimer's disease, the evidence is weak or nonexistent. No large well-controlled studies on humans have been done. High doses of lecithin can produce side effects such as nausea, nerve disorders, and depression.

## CHOLESTEROL (STEROLS)

The remaining 5% of body fat is composed of substances such as cholesterol, which may accumulate on the inner walls of arteries and narrow the channel through which blood flows. Understanding the role of fats in the body means understanding their relationship to cholesterol. The human body produces 800 to 1,500 milligrams of cholesterol each day. **Cholesterol** is required for metabolism and production of certain hormones, including the sex hormones estrogen, progesterone, and androgen. Cholesterol also aids in digestion, helps produce vitamin D (a major component of cell membranes), and protects the nerve fibers.

Cholesterol is present only in animal products such as egg yolks, cheese, milk, and meat. It is found primarily in the liver, kidneys, spinal cord, adrenal glands, and brain. The liver manufactures about 80% of total cholesterol found in the blood and tissues; dietary sources furnish the other 20%.

Fats first must be combined with protein. When they travel through the body in this form they are **lipoproteins,** which are the transport facilitators for cholesterol in the blood. The molecules of **low-density lipoprotein (LDL),** or "bad" cholesterol, contain large amounts of cholesterol and transport cholesterol to the body cells. The HDL or "good" cholesterol molecule has a high concentration of protein. These molecules remove other cholesterol from the walls of the arteries and transport it to the liver for metabolism and elimination from the body.

There is controversy concerning which type of unsaturated fat is most beneficial. Monounsaturated (MUFA)

fats tend to lower LDL cholesterol levels, may lower blood pressure and the blood sugar level, increase HDL levels, and seem to be the least harmful of the fats. MUFAs are resistant to oxidation, a process that leads to cell and tissue damage. Many nutritional researchers believe that polyunsaturated (PUFA) fats may decrease beneficial HDL levels while reducing LDL levels.

Current research indicates that the actual amount of circulating cholesterol is not as important as is the ratio of total cholesterol to a group of compounds called high-density lipoproteins (HDLs). Most research indicates that HDL cholesterol is determined by heredity and decreases with age. Women tend to have higher levels than men do, and most African-Americans have lower levels than Caucasians. Low levels of HDL cholesterol may be the best predictors of coronary heart disease, more significant than the total cholesterol values. People with a high percentage of HDLs appear to be at lower risk for developing cholesterol-clogged arteries. Because HDL cholesterol rids the body of cholesterol, a high HDL cholesterol level is desirable. Regular vigorous exercise is an important part in reducing cholesterol by increasing HDLs. Limiting the saturated fat content of foods helps reduce the production of cholesterol in the body. To see a significant effect in lowering LDL cholesterol, total fat consumption should be less than 30% of total daily caloric intake.

### KEY TERMS

**Lecithin** fatlike substance occurring in foods such as liver, eggs, peanuts, and soybeans

**Cholesterol** yellow, waxy substance produced by the liver and found in animal products; used by the body for metabolism and production of certain hormones

**Lipoprotein** form of cholesterol combined with protein when traveling through the body

**Low-Density Lipoprotein (LDL)** "bad cholesterol" molecule containing large amounts of cholesterol

---

**Tips for Action** A Formula for Fat

Here is a handy formula for figuring how many fat calories a day you should have.

Your total calories per day = _____

multiplied by .30 = _____ fat calories per day

divided by 9 (1 gram of fat has 9 calories) = _____ grams of total fat allowable per day

---

At least 26 million Americans are taking drugs to lower their blood cholesterol. The *Journal of the American Medical Association* has suggested that some of these drugs might, over the long term, cause cancer. The two most widely used types are fibrates (gemfibrozil and clofibrate) and statins (lovastatin and pravastatin). Lab studies conducted before the FDA approved the drugs show that both types had caused cancer in rats. The American Heart Association, however, stated that human studies never have shown these drugs to cause cancer and that they are extremely valuable in preventing and treating coronary artery disease.

These drugs generally are not recommended for men under age 45 and women under 55, except those who appear to have a very high risk of heart attack. A high blood cholesterol level is a significant risk factor for heart attack. Therefore, your doctor could discuss all your risk factors with you before deciding to put you on drugs.

Cholesterol-lowering drugs are only for those who have been unable to lower their cholesterol by any other means, those who have symptoms or high-risk factors for heart disease, and those who have had a heart attack. Others with high cholesterol levels should try changing their lifestyle habits before taking drugs.

## TRIGLYCERIDES

**Triglycerides** make up 95% of total body fat and are the most common form of fat circulating in the blood. These fatty acids are carried in the bloodstream primarily by **very low-density lipoproteins (VLDL)** and chylomicrons and cannot travel in the bloodstream without the phospholipids. Combined with cholesterol, triglycerides speed formation of plaque in the arteries. Triglycerides should be less than 125 milligrams per deciliter (mg/dL) of blood, and less than 100 mg/dL is ideal. As triglyceride levels increase, HDL cholesterol levels decrease.

Triglycerides are present in most sources of dietary fat (meat, dairy fat, shellfish, poultry skin) and are manufactured mainly in the liver from refined sugars, starches, and alcohol. Diets high in sugars and alcohol raise triglyceride levels. In addition, you will make triglyceride fat for storage when you eat anything in excess of your caloric needs. For some people with high triglycerides, decreasing alcohol and concentrated sweets is recommended because they both can raise triglyceride levels. The first strategy is to reduce dietary fat to 30% of calories.

Research has shown that **omega-3 oils** reduce triglycerides but do not alter cholesterol. Eskimos' traditional diet consists of 40% fat, but they have a low rate of heart disease. This may be attributable to a diet replete with fish. Fish oils are rich in omega-3 fatty acids, which make molecules such as prostaglandins that enhance cardiovascular health. These oils improve healthy blood lipid levels (fats), prevent blood clots, ward off the age-related vision problem called macular degeneration, and may lower blood pressure especially in people with hypertension or atherosclerosis. Most college students do not consume enough omega-3 fatty acids. However, a new epidemiological study indicates that high levels of omega-3s could increase the risk for neurological disorders. Consuming moderate amount of foods high in omega-3s can be beneficial to your health. Omega-3 oils are found in foods such as sardines, salmon, tuna, herring, and mackerel. Studies indicate that fish-oil capsules are not as effective as eating fish three times a week. **Fat substitutes** mimic the taste of fat and contain a small percentage of calories, fat, and cholesterol. They can be found in yogurt, ice cream, sour cream, and salad dressing, among other foods.

## CHOLESTEROL TESTING

After a person has an initial normal baseline test, a blood lipid analysis should be done every three to four years prior to age 35 and every year after age 35 in conjunction with a regular medical physical examination. Your cholesterol level is not affected as much by the cholesterol you eat as by the overall percentage of fat in your diet. Of the 30%, less than one-third should come from saturated fats, the rest from monounsaturated fats.

The American Heart Association advises that the intake of cholesterol be limited to 300 mg/dL per day. The National Cholesterol Education Program recommends keeping serum (blood) cholesterol levels below 200 mg/dL per day. Other researchers recommend that for individuals age 30 and younger, total cholesterol should not be higher than 180 mg/dL per day, and for preteens the level should be below 170 mg/dL per day.

The ratio of total cholesterol to HDL cholesterol can be determined by dividing the total cholesterol level by the value for HDL cholesterol. For example:

Total cholesterol    200 mg/dL
HDL                  ÷ 45 mg/dL = 4.4

**Tips for Action** To Raise HDL (Good) Cholesterol Levels

- Exercise, especially aerobic exercise (five times per week; 45–60 minute sessions).

- Maintain proper body weight or lose weight.

- If you smoke, quit.

- Do not take anabolic steroids.

- Substitute monounsaturated oils for saturated fat in your diet, and do not exceed 30% of all calories from fat.

- Take cholesterol medications (only if necessary and prescribed by your physician).

The recommended ratio of HDL cholesterol to total cholesterol should be less than 4.5 for men and less than 4.0 for women. Before menopause, women tend to have higher levels of HDL cholesterol.

## PROTEINS

**Proteins** comprise about 16% of body weight and supply 4 calories of energy per gram. They consist of chains of **amino acids** that are the building blocks of body tissues. Proteins are essential to growth and repair tissues such as blood, bones, muscles, skin, hair, nails, and internal organs. They regulate the body's chemical processes, carry nutrients to body cells, form enzymes, formulate hormones, and protect against disease because they are the major ingredient in antibodies. Nutrients, oxygen, and iron are transported to the cells of the body through protein.

The 20 amino acids are classified as either essential or nonessential. The nine essential amino acids cannot be synthesized by the body and must be obtained by the diet. The 11 nonessential amino acids can be synthesized by the body. Complete proteins are those foods that contain all nine essential amino acids in proper balance. These high-quality concentrated proteins tend to come from animal sources such as meat, fish, poultry, cheese, eggs, and milk. Some researchers have linked high intake of animal protein with increased risk of heart disease, osteoporosis, kidney damage, and some cancers (such as **colon** and prostate).

Incomplete proteins come from nonanimal sources (grains, cereals, green vegetables, **legumes,** nuts, and seeds) and contain only some of the essential amino acids. People who get their protein from plants are generally healthier and have a lower risk of heart disease, as vegetarian sources of protein usually are low in fat and high in fiber and other beneficial substances. The form of protein in plant foods (except soybeans), however, is incomplete. Thus, it has low and sometimes insufficient amounts of one or more of the nine essential amino acids.

As protein intake rises, so does the amount of calcium excreted in urine. A high-protein diet may have a diuretic effect and cause kidney damage. A lack of calcium

**FYI** | **LEANEST CUTS OF MEAT**

| Meat (select grade, visible fat removed) | Fat content (grams per 4 oz.) |
|---|---|
| Skinless turkey breast | 1 |
| Skinless chicken breast | 4 |
| Veal leg | 4 |
| Skinless turkey drumstick | 4 |
| Beef eye of round, minute steak | 5 |
| Skinless chicken drumstick | 6 |
| Beef top round, London broil | 6 |
| Pork tenderloin | 7 |
| Beef top loin, strip steak | 7 |
| Veal shoulder, loin, or sirloin | 7 |
| Lamb shank | 8 |
| Pork chop | 8 |
| Beef sirloin | 9 |

*Note:* For comparison, 4 ounces of some cuts of untrimmed prime beef contain 30+ grams of fat.

may affect bone density and thus may hasten the development of osteoporosis (bone thinning). The body should preserve, not excrete, calcium.

### KEY TERMS

**Triglycerides** the most common fatty substance in the blood

**Very Low-Density Lipoprotein (VLDL)** largest of the lipoproteins; allows cholesterol to circulate in bloodstream

**Omega-3 oils** oils found in fish

**Fat substitutes** substances that taste like fat and contain fewer calories, fat, and cholesterol

**Proteins** chains of amino acids

**Amino acids** chemical compounds that contain carbon, oxygen, hydrogen, and nitrogen

**Colon** large intestine where wastes are processed

**Legumes** vegetables such as peas and beans that are high in fiber and are also important sources of protein

- Males and females get similar percentages of their calories from protein.
- Various ethnic groups get similar percentages of their calories from protein but their sources are different.
- African-Americans eat a higher percentage of poultry and pork protein and a lower percentage of dairy protein than do whites and Mexican Americans.

- Mexican Americans consume a higher percentage of legume and egg protein than do whites and African-Americans.
- Whites consume a higher percentage of grain protein than do Mexican Americans and African-Americans.

Proteins constantly are being broken down by the body. Most of the amino acids are reused, but those that are lost must be regularly replaced. Excess protein is broken down in the body and burned for energy or is stored as fat. Therefore, all meats should be limited to no more than 6 ounces per day. Females who are pregnant and those who are breast-feeding need more protein.

The daily Recommended Dietary Allowance (RDA) for protein is the amount the average person needs to stay healthy. Based on age and weight, it usually is about 12%–15% of daily calories. The recommended protein intake for the average man is only 63 grams, and the average woman needs only 50 grams. For a 2,000-calorie diet, about 10% of calories should come from protein. The protein sources should be low in fat, and when we eat more than the recommended amounts, the extra calories contribute to weight gain. The RDA for adults is 0.8 grams of protein for each kilogram (2.2 pounds) of body weight. This adds up to 64 grams (about 2 ounces) of pure protein for a 175-pound man and 47 grams for a 130-pound woman. To estimate your protein requirement, use the following equation (Figure 9.6).

Overweight persons may need less protein. Children under age 18 and pregnant or lactating women need slightly more protein per pound of body weight than others.

According to the National Research Council, the upper bound for protein is twice the RDA. Consuming more than that over the long term increases the risk of chronic disease and is not recommended. Several studies have found that elderly people need a little more protein than the RDA, because the body uses protein less efficiently as it ages. By consuming more protein from plants, individuals will get less fat and cholesterol and more of the good things found in grains, beans, and vegetables.

## The Regulatory Nutrients

### WATER

Water is the most important nutrient. Approximately 60% of the body's weight is made up of water apportioned among body tissues. Bones, for example, consist of about

**FIGURE 9.6** ▶ Calculating Your Protein RDA (Recommended Dietary Allowance)

| Calculating Your Protein RDA | Example |
|---|---|
| 1. Determine your body weight. | 1. Weight = 150 lbs |
| 2. Convert pounds to kilograms (lb ÷ 2.2 lb/kg = kilograms). | 2. 150 ÷ 2.2 lbs/kg = 68.2 |
| 3. Multiply by 0.8 g/kg (average adult RDA) to get an RDA in kilograms per day | 3. 68.2 x 0.8 g/kg average adult = 54.6 (rounded to 55) |
| | Results: a 150 lb person would have an RDA of 55 g of protein. |

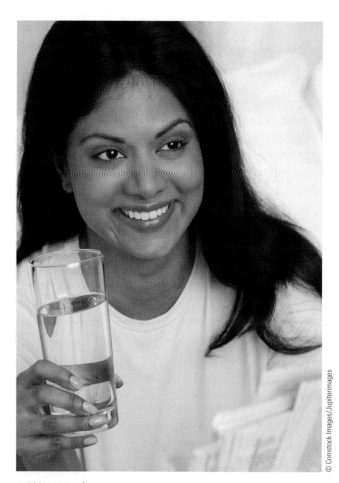

▲ *Water is the most important nutrient*

20% water, blood is about 85% water, muscle is about 70% water, and brain tissue is about 75% water.

The body's need for water depends upon the individual person and factors such as sweat loss, activity patterns, body weight, loss through expired air and urine, and the amount of liquid consumed in foods and drinks. The adult body contains approximately 10 gallons of water. The percentage of water may be as low as 40% in obese individuals and as high as 70% in muscular individuals, because fat tissue is low in water content and muscle tissue is high in water content.

Water is essential to digest and absorb nutrients, regulate body temperature (particularly during exercise in the heat), lubricate the joints, remove waste products through urine, transport oxygen and nutrients, and build and rebuild cells. Water also contributes to the production of sweat, which evaporates from the skin to cool the body. Research has correlated high fluid intake with a lower risk of colon cancer, kidney stones, and bladder cancer. You lose about 64 to 80 ounces of water a day, the equivalent of eight to 10 8-ounce glasses, through urination, bowel movements, perspiration, and normal exhalation. A loss of 5% body water causes **dehydration,** dizziness, fatigue, headache, and weakness. A 15%–20% loss can be

harmful or even fatal. A person can survive only three days without drinking water. You lose water faster if you live in a hot, dry climate, live at a high altitude, are ill, drink excessive amounts of caffine or alcohol (increases urination), skip meals, travel on an airplane, and exercise. A person should drink before becoming thirsty—approximately a half cup every 30–45 minutes. Before and during exercise, people should drink water to prevent dehydration—one or two 8-ounce glasses of water 30 minutes to an hour before exercising and half to three-quarters of a glass of water every 10 to 20 minutes during a workout. Liquids containing dissolved sugars or sodium stay in the stomach longer, delaying the usefulness of the fluids. Plain water is absorbed faster in the stomach and gets into the bloodstream more quickly. Cool water is best because it cools the body and leaves the digestive tract rapidly to enter tissues where it is needed.

A pale yellow urine output at least four times a day is a good indicator of hydration, that water is being added to tissue. Dark yellow urine indicates that the kidneys had to concentrate waste material into a smaller volume of water.

Although most foods provide water to the body, fruits and vegetables are the best sources because of their high water content—lettuce (96%), tomatoes (94%), apples (84%), and oranges (86%). Foods such as bread and meat contain from 33% to 50% water. As a general guideline, individuals should consume at least 64 ounces of water each day (tea, coffee, and alcoholic beverages do not count). This amount is needed to maintain adequate water balance in the body. Consuming sugar and protein (waste from proteins builds up in the kidneys) also increases the need for water.

College students tend to reuse plastic water bottles and reuse plastic containers in the microwave. Reusable plastic water bottles and/or microwave containers can collect harmful bacteria by backwashing germs into the water or container and providing them with a warm, wet place to grow. Reusable Nalgene bottles (bright, hard plastic bottles) can cause brain damage. Bisphenol A (BPA) is a chemical that mimics the hormone estrogen and is used to make Nalgene bottles and other hard plastic projects. BPA seeps into the body and can, in certain doses, change the function of the brain.

**Energy Replacement Options.** For most exercisers, water is the ideal fluid replacement. During strenuous activity lasting more than an hour, slightly sugared beverages may help the body conserve its carbohydrate stores, maintain normal blood sugar levels, and delay fatigue. Nutritional sports drinks are similar to diluted juice or soft drinks but are more expensive. Sports nutritionist Nancy

---

## KEY TERMS

**Dehydration** abnormal depletion of body fluids

**TABLE 9.4** ▶ Sources and Functions of Vitamins

| VITAMIN/RECOMMENDED INTAKE PER DAY | SIGNIFICANT SOURCES | CHIEF FUNCTIONS | SIGNS OF SEVERE, PROLONGED DEFICIENCY | SIGNS OF EXTREME EXCESS |
|---|---|---|---|---|
| **FAT-SOLUBLE VITAMINS** | | | | |
| **Vitamin A**<br>Males 19–50: 900 µg<br>Females 19–50: 700 µg | Fortified milk, cheese, cream, butter, fortified margarine, eggs, liver; spinach and other dark, leafy greens, broccoli, deep orange fruits (apricots, cantaloupes) and vegetables (carrots, sweet potatoes, pumpkins) | Antioxidant; needed for vision, health of cornea, epithelial cells, mucous membranes, skin health, bone and tooth growth, reproduction, immunity | Anemia, painful joints, cracks in teeth, tendency toward tooth decay, diarrhea, depression, frequent infections, night blindness, keratinization, corneal degeneration, rashes, kidney stones | Nosebleeds, bone pain, growth retardation, headaches, abdominal cramps and pain, vomiting, diarrhea, weight loss, overreactive immune system, blurred vision, fatigue, irritability, hair loss, dry skin |
| **Vitamin D**<br>Males 19–50: 5 µg<br>Females 19–50: 5 µg | Fortified milk or margarine, eggs, liver, sardines; exposure to sunlight | Mineralization of bones (promotes calcium and phosphorus absorption) | Abnormal growth, misshapen bones (bowing of legs), soft bones, joint pain, malformed teeth | Raised blood calcium, excessive thirst, headaches, irritability, loss of appetite, weakness, nausea, kidney stones, deposits in arteries |
| **Vitamin E**<br>Males 19–50: 15 mg<br>Females 19–50: 15 mg | Polyunsaturated plant oils (margarine, salad dressings, shortenings), green and leafy vegetables, wheat germ, whole-grain products, nuts, seeds | Antioxidant; needed for stabilization of cell membranes, regulation of oxidation reactions | Red blood cell breakage, anemia, muscle degeneration, difficulty walking, leg cramps | Augments the effects of anticlotting medication; general discomfort; blurred vision |
| **Vitamin K (Menadione)**<br>Males 19–50: 120 µg<br>Females 19–50: 90 µg | Green leafy vegetables, cabbage-type vegetables, soybeans, vegetable oils | Synthesis of blood-clotting proteins and proteins important in bone mineralization | Hemorrhage | Interference with anticlotting medication; jaundice |
| **WATER-SOLUBLE VITAMINS** | | | | |
| **Vitamin B$_6$ (Pyridoxine)**<br>Males 19–50: 1.3 mg<br>Females 19–50: 1.3 mg | Meats, fish, poultry liver, legumes, fruits, whole grains, potatoes, soy products | Part of a coenzyme used in amino acid and fatty acid metabolism, helps make red blood cells | Anemia, depression, abnormal brain wave pattern, convulsions, skin rashes | Impaired memory, irritability, headaches, numbness, damage to nerves, difficulty walking, loss of reflexes |
| **Vitamin B$_{12}$**<br>Males 19–50: 2.4 µg<br>Females 19–50: 2.4 µg | Animal products (meat, fish, poultry, milk, cheese, eggs) | Part of a coenzyme used in new cell synthesis, helps maintain nerve cells | Anemia, nervous system degeneration progressing to paralysis, hypersensitivity | None known |

Clark suggests a homemade recipe: In a glass dissolve 1 tablespoon of sugar and a pinch (1/6 teaspoon) of salt in a little hot water. Add 1 tablespoon of orange juice or 2 tablespoons of lemon juice and 7 1/2 ounces of ice water.

## VITAMINS

**Vitamins** are needed in relatively small amounts to carry out a variety of metabolic and nutrition functions. Vitamins help put proteins, fats, and carbohydrates to use.

Vitamins produce the chemical reactions involved in manufacturing hormones and blood cells, enable good vision, promote strong bones and teeth, and ensure proper functioning of the nervous system and the heart. The 13 vitamins are divided into two types: fat-soluble (A, D, E, and K) and water-soluble (B-complex and C). Vitamin K is toxic in large amounts. The animal form of vitamin A, not beta-carotene, is potentially toxic and may cause birth defects if used during pregnancy. Table 9.4 summarizes the sources and functions of the vitamins

**TABLE 9.4 ▶** Sources and Functions of Vitamins—*(Continued)*

| VITAMIN/RECOMMENDED INTAKE PER DAY | SIGNIFICANT SOURCES | CHIEF FUNCTIONS | SIGNS OF SEVERE, PROLONGED DEFICIENCY | SIGNS OF EXTREME EXCESS |
|---|---|---|---|---|
| **Vitamin C** Males 19–50: 90 mg Females 19–50: 75 mg | Citrus fruits, cabbage-type vegetables, dark green vegetables, cantaloupe, strawberries, peppers, lettuce, tomatoes, potatoes, papayas, mangoes | Antioxidant, collagen synthesis (strengthens blood vessel walls, forms scar tissue, matrix for bone growth), amino acid metabolism, strengthens resistance to infection, aids iron absorption | Anemia, pinpoint hemorrhages, frequent infections, bleeding gums, loosened teeth, muscle degeneration and pain, joint pain, blotchy bruises, failure of wounds to heal | Nausea, abdominal cramps, diarrhea, excessive urination, headache, fatigue, insomnia, rashes, deficiency symptoms may appear at first on withdrawal of high doses |
| **Thiamin (B$_1$)** Males 19–50: 1.2 mg Females 19–50: 1.1 mg | Pork, ham, bacon, liver, whole grains, legumes, nuts; occurs in all nutritious foods in moderate amounts | Part of a coenzyme used in energy metabolism, supports normal appetite and nervous system function | Edema, enlarged heart, nervous/muscular system degeneration, difficulty walking, loss of reflexes, mental confusion | None reported |
| **Riboflavin (B$_2$)** Males 19–50: 1.3 mg Females 19–50: 1.1 mg | Milk, yogurt, cottage cheese, meat, leafy green vegetables, whole-grain or enriched breads and cereals | Part of a coenzyme used in energy metabolism, supports normal vision and skin health | Cracks at corner of mouth, magenta tongue, hyper-sensitivity to light, reddening of cornea, skin rash | None reported |
| **Niacin** Males 19–50: 16 mg Females 19–50: 14 mg | Milk, eggs, meat, poultry, fish, whole-grain and enriched breads and cereals, nuts, and all protein-containing foods | Part of a coenzyme used in energy metabolism | Diarrhea, black smooth tongue, irritability, loss of appetite, weakness, dizziness, mental confusion, flaky skin rash on areas exposed to sun | Nausea, vomiting, painful flush and rash, sweating, liver damage |
| **Folate** Males 19–50: 400 μg Females 19–50: 400 μg | Leafy green vegetables, legumes, seeds, liver, enriched breads, cereal, pasta, and grains | Part of a coenzyme needed for new cell synthesis | Anemia, heartburn, frequent infections, smooth red tongue, depression, mental confusion | Masks, vitamin B$_{12}$ deficiency |
| **Pantothenic acid** Males 19–50: 5 mg Females 19–50: 5 mg | Widespread in foods | Part of a coenzyme used in energy metabolism | Vomiting, intestinal distress, insomnia, fatigue | Water retention (rate) |
| **Biotin** Males 19–50: 30 μg Females 19–50: 30 μg | Widespread in foods | Used in energy metabolism, fat synthesis, amino acid metabolism, and glycogen synthesis | Abnormal heart action, loss of appetite, nausea, depression, muscle pain, drying of facial skin | None reported |

*Source:* Adapted from Sizer, Frances and Ellie Whitney. *Nutrition: Concepts and Controversies*, 10th ed. (Belmont, CA: Wadsworth, 2006).

and gives the best sources for each, as well as the symptoms of deficiency.

Fat-soluble vitamins are absorbed through the intestinal tract with the help of fats, and are found in foods associated with fats (lipids). They are stored in the body and normally are not excreted in the urine but, instead, tend to remain stored in the liver and fatty tissues until they are needed. Since fat-soluble vitamins tend to be stored in the body, toxic accumulations in the liver may cause cirrhosis-like symptoms. The body does not require an everyday supply, and overdoses can interfere with or disrupt the action of other nutrients.

Most vitamins must be ingested, whereas some vitamins, such as vitamin D, are produced within the body. Vitamin D is manufactured in the skin after exposure to

### KEY TERMS

**Vitamins** organic substances essential for normal growth

sunlight, and it then changes to an active form through processes in the liver and the kidney. African-Americans may not get enough vitamin D because their darker skin screens out the vitamin D-activating property of sunlight.

Water-soluble vitamins (B complex and C complex) are dissolved easily in water and are absorbed directly into the blood and then used up or washed out of the body in urine and sweat. These vitamins are not stored in the body in large quantities. In addition, they can be lost or destroyed in varying amounts through heat (when the water in which food is cooked or soaked is discarded), age, and other environmental conditions. Water-soluble vitamins must be replaced daily.

Large doses of some vitamins may be harmful. For example, vitamins A and D can build up in the body, causing serious complications, such as damage to the kidneys, liver, or bones. High doses of the B vitamins may be harmful. For example, $B_6$ (pyridoxine), often used to relieve premenstrual bloating, can cause neurological damage, such as numbness in the mouth and tingling in the hands. High doses of vitamin C can produce stomachaches and diarrhea. Niacin, often taken in high doses to lower cholesterol, can cause jaundice, liver damage, and irregular heartbeats as well as severe, uncomfortable flushing of the skin.

Generally, Americans do not suffer from true vitamin deficiencies if they eat a diet containing all of the food groups at least part of the time. Vitamin supplements are usually unnecessary and may even be harmful. Overusing them can lead to a toxic condition known as **hypervitaminosis.**

**Folic Acid.** Beginning in 1998, the FDA required all enriched grain products to be fortified with the B vitamin folacin, folate, or folic acid. Insufficient levels of folic acid increase the risk of neural tube defects (abnormalities of the spinal cord and brain), such as spina bifida (a piece of the spinal cord protrudes from the spinal column). Neural tube defects occur in about 4,000 pregnancies each year; 50% to 70% could be prevented with a daily intake of 4,000 micrograms of folic acid. Folate can be obtained from supplements as well as from a diet high in citrus fruits and vegetables.

The fortification requirement affects flour, cornmeal, pasta, rice, enriched breads, and many other grain products. Whole-grain products already contain some natural folacin and therefore are not affected.

The FDA supports a low level of fortification because of the concern that high intakes of folacin make it hard to diagnose vitamin $B_{12}$ deficiency, which can lead to anemia and damage to the nervous system, especially in elderly people.

In summary, folacin protects against heart disease, along with other B vitamins such as $B_{12}$ and $B_6$, and it also protects some women against cervical cancer, particularly those infected with certain forms of human papillomavirus. Preliminary evidence indicates that folacin may help protect against colorectal and lung cancer and prevents birth defects including spina bifida, anencephaly (fatal defect in which most of the brain never develops), and oral and facial defects such as cleft palate. Folic acid is also useful to men because it may cut the risk of heart disease, stroke, and colon cancer.

The latest research shows an additional benefit of folic acid in preventing atherosclerosis by lowering the level of plasma **homocysteine.** Research shows that increasing dietary folic acid to an optimum level could prevent deaths from cardiovascular disease.

Folic acid converts homocysteine to **methionine,** an essential amino acid. Individuals with low folic acid intakes tend to have low homocysteine levels. Most Americans do not meet the RDA for folic acid of 200 µg/day. Most multivitamins contain folic acid. The best foods are green peas, avocados, brussels sprouts, sunflower seeds, wheat germ, chickpeas, beets, oatmeal, broccoli, black-eyed peas, asparagus, lentils, breakfast cereals, fortified brewer's yeast, spinach, pinto beans, lima beans, navy beans, kidney beans, peanuts, liver, whole grains, and green leafy vegetables.

**Antioxidants.** Electrons—electrically charged atomic particles—always are being released and shifted around in the body. During this process **free radicals** are born. External factors such as exposure to smoking, pollution, radiation, or ozone, for example, can intensify free radical activity. Stress may also intensify free radical activity. Free radicals can damage the basic structure of cells, leading to chronic disease including various forms of cancer and heart disease. They also accelerate the aging process.

To protect against free radicals the body produces **antioxidants**—"good guy" substances that prevent the harmful effects caused by oxidation within the body, and these chemicals quench or mop up free radicals and help repair damage to cells. The cells themselves manufacture some antioxidants, and others come from nutrients in food. Table 9.5 lists the antioxidants and good food sources for them. Antioxidant vitamins, beta-carotene (a form of vitamin A), vitamin C, vitamin E, and compounds such as carotenoids and flavonoids have many health benefits. Diets high in antioxidant-rich fruits and vegetables have been linked with lower rates of lung, colon, esophageal, and stomach cancer. Scientific studies have not proved conclusively that antioxidants, particularly in supplement form, can prevent cancer.

**Carotenoids.** About 400 **carotenoids** have been chemically identified and named, including **beta-carotene.** People who consume foods rich in beta-carotene have a lower risk for heart disease, cancer, and certain eye disorders. Beta-carotene helps foster resistance to infection and keeps skin, hair, teeth, gums, and bones healthy. People who have a high blood level of beta-carotene likely eat many fruits and vegetables. Carotenoids act in unison with other nutrients to confer protection, and beta-carotene may

**TABLE 9.5 ▶** Antioxidants and Their Sources

| ANTIOXIDANT NUTRIENT | PRIMARY FOOD SOURCES |
|---|---|
| Vitamin C (ascorbic acid) | Papaya, cantaloupe, cauliflower, melons, citrus fruits, tomatoes, dark green vegetables, grapefruit, green and red peppers, strawberries, raspberries, asparagus, broccoli, cabbage, collard greens, orange juice, tomato juice, brussels sprouts, kiwi fruit |
| Vitamin E | Vegetable oils (safflower, corn, cottonseed, sunflower), nuts and seeds, legumes, egg yolk, liver, dried beans, yellow and green leafy vegetables, sunflower seeds, almonds, wheat germ, 100% whole-wheat bread, 100% whole-grain cereals, oatmeal, hazelnuts, mayonnaise, sweet potatoes |
| Carotenoids (including beta-carotene) | Yellow, orange, and dark green leafy vegetables and fruits (sweet potatoes, carrots, squash, tomatoes, mango, cantaloupe, pumpkin, asparagus, broccoli, apricots, peaches, spinach, romaine lettuce, papaya) |
| Vitamin A | Fortified milk, egg yolk, cheese, liver, butter, fish oil, dark green, yellow and orange vegetables and fruits, (carrots, sweet potatoes, cantaloupe) |
| Flavonoids | Purple grapes, apples, berries, peas, beets, onions, garlic, green tea, red wine |
| Selenium (mineral) | Lean meat, nonfat milk, seafood, kidney, liver, 100% whole-grain cereal, 100% whole-wheat bread, dairy products, skinless chicken |

## FYI | E. COLI IN YOUR VEGGIES

Contaminated bag salads which are cut and ready to eat may have a risk of being infected with *E. coli*. Six million bags of salad are sold every day in the United States.

Next to ground beef, lettuce is the most commonly implicated food item for *E. coli* infections.

### Safety Tips:

■ Wash your hands before handling lettuce or any raw produce, especially if you have handled any raw meat. Clean counter tops/utensils with warm soap and water before reusing with another food.

■ Keep the salad refrigerated.

■ Check the expiration date before you purchase.

■ Even if lettuce looks good, *E. coli* can grow quickly.

be a marker for other beneficial substances in fruits and vegetables.

**Vitamin C.** Vitamin C speeds healing, prevents scurvy, may reduce the risk of cataracts by as much as 80%, and strengthens resistance to infection. Citrus fruits, cabbage-type vegetables, dark green vegetables, strawberries, cantaloupe, lettuce, tomatoes, potatoes, papayas, and mangoes are examples of excellent sources of vitamin C.

**Vitamin E.** Vitamin E was once thought to provide enormous health benefits with little risk. In a 12-year study of nearly 40,000 women, vitamin E failed to show any protective effects against cardiovascular problems or breast, lung, and colon cancer. It has not been proven if it may be beneficial for men. Super-high doses of vitamin E have not

helped people with mild cognitive impairment, an early stage of Alzheimer's disease. Certain antioxidants can interfere with the efficacy of cholesterol-lowering medications. High doses of vitamin E may increase the chances of earlier death. Those taking large doses had in increased risk of a new cancer.

Tolerable levels of intake for selected nutrients are listed in Table 9.6.

**Phytochemicals.** Phyto refers to plant processes, and **phytochemicals** thus are derived naturally from plant sources. Phytochemicals help plants to protect themselves from disease and bacteria. For example, solanine, an insect-repelling chemical found in the leaves and stalks

## KEY TERMS

**Hypervitaminosis** a toxic condition caused by overuse of vitamin supplements

**Homocysteine** an amino acid not produced in the body and not present in foods; plays a role in methionine metabolism

**Methionine** an essential amino acid

**Free radicals** unstable molecules produced when the body burns fuel for energy; can damage body cells and lead to heart disease, a weakened immune system, and other serious illnesses

**Antioxidants** disease-fighting vitamins that protect the body from the harmful effects of free radicals

**Carotenoids** a nutrient occurring in plants, which lowers the risks for heart disease, cancer, and other chronic diseases

**Beta-carotene** plant source of vitamin A; helps guard against free radicals

**Phytochemicals** compounds found in vegetables and fruits; have antioxidant properties

**TABLE 9.6** ▶ Tolerable Upper Intake Levels (UL) of Selected Nutrients for Adults 19–70 Years Old

| NUTRIENT | UL PER DAY |
|---|---|
| Calcium | 2.5 gr |
| Phosphorus | 4.0 gr* |
| Magnesium | 350 mg |
| Vitamin D | 50 mcg |
| Fluoride | 10 mg |
| Niacin | 35 mg |
| Vitamin B$_6$ | 100 mg |
| Folate | 1,000 mcg |
| Choline | 3.5 gr |
| Vitamin C | 2,000 mg |
| Vitamin E | 1,000 mg |
| Selenium | 400 mcg |

*Source:* W. W. K. Hoeger and S. A. Hoeger, *Principles and Labs for Physical Fitness*, 3rd ed. (Belmont, CA: Wadsworth, 2002), p. 58.

*3.5 gr per day for pregnant women 19 years of age and older.

**TABLE 9.7** ▶ Phytochemical Foods

| PHYTOCHEMICAL | FOODS |
|---|---|
| Capsaicin | Hot peppers |
| Coumarins | Citrus fruit, tomatoes |
| Flavonoids | Berries, citrus fruits, carrots, peppers, tomatoes |
| Genistein | Lentils, beans, peas |
| Indoles | Broccoli, cabbage family |
| Isothiocyanates | Broccoli, mustard, cabbage, horseradish |
| Ligands | Barley, wheat, flaxseed |
| Lycopene | Pink grapefruit, tomatoes |
| S-allyl cysteine | Garlic, onions, chives |
| Triterpenoids | Citrus fruits, licorice root |

of potato plants, is a natural toxin. Other phytochemicals are associated with a reduced risk of heart disease, age-related macular degeneration, certain cancers, adult-onset diabetes, stroke, and other diseases. Also, some phytochemicals act as antioxidants and repair and limit damage caused by free radicals. Among the many phytochemicals are **flavonoids** (apples, strawberries, grapes, onions, green and black tea, and red wine), which may decrease atherosclerotic plaque and DNA damage related to cancer development and have been shown to inhibit the growth of cancer cells. However, research has shown neither an increase nor decrease in breast cancer with consumption of phytochemicals. Carotenoids (beta-carotene, lutein, zeaxanthin, lycopene, cryptoxanthin) protect the eye from harmful oxidation reactions. Lignans (seaweed, soybeans, bran, flaxseed, dried beans) are phytoestrogens that interfere with the action of the sex hormone estrogen and may help prevent hormone-related cancers, slow the growth of cancer cells, and lower the risk of heart disease (see Table 9.7).

## MINERALS

Many **minerals** are essential to life. Vitamins cannot be assimilated without the aid of minerals. And, though the body can manufacture a few vitamins, it cannot manufacture a single mineral. Among their functions, they

- Build bones and teeth
- Maintain the acid–base balance of the blood
- Promote normal blood clotting
- Promote normal heart rhythm
- Transmit messages of the nervous system
- Maintain water balance
- Regulate muscular contraction and metabolic processes

Table 9.8 outlines the features of the most important minerals. The two basic types of minerals are macrominerals and trace minerals. **Macrominerals,** or major minerals, are the seven minerals the body needs in relatively large quantities daily—a 10th of a gram (100 mg or more per day). In order of importance to the human body, these are calcium, phosphorus, potassium, sulfur, sodium, chloride, and magnesium. Most of these minerals are acquired by eating a variety of foods.

**Calcium.** Of the **calcium** in the body, 98% is found in the skeleton. Calcium is needed because the body breaks down and rebuilds bone tissue constantly. Healthy adults replace approximately one-fifth of their bone tissue each year. Every cell in the body requires calcium. Without it the nerve cells cannot conduct impulses, the heart cannot beat, and the brain cannot function. In addition, calcium may help control high blood pressure and prevent colon cancer in adults.

If the diet does not contain sufficient calcium, the body takes it from the bones. Teens who eat the typical American meat-based diet should be especially careful to get enough calcium—four or more servings of calcium-rich foods every day. Bone mass is built primarily between ages 11 and 25.

Calcium may be the most common supplement. It often is suggested for postmenopausal women. Also, pregnant women who take calcium supplements are less likely to develop high blood pressure and preeclampsia. Breast-feeding women, however, are advised that calcium supplementation is not necessary. Anyone who is taking more than 500 milligrams a day of calcium supplements should distribute these throughout the day to enhance absorption and reduce the chances of constipation. The Cooper Institute for Aerobics Research and the National Institutes of Health recommend 1,000 mg/day for adult men and women and 1,500 mg/day for postmenopausal women not taking estrogen. RDA established that Americans should consume 1,200 mg of calcium per day.

It is best to take calcium throughout the day and consume it with foods containing protein, vitamin D, and vitamin C for optimum absorption. Not all calcium

**Tips for Action** If You Need to Take Calcium Supplements . . .

■ Look for a label saying the pill meets the standards set by U.S. Pharmacopeia, a nonprofit organization that sets standards for drugs. Put a tablet in a glass of white vinegar for a half-hour, stirring every few minutes. If the tablet breaks up or dissolves, it will do the same thing in your stomach (chewable calcium need not be tested this way).

■ Test every new supply, as even the same brand will dissolve differently from lot to lot.

**FIGURE 9.7** ▶ Diet Soda versus Fat-Free Milk

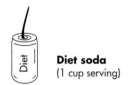

**Diet soda**
(1 cup serving)

**1 calorie**
**0 fat grams**

| | % Daily Value |
|---|---|
| Protein | <1% |
| Calcium | <1% |
| Potassium | <1% |
| Riboflavin | <1% |
| Niacin | 0% |
| Vitamin A | 0% |
| Vitamin B₁₂ | 0% |
| Vitamin D | 0% |
| Phosphorus | 2% |

**Fat-free milk**
(1 cup serving) fortified with vitamin D

**80 calories**
**0 fat grams**

| | % Daily Value |
|---|---|
| Protein | 16% |
| Calcium | 30% |
| Potassium | 11% |
| Riboflavin | 24% |
| Niacin | 10% |
| Vitamin A | 10% |
| Vitamin B₁₂ | 13% |
| Vitamin D | 25% |
| Phosphorus | 20% |

supplements are recommended. For example, supplements derived from oyster shells and dolomite have been found to be contaminated with heavy metals and are not absorbed well. Citrate and aspartate salts of calcium are often recommended. Women using the birth control method Depo-Provera® need calcium also. Postmenopausal women with deficient calcium intake and limited physical activity are at risk for osteoporosis, a bone-weakening disease that strikes one in every four women over age 60. It is more common in older women than arthritis, diabetes, heart attacks, and breast cancer and is characterized in later stages by a hunched-over appearance. New prescription medicines used to treat or prevent osteoporosis in postmenopausal women include Boniva® (ibandronate sodium). Boniva® may reverse bone loss by stopping further loss of bone and increasing bone mass. Most women who take this once-monthly osteoporosis therapy are not able to see or feel a difference. Boniva® may also help lower the incidence of bone fractures. Osteoporosis is addressed more fully in Chapter 14.

Calcium depletion also is found in people who eat a high-protein diet, large quantities of refined sugars, and phosphorus-rich junk foods, such as carbonated beverages (soft drinks) and potato chips. Foods rich in vitamins A and D help the body absorb calcium, whereas caffeine, alcohol, and phosphates (soda) cause the body to excrete calcium. Good primary sources of calcium include low-fat milk, yogurt, low-fat cheese, green leafy vegetables, sardines, and salmon. Calcium and potassium, which protect against heart disease, are of special concern for African-Americans, who have a higher risk for high blood pressure and obesity than the rest of the population. African-Americans consume fewer than one serving of dairy foods a day, and more than 80% fail to get their daily recommended amount of calcium. Refer to Figure 9.7 for a comparison of diet soda and fat-free milk.

## KEY TERMS

**Flavonoids** phytochemicals that have anticlotting properties

**Minerals** inorganic substances that make up 4% of body weight and are vital to mental and physical functioning

**Macrominerals** the seven major minerals the body needs in relatively large quantities daily (100 mg or more per day)

**Calcium** an essential mineral needed for growth and maintenance of strong bones and teeth

**TABLE 9.8 ▶** Major Sources and Functions of Minerals

| MINERAL | SIGNIFICANT SOURCES | CHIEF FUNCTIONS | SIGNS OF SEVERE, PROLONGED DEFICIENCY | SIGNS OF EXTREME EXCESS |
|---------|---------------------|-----------------|---------------------------------------|--------------------------|
| **MAJOR MINERALS** | | | | |
| Sodium | Salt, soy sauce, processed foods | Needed to maintain fluid balance and acid–base balance in body cells; critical to nerve impulse transmission | Mental apathy, poor appetite, muscle cramps | High blood pressure |
| Potassium | All whole foods; meats, milk, fruits, vegetables, grains, legumes | Needed to maintain fluid balance and acid–base balance in body cells; needed for muscle and nerve activity | Muscle weakness, mental confusion, paralysis | Irregular heartbeat, heart attack; muscular weakness |
| Chloride | Salt, soy sauce, processed foods | Aids in digestion; needed to maintain fluid balance and acid–base balance in body cells | Muscle cramps, apathy, poor appetite, growth failure in children | Vomiting |
| Calcium | Milk and milk products, oysters, small fish (with bones), tofu, greens, legumes | Components of bones and teeth, needed for muscle and nerve activity, blood clotting | Stunted growth in children, adult bone loss (osteoporosis) | Constipation, calcium deposits in kidneys, liver, and other tissues, decreased absorption of other minerals |
| Phosphorus | All animal tissues | Component of bones and teeth, energy formation, needed to maintain cell membranes | Loss of appetite, muscle weakness, impaired growth | Loss of calcium from bones |
| Magnesium | Nuts, legumes, whole grains, dark green vegetables, seafoods, chocolate, cocoa | Component of bones and teeth, nerve activity, energy and protein formation | Stunted growth in children, weakness, muscle spasms, personality changes | Diarhea, dehydration, impaired nerve activity |
| Sulfur | All protein-containing foods | Component of certain amino acids; stabilizes protein shape | None known: protein deficiency would occur first | Depresses growth in animals |
| **TRACE MINERALS** | | | | |
| Iron | Red meats, fish, poultry, shellfish, eggs, legumes, dried fruits | Aids in transport of oxygen, component of myoglobin, energy formation | Anemia, weakness, fatigue, pale appearance, reduced attention span, development delays in children | "Iron poisoning," vomiting, abdominal pain, blue coloration of skin, shock, heart failure, diabetes, decreased zinc absorption |

**Sodium.** Sodium is found naturally in food, and manufacturers add it as a food preservative. It is most often consumed in the form of table salt. Table salt accounts for only 15% of sodium intake; the remainder comes from water and highly processed foods that are infused with sodium to enhance flavor (salty snack foods, processed cheeses, pickles, breads and bakery products, smoked meats/sausages, and many fast food and convenience foods). An abundance of salt without adequate water draws fluids from the cells and increases urination and loss of potassium. Some sodium, however, is useful to retain fluid inside blood vessels and thus maintain blood pressure. It is essential for muscle function and nerve conduction. People usually get all the sodium they need from unprocessed fruits, vegetables, and meats.

Approximately 10% to 15% of all people, especially African-Americans, are sensitive to sodium. In these salt-sensitive individuals, salt draws fluid into the circulatory system. This produces high blood pressure and increases the risk of stroke, heart attacks, and kidney disease. Limiting salt intake reduces hypertension in salt-sensitive individuals. African-Americans have a higher rate of high blood pressure and diseases related to hypertension, such as stroke and kidney failure and tend to be more sensitive to salt than nonblacks. African-Americans and middle-age and older adults should consume no more than 1,500 milligrams of sodium and increase potassium to at least 4,700 mg. Potassium reduces the effect of sodium on blood pressure, may decrease bone loss, and reduces the risk of kidney stones.

Because identifying individuals who may be sensitive to salt is difficult, the average adult should limit sodium intake to 500 milligrams (equivalent to about 1/4 teaspoon) per day. The average American consumes

**TABLE 9.8 ▶** Major Sources and Functions of Minerals—*(Continued)*

| MINERAL | SIGNIFICANT SOURCES | CHIEF FUNCTIONS | SIGNS OF SEVERE, PROLONGED DEFICIENCY | SIGNS OF EXTREME EXCESS |
|---------|---------------------|-----------------|---------------------------------------|-------------------------|
| Zinc | Protein-containing foods; fish, shellfish, poultry, grains, vegetables | Protein reproduction, component of insulin | Growth failure, delayed sexual maturation, slow wound healing | Nausea, vomiting, weakness, fatigue, susceptibility to infection, copper deficiency, metallic taste in mouth |
| Selenium | Meats and seafood, eggs, grains | Acts as an antioxidant in conjunction with vitamin E | Anemia, muscle pain and tenderness, heart failure | Hair and fingernail loss, weakness, liver damage, garlic or metallic breath |
| Molybdenum | Dried beans, grains, dark green vegetables, liver, milk and milk products | Aids in oxygen transfer from one molecule to another | Rapid heartbeat and breathing, nausea, vomiting, coma | Loss of copper from the body, joint pain, growth failure, anemia, gout |
| Iodine | Iodized salt, milk and milk products, seaweed, seafood, bread | Component of thyroid hormones that helps regulate energy production and growth | Goiter, cretinism in newborns (mental retardation; hearing loss, growth failure) | Pimples, goiter, decreased thyroid function |
| Copper | Organ meats, whole grains, nuts and seeds, seafood, drinking water | Component of enzymes involved in the body's utilization of iron and oxygen | Anemia, nerve and bone abnormalities in children, growth retardation | Wilson's disease (excessive accumulation of copper in the liver and kidneys); vomiting, diarrhea, liver disease |
| Manganese | Whole grains, coffee, tea, dried beans, nuts | Formation of body fat and bone | Weight loss; rash, nausea and vomiting | Infertility in men, disruptions in the nervous system, muscle spasms |
| Fluoride | Fluoridated water, foods and beverages; tea; shrimp; crab | Component of bones and teeth (enamel) | Tooth decay and other dental diseases | Fluorosis, brittle bones, mottled teeth, nerve abnormalities |
| Chromium | Whole grains, liver, meat, beer, wine | Glucose utilization | Poor blood glucose control, weight loss | Kidney and skin damage |

*Source:* Adapted from Brown, Judith E. *Nutrition Now,* 3rd ed. (Belmont, CA: Wadsworth, 2002); Sizer, Frances, and Ellie Whitney. *Nutrition: Concepts and Controversies,* 10th ed. (Belmont, CA: Wadsworth, 2006).

6,000 to 12,000 milligrams per day. Most professional groups recommend restricting sodium to 1,100 to 2,300 milligrams per day.

Salt substitutes are not for everyone, particularly people with diabetes. Some substitutes to avoid or use sparingly are onion, celery, or garlic salt, seasoned salt, meat tenderizer, bouillon, monosodium glutamate (MSG), soy sauce, Worcestershire sauce, dill pickles, sauerkraut, and tomato juice. Suggestions to limit salt include:

Look for labels that say "low sodium." They contain 140 mg or less of sodium per serving.

Use fewer condiments such as soy sauce, olives, ketchup, pickles, and mustard, which can add a lot of salt to food.

Always check the amount of sodium in processed foods, such as frozen dinners, packaged mixes,

salad dressing, sauces, and cereals. The amount in different types and brands can vary widely. Learn to use spices and herbs rather than salt to enhance the flavor of food.

**Trace Minerals. Microminerals** or **trace minerals** are those the body requires in small daily amounts of a hundredth of a gram (10 mg) or less. Serious problems may result if excesses or deficiencies occur. These include iron (more for premenopausal women), zinc, iodine, fluoride,

---

**KEY TERMS**

**Microminerals** or **trace minerals** those the body requires daily in minute quantities (100 mg or less per day)

## Tips for Action Watch Your Salt

- Check the labels of processed foods. Gelatin, instant potatoes, and American cheese are some of the worst offenders.
- Taste food before salting it.
- Take the saltshaker off the table.
- Flavor cooking water with bay leaf or other herbs and spices.
- Use onion or garlic powder (not onion salt or garlic salt) for flavoring.

- Substitute pepper, lemon, herbs, or spices for salt.
- Eat fresh fruits and vegetables instead of canned foods.
- Avoid processed soups that do not claim to be low-sodium.
- Avoid salty processed foods such as bacon, lunchmeats, hams, and sausage.

selenium, copper, cobalt, chromium, manganese, and molybdenum.

Mineral deficiency has been linked to high blood pressure, cancer, diabetes, tooth decay, **anemia,** and osteoporosis. A nutritious, balanced diet should supply enough of the essential minerals.

**Iron.** Iron deficiency is the most common nutrient deficiency, affecting more than 1 billion people worldwide. Iron is an essential ingredient of **hemoglobin,** which transports oxygen from the lungs to the body tissues. Males aged 19 to 50 need about 10 mg per day, whereas females need about 18 mg. Many women of childbearing age have an iron deficiency because of the loss of blood during menstruation. Pregnant, nursing, and premenopausal women need more iron. In addition, exercisers may have an iron deficiency, because exercise increases the rate of iron loss through the gastrointestinal tract, urine, and possibly sweat as well. Other factors, such as a high-fiber diet, dietary iron deficiency, or consuming a large amount of caffeine (coffee or tea [tannin]), may place a person at risk. Fiber and caffeine can decrease the absorption rate of iron. A person should not drink more than three cups of tea or coffee a day, and preferably not with a meal.

Symptoms of iron deficiency include shortness of breath, depression, sleeplessness, susceptibility to colds and infections, sensitivity to cold, faintness, pallor (in light-skinned individuals), loss of appetite, loss of vision, shortened attention span, chronic fatigue, and constipation or diarrhea. By comparison, excessive iron can cause severe constipation, infections, liver damage, and tissue damage. Anemia is a problem resulting from the body's inability to produce hemoglobin, the bright red, oxygen-carrying component of the blood. In America, iron-deficiency anemia occurs less frequently than in most countries but still affects 10% of toddlers, adolescent girls, and women of childbearing age. Generally women eat less than men, their diets contain less iron, and some have heavy menstrual flow; therefore, these women are more likely to develop iron-deficiency problems. **Hemochromatosis,** or iron toxicity due to ingesting too many iron-containing supplements,

remains the leading cause of accidental poisoning in small children in America. Symptoms of iron toxicity include nausea, diarrhea, rapid heartbeat, vomiting, weak pulse, dizziness, shock, and confusion. Fewer than five iron tablets containing as little as 200 mg of iron have killed dozens of children in America.

Do not take supplements unless you are under a physician's care and have had a blood test that indicates you should. Good plant sources of iron are iron-fortified cereals, soybeans, red kidney beans, legumes, whole-grain cereals, and broccoli. Adding foods rich in vitamin C will increase iron absorption from plant foods as much as two or three times. Do not drink tea with your meal, because the tannin in it may interfere with iron absorption. Animal sources, heme iron, are absorbed best. These include lean red meats (the richest form), which the body utilizes best, iron-rich organ meats such as liver, and oysters. Because organ meats are high in fat content, intake should be limited to once or twice a month. Cooking foods in cast-iron cookware leaches iron that the body can utilize.

## Nutritional Guidelines for Health

Scientific and governmental agencies have established numerous nutritional guidelines to assist consumers in planning a nutritional lifestyle. Historically, the Recommended Dietary Allowances (RDAs) were developed to reduce the public risk of diseases from nutrient deficiency. These guidelines have provided Americans and Canadians with recommended intake levels necessary to meet the nutritional needs for about 97% of healthy individuals. Recently, the U.S. Food and Nutrition Board replaced and expanded upon the RDAs by creating new **Dietary Reference Intakes (DRIs),** a list of 26 nutrients essential to maintaining health. The DRIs identify recommended and maximun safe intake levels for healthy people and established the amount of a nutrient needed to prevent deficiencies or to reduce the risk of chronic disease. These DRIs are the guidelines under which the following categories fall:

**United States Recommended Daily Allowances (USRDAs)**—Dietary guidelines developed by the FDA and USDA.

**Adequate Intake (AI)**—The recommended average daily nutrient intake level of a nutrient by healthy people when there is not enough research to determine the full RDA.

**Tolerable Upper Intake Level (UL)**—The highest amount of a nutrient an individual can consume daily without the risk of adverse health effects.

## 2005 DIETARY GUIDELINES FOR AMERICANS

The 2005 Dietary Guidelines represent a synthesis of current knowledge about nutrition, presented as general recommendations for diet and physical activity. The guidelines are designed to address two major concerns: the role of poor diet and a sedentary lifestyle, major causes of disease and death in the United States, and the role of these same factors in the increase in overweight and obesity in this country. MyPyramid was developed as a graphic to help people apply the guidelines and the DRIs to their daily meal planning.

The nine guidelines in the document are made both for the general population and for specific population groups, such as people over 50, people who need to lose weight, and women of childbearing age. These guidelines address the following areas.

- Adequate Nutrients within Calorie Needs:

—Consume a variety of nutrient-sense foods and beverages within and among the basic food groups while choosing foods that limit the intake of saturated and trans fats, cholesterol, added sugars, salt, and alcohol.

—Meet recommended intakes within energy needs by adopting a balanced eating pattern, such as the USDA Food Guide or the DASH Eating Plan.

- Weight Management:

—To maintain body weight in a healthy range, balance calories from foods and beverages with calories expended.

—To prevent gradual weight gain over time, make small decreases in food and beverage calories and increase physical activity.

- Physical Activity:

—Engage in regular physical activity and reduce sedentary activities to promote health, psychological well-being, and a healthy body weight.

—To reduce the risk of chronic disease in adulthood: Engage in at least 30 minutes of moderate-intensity physical activity, above usual activity, at work or home on most days of the week.

—For most people, greater health benefits can be obtained by engaging in physical activity of more vigorous intensity or longer duration.

—To help manage body weight and prevent gradual unhealthy body weight gain in adulthood: Engage in approximately 60 minutes of moderate-to-vigorous-intensity activity on most days of the week while not exceeding caloric intake requirements.

—To sustain weight loss in adulthood: Participate in at least 60 to 90 minutes of daily moderate-intensity physical activity while not exceeding caloric intake requirements. Some people may need to consult with a health care provider before participating in this level of activity.

—Achieve physical fitness by including cardiovascular conditioning, stretching exercises for flexibility, and resistance exercises or calisthenics for muscle strength and endurance.

- Food Groups to Encourage:

—Consume a sufficient amount of fruits and vegetables while staying within energy needs. Two cups of fruit and 2.5 cups of vegetables per day are recommended for a reference 2,000 calorie intake, with higher or lower amounts depending on the calorie level.

—Choose a variety of fruits and vegetables each day. In particular, select from all five vegetable subgroups (dark green, orange, legumes, starchy vegetables, and other vegetables) several times a week.

—Consume 3 ounce servings or more of whole-grain products per day, with the rest of the recommended grains coming from enriched or whole-grain products. In general, at least half the grains should come from whole grains.

—Consume 3 cups per day of fat-free or low-fat milk or equivalent milk products.

---

## KEY TERMS

**Anemia** a deficiency in the oxygen-carrying material in the red blood cells

**Hemoglobin** the protein that makes the blood red and transports oxygen from the lungs to the rest of the body

**Hemochromatosis** iron toxicity due to ingesting too many iron-containing supplements

**Dietary Reference Intake (DRI)** a set of nutritional values, new combined listing, including more than 26 essential vitamins and minerals, which apply to healthy people

**United States Recommended Daily Allowances (USRDAs)** dietary guidelines developed by the FDA and USDA

**Adequate Intake (AI)** the recommended average daily nutrient intake level of a nutrient by healthy people when there is not enough research to determine the full RDA

**Tolerable Upper Intake Level (UL)** the highest amount of a nutrient an individual can consume daily without the risk of adverse health effects

**TABLE 9.9 ▶** Nutrient Contributions of Each Food Group

| FOOD GROUP | MAJOR CONTRIBUTION(S)[1] | SUBSTANTIAL CONTRIBUTION(S) (>10% OF TOTAL)[2] | | |
|---|---|---|---|---|
| **Fruit Group** | Vitamin C | Thiamin<br>Vitamin B<br>Folate | Copper<br>Potassium<br>Carbohydrate | Magnesium<br>Fiber |
| **Vegetable Group** | Vitamin A<br>Potassium | Vitamin E<br>Vitamin C<br>Thiamin<br>Niacin<br>Vitamin B | Magnesium<br>Iron<br>Zinc<br>Copper<br>Carbohydrate | Folate<br>Calcium<br>Phosphorus<br>Fiber<br>Alpha-linolenic acid |
| **Vegetable Subgroups** | | | | |
| Dark green vegetables | | Vitamin A<br>Vitamin C | | |
| Orange vegetables | Vitamin A | | | |
| Legumes | | Folate<br>Copper | Fiber | |
| Starchy vegetables | | Vitamin B<br>Copper | | |
| Other vegetables | | | Vitamin C | |
| **Grain Group** | Thiamin<br>Folate<br>Magnesium<br>Iron<br>Copper<br>Carbohydrate<br>Fiber | Vitamin A<br>Riboflavin<br>Niacin<br>Vitamin B$_6$<br>Vitamin B$_{12}$<br>Calcium | Phosphorus<br>Zinc<br>Potassium<br>Protein<br>Linoleic acid<br>Alpha-linolenic acid | |
| **Grain Subgroups** | | | | |
| Whole grains | Folate (tie)<br>Magnesium<br>Iron<br>Copper<br>Carbohydrate (tie)<br>Fiber | Thiamin<br>Riboflavin<br>Niacin<br>Vitamin B$_6$ | Vitamin B$_{12}$<br>Phosphorus<br>Zinc<br>Protein | |
| Enriched grain | Folate (tie)<br>Thiamin<br>Carbohydrate (tie) | Riboflavin<br>Niacin | Iron<br>Copper | |
| **Meat, Poultry, Fish, Eggs, and Nuts Group** | Niacin<br>Vitamin B$_6$<br>Zinc<br>Protein | Vitamin E<br>Thiamin<br>Riboflavin<br>Vitamin B$_{12}$<br>Phosphorus | Magnesium<br>Iron<br>Copper<br>Potassium<br>Linoleic acid | |
| **Milk Group** | Riboflavin<br>Vitamin B$_{12}$<br>Calcium<br>Phosphorus | Vitamin A<br>Thiamin<br>Vitamin B$_6$<br>Magnesium | Zinc<br>Potassium<br>Carbohydrate<br>Protein | |
| **Oils and Soft Margarines** | Vitamin<br>Linoleic acid<br>Alpha-linolenic acid | | | |

1. *Major contribution* means that the food group or subgroup provides more of the nutrient than any other single food group average over all calorie levels. When two food groups or subgroups provide equal amounts, it is noted as a tie.

2. A *substantial contribution* means that the food group or subgroup provides 10% or more of the total amount of the nutrient in the food patterns, averaged over all calorie levels.

*Source: Dietary Guidelines for Americans, 2005. USDHHS, USDA. www.healthlerus.gov/dietaryguidelines.*

- Fats:
  - —Consume less than 10% of calories from saturated fatty acids and less than 300 mg/day of cholesterol, and keep trans-fatty acid consumption as low as possible.
  - —Keep total fat intake between 20% and 35% of calories, with most fats coming from sources of polyunsaturated and monounsaturated fatty acids, such as fish, nuts, and vegetable oils.
  - —When selecting and preparing meat, poultry, dry beans, and milk or milk products, make choices that are lean, low-fat, or fat-free.
  - —Limit intake of fats and oils high in saturated and/or trans-fatty acids, and choose products low in such fats and oils.

- Carbohydrates:
  - —Choose fiber-rich fruits, vegetables, and whole grains often.
  - —Choose and prepare foods and beverages with little added sugars or caloric sweeteners, such as amounts suggested by the USDA Food Guide and the DASH Eating Plan. (Note: MyPyramid has replaced the Food Guide Pyramid, as discussed later in this section.)
  - —Reduce the incidence of dental caries by practicing good oral hygiene and consuming fewer sugar- and starch-containing foods and beverages.

- Sodium:
  - —Consume fewer than 2,300 mg (approximately 1 tsp of salt) of sodium per day.
  - —Choose and prepare foods with little salt. At the same time, consume potassium-rich foods, such as fruits and vegetables.

- Alcoholic Beverages:
  - —Those who choose to drink alcoholic beverages should do so sensibly and in moderation—defined as the consumption of up to one drink per day for women and up to two drinks per day for men.
  - —Alcoholic beverages should not be consumed by some individuals, including those who cannot restrict their alcoholic intake, women of childbearing age who may become pregnant, pregnant and lactating women, children and adolescents, individuals taking medication that can interact with alcohol, and those with specific medical conditions.
  - —Alcoholic beverages should be avoided by individuals engaging in activities that require attention, skill, or coordination, such as driving or operating machinery.

- Food Safety (to avoid microbial food-borne illness):
  - —Clean hands, food contact surfaces, and fruits and vegetables with soap and water. Meat and poultry should not be washed and rinsed.
  - —Separate raw, cooked, and ready-to-eat foods while shopping, preparing, or storing foods.
  - —Cook foods to a safe temperature to kill microorganisms.
  - —Chill (refrigerate) perishable food promptly and defrost foods properly.
  - —Avoid raw (unpasteurized) milk or any products made from unpasteurized milk, raw or partially cooked eggs or foods containing raw eggs, raw or undercooked meat and poultry, unpasteurized juices, and raw sprouts.

## MYPYRAMID

The Food Guide Pyramid underwent a landmark overhaul in 2005 in order to better account for the variety of different nutritional needs throughout the United States population (Figure 9.8). This new pyramid, called the **MyPyramid Plan,** replaces the former Food Guide Pyramid that had been promoted since 1993 by the USDA and incorporates the 2005 Dietary Guidelines for Americans, released in January 2005.

**Goals of the MyPyramid Plan.** MyPyramid Plan is meant to promote personalized dietary and exercise recommendations based upon individual needs and to encourage consumers to make healthier food choices and to be active every day. These guidelines can help you eat smart and stay well. The key themes of MyPyramid are:

- Variety is represented by the six color bands of the five food groups—grains, vegetables, fruits, milk, and meat and beans. It is important to eat foods from each group and subgroups every day in order to receive the proper nutrients for overall health.

- Proportionality is symbolized by the varying width of each color band. A wider band generally suggests you should choose more foods from that group (fruits, vegetables, whole grains, fat-free or low-fat milk products), while a narrow band suggests you limit your intake of foods high in saturated or trans fats, salt, added sugars, cholesterol, and alcohol.

- Moderation of food intake is represented by the narrowing of each color band from bottom to top. You should select foods that limit intake of saturated or trans fats, added sugars, cholesterol, alcohol, and salt.

- Physical activity, represented by the person climbing steps, reminds individuals about the importance of being physically active each day and in maintaining

**KEY TERMS**

**MyPyramid Plan** grouping of foods into five groups plus oils indicating serving sizes for each

**FIGURE 9.8 ▶** MyPyramid: Steps to a Healthier You

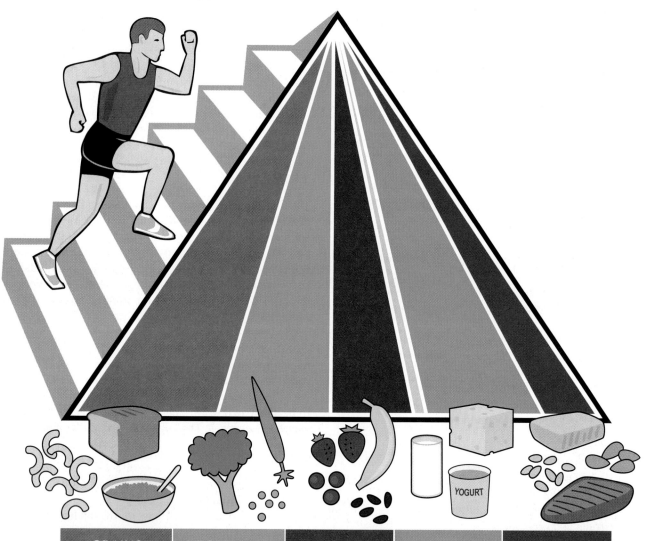

| GRAINS | VEGETABLES | FRUITS | MILK | MEAT & BEANS |
|---|---|---|---|---|
| Make half your grains whole | Vary your veggies | Focus on fruits | Get your calcium-rich foods | Go lean with protein |
| Eat at least 3 oz. of whole-grain cereals, breads, crackers, rice, or pasta every day<br><br>1 oz. is about 1 slice of bread, about 1 cup of breakfast cereal, or ½ cup of cooked rice, cereal, or pasta | Eat more dark-green veggies like broccoli, spinach, and other dark leafy greens<br><br>Eat more orange vegetables like carrots and sweet potatoes<br><br>Eat more dry beans and peas like pinto beans, kidney beans, and lentils | Eat a variety of fruit<br><br>Choose fresh, frozen, canned, or dried fruit<br><br>Go easy on fruit juices | Go low-fat or fat-free when you choose milk, yogurt, and other milk products<br><br>If you don't or can't consume milk, choose lactose-free products or other calcium sources such as fortified foods and beverages | Choose low-fat or lean meats and poultry<br><br>Bake it, broil it, or grill it<br><br>Vary your protein routine — choose more fish, beans, peas, nuts, and seeds |

For a 2,000-calorie diet, you need the amounts below from each food group. To find the amounts that are right for you, go to MyPyramid.gov.

| Eat 6 oz. every day | Eat 2½ cups every day | Eat 2 cups every day | Get 3 cups every day; for kids aged 2 to 8, it's 2 | Eat 5½ oz. every day |
|---|---|---|---|---|

**Find your balance between food and physical activity**
- Be sure to stay within your daily calorie needs.
- Be physically active for at least 30 minutes most days of the week.
- About 60 minutes a day of physical activity may be needed to prevent weight gain.
- For sustaining weight loss, at least 60 to 90 minutes a day of physical activity may be required.
- Children and teenagers should be physically active for 60 minutes every day, or most days.

**Know the limits on fats, sugars, and salt (sodium)**
- Make most of your fat sources from fish, nuts, and vegetable oils.
- Limit solid fats like butter, stick margarine, shortening, and lard, as well as foods that contain these.
- Check the Nutrition Facts label to keep saturated fats, *trans* fats, and sodium low.
- Choose food and beverages low in added sugars. Added sugars contribute calories with few, if any, nutrients.

*Source:* U.S. Department of Agriculture graphic.

© IT Stock Free/Jupiterimages

## FYI GOVERNMENT-ACCEPTED DEFINITIONS

- **Light (lite).** May refer to calories, fat, or sodium. Contains one-third fewer calories, or no more than half the fat of the higher-calorie, higher-fat version; or no more than half the sodium of the higher-sodium version.
- **Calorie-free.** Fewer than 5 calories per serving.
- **Fat-free.** Contains less than 0.5 gram of fat per serving.
- **Low fat.** Contains 3 grams of fat (or less) per serving.
- **Reduced or less fat.** At least 25% less fat per serving than the higher-fat version.
- **Lean.** Less than 10 grams of fat, 4 grams of saturated fat, and 95 milligrams of cholesterol per serving.
- **Extra lean.** Less than 5 grams of fat, 2 grams of saturated fat, and 95 milligrams of cholesterol per serving.
- **Cholesterol-free.** Contains less than 2 milligrams of cholesterol and 2 grams (or less) of saturated fat per serving.
- **Low cholesterol.** Contains 20 milligrams of cholesterol (or less) and 2 grams of saturated fat (or less) per serving.
- **Reduced cholesterol.** At least 25% less cholesterol than the higher-cholesterol version and 2 grams (or less) of saturated fat per serving.
- **Sodium-free.** Less than 5 milligrams of sodium per serving and no sodium chloride (NaCl) in ingredients.
- **Very low sodium.** Contains 35 milligrams of sodium (or less) per serving.
- **Low sodium.** Contains 140 milligrams (or less) per serving.
- **Sugar-free.** Less than 0.5 gram of sugar per serving.
- **High-fiber.** Contains 5 grams of fiber (or more) per serving.
- **Good source of fiber.** Contains 2.5 to 4.9 grams of fiber per serving.

a healthy weight and improving overall health and disease prevention.

- Personalization is demonstrated by the MyPyramid website, www.MyPyramid.gov. The website offers personalized recommendations of the kinds and amounts of food to eat each day, tips and ideas for achieving a healthy diet, and interactive assessments based on an individual's gender, age, and activity level. Go online and fill in your age, gender, and typical level of activity. You will be linked to one of 12 versions of the pyramid,

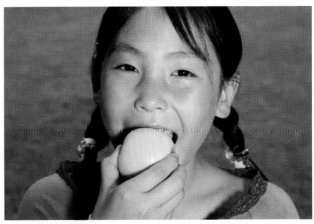

▲ *Fruit is essential to a healthy diet*

ranging from 1,000 to 3,200 daily calories. Print out your customized pyramid and use it as a dietary guide. Keep a record of your eating habits for a week and compare it with the recommendations and get specific suggestions from this website.

- Gradual improvement encourages individuals to take small steps to improve their diet and lifestyle each day.

The Mediterranean pyramid (Figure 9.9) was developed from the diet typical of the region in southern Europe, including Italy and Greece. Like MyPyramid, the Mediterranean pyramid emphasizes grains, fruits, and vegetables, but it also recommends daily servings of beans, legumes, and nuts and foods that are high in protein, fiber, and fats. It encourages the use of olive oil over other oils. Although rates of heart disease and cancer are lower in Mediterranean countries, the prevalence of stroke is almost double that in the United States. This may be explained by lifestyle factors other than diet, such as smoking and level of physical activity.

**Vegetarians.** Between 5% and 15% of all Americans today claim to be vegetarians. These Americans follow a **vegetarian** diet because of religious beliefs, aesthetic, animal rights, economic, personal, health, cultural, ethical, or philosophical reasons, or they think foods of plant origin provide more natural nourishment for the body. The styles of vegetarians are

- **Lacto-vegetarian.** One who consumes dairy products (milk, milk products, and cheese) as well as

## KEY TERMS

**Vegetarian** person who eats foods of plant origin and not meat

**Lacto-vegetarian** a vegetarian who includes milk and cheese products in the diet

**Tips for Action** Vegetarian Diet Planning

Vegetarian diets can be healthy if they are carefully designed to include adequate amounts of all the essential nutrients. Vegetarians, especially vegans, need to pay careful attention to the following nutrients:

■ **Protein** Some vegetarians can get their protein from dairy products, eggs, fish, or poultry. Vegans can get all of the essential and nonessential amino acids by eating a variety of plant food—whole grains, legumes, seeds and nuts, and vegetables—and consuming foods from two or more of these categories over the course of a day. Soy protein provides all the essential amino acids and can be the sole protein source in a diet.

■ **Vitamin D** This vitamin is found in eggs, butter, and fortified dairy products. Sunlight transforms a provitamin into a substance that the body can use to make vitamin D. Vegans who don't get much sunlight may need a vitamin D supplement (but supplementation should not exceed the RDA).

■ **Iron** Nonvegetarians get much of their iron from red meat and eggs. Good plant sources of iron are prune juice, dried beans and lentils, spinach, dried fruits, molasses, brewer's yeast, and enriched products, such as enriched flour. Cooking in iron cookware (cast iron pans) also provides iron in the diet.

■ **Calcium** Calcium is plentiful in dairy products, molasses, leafy green vegetables like kale and mustard greens, broccoli, tofu and other soy products, and some legumes. (The

calcium in some foods, including spinach, chocolate, and wheat bran, is poorly used in the body.) Studies show that vegetarians absorb and retain more calcium from foods than nonvegetarians do.

■ **Vitamin B$_2$** (riboflavin) Good sources of this vitamin are dairy products, nutritional yeast, leafy green vegetables (collard greens, spinach), broccoli, mushrooms, and dried beans.

■ **Zinc** Good sources of this essential mineral are legumes, whole grains, soy products, peas, spinach, and nuts. It is also abundant in dairy products and shellfish. Take care to select supplements containing no more than 15–18 milligrams (mg) of zinc. Supplements containing 50 mg or more may lower HDL ("good") cholesterol in some people.

■ **Vitamin B$_{12}$** This vitamin is found naturally only in animal sources, especially meat and dairy products, so it is particularly important for vegans to make sure it is present in their diets. It can be found in some fortified (not enriched) breakfast cereals, fortified soy beverages, and some brands of nutritional (brewer's) yeast, and other foods (check the labels), as well as vitamin supplements.

■ **Calories** Plant foods have fewer calories than animal foods, so vegetarians should make sure they are consuming enough calories to meet their bodies' energy needs.

*Source:* Adapted from "Vegetarian Diets," American Heart Association, 2004, www.americanheart.org

**FIGURE 9.9** ▶ Mediterranean Diet Pyramid

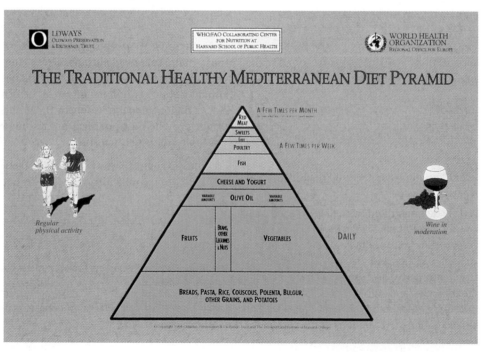

**FIGURE 9.10 ▶** Vegetarian Food Combinations That Supply Complete Protein

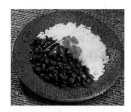
*Rice and black beans*

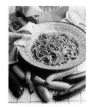
*Wheat pasta and squash*

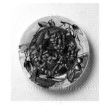
*Bean soup*

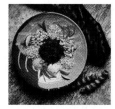
*Nuts, lentils, bulgur*

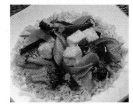
*Tofu and rice*

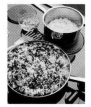
*Spinach, pine nuts, and rice*

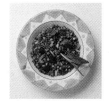
*Lentil soup*

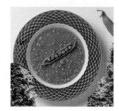
*Pea soup and bread*

*Source:* From Judith E. Brown, *Nutrition Now* (Belmont, CA: Wadsworth, 1999).

plant foods (fruits, vegetables, and grains) but does not eat meat, poultry, seafood, or eggs.

- **Lacto-ovo-vegetarian.** One who eats eggs, dairy products, and plant foods (fruits and vegetables) but does not eat meat, poultry, or seafood.

- **Vegan.** A pure vegetarian, one who eats only plant foods and often takes vitamin $B_{12}$ supplements because this vitamin normally is found only in animal products. They abstain from wearing wool, silk, and leather.

- **Partial vegetarian, semivegetarian,** or **pesco-vegetarian.** One who eats plant food, dairy products, eggs, and usually a small selection of poultry, fish, and other seafood, but not red meat (beef or pork). Some people in this category prefer to call themselves "non-red-meat eaters."

Vegetarians must obtain sufficient amounts of protein, iron, vitamin $B_{12}$, vitamin D, and calcium from fewer food sources. Research studies show that vegetarians have lower cholesterol levels, fewer problems with irregular bowel movements (constipation and diarrhea), and a lower risk of heart disease than do nonvegetarians. They have lower incidences of breast, colon, and prostate cancers, lower blood pressure, less kidney disease, and less osteoporosis. Vegetarians usually are not overweight.

Eating a wide variety of foods is necessary to ensure that all nutritional needs are met. Careful planning and time should be devoted to selecting a proper vegetarian diet. By combining complementary protein sources you can get the necessary nonanimal protein. Complete proteins (meat, poultry, fish, eggs, and dairy products) provide the nine essential amino acids (substances containing carbon, hydrogen, oxygen, and nitrogen that the human body cannot produce). Incomplete proteins (legumes or nuts) are relatively low in one or two essential amino acids but have high levels of others (see Figure 9.10). Vegan diets may be deficient in vitamins $B_2$ (riboflavin), $B_{12}$, and D. Vitamin $B_2$ is found mainly in meat, eggs, and dairy products, but broccoli, asparagus, almonds, and fortified cereals are also good sources. Vitamins $B_{12}$ and D are found only in dairy products and fortified products such as soy milk. Examples of complementary combinations are corn with beans and peanut butter with whole-grain bread. Eating a full variety of grains, legumes, fruits, vegetables, and seeds each day will keep the vegetarian in excellent health.

**MyPyramid Adapted for Vegetarians.** Vegetarians can meet all the recommendations for nutrient needs. By focusing on nonmeat sources such as protein, calcium, zinc, iron, and vitamin $B_{12}$, following the physical activity guidelines, and personalized serving size, vegetarians can be just as healthy as omnivores.

### KEY TERMS

**Lacto-ovo-vegetarian** a vegetarian who eats no meat, poultry, or fish but does eat eggs and milk products

**Vegan** a vegetarian who eats no animal products at all

**Partial vegetarian, semivegetarian,** or **pesco-vegetarian** a vegetarian who includes eggs, dairy products, and small amounts of poultry and seafood in the diet

**FIGURE 9.11 ▶** Understanding Nutrition Labels

Serving size. The new labels reflect more realistic portions than on previous labels. Serving sizes, which have been defined for approximately 150 food categories, must be the same for similar products (for example, different brands of potato chips) and for similar products within a category (snack foods such as potato chips, pretzels, and popcorn). This makes it simple to compare the nutritional content of foods.

Calories. The Nutrition Facts Label lists two numbers for calories: calories per serving and calories from fat per serving, which allows people to calculate how many calories they will consume and to determine the percentage of fat in an item.

Percent Daily Values (% DVs). A full day's diet should consist of selected foods that add up to 100% of the DVs. The % DVs show how a particular food's nutrient content fits into a 2,000-calorie diet. If people consume fewer than 2,000 total calories a day, they must lower their % DVs for total fat, saturated fat, and carbohydrates. Individuals consuming more than 2,000 calories per day should adjust the DVs upward by 10% and those consuming fewer than 2,000 calories should lower the DVs by 10%.

Daily Values (DVs). DVs refer to the total amount of a nutrient that the average adult should aim to get or not exceed on a daily basis. The DVs for cholesterol, sodium, vitamins, and minerals are the same for all adults. The DVs for total fat, saturated fat, carbohydrate, fiber, and protein are based on a 2,000-calorie daily diet, the amount of food ingested by many American men and active women.

Calories per gram. The bottom of the food label lists the number of calories per gram for fat, carbohydrates, and protein.

The name and address of the manufacturer, packer, or distributor

The common or usual product name

Approved nutrient claims if the product meets specified criteria

The net contents in weight, measure, or count

Approved health claims stated in terms of the total diet

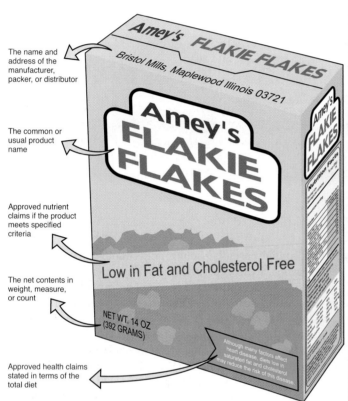

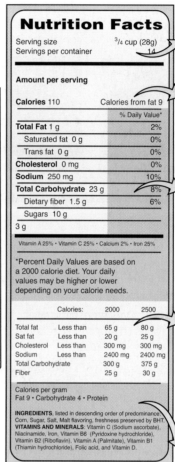

## Nutrition Facts

| Serving size | ³/₄ cup (28g) |
|---|---|
| Servings per container | 14 |

**Amount per serving**

| **Calories** 110 | Calories from fat 9 |
|---|---|

| | % Daily Value* |
|---|---|
| **Total Fat** 1 g | 2% |
| Saturated fat 0 g | 0% |
| Trans fat 0 g | 0% |
| **Cholesterol** 0 mg | 0% |
| **Sodium** 250 mg | 10% |
| **Total Carbohydrate** 23 g | 8% |
| Dietary fiber 1.5 g | 6% |
| Sugars 10 g | |
| 3 g | |

Vitamin A 25% • Vitamin C 25% • Calcium 2% • Iron 25%

*Percent Daily Values are based on a 2000 calorie diet. Your daily values may be higher or lower depending on your calorie needs.

| | Calories: | 2000 | 2500 |
|---|---|---|---|
| Total fat | Less than | 65 g | 80 g |
| Sat fat | Less than | 20 g | 25 g |
| Cholesterol | Less than | 300 mg | 300 mg |
| Sodium | Less than | 2400 mg | 2400 mg |
| Total Carbohydrate | | 300 g | 375 g |
| Fiber | | 25 g | 30 g |

Calories per gram
Fat 9 • Carbohydrate 4 • Protein

**INGREDIENTS**, listed in descending order of predominance: Corn, Sugar, Salt, Malt flavoring, freshness preserved by BHT. **VITAMINS AND MINERALS**: Vitamin C (Sodium ascorbate), Niacinamide, Iron, Vitamin B6 (Pyridoxine hydrochloride), Vitamin B2 (Riboflavin), Vitamin A (Palmitate), Vitamin B1 (Thiamin hydrochloride), Folic acid, and Vitamin D.

A container with fewer than 40 square inches of surface area can present fewer facts in this format.

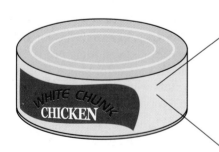

## Nutrition Facts

Serv.Size ¹/₃ cup (85g)**
Servings 2
Calories 111
Fat Cal. 27
* Percent Daily Values (DV) are based on a 2000 calorie diet.
** Drained solids only.

| Amount/serving | | %DV* | Amount/serving | | %DV* |
|---|---|---|---|---|---|
| Total Fat | 3g | 5% | Total Carb. | 0g | 0% |
| Sat. Fat | 1g | 5% | Fiber | 0g | 0% |
| Trans Fat | 0g | | | | |
| Cholest. | 60mg | 20% | Sugars | 0g | |
| Sodium | 200mg | 8% | Protein | 21g | |

Vitamin A 0% • Vitamin C 0% • Calcium 0% • Iron 2%

Packages with fewer than 12 square inches of surface area need not carry nutrition information, but they must provide an address or telephone number for obtaining information.

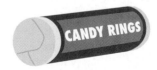

## NUTRITION FACTS ON FOOD LABELS

Since May 8, 1993, the federal government has required food manufacturers to include accurate nutritional information on their product labels. Perhaps by reading and understanding food labels, you can make wiser decisions at the supermarket, fast-food restaurants, and the dinner table. The FDA and the U.S. Department of Agriculture (USDA) developed the **Reference Daily Intakes (RDIs)** and **Daily Reference Values (DRVs)** in order to help consumers determine the nutritional values of foods. RDIs are the recommended amounts of 19 vitamins and minerals, also known as micronutrients (trace), and DRVs are the recommended amounts of macronutrients, such as total fat, saturated fat, cholesterol, total carbohydrates, dietary fiber, sodium, potassium, and protein. The RDIs and DRVs make up the **Daily Values (DVs)** that you will find on food and supplement labels listed as percentage (% DV; Figure 9.11). In addition to the percentage of nutrients found in a serving of food, labels also include information on the serving size, calories, and calories from fat per serving, and percentage of trans fats in a food.

The food label (Figure 9.11) represents an attempt to assist consumers in making healthful food choices and focuses on those nutrients most clearly associated with disease risk and health: total fat, saturated fat, cholesterol, sodium, total carbohydrate, dietary fiber, sugar, and protein.

The following are useful items to look for on food labels if people are watching their weight or if they have food allergies.

**Calories from fat.** Calculate the percentage of fat calories in a food before buying or eating it.

**Total fat.** Saturated and trans-fat numbers deserve special attention because of their reported link to several diseases.

**Cholesterol.** Cholesterol is made by and contained in products of animal origin only. Many high-fat products, such as potato chips, contain 0% cholesterol because they're made from plants and are cooked in vegetable fats. However, if the vegetable fats are hydrogenated, the resulting trans fat is more harmful to the heart than cholesterol.

**Sugars.** Daily Value on sugars does not exist since health experts have yet to agree on a daily limit. The figure on the label includes naturally present sugars, such as lactose in milk and fructose in fruit, as well as those added to the food, such as table sugar, corn syrup, or dextrose.

**Fiber.** A "high-fiber" food has 5 or more grams of fiber per serving. A "good" source of fiber provides at least 2.5 grams. "More" or "added" fiber means at least 2.5 grams more per serving than similar foods, 10% more of the DV for fiber.

**Calcium.** "High" equals 200 milligrams (mg) or more per serving. "Good" means at least 100 mg, whereas "more" indicates that the food contains at least 100 mg more calcium, 10% more of the DV, than the item usually would have.

**Sodium.** Read the labels carefully to avoid excess sodium, which can be a health threat.

**Vitamins.** A Daily Value of 10% of any vitamin makes a food a "good" source; 20% qualifies it as "high" in a certain vitamin.

Nutrition labeling for fresh produce, fish, meat, and poultry remains voluntary. In the case of packages too small for a full-size label, the manufacturer must provide an address or phone number so consumers can obtain nutrition information.

Some of the names for added sugars that may be in processed foods and listed on the food label ingredients list include:

| | |
|---|---|
| Brown sugar | Invert sugar |
| Corn sweetener | Lactose |
| Corn syrup | Maltose |
| Dextrose | Malt syrup |
| Fructose | Molasses |
| Fruit juice concentrates | Raw sugar |
| Glucose | Sucrose |
| High-fructose corn syrup | Sugar |
| Honey | Syrup |

## PORTIONS AND SERVINGS

A **serving** is the recommended amount you should consume, while a **portion** is the amount you choose to eat at any one time and may be more or less than a serving on food labels. According to nutritionists, "marketplace portions," the actual amounts served to customers, are two to eight times larger than the standard serving sizes defined by the USDA. Fast-food chains provide portions two to five times larger than the original sizes (Table 9.10). People presented with larger portions eat 30% to 50% more than they otherwise would eat. Watch the size of your portions if you are trying to control your weight. Make sure that you do not exceed the recommended servings. For example, a half cup of ice cream is about the size of a racquet ball (Figure 9.13). If you eat more, count it as more than one serving.

How many servings do you need each day? The number of servings that will be right for you depends on how

---

### KEY TERMS

**Reference Daily Intake (RDI)** Recommended amounts of 19 vitamins and minerals, also known as micronutrients.

**Daily Reference Values (DRVs)** Recommended amounts of macronutrients such as total fat, saturated fat, and cholesterol

**Daily Values (DVs)** The RDIs and DRVs together make the Daily Values seen on food and supplement labels

**Serving** Recommended amount you should consume

**Portion** Amount one chooses to eat at any one time and may be more or less than a serving on food labels.

**TABLE 9.10 ▶** Supersizing Portions

| FOOD ITEM | CALORIES PER PORTION | |
| --- | --- | --- |
| | 20 YEARS AGO | TODAY |
| Bagel | 140 Calories (3-in. diameter) | 350 calories (6-in. diameter) |
| Fast-food cheeseburger | 333 calories | 590 calories |
| Spaghetti and meatballs | 500 calories (1 cup of spaghetti with sauce and 3 small meatballs) | 1,025 calories (2 cups of spaghetti and 3 large meatballs) |
| Bottle of soda | 85 calories (6.5 oz.) | 250 calories (20 oz.) |
| Fast-food french fries | 210 calories (2.4 oz.) | 610 calories (6.9 oz.) |
| Turkey sandwich | 320 calories | 820 calories (10-in. sub) |

*Source: Dietary Guidelines for Americans 2005*, USDHHS, USDA, www.healthierus.gov/dietaryguidelines. Adapted from the Portion Distortion Quiz, National Heart, Lung and Blood Institute, www.nhibl.nih.gov.

many calories you need, which in turn depends on your age, sex, size, and activity level. Almost everyone should have at least the lowest number of servings in each food group. Do you need to measure servings? Servings should be used only as a general guide. For mixed foods you should do the best you can to estimate the food group servings of the main ingredients. For example, a generous serving of pizza counts in the bread group (crust), milk group (cheese), and vegetable group (tomato); a helping of beef stew counts in the meat group and the vegetable group. Both examples have some fat (in the cheese on the pizza and in the beef in the stew). A serving adds up more quickly than you think. Examples of one serving from each food group in MyPyramid are listed below.

—Grains
   1 slice of bread or ½ English muffin
   ½ cup cooked rice, pasta, or hot cereal
   1 cup ready-to-eat cereal

—Fruits
   1 small apple or 1 large banana
   1 cup of raw, cooked, or canned fruit
   1 cup of fruit juice
   ½ cup dried fruit

—Vegetables
   1 cup raw greens or 2 cups cooked greens
   1 cup beans, peas, or carrots (raw or cooked)
   1 medium baked potato

—Meat and Beans
   1 ounce lean meat, poultry, or fish
   1 tablespoon peanut butter
   ¼ cup tofu or cooked beans
   1 egg

—Milk
   1 cup milk or yogurt
   1½ ounces natural cheese or ⅓ cup shredded cheese
   2 ounces processed cheese

**FIGURE 9.12 ▶** Easy Estimates of Portion Sizes

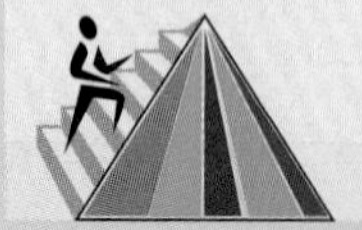

| | 1,200 | 1,400 | 1,600 | 1,800 | 2,000 | 2,200 | 2,400 | 2,600 | 2,800 | 3,000 |
| --- | --- | --- | --- | --- | --- | --- | --- | --- | --- | --- |
| Fruits | 1 cup | 1.5 cups | 1.5 cups | 1.5 cups | 2 cups | 2 cups | 2 cups | 2 cups | 2.5 cups | 2.5 cups |
| Vegetables | 1.5 cups | 1.5 cups | 2 cups | 2.5 cups | 2.5 cups | 3 cups | 3 cups | 3.5 cups | 3.5 cups | 4 cups |
| Grains | 4 oz.-eq. | 5 oz.-eq. | 5 oz.-eq. | 6 oz.-eq. | 6 oz.-eq. | 7 oz.-eq. | 8 oz.-eq. | 9 oz.-eq. | 10 oz.-eq. | 10 oz.-eq. |
| Meat and Beans | 3 oz.-eq. | 4 oz.-eq. | 5 oz.-eq. | 5 oz.-eq. | 5.5 oz.-eq. | 6 oz.-eq. | 6.5 oz.-eq. | 6.5 oz.-eq. | 7 oz.-eq. | 7 oz.-eq. |
| Milk | 2 cups | 2 cups | 3 cups | 3 cups | 3 cups | 3 cups | 3 cups | 3 cups | 3 cups | 3 cups |
| Oils | 4 tsp | 4 tsp | 5 tsp | 5 tsp | 6 tsp | 6 tsp | 7 tsp | 8 tsp | 8 tsp | 10 tsp |
| Discretionary calorie allowance | 171 | 171 | 132 | 195 | 267 | 290 | 362 | 410 | 426 | 512 |

**TABLE 9.11** ▶ Fruits, Vegetables, and Legumes (Dry Beans) That Contain Vitamin A (Carotenoids), Vitamin C, Folate, and Potassium

**Sources of vitamin A (Carotenoids)**
- Bright orange vegetables like carrots, sweet potatoes, and pumpkin
- Tomatoes and tomato products, red sweet pepper
- Leafy greens such as spinach, collards, turnip greens, kale, beet and mustard greens, green leaf lettuce, and romaine
- Orange fruits like mango, cantaloupe, apricots, and red or pink grapefruit

**Sources of vitamin C**
- Citrus fruits and juices, kiwi fruit, strawberries, guava, papaya, and cantaloupe
- Broccoli, peppers, tomatoes, cabbage (especially Chinese Cabbage), Brussels sprouts, and potatoes
- Leafy greens such as romaine, turnip greens, and spinach

**Sources of folate**
- Cooked dry beans and peas
- Orange and orange juice
- Deep green leaves like spinach and mustard greens

**Sources of potassium**
- Baked white or sweet potatoes, cooked greens (such as spinach), winter (orange) squash
- Bananas, plantains, many dried fruits, oranges and orange juice, cantaloupe, and honeydew melons
- Cooked dry beans
- Soybeans (green and mature)
- Tomato products (sauce, paste, puree)
- Beet greens

Many of the fruits, vegetables, and legumes (beans) are considered to be important sources of vitamin A (as carotenoids), vitamin C, and potassium in the adult population. Intakes of these nutrients, based on dietary intake data or evidence of public health problems, may be of concern. Also listed are sources of naturally occurring folate, a nutrient considered to be of concern for women of childbearing age and those in the first trimester of pregnancy. Folic acid-fortified grain products, not listed in this table, are also good sources.

—Oil

1 tablespoon margarine or mayonnaise equals 2½ teaspoons of oil

½ avocado equals 3 teaspoons of oil

2 tablespoons Italian dressing equals 2 teaspoons oil

(See Appendix B: Fruits and Veggies to calculate your Fruit and Vegetable needs.)

## FUNCTIONAL FOODS

As the American Dietetic Association has noted, all foods are functional at some physiological level. However, the term **functional foods** applies generally to a food specifically created to have health-promoting benefits. The International Food Information Council defines functional foods as those "that provide health benefits beyond basic nutrition." Some manufacturers are adding biologically active components such as beta-carotene to food products and promoting them as functional foods. However, the amounts added are often too low to have any effect, and many such foods are high-sugared drinks and snack foods. More research should be done to evaluate their claims of health benefits.

## DISCRETIONARY CALORIES

Discretionary calories are those obtained from foods that do not provide a significant source of nutritional value. Suppose you have eaten wisely all day, choosing whole grains, low-fat, and low-sugar food items and your calorie balance for the day is 1,800 on a 2,000-calorie food plan. This means you can spend the remaining 200 calories on what you might consider a luxury food reward such as soda, small serving of ice cream or cake, higher fat meat or cheese than you would normally consume. Enjoy your food and start the next day with foods of nutritional value.

## ETHNIC CUISINES

America's diversity is reflected in its ethnic foods, ranging from Chinese to Korean to Italian. As people migrate from other countries, they bring with them their customs and traditions, different types of foods grown in different climates and terrains, eating practices, and manner of preparing foods.

African-Americans brought some of their food traditions from West Africa—foods such as peanuts, black-eyed peas, and okra—and these foods were combined with Native

**KEY TERMS**

**Functional foods** foods that may help prevent disease, usually because health-promoting ingredients have been added to them.

**FIGURE 9.13 ▶** Nutritional Needs for Different Groups

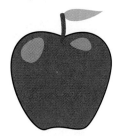
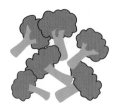

1 medium fruit is about the size of a baseball.

1 c cooked vegetables is about the size of your fist.

1/2 c ice cream is about the size of a racquetball.

3 oz. of meat is about the size of a deck of cards.

1 1/2 oz. cheese is about the size of six stacked dice.

1/4 c dried fruit is about the size of a golf ball.

2 tbs. peanut butter is about the size of a marshmallow.

4 small cookies are about the size of 4 poker chips.

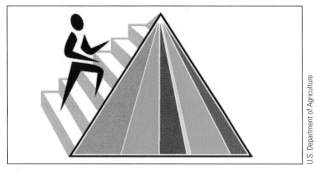

U.S. Department of Agriculture

▲ *MyPyramid recommends 2 cups of fruits and 2 1/2 cups of vegetables daily*

American foods including sweet potatoes, wild game, fish, and greens. Vegetables, collard greens, and sweet potatoes, as well as legumes, make up their diet. Some dishes include high-fat food products such as peanuts and pecans and involve frying, sometimes in saturated fat.

Mexican cuisine features rice, corn, and beans, which are low in fat and high in nutrients. The American Mexican dishes are less healthful. For example, burritos, when topped with cheese and sour cream, are very high in fat. Guacamole has a high fat content and contains mostly monounsaturated fatty acids, a better form of fat.

The traditional Japanese diet is very low in fat, cheese, and meats, which may account for the low incidence of heart disease in Japan. Dietary staples include soybean products, seafood (fish), vegetables, noodles, and rice. A variety of fruits and vegetables are also included in many dishes. The Japanese diet is high in salted, smoked, and pickled foods. Use caution with deep-fried dishes such as tempura and salty soups and sauces.

Considered to be one of the healthiest in the world, mainland Chinese cuisine is plant-based, high in carbohydrates, and low in fats and animal protein. However, Chinese restaurants in America serve more meat and sauces than are generally eaten in China. According to laboratory tests of typical take-out dishes from Chinese restaurants, many have more fats and cholesterol than hamburgers or egg dishes from fast-food chains.

Korean dishes consist primarily of rice, and the most popular main dishes are bulgogi (beef) and galbi (beef ribs), samgetang (small young whole chicken boiled in an individual pot with ginseng, an herb). Kimchi (pickled cabbage) and beef, fish, or vegetable soup are included in Korean diets. Noodles and fermented yogurt are also popular. Fish of choice include brims, eels, pollack, and cod. Sauces include bean paste and hot, soy, and sesame oil. The drink of choice is barley tea and milk, with yogurt added occasionally. Seasonal fruits include melons, plums, pears, and apples. Miyokguk (seaweed and beef soup) is served to the mother of a newborn and is also a special dish for birthdays. The Korean diet is very limited in saturated fat. The boiling and steaming methods of cooking are preferred over frying. Sesame, vegetable, cottonseed, and peanut oils are used to prepare Korean dishes.

Indian dishes, which are healthy and high in protein, include ingredients such as vegetables and legumes (beans and peas). Many use ghee (a form of butter) or coconut oil; both are rich in harmful saturated fats. Too much saturated fat in these foods can cancel some of the benefits. When dining at an Indian restaurant, it is a good idea to ask how each dish is prepared. Good choices include daal or dal (lentils), karbi or karni (chickpea soup), and chapati (tortilla-like bread).

French cuisine includes rich, high-fat sauces and dishes that may not be considered healthful. Yet nutritionists have been hard pressed to explain the so-called French paradox: Despite eating foods high in saturated fats, the French have one of the lowest rates of coronary artery disease in the world. The French diet increasingly resembles the American diet, but French portions tend to be one-third to one-half the size of American portions.

As a result of a deficiency in the digestive enzyme lactase, some people cannot digest milk sugar. After ingesting dairy products, they develop abdominal cramps, gas pains, and diarrhea. Among ethnic groups, lactose intolerance is present at birth or develops in as many as three-fourths of African-Americans, American Indians, and Jewish people.

The only treatment for lactose intolerance is to control the symptoms, as lactose production in the digestive system cannot be stimulated. Some over-the-counter products contain the natural lactase enzyme to counteract the unpleasant symptoms.

Large health-food stores and supermarkets stock an impressive array of frozen ethnic foods, including Indian, Moroccan, Greek, Chinese, Italian, Japanese, Korean, and Mexican, among many others. Ethnic cuisines are being promoted as the new healthy way of eating. Shoppers are encouraged to adopt the eating habits of the Mediterranean basin, China, and the Pacific Rim. Ethnic dishes each have their pros and cons; however, many ethnic cuisines are semivegetarian and, thus, low in fat and high in fiber. Meals are centered on vegetables, legumes, grains, and fruits, with small amounts of fish, poultry, and occasionally some red meat. Two main concerns arise concerning frozen ethnic foods.

1. The Americanized versions of ethnic dishes prepared for export to the United States include more meat and fewer grains and vegetables. The result is a much higher fat content than in the original.

2. Frozen ethnic food, until recently, has tended to be a nutritional wasteland of salty, fatty dinners with a smidgen of mushy vegetables. Now the consumer can select better options for a healthy diet. When reading labels, notice the serving size. One 3-ounce egg roll or 4-ounce empañada may be called a serving but is not much more than a snack. In addition, check the sodium content, which ideally should be lower than 800 milligrams (one-third the recommended daily maximum).

Many ethnic dishes are easy to prepare at home and are cheaper. They require brown rice, a variety of vegetables and beans, plus spices and condiments. The presence of international students on many college campuses offers an opportunity for seeking new friends, sharing different cultures, and learning how to prepare and enjoy various ethnic cuisines.

## NUTRITION AND GENDER

Men and women have different needs for most nutrients given that they differ in body composition, size, age, level of fitness, and overall metabolic rates. For example, from menarche to menopause, women require different nutritional needs due to their metabolism and nutritional needs such as iron, calcium, and folate nutrients. It has been reported that some women have food cravings that may cause them to overconsume during their menstrual cycle. As one grows older with the depletion of the hormone estrogen, the body's need for calcium to combat bone deterioration (osteoporosis) is pronounced. Slower metabolism means you need fewer calories to maintain a healthy weight.

Men do not have the same cyclical patterns and dietary needs as women do. However, they engage in dietary excess that is difficult to change. Men who eat excessive red meat are more than twice as likely to get prostate cancer and nearly five times more likely to get colon cancer. For every three servings of fruits or vegetables per day men can expect a 22% lower risk of stroke. The fastest rising malignancy in the United States is cancer of the lower esophagus (especially in white men); while obesity seems to be a factor, fruits and vegetables serve as protectors. The average American male eats fewer than three servings per day of fruits and vegetables; women average three to seven servings per day. The recommended servings per day is fruit (2 cups) and vegetables (2½ cups). Men who eat red meat as a main dish five or more times a week have four times the risk of colon cancer of men who eat red meat less than once a month.

## EATING FOR THE COLLEGE STUDENT

Eating healthy in college is a challenge because some students live in dorms and do not have their own cooking and refrigeration facilities. Others live in apartments with limited space, while others eat at university food services where food choices are generally limited. It is a balancing act to select proper nutrition when finances, as well as having time to buy and prepare nutritious foods, are limited.

Eating breakfast and lunch are important in order to keep energy levels high and get the most out of your classes. Most campuses are moving toward fast-food restaurants in student unions in order to fit students' needs for a fast bite of food at a reasonable price between classes. You should fit meals into your daily schedule. For example, a complete breakfast includes complex carbohydrates and

**African-American** African-American cooking centers on peanuts, pecans, okra, black-eyed peas, fish, game, collard greens, sweet potatoes, legumes, gumbos, red beans, seafood, and sausage. Some dishes are high in fat, such as peanuts and pecans, and involve frying, often in saturated fat. Bake or broil selected foods instead of frying.

**Asian** The emphasis in Asian meals is placed on rice, grains, fruits, vegetables, legumes, nuts, seeds, and vegetable oils. Daily options include dairy, fish, and shellfish. Sweets, eggs, and poultry are suggested weekly, and meats, monthly.

**Chinese** The Chinese diet is plant-based, high in carbohydrates, and low in fats and animal protein. It features boiled, steamed, or stir-fried dishes and entrées mixed with steamed rice. The mainland Chinese diet is considered one of the healthiest; however, Chinese food prepared in America is not the same. More meat and sauces are typically used in America. Watch out for high sodium content of soy and sauces. Individuals prone to high blood pressure beware of MSG (monosodium glutamate). Most restaurants offer some MSG-free dishes.

**French** Traditional French cuisine includes rich, high-fat sauces and dishes even though the French have had one of the lowest rates of coronary artery disease in the world. Fat consumption has increased, and the French are eating more meat, fast foods, and snacks, and they are exercising less and drinking more wine. Researchers report that French people are getting fatter, and most likely their rates of heart disease will rise. French portions tend to be one-third to one-half the size of American portions.

**Indian** Indian dishes include vegetables, legumes (beans and peas), daal or dal (lentils), chapati (tortilla-like bread), and karbi or karni (chickpea soup). Often ghee (a form of butter) or coconut oil (saturated fats) is used when preparing meals. Bhatura (fried bread), samosas (fried meat or vegetables in dough), and coconut milk should be used sparingly.

**Japanese** The Japanese diet is low in fat (heart disease is low in Japan) and includes soybean products, noodles, rice, fish, and a variety of fruits and vegetables. Japanese cuisine is high in smoked, pickled, and salted foods. Deep-fried dishes such as tempura and salty soups and sauces should be used sparingly. Order broiled entrées or nonfried dishes made with tofu (a soybean curd protein), which has no cholesterol.

**Korean** The low-fat Korean dishes consist of rice, bulgogi (beef) and galbi (beef ribs), samgetang (small young whole chicken boiled in an individual pot with ginseng, an herb), kimchi (pickled cabbage), beef, fish, or vegetable soups, and fish including brims, eels, pollack, and cod. Sauces include bean paste and hot, soy, and sesame oil. Noodles and fermented yogurt are popular. Cooking methods are mainly boiling and steaming. The drink of choice is barley tea and milk, with yogurt added occasionally. Seasonal fruits include melons, plums, pears, and apples. Sesame, vegetable, cottonseed, and peanut oils are used to prepare Korean dishes.

**Latin American** In the Latin American diet, fruits, vegetables, beans, grains, and nuts are to be eaten at every meal, while fish and shellfish, plant oils, dairy, and poultry are to be eaten daily or less frequently. Eggs, meats, and sweets are to be eaten on occasion or in small quantities.

**Mexican** The traditional Mexican diet includes rice, beans, and corn, which are low in fat and high in nutrients. In America the dishes are less nutritious. For example, burritos (topped with cheese and sour cream) are high in fat. Guacamole, although it has a high fat content, is high in monounsaturated fatty acids (best form of fat). When dining in a Mexican restaurant, order cheese and sour cream on the side. Avoid refried beans (usually cooked in lard). Limit quesadillas, guacamole, and enchiladas. Better food choices include beans, rice, and shrimp or chicken tostadas on unfried cornmeal tortillas.

**Southeast Asian** The Southeast Asian diet is rich in a variety of fruits and vegetables (bok choy, bamboo shoots, cabbage, papayas, mangoes, and cucumbers). Fat is low because most foods are broiled or stir-fried. Coconut oil and milk (used in sauces) are high in fat. MSG and pickled foods increase the sodium content. Choose salads (larb is a chicken salad with mint) or seafood soup (po tak) at Thai or Vietnamese restaurants.

**Mediterranean** The Mediterranean diet depicted in Figure 9.9 is modeled after the typical eating pattern of men in the Mediterranean region around 1960. This population had notably low rates of diet-linked diseases and a longer life expectancy. Like the MyPyramid plan, this one recommends high consumption of complex carbohydrates and fruits and vegetables, legumes, nuts, and grains. Red meat (eaten a few times per month) is used mainly as a condiment, not as a main course, and fish, yogurt, and low-fat feta cheese are the predominant animal foods. It differs, however, in its recommendation of olive oil, which is high in monounsaturated fat and is suggested for use sparingly in MyPyramid. Another major difference is the recommendation: "Exercise daily, wine in moderation." The recognition of exercise is not debatable. Some researchers reported that wine's effect on blood platelets in men with heart disease differs according to whether they are eating a Mediterranean or a Western diet. Critics of the Mediterranean diet, however, believe that wine drinking could lead to alcohol abuse and liver damage and should not be encouraged. Proponents counter them by citing studies that show a glass or two of wine a day may prevent certain cardiovascular diseases. While the verdict is still out, the Greeks may have the best advice: moderation in all things.

## Tips for Action Nutrition and the College Student

- Shop with coupons and watch for specials.
- Shop at a discount warehouse food store.
- Plan meals, avoid extra trips to the store, and make a list and stay with it.
- Purchase fruits and vegetables in season (lower cost, higher nutrient quality, larger variety).
- Cook larger meals; freeze smaller portions.
- Drain off extra fat after cooking.

- Save leftovers for soups.
- Purchase meats and other products in volume, freezing portions for later.
- Purchase smaller portions of meats and combine them with plant proteins and beans (lower cost, calories, and fat).
- When visiting home during the weekend or on special holidays, ask for leftovers to take back to campus.

protein. Supplement meals with a small healthy snack such as carrots, an apple, or even a small sandwich on whole-grain bread that can be brought to class. If you must eat fast food, follow the tips in the section Fast Food and Junk Food for more ideas on eating healthy while eating out.

## FAST FOOD AND JUNK FOOD

The consumption of junk food is on the rise. Every day millions of people line up at or drive through the thousands of fast-food restaurants in the United States. Fast food has become a mainstay in the diets of children, adolescents, and college students. In fact, one in three children will eat fast food today. Not all fast foods are low in nutritional value, but most fast foods are high in total calories, fat, sugar, and salt and are low in nutrients and fiber. Three of the fastest-growing sales are hamburgers, french fries, and chicken nuggets. Fast-food restaurants are discontinuing low-fat items. The first to go was Taco Bell's Border Lights. Then McDonald's discontinued its much-advertised McLean Deluxe, which premiered five years earlier. Meanwhile, the new Pizza Hut Triple-Decker Pizza is selling like hotcakes. Restaurants have tried to promote lower-fat products, but they have failed miserably.

The fat content of many items is very high. For example, a McDonald's Sausage McMuffin with egg has 517 calories and 33 grams of fat, 13 grams from saturated fat. A Burger King Whopper with cheese contains 723 calories and 48 grams of fat, 18 grams from saturated fat. Because of the criticism of consumers and health professionals, many fast-food restaurants have added lighter menu items such as grilled chicken sandwiches on whole-grain buns, salads, and nonfat yogurt. Also, in response to public demand, these restaurants are reducing sodium, eliminating additives from fish breading, and removing MSG from sausages. At restaurants, you can request that your entrée be baked or broiled without fat and vegetables be steamed without salt or butter, or order appetizers and side dishes (soup, salad, or vegetables) instead of the usual entrée. Request low-fat salad dressing on the side or make your own dressing with vinegar and lemon juice.

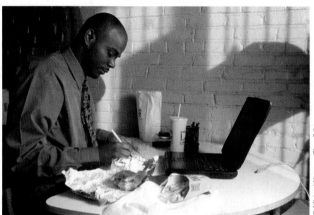

© Michael Newman/PhotoEdit

▲ *Fast food should be limited in your diet*

Consumers are still not eating more of the ever-increasing variety of nutritional low-fat foods on supermarket shelves. According to a study published in the *American Journal of Public Health* (2005), researchers found that three to four times as many fast-food restaurants were located within walking distance (approximately one mile) of a Chicago-area school as in other areas of the city.

## SUGGESTIONS

Rather than give up chocolate-chip cookies for fruits and vegetables, many people opt for low-fat brands such as Snackwell's and think this makes them health-conscious. Furthermore, they eat the whole box instead of three or four cookies. Sales of low-fat frozen dinners are flat.

Fast-food restaurants still offer lighter menu items such as salads, grilled chicken sandwiches, and nonfat yogurt. Many states require fast-food restaurants to post nutritional information about their foods. Making good food choices is difficult. Advertising claims are confusing, and it is difficult to sort out which to believe. Food can and should be pleasurable and satisfying. Making smart choices in foods will enable you to eat well and feel well. Tips for eating healthy at fast-food chains include:

**TABLE 9.12** ▶ Calories in Variations of Milk

| MILK (1 CUP) | CALORIES | GRAMS OF FAT | TOTAL CALORIES FROM FAT | PERCENT OF CALORIES FROM FAT |
|---|---|---|---|---|
| Whole milk (3.3%) | 150 | 8.5 | 76.5 | 76.5 ÷ 150 = 51 |
| 2% milk (low fat) | 120 | 4.7 | 42.3 | 42.3 ÷ 120 = 35 |
| 1% milk (low fat) | 100 | 0.5 | 4.5 | 4.5 ÷ 100 = 4.5 |
| Skim (nonfat) milk | 85 | 0.4 | 3.6 | 3.6 ÷ 85 = 4.2 |
| Nonfat buttermilk | 80 | Trace | Trace | Trace |
| Chocolate (2%) | 170 | 4 | 36 | 36 ÷ 170 = 21 |

—Ask fast-food chains for nutritional analysis of items.

—Order salads but watch the dressing you add. Try vinegar and oil or low-fat dressings. Stay away from eggs and other high-fat add-ons such as bacon bits.

—Order a salad rather than onion rings or french fries.

—Forgo junk foods such as sodas, chips, dips, candy, and cookies.

—Order a plain burger rather than a bacon cheeseburger.

—Eat whole-grain cereal with fruit and low-fat milk instead of an egg-and-sausage sandwich.

Now it is time for you to design your own goals for more nutritious choices; go to the websites listed at the end of this chaper for more information.

## DIETARY SUPPLEMENTS

The sales of dietary supplements in 2002 increased to nearly $20 billion with predictions that a rapid increase over the next decade would continue. Dietary supplements are usually vitamins and minerals taken by mouth and are intended to supplement existing diets. They come in capsule, liquid tablet, or other forms. Currently, there are no formal guidelines for their sale and safety, and supplement manufacturers are responsbile for self-monitoring their activities. The FDA is developing guidelines for their sale. Supplementing the diet may have significant health benefits for some people. For example, the U.S. Public Health Service recommended a vitamin supplement—folic acid—for all women of childbearing age. This vitamin may play a protective role in preventing birth defects and may help prevent cervical and other cancers by strengthening the chromosomes.

The *Journal of the American Medical Association* (JAMA) recommended that "a vitamin/mineral supplement a day just might be important in keeping the doctor away, particularly for some groups of people." The article indicated that vegans, elderly people, alcohol-dependent individuals, and patients with malabsorption problems may be at particular risk of deficiency of several vitamins. Even though the study acknowledged a possible risk of overdosing on fat-soluble vitamins, it noted that preliminary research has linked inadequate amounts of nutrients such as vitamins $B_6$, $B_{12}$, D, E, and lycopene to chronic diseases, including coronary heart disease, cancer, and osteoporosis. JAMA advised that all adults should take a basic multivitamin and there is no substitute for a well-balanced diet consisting of healthy meals. A multivitamin added to a balanced diet is likely to do more good than harm. Beware of megadoses, overdosing on ultravitamin supplements, and possible interactions of your supplement with any drugs you may be taking.

## VITAMINS AND MINERALS

According to the National Research Council's report *Diet and Health*, "The desirable way for the general public to obtain recommended levels of nutrients is by eating a variety of foods." The report also suggests several instances in which supplements may be appropriate. Those who might benefit from nutrient supplements include

■ Pregnant and breast-feeding women, who have hard-to-meet needs for nutrients such as folate, iron, and calcium

■ Women who have excessive menstrual bleeding (may need iron to help replenish iron stores lost in blood)

■ Individuals on very low calorie diets or strict vegetarian regimens, which often lack sufficient zinc, calcium, iron, and vitamin $B_{12}$

■ Individuals who have chronic illnesses or diseases or take medications that interfere with appetite or the way the body handles certain nutrients

■ People who smoke, drink a considerable amount of alcohol, or take drugs such as aspirin and oral contraceptives.

People at risk of heart attack, elderly people, and high-performance athletes may also need to take a supplement. African-Americans may not get enough vitamin D because their darker skin screens out the vitamin

## Tips for Action For Families

### Eat Right

1. Make half your grains whole. Choose whole-grain foods, such as whole-wheat bread, oatmeal, brown rice, and lowfat popcorn, more often.

2. Vary your veggies. Go dark green and orange with your vegetables—eat spinach, broccoli, carrots, and sweet potatoes.

3. Focus on fruits. Eat them at meals, and at snack time, too. Choose fresh, frozen, canned, or dried, and go easy on the fruit juice.

4. Get your calcium-rich foods. To build strong bones serve low-fat and fat-free milk and other milk products several times a day.

5. Go lean with protein. Eat lean or low-fat meat, chicken, turkey, and fish. Also, change your tune with more dry beans and peas. Add chickpeas, nuts, or seeds to a salad: pinto beans to a burrito; or kidney beans to soup.

6. Change your oil. We all need oil. Get yours from fish, nuts, and liquid oils such as corn, soybean, canola, and olive oil.

7. Don't sugarcoat it. Choose foods and beverages that do not have sugar and caloric sweeteners as one of the first ingredients. Added sugars contribute calories with few, if any, nutrients.

### Exercise

1. Set a good example. Be active and get your family to join you. Have fun together. Play with the kids or pets. Go for a walk, tumble in the leaves, or play catch.

2. Take the President's Challenge as a family. Track your individual physical activities together and earn awards for active lifestyles at www.presidentschallenge.org.

3. Establish a routine. Set aside time each day as activity time—walk, jog, skate, cycle, or swim. Adults need at least 30 minutes of physical activity most days of the week; children 60 minutes everyday or most days.

4. Have an activity party. Make the next birthday party centered on physical activity. Try backyard Olympics, or relay races. Have a bowling or skating party.

5. Set up a home gym. Use household items, such as canned foods, as weights. Stairs can substitute for stair machines.

6. Move it! Instead of sitting through TV commercials, get up and move. When you talk on the phone, lift weights or walk around. Remember to limit TV watching and computer time.

7. Give activity gifts. Give gifts that encourage physical activity—active games or sporting equipment.

---

D-activating property of sunlight. People who are taking supplements because of an illness or drug therapy should be under professional guidance because some vitamins and minerals counteract certain medications.

Maintaining a balance between vitamin and mineral supplements is necessary to lessen the chances of competition between the two. For example, a high amount of folate can hide the symptoms of a vitamin $B_{12}$ deficiency, and a high amount of copper can inhibit zinc absorption. The main consideration is to keep vitamin supplementation reasonable. Megadoses can be unhealthy.

## LIQUID SUPPLEMENTS

Whole foods have no substitute. Supplements such as Ensure, Boost, and Sustacal originally were designed for people too sick or weak to manage solid food and for obese people (especially diabetics) in doctor-supervised weight-loss programs.

Nutrament originally was targeted at athletes who wanted high-energy supplements. Now liquid meals such as Nutrament are being marketed aggressively to the general public. Most people do not need them, even though they constitute healthier snacks than a bag of chips or a candy bar.

Liquid nutritional supplements are simply skim milk, water, sugars, vegetable oil, thickeners, and flavoring agents, plus added vitamins and minerals. Claims of these supplements include the following.

- "Energy drink"—"Energy" simply means calories. The drinks have anywhere from 200 to 360 calories per can.

- "Low-fat"—Most are relatively low in fat, but a few have 9 or more grams per cup.

- "High-protein"—Each can (8 to 12 ounces) contains 10 to 16 grams of protein, compared with 8 grams in a cup of milk. The average person usually gets more than enough protein, and protein by itself will not build muscle.

- "Complete nutrition"—A can typically supplies 15% to 50% of most vitamins and minerals. Most brands contain no fiber (though one or two do contain some added fiber).

- "Easy and convenient"—Grabbing a cup of low-fat yogurt, fruit juice, or a banana is just as easy.

**FIGURE 9.14 ▶** Food Pyramid for Kids

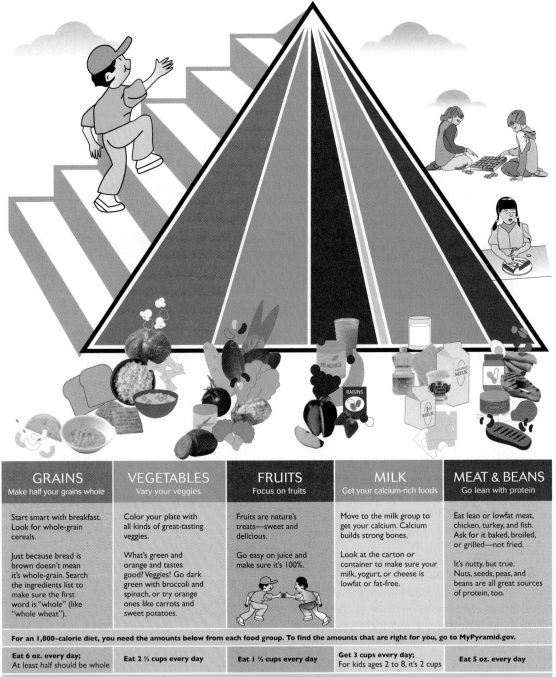

| GRAINS | VEGETABLES | FRUITS | MILK | MEAT & BEANS |
|---|---|---|---|---|
| Make half your grains whole | Vary your veggies | Focus on fruits | Get your calcium-rich foods | Go lean with protein |
| Start smart with breakfast. Look for whole-grain cereals. Just because bread is brown doesn't mean it's whole-grain. Search the ingredients list to make sure the first word is "whole" (like "whole wheat"). | Color your plate with all kinds of great-tasting veggies. What's green and orange and tastes good? Veggies! Go dark green with broccoli and spinach, or try orange ones like carrots and sweet potatoes. | Fruits are nature's treats—sweet and delicious. Go easy on juice and make sure it's 100%.  | Move to the milk group to get your calcium. Calcium builds strong bones. Look at the carton or container to make sure your milk, yogurt, or cheese is lowfat or fat-free. | Eat lean or lowfat meat, chicken, turkey, and fish. Ask for it baked, broiled, or grilled—not fried. It's nutty, but true. Nuts, seeds, peas, and beans are all great sources of protein, too. |

**For an 1,800-calorie diet, you need the amounts below from each food group. To find the amounts that are right for you, go to MyPyramid.gov.**

| Eat 6 oz. every day; At least half should be whole | Eat 2 ½ cups every day | Eat 1 ½ cups every day | Get 3 cups every day; For kids ages 2 to 8, it's 2 cups | Eat 5 oz. every day |
|---|---|---|---|---|

**Oils**  Oils are not a food group, but you need some for good health. Get your oils from fish, nuts, and liquid oils such as corn oil, soybean oil, and canola oil.

**Find your balance between food and fun**
- Move more. Aim for at least 60 minutes everyday, or most days.
- Walk, dance, bike, rollerblade—it all counts. How great is that!

**Facts and sugars—know your limits**
- Get your fat facts and sugar smarts from the Nutrition Facts label.
- Limit solid fats as well as foods that contain them.
- Choose food and beverages low in added sugars and other caloric sweeteners.

*Note:* Graphic depicts daily servings for two- to six-year-olds as recommended by the U.S. Department of Agriculture.

- "Delicious"—Individuals may be able to find a brand or flavor they like, but most will find the drinks overly sweet and oily and sometimes medicinal tasting.

- "Doctor-recommended"—Doctors may recommend these drinks if the person is in a hospital and cannot eat enough food, has AIDS, or is undergoing chemotherapy. Rarely are they recommended for other people.

If you do take supplements, there are several things to keep in mind.

- Notice the expiration date and buy ones that will last a while.
- Keep them in a cool, dark, dry place, such as the refrigerator.
- Buy vitamin C separately. Multivitamins containing large doses of vitamin C usually are expensive.
- Check to be certain that multivitamins contain folic acid.
- Select a supplement that does not contain additives.

> **VIEWPOINT** *While taking some vitamin and mineral supplements is encouraged, most do not seem to provide additional benefits for healthy people who eat a balanced diet. They do not help people run faster, jump higher, relieve stress, improve social prowess, cure the common cold, or boost energy levels. Are vitamin and mineral supplements right for you?*

## FOOD ADDITIVES AND FOOD ALLERGIES

Today, more than 2,800 substances are added to foods to improve their nutritional quality, maintain freshness, aid in processing or preparation, or alter the taste or appearance. The average American consumes approximately 160 pounds of food additives per year: 140 pounds of sweeteners, 15 pounds of table salt, and 5 to 10 pounds of other additives. The most widely used additives are sugar, salt, and corn syrup. Others include citric acid, baking soda, vegetable colors, mustard, and pepper.

If the additive is known to cause cancer in animals, the FDA will not approve it in foods for humans. Negative health consequences from food additives are minimal for people who eat sensibly.

Additives can enhance nutrient value. For example, milk is fortified with vitamin D, folate is added to grain products, and meats are cured with nitrates to reduce the risk of food-borne illness.

Monosodium glutamate is a flavor enhancer that has met with claims of severe, even life-threatening, reactions. MSG consists of about 12% sodium and 78% glutamic acid and occurs naturally in some foods.

Asian cooks have used MSG for centuries. It can be extracted from seaweed, but today it usually is fermented from molasses, sugar beets, or sugar cane. It is fairly flavorless until it is added to foods. Certain foods such as tomatoes, parmesan cheese, and soy sauce contain a considerable amount of natural glutamate. MSG can produce in some people a combination of unpleasant but temporary symptoms such as headache, nausea, drowsiness, weakness, and burning sensations. Asthmatics may incur breathing difficulties.

The FDA is preparing new labeling regulations for foods containing a significant amount of free glutamate for people with severe asthma. Avoiding free glutamate entirely would be difficult; it is present in all types of foods, such as peas, chicken, soy, corn, milk, and tomatoes. Hydrolyzed vegetable protein (from soy, wheat, or corn) also is high in free glutamate; therefore, it also must be listed on labels. Sulfites, used to prevent browning, can produce severe, even fatal, allergic reactions in some individuals. Therefore, the FDA has required the labeling of sulfites in packaged foods and has banned the use of sulfites on fresh fruits and vegetables (including those in salad bars). Nitrates used in sausages, bacon, and luncheon meats to delay spoilage, prevent botulism, and add color can react with substances in your body or in the food to form cancer-causing agents known as nitrosamines. Nitrates have been reduced in foods by the food industry but can be dangerous to some individuals. Indirect food additives are substances that inadvertently get into food products from handling or packaging. For example, dioxins are found in coffee filters, frozen foods,

**TABLE 9.13 ▶** Food Additives

| | |
|---|---|
| Antimicrobial agents | Substances such as salt, sugar, nitrates, and others that tend to make foods less hospitable for microbes |
| Antioxidants | Preserve color and flavor by reducing loss due to exposure to oxygen. Vitamins C and E are among those antioxidants believed to play a role in reduced cancer and cardiovascular disease. Additives BHA and BHT are also antioxidants |
| Artificial colors, nutrient additives, and flavor enhancers | MSC (monosodium glutamate) salt, mustard, pepper, vegetable colors |
| Sulfites | Used to preserve vegetable color; some people have severe allergic reactions to them |
| Dioxins | Coffee filters, milk container, and frozen foods |
| Methylene chloride | Decaffeinated coffee |
| Hormones | Bovine growth hormone (BGH) found in animal meat |

## Tips for Action When Eating Out

- Select plain scrambled eggs, pancakes without butter or syrup, or English muffins.

- Select plain hamburgers (no cheese) or roast beef (leaner than hamburger, lower in fat and calories). Skip the mayonnaise (and save 100–150 calories), bacon, and cheese (save 200 calories from saturated fat and cholesterol).

- Avoid fried foods, foods prepared with sauces, gravies, or sauteed in butter. Avoid fried chicken and processed chicken, which contains fatty, ground-up skin. Be cautious of fish sandwiches (trapped oil in breading) and creamy tartar sauce (high in fat and calories).

- Request unsalted items.

- Include dairy products for additional calcium.

- Include fresh fruits and vegetables for vitamins A, C, and fiber.

- Eat a baked potato instead of french fries, and skip toppings made with sour cream, melted cheese, or butter.

- At the salad bar be cautious of mayonnaise, oily vegetable salads, and rich dressings. Get salad dressing on the side. Use low-calorie dressing in moderation (two small ladles can contain nearly as much fat as a large burger, even though the fat is largely unsaturated). At home, make your own salad dressing using lemon juice or vinegar as basic ingredients.

- Avoid frosted desserts and cakes. Choose fruit or sherbet.

---

and milk containers; methylene chloride, in decaffeinated coffee; and hormones, including bovine growth hormone (BGH), in animal meat.

Approximately 12% to 20% of adults have some type of food allergy, or hypersensitivity, an adverse reaction to a particular food. Women are more likely to report hypersensitivity or food allergies than men. Food allergies occur when a person's body views a specific food (usually a protein) as a threat or an invader. Symptoms may include vomiting, diarrhea, headaches, sneezing, rash or hives, rapid heartbeat, or dizziness. Symptoms may vary and not develop for up to 72 hours, making it difficult to identify the particular food causing the allergy. Researchers disagree about which foods may trigger allergies. Common foods include eggs, peanuts, soybeans, tree nuts (walnuts), seeds, seafood (shrimp, crayfish, lobster, crab, fish, shellfish), wheat, chocolate, and cow's milk. With children, food allergens that cause the most problems are milk, eggs, and peanuts. Avoid the food causing your allergy once you have identified it. Refer to a physician with specialized training in allergy diagnosis if you think you have a food allergy.

> **VIEWPOINT** *How many times per week do you eat out at a fast-food restaurant? What types of fast foods do you eat? Junk foods? What foods could you have selected from MyPyramid that would have cost you less and been healthier? Approximately how much money did you spend during the week while eating out? Approximately how much could you have saved if you prepared the meals at home?*

## FOOD INTOXICATION

The World Health Organization describes food as "the major source of exposure to disease-causing agents—biological and chemical—from which no one in either the developing or developed countries is spared." Food-borne infections usually produce vomiting, diarrhea, and nausea from 12 hours to five days after infection. The symptoms depend on the microorganism and the person's overall health. It can be fatal to those individuals who are not in good health or whose immune systems are impaired (see Table 9.14).

The Centers for Disease Control and Prevention (CDC) estimates 40,000 reported cases of *Salmonella* poisoning a year. *Salmonella* is a bacterium that contaminates many foods such as undercooked chicken, eggs, and sometimes processed meat. Eating these foods may result in *Salmonella* poisoning, which causes diarrhea and vomiting.

Another bacterium, *Campylobacter jejuni*, may cause more stomach infections than *Salmonella*. This bacterium is found in milk, water, and some foods. It causes severe diarrhea and has been implicated in the growth of stomach ulcers.

*Staphylococcus* is a bacterium that can produce toxins in food. When cooked foods are cross-contaminated with the bacteria from raw foods and not stored properly, staph infections can result, causing nausea and abdominal pain from 30 minutes to eight hours after ingestion.

The FDA has urged consumers to avoid eating raw sprouts because of the risk of illness. Sprouts, alfalfa, and clover can be contaminated by *Salmonella* or *E. coli* bacteria, which can cause nausea, diarrhea, and cramping in healthy adults. Children and seniors can experience serious symptoms that lead to kidney failure and compromised immune systems.

**TABLE 9.14 ▶** Food-Borne Illness

| | SOURCE | SYMPTOMS | ONSET | PREVENTION |
|---|---|---|---|---|
| **Bacterial** | | | | |
| *Campylobacter jejuni* | Meat or milk from poultry, cattle, and sheep | Diarrhea, abdominal cramping, fever and bloody stools | Two to five days | Cook foods thoroughly; drink pasteurized milk |
| *Escherichia coli (E. coli)* | Water, raw or undercooked meat, and cross-contaminated foods | Watery or bloody diarrhea, abdominal cramps, or vomiting | 10 to 72 hours | Cook foods thoroughly; wash hands well |
| *Listeria* | Deli meats, hot dogs, soft cheese, raw meat, and unpasteurized milk | Headache, fever, and nausea | 24 hours to 12 days | Cook meats thoroughly; buy pasteurized milk; wash hands well |
| *Salmonella* | Raw or undercooked meat, poultry, or eggs, and unpasteurized milk | Fever, muscle aches, nausea, abdominal cramps, diarrhea, fever, and headache | Five hours to four days | Cook meats and leftovers thoroughly; wash hands well |
| *Staphylococcus aureus* | Food left too long at room temperature, including meat, poultry, or egg products, tuna, potato salad, and cream-filled pastries. Unlike other bacteria, staphylococci grow well in foods that are high in sugar or salt; any food can be contaminated by infected food handlers | Vomiting, nausea, diarrhea, abdominal pain, and cramps | 30 minutes to eight hours | Cook foods thoroughly; refrigerate leftovers immediately; wash your hands before and after handling food |
| **Nonbacterial** | | | | |
| Hepatitis A virus | Oysters, clams, mussels, or scallops that come from waters polluted with untreated sewage, and improper food handling with unwashed hands | Weakness, appetite loss, nausea, vomiting, and fever; jaundice may develop | 15 to 50 days | Buy seafood from reputable markets; wash hands well |
| *Trichinella spiralis* | Raw or undercooked pork or carnivorous animals | Muscle pain, swollen eyelids, and/or fever; can be fatal | Eight to 15 days | Cook meat thoroughly |

Botulism caused by the *Clostridium botulinum* organism can be a fatal form of food poisoning. Improper home-canning procedures are the most common cause of this potentially fatal problem.

*Listeria*, commonly found in deli meats, hot dogs, soft cheese, raw meat, and unpasteurized milk, can be life-threatening. It is of greatest risk to pregnant women, infants, and those with weakened immune systems. Decrease your risk by cooking meats and leftovers and washing everthing that may come into contact with raw meat.

Verotoxigenic *E. coli* or VTEC is commonly known as the barbecue syndrome. Consumers report that they consumed ground beef hamburgers prior to getting ill. Other kinds of undercooked meat and poultry, as well as drinking unpasteurized milk or unchlorinated water are also dangerous. Symptoms ranging from mild to life-threatening usually develop within two to 10 days and include severe stomach cramps, mild fever, and vomiting. Recovery is usually within seven to 10 days. Proper handling and cooking food thoroughly can practically eliminate hamburger disease. More than 30% of food-borne illness results from unsafe handling of food at home.

Steps to protect yourself from food poisoning include:

—Wash hands by scrubbing together vigorously for 10–15 seconds with liquid or clean bar soap and hot water before handling food.
—Wash countertop/cutting boards with soap and hot water particularly after handling meat, fish, or poultry.
—Wipe spills immediately. Do not allow liquids to touch or drip onto other items such as surfaces, other foods, and utensils during shopping, in the refrigerator, or during preparation.
—When preparing fresh fruits and vegetables, discard outer leaves, wash under running water, and scrub when possible with a clean brush or hands. Do not wash meat or poultry.

■
**KEY TERMS**

**Food intoxication** a kind of food poisoning in which a food is contaminated by natural toxins or by microbes that produce toxins.

## Tips for Action Supermarket Shopping Suggestions

- Take your time in reading the labels.
- Make a shopping list so you will buy only items you need.
- Shop early in the morning or whenever the store has the fewest people.
- Never shop on an empty stomach. You will purchase more junk foods when you are hungry.
- For healthy shopping, look high and look low. The healthiest and least expensive foods are placed on the top and bottom shelves. Less healthful and more expensive foods often are positioned at eye level.
- Shop around the perimeter of the store, where fresh produce and dairy products generally are located.

Processed and packaged foods usually are displayed in the inner aisles.

- Check sell-by and use-by dates on packages. Purchase products with the most distant date, which usually are located in the back of the shelf.
- Avoid wilted vegetables and bruised fruits, even if they are less expensive. This produce does not contain as much nutritional value as fresh produce.
- Select refrigerated and frozen food and hot deli items last—right before checkout.
- Select fresh or frozen produce, and shop twice a week for the former, as it loses nutritional value quickly. Avoid prepackaged fruits and vegetables.

## FYI  FOOD ALLERGIES

Many people who believe they are allergic to certain foods do not have a true food allergy. In an allergic reaction the body erroneously reacts to a harmless substance and produces histamines, which evoke the symptoms of an allergy. The most common symptoms are rash or hives, swelling body parts, and nausea and vomiting. In the most severe cases, if untreated, disruption of normal breathing and heartbeat can lead to death. The foods that most commonly provoke an allergic reaction are soybeans, shellfish, legumes (beans), wheat, and milk.

—Throw out leftovers stored for 3–4 days and regularly clean your refrigerator.
—Never thaw frozen foods at room temperature.
—Never leave cooked food standing on the stove or table for more than two hours.
—Keep hot foods hot (140°F or above) and cold foods cold (40°F or below).
—When shopping for fish, buy from markets that get their supplies from state-approved sources. Cleanliness at the salad bar and meat and fish counters should be checked.
—Fish is done when the thickest part becomes opaque and the fish flakes easily when poked with a fork.
—When freezing food such as chicken, make sure juices can't spill over into ice cubes or into other areas of the refrigerator.

—A meat thermometer should be used so that meats are completely cooked to kill bacteria.
—Use different cutting boards for raw meat and poultry, produce, and ready-to-eat foods. Keep all boards thoroughly clean.

## PESTICIDES AND IRRADIATION

Commercial pesticides save billions of dollars of valuable crops from pests, but they also may endanger human health and life. Plants and animals naturally produce compounds that act as pesticides to aid in their survival, and the vast majority of the pesticides consumed are natural, not added by farmers or food processors. Since there may be risk in pesticides, consumers are purchasing organic foods (see the section Organic Foods).

**Food irradiation** is the use of radiation, either from radioactive substances or from devices that produce x-rays, on food. The food is not radioactive, but irradiation's primary benefit is to prolong the shelf life of food. Irradiation can kill all the microorganisms that might grow in a food, and the sterilized food can be stored for years in sealed containers at room temperature without spoiling. Safety concerns have been raised by environmentalists and consumer groups; and although the data do not conclusively show that irradiated foods are safe to eat, the facts appear to support the use of irradiation. Foods that are irradiated include fruits, vegetables, dried spices, meat and poultry, and some prepackaged foods. Look for the food irradiation symbol to know if food has undergone this process.

## ORGANIC FOODS

The term organic refers to foods produced without the use of commercial chemicals at any stage. As of 2002, foods sold as organic has to meet criteria set by the USDA under the

**FIGURE 9.15 ►** USDA Label for Certified
Organic Foods

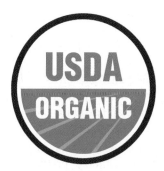

National Organic Rule and can carry a new USDA seal verifying products as "certified organic" (Figure 9.15). Under this rule, something that is certified may carry one of the following terms: 100% Organic (100% compliance with organic criteria), Organic (must contain at least 95% organic materials), Made with Organic Ingredients (must contain at least 70% organic ingredients), or Some Organic Ingredients (contains less than 70% organic ingredients (usually listed individually). In order to use any of the above terms, the foods must be produced without hormones, antibiotics, herbicides, insecticides, chemical fertilizers, genetic modification, or germ-killing radiation. The food that you buy at a grocery or health-food store is not guaranteed to be more nutritious than other produce. But buying organic foods is the only way to have a healthier environment.

## GENETICALLY MODIFIED FOODS

Scientists, farmers, and breeders have been for years modifying the genetic makeup of plants and animals to breed organisms with desirable traits, a process known as selective breeding. Selective breeding is an old technology, slow and imprecise when compared to modern techniques. Using biotechnology to produce **genetically modifed (GM) organisms** is a faster and more refined process. Genetic modification involves the addition, deletion, or reorganization of an organism's genes in order to change the organism's protein production. Research on genetic modification in agriculture has focused on three areas:

—new strains of crops and animals with improved resistance to disease and pests (corn plants that resist blights)

—strains of microorganisms that produce specific substances that occur in small amounts or not at all in nature (bovine somatotropin, a growth hormone used in cattle to produce more meat)

—crops that resist destruction by herbicides (soybean plants that can survive herbicides used to kill weeds). Sixty percent of processed foods currently sold in supermarkets contain one or more GM ingredients.

The safety of food products produced by biotechnology is assessed by the FDA's new National Center for Food Safety and Technology. As of this date, the center has held that GM foods do not require any special safety testing, nor do they have to be labeled as GM foods, unless they differ significantly from foods already in use. Consumer advocacy groups have called for all foods containing GM ingredients to be labeled. One concern is that genetic material added to a food could cause allergic reactions (genes from peanuts added to GM soybeans, for example). Also, people with religious objections to certain foods might unknowingly consume them in GM foods (a person maintaining a kosher kitchen might purchase a food containing genes normally found in pork). The American Dietetic Association and various scientific organizations support the FDA position on GM foods, citing the potential benefits.

## NUTRITION FRAUD

U.S. representative Claude Pepper defined a quack as "anyone who promotes medical schemes or remedies known to be false, or which are unproven, for a profit." People with chronic or life-threatening diseases (such as AIDS, cancer, and arthritis), elderly people, and young parents are favored targets. If the promises of a nutritional claim sound too good to be true—they probably are.

Consumers should ask questions such as the following:

■ What are your credentials and professional association for you to give nutritional advice? (Check these credentials with your local chapter of the American Dietetic Association to see if they are legitimate.)

■ Can you supply data from controlled scientific studies to support your claims?

Responses that should make one suspicious include the following.

■ Use of unfamiliar credentials and degrees such as D.M. (doctor of metaphysics); neither does M.D. nor Ph.D. automatically confer legitimacy

■ Certification or accreditation from unfamiliar (often nonexistent) or mail-order institutions

■ Use of discredited tests such as hair analysis or computerized questionnaires to diagnose nutritional deficiencies

■ Promotion of books or pamphlets tied to exclusive products available only from the author or self-styled nutritionist

### KEY TERMS

**Food irradiation** process that exposes food to gamma rays to destroy contaminants

**Genetically modified (GM) organisms** organisms whose genetic makeup has been changed to produce desirable traits.

- Nutritional products and treatments not endorsed by registered dietitians and physicians trained in nutrition science

## Summary

- The two major types of nutrients are the energy nutrients (carbohydrates, fats, and proteins) and the regulatory nutrients (water, vitamins, and minerals).

- The process of digestion begins when the food enters the mouth. Then the food moves through the esophagus to the stomach, small and large intestines, and exits through the rectum and anus.

- Dietary fats are either saturated fats (animal products, coconut oil, palm oil, palm kernel oil) or unsaturated fats (which are separated further into monounsaturated and polyunsaturated fats).

- Lipoproteins (fats combined with protein) are low-density lipoprotein (LDL, or bad cholesterol) and high-density lipoprotein (HDL, or good cholesterol).

- Complete proteins (usually from animal sources) contain the nine essential amino acids; incomplete proteins (from vegetable sources) contain only some of the essential amino acids.

- Water is the most important nutrient, as it is needed in all bodily functions. Without it, the individual will die in less than a week.

- Vitamins are of two major types: fat-soluble (associated with lipids) and water-soluble (cannot be stored long in the body).

- Some essential minerals that the body needs daily are calcium, iron, and sodium (salt).

- MyPyramid is the standard that replaced the Food Guide Pyramid.

- The Mediterranean Diet Pyramid recommends high consumption of complex carbohydrates, fruits, and vegetables.

- The styles of vegetarians (plant food eaters) are lacto-vegetarian, lacto-ovo-vegetarian, vegan, and partial—semivegetarians or pesco-vegetarians—based on whether dairy products and eggs are included.

- Men and women have different nutritional needs because their hormones, body size, and body composition are different.

- College students find it difficult to eat nutritionally in the dorm or in their apartment because funds are limited and preparing food is time-consuming.

- Some people need vitamin and mineral supplements for specific purposes, but a balanced nutritional diet should preclude a blanket recommendation for supplementation.

- Food substitutes and additives should be used advisedly. Also, people should be on the alert for nutrition fraud.

- Food-borne illness, food allergies, and food safety are important to prevent problems as part of a sound nutritional plan.

- Fast foods and junk foods are generally unhealthy. Wise health consumers choose nutritional foods in any marketplace and restaurant.

- Like the American menu, all ethnic foods include good and poor choices, usually based on the fat and salt content and method of preparation.

- Using biotechnology to produce genetically modified (GM) organisms is a faster and more refined process in producing foods.

- Fraud and quackery are rampant in nutrition. People should be alert to schemes that seem too good to be true.

## Personal Health Resources

**ThomsonNOW** Visit the ThomsonNOW website at http://thomsonedu.com/thomsonnow for valuable resources that will:

- Help you evaluate your knowledge of the material.

- Guide you through tutorials to help you understand and apply the material.

- Allow you to take an exam-prep quiz to better prepare for class tests.

**CyberDiet's Eating Out Guidelines.** This site includes information on healthy food selections from the following cuisines: China, France, Greece, India, Italy, Japan, Mexico, Thailand, and the United States.

**www.CyberDiet.com/foodfact/eatguide.html**

**Cyberkitchen.** This site helps you discover how much you are really eating with an activity on comparing standard serving sizes versus real serving sizes. It also provides personal information regarding your age, gender, height, weight, and activity level, and provides you with a healthy diet plan to meet your weight management goals.

**www.nhlbi.nih.gov/chd/Tipsheets/cyberkit.htm**

**Diet Analysis Website.** With this site you may receive a complete nutritional review of your diet based on the Recommended Dietary Allowances and your age and gender.

**www.dawp.anet.com/cgi-bin-w3-msql-dawp.html**

**Nutrition Quizzes.** Test yourself on vitamins and safe foods, rate your diet, or take the "Fat or Fiction" Nutrition Action Fat Quiz. These tests are sponsored by the Center for Science in the Public Interest.

**www.cspinet.org/quiz**

**Ask the Dietitian.** This site provides information from a registered dietitian. Topics include vitamins, food supplements, fast food, fiber and constipation, junk foods, food safety, diets, sports nutrition, and tips on how to spot nutrition quackery.

**www.dietitian.com**

**Dietary Guidelines from the Food and Nutrition Information Center.** This site features the 2005 American Dietary Guidelines and has links to historical dietary guidelines and dietary guidelines from 20 countries.

**www.nal.usda.gov/fnic/dga/index.html**

**USDA Center for Nutrition Policy and Promotion.** This site features the Interactive Health Eating Index, an online dietary assessment that enables you to receive, on a daily basis, a personalized score on the overall quality of your diet, total fat, cholesterol, sodium, and other nutrients.

**www.usda.gov/cnpp/**

**Dietary Supplements.** This site includes information from the Food and Drug Administration Center for Food Safety and Applied Nutrition.

**www.vm.cfsan.fda.gov/-dms/supplmnt.htm/**

**Fast Food Finder.** A selection of fast-food items from numerous chain restaurants with information regarding food calories, cholesterol, sodium, and fat content.

**www.olen.com/food**

**MyPyramid.** Offers personalized recommendations of the kinds and amounts of food to eat each day, tips and ideas for achieving a healthy diet, and interactive assessments based on an individual's gender, age, and activity level.

**www. mypyramid.gov**

**InfoTrac College Edition Activities.** An online library of more than 900 journals and publications. Follow the instructions for accessing InfoTrac College Edition that were packaged with your textbook; then search for articles using a keyword search. For additional links, resources, and suggested readings on the InfoTrac College Edition, visit our Health and Wellness Resource Center at www. health.wadsworth.com.

## It's Your Turn For Study and Review

1. What are the major food groups on the MyPyramid system? Which group is the most difficult to prepare? The least? What actions can you take as a college student to increase or decrease your intake of these groups? What problems have you encountered?

2. How did you and your family eat when you were growing up? Did your diet consist mainly of dairy products and red meats? Today, do you follow approximately the same diet as you did when you were young?

3. Discuss the types of vegetarians. What are some health benefits and risks from these alternative diets?

4. Discuss the three essential energy nutrients. What is their purpose?

5. Discuss the major regulatory nutrients. What is their purpose?

6. Do you take vitamin supplements? If so, which ones? What is your purpose of taking these supplements?

7. When eating out, which foods do you mostly likely choose? Least likely? Why?

8. Do you often eat different ethnic foods? Which ethnic diet do you think would be the simplest to prepare? Which one has the most nutritional food choices?

9. What are the major risks for food-borne illnesses, and what steps can you take to protect yourself?

10. After reading this chapter, are you planning to take action to make sure your nutritional intake is sufficient? What actions will you take?

## Thinking about Health Issues

■ Are vitamins necessary as a dietary supplement?

Martha Miller, "Getting Your Vitamins," *Better Homes and Gardens*, February 2001, p. 206.

1. What is the recommendation of nutrition researchers about taking vitamins and dietary supplements of antioxidants? Why?

2. What is the controversy concerning antioxidants and the prevention of cancer and heart disease?

## Selected Bibliography

"American Heart Association Position Statement," 2005, www.americanheart.org.

American Medical Association, "Diagnosis and Management of Foodborne Illness: A Primer for Physicians and Other Health Care Professionals," 2004, www.ama-assn.org/ama/org.

Applegate, L. "Ethnic Food Options." *Runner's World*, October 1992, pp. 26–29.

Applegate, L. "Liquid Energy." *Runner's World*, July 2001, pp. 24–26.

Black, B. "Healthgate: Just How Much Food Is on the Plate? Understanding Portion Control," 2004, www.community. healthgate.com/getcontent.asp?siteid=contentupdate&docid=/healthy.

Centers for Disease Control and Prevention, "Behavioral Risk Factor Surveillance System," 2004, www.cdc.gov.

Centers for Disease Control and Prevention, "Food Borne Illnesses," 2002, www.cdc.gov.

Clark, N. "Fats Facts and Fads," *Runner's World*, July 27, 2005.

Department of Health and Human Services and the Department of Agriculture, "Dietary Guidelines for American Government 2005," Washington, DC: Government Printing Office.

Floyd, P. A., and Parke, J. E. *Walk, Jog, Run for Wellness Everyone*, 5th ed. Winston-Salem, NC: Hunter Textbooks, 2006.

Hales, D. *An Invitation to Health*, 12th ed. Belmont, CA: Wadsworth, 2007.

Hasler, C. M., et al. "Position Statement of the American Dietetic Association: Functional Foods," *Journal of the American Dietetic Association*, 104:5, 2004, pp. 814–818.

Hoeger, W. W. K., and Hoeger, S. A. *Principles and Labs for Physical Fitness*, 3rd ed. Belmont, CA: Wadsworth, 2002.

Institute of Medicine, "Dietary Reference Intake for Water, Potassium, Sodium, Chloride, and Sulfate," March 4, 2004, www.nap.edu.

Lowrey, L. "Dietary Fat and Sports Nutrition: A Primer," *Journal of Sports Science and Medicine*, 3, 2004, pp. 106–107.

MUFAs and PUFAs. *Food and Fitness Advisor*, September 2002, www.foodandfitnessadvisor.com.

National Institute of Allergy and Infectious Diseases, "Fact Sheet: Food Allergy and Intolerances," 2002, www.niaid.nih.gov/

Pereira, M., et al. "Dietary Fiber and Risk of Coronary Heart Disease: A Pooled Analysis of Cohort Studies," *Archives of Internal Medicine*, 164:4, 2004, pp. 370–376.

Pinkowish, M. "Effects of the Mediterranean Diet in MI Prevention." *Patient Care*, 33, 1999, p. 7.

Sandler, R. "Gastrointestinal Symptoms in 3,181 Volunteers Ingesting Snack Foods Containing Olestra or Triglycerides: A 6-Week Randomized, Placebo-Controlled Trial." *Journal of the American Medical Association*, 281, 1999, p. 20.

Schulz, M. and Hu, F. "Primary Prevention of Diabetes: What Can Be Done and How Much Can Be Prevented?" *Annual Review of Public Health*, 26, 2005, pp. 445–467.

"Special Report: Irradiation Plants Geared to 'Zap' Meat and Poultry—Is It Safe?" *Tufts University Health and Nutrition Letter*, 18:1, 2000, pp. 4–7.

Thompson, J. and Manore, M. Nutrition: *An Applied Approach*. San Francisco: Benjamin Cummings, 2005, pp. 36–38.

United States Department of Agriculture, "Johanns Reveals USDA's Steps to a Healthier You," Press Release, April 19, 2005.

World Health Organization, "Micronutrient Deficiencies: Battling Iron Deficiency Anemia, 2003," August 2005, www.who.int.

Young, G. and Conquer, J. "Omega-3 Fatty Acids and Neuropsychiatric Disorders," *Reproduction Nutrition Development*, 45, 2005, pp. 1–28.

Name _____    Course _____

Date _____    Section _____

MyPyramid will help you focus on the necessary nutrients you need daily in your diet. Fill in the appropriate space of each of the categories.

# Self Assessment 9.2 Healthy Nutrition Analysis

Name _____     Course _____

Date _____     Section _____

MyPyramid provides a general outline of what to eat each day for a healthful diet. The pyramid suggests eating a variety of foods to get the required nutrients your body needs and to get the right amount of calories to maintain a healthy weight. Your choice of foods within each of the recommended groups of the MyPyramid are factors to consider when evaluating your nutrition dietary habits. This lab will assist you in evaluating your dietary habits. Answer the following question with "yes" (Y) or "no" (N). A "no" answer indicates a behavior you should consider changing.

_____ **1.** I eat a wide variety of foods each day.

_____ **2.** I read food labels carefully when shopping for groceries.

_____ **3.** I have a minimum of two cups of the fruit group each day.

_____ **4.** I have a minimum of 2½ cups of the vegetable group each day.

_____ **5.** I have a minimum of 3 cups of the milk, yogurt, and cheese group each day.

_____ **6.** I have a minimum of 5½ ounces of the meat, poultry, fish, dry beans, eggs, and nuts group each day.

_____ **7.** I select whole-grain breads instead of white breads.

_____ **8.** I steam vegetables; I do not boil them.

_____ **9.** I remove the skin and fat before cooking meat, poultry, or fish.

_____ **10.** I broil, boil, or bake, instead of fry, the meat, fish, and poultry that I eat.

_____ **11.** I eat cereals that are high in fiber.

_____ **12.** I eat crackers, bread, cereals, and foods that are low in fat and added sugar.

_____ **13.** I eat fresh fruits and vegetables instead of canned when at all possible.

_____ **14.** I choose nonfat or low-fat milk and milk products.

_____ **15.** I choose foods often that are unprocessed.

_____ **16.** I cook with vegetable oil instead of margarine or butter.

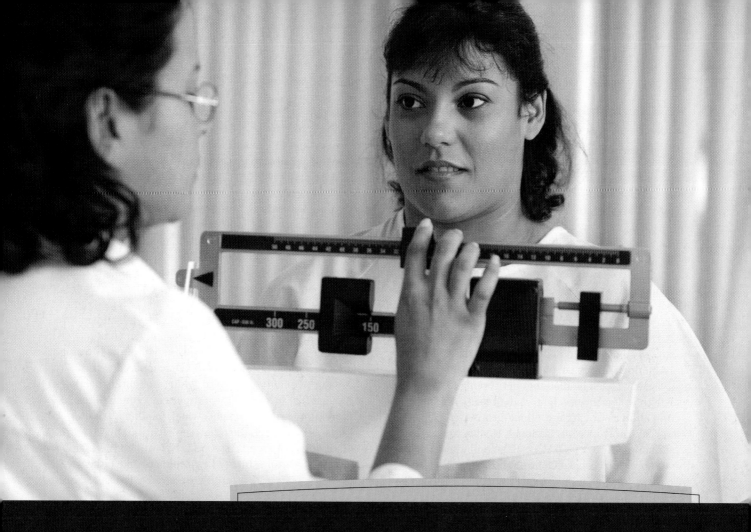

# Chapter Ten Weight Management

**OBJECTIVES** ■ Explain body composition and metabolic rate.
■ Differentiate overweight and obesity, and describe their relationship
to major health problems. ■ Explain three unhealthy eating disorders
and the differences between them. ■ Identify three aids to determine
if you are overweight or underweight. ■ Describe three methods for
assessing body composition. ■ Assess various approaches to weight
loss. ■ Explain the most effective strategies for losing weight.

ThomsonNOW™  Log on to ThomsonNOW at http://thomsonedu.com/
thomsonnow to access and explore self-assessments, interactive
tutorials, and practice quizzes.

The basic premise of weight management is

- Calories in = calories out (weight maintenance)
- Calories in > calories out (weight gain)
- Calories in < calories out (weight loss)

Many underweight Americans wish to gain weight while others are constantly seeking means to lose those unwanted pounds. The ultimate message within this chapter is that life is an all-you-can-eat buffet. It is important to "eat to live" and not "live to eat," therefore enjoying each and every moment that life shares with us to make our lives healthier and more stress free. Some of you may wish to maintain, gain, or lose weight and you will find valuable information in this chapter that will help you achieve or maintain a healthy lifestyle. Since overweight and obesity are major issues and risk factors in today's health, these topics will be strongly emphasized in this chapter.

Americans' love of junk foods and lack of regular exercise have been blamed for contributing to the nation's rise in obesity. Overweight and obesity are prevalent among all ages, racial and ethnic groups, and both genders. The most recent National Health and Nutrition Examination Survey (NHANES III), conducted in 2003 by the Centers for Disease Control and Prevention, reports that 61% of U.S. adults are either overweight or obese, which is an increase of more than 5% over the past decade. The economic cost of obesity in the United States exceeds $123 billion in lost productivity and medical expenses. Officials estimate that between 300,000 and 500,000 lives are lost each year to conditions directly related to obesity. Associated health risks include coronary heart disease, diabetes, gallstones, hypertension, osteoarthritis, sleep apnea, numerous cancers, and psychosocial development

including self-esteem. Obesity in the United States is depicted in Figure 10.1, which shows that the southern states have the highest concentration of obese residents.

Research suggests that the sheer variety of high-calorie foods and the lack of a routine exercise program may be pushing people to go on a number of diets to lose those unwanted pounds. One reason for the low success rate is that Americans find it hard to believe in this age of medical miracles and scientific innovations that an effortless weight-loss method still does not exist. So they invest their hopes, dreams, and money in quick-fix claims such as "Eat All You Want and Still Lose Weight!" or "Melt Fat Away While You Sleep!" People invest in pills, gadgets, potions, and programs that hold the promise of a slimmer, happier future. The United States is a supersized nation, and obesity crosses all barriers—age, gender, and culture. For example, there are more obese adult women (38%) than obese men (28%); and non-Hispanic black women have the highest obesity rate (50%), compared with 40% of Hispanic women and 30% of white women. It has been reported that in some Native American communities 70% of all adults are overweight, which may be attributed to differences in metabolic rates (see Figure 10.2). The problem of obesity extends beyond U.S. borders; it is a global epidemic with an estimated 1.1 billion people either overweight or obese. The International Obesity Task Force reports that more than 115 million people in developing countries suffer from obesity-related problems. While people living in cities are obese, those living in rural areas remain underweight and malnourished. It is estimated that one in two Germans, Italians, and Britons, seven in 10 Spanish and Dutch, and two in three Americans and Canadians are overweight or obese. In Europe, excess weight is the most common childhood disorder. In 2004,

**FIGURE 10.1 ▶** Obesity in the United States

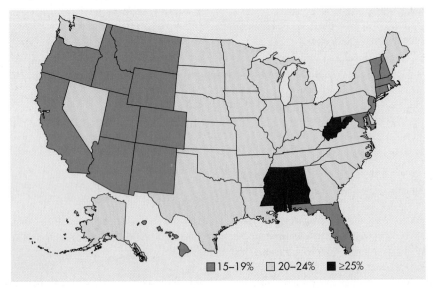

*Source:* Data from National Center for Chronic Disease Prevention & Health Promotion, 2002.

**FIGURE 10.2** ▶ Weight Problems by Race/Ethnic Group & Gender

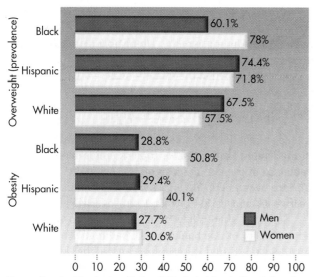

Source: America Obesity Association, "Obesity in Minority Populations," www.obesity.org

**FIGURE 10.3** ▶ Typical Body Composition of an Adult Man and Woman

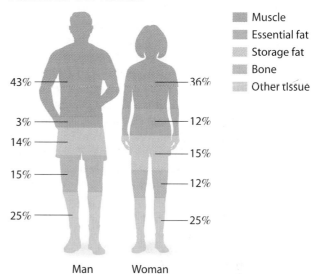

Source: W. W. K. Hoeger and S. A. Hoeger, *Principles and Labs: For Physical Fitness*, 3rd ed. (Belmont, CA: Wadsworth, 2002), p. 93.

the World Health Organization adopted its first global diet, exercise, and health strategy to combat obesity. It recommends that governments promote public knowledge about exercise, diet, and health; offer information that makes healthy choices easier for consumers to make; and require accurate, comprehensible food labels.

According to the *Surgeon General's Call to Action Report*, overweight and obesity result from an imbalance involving excessive calorie consumption or inadequate physical activity or both. For each individual, body weight is the result of a combination of genetic, metabolic, behavioral, environmental, cultural, and socioeconomic influences. The typical body composition of an adult male and female is depicted in Figure 10.3.

In 2004, Tommy Thompson, Secretary of Health and Human Services, declared a national war on excess weight. Deaths due to poor diet and physical inactivity rose by 33% over the past decade with only tobacco causing more preventable deaths. By middle age, 70% of Americans are overweight or obese. Americans spend billions each year on all types of diet programs and products, including diet snacks, food, pills, drinks, and exercise/nutrition CDs.

## The Image of Healthy Weight

In the past, a larger body was considered better. Many cultures still regard a full figure as more desirable than a thin figure. Studies show that men do not consider the slimmest women the most attractive. African-American women often feel satisfied with their weight and see their heavier selves as more attractive than being thin. White

women grow up thinking that thin is better. The older population (both men and women) feels less positive about their facial appearance, but older women are more satisfied than younger women with their weight. Throughout life generally men have a more positive attitude about their body changes, but this gender difference lessens with age.

## OVERWEIGHT OR OBESE

The federal government developed clinical guidelines from scientific evidence that changed the meaning of what it means to be overweight or obese. The federal guidelines moved away from using **height and weight tables** to using body mass index, waist circumference, and individual risk factors for diseases and conditions associated with obesity.

Definitions of overweight and obesity in adults are based on findings from the National Heart, Lung, and Blood Institute of the National Institutes of Health. Body mass index is used to classify overweight (BMI 25.0–29.9) and obesity (BMI greater than or equal to 30.0) in adults. A person with a BMI of 30 is about 30 pounds overweight, the equivalent of 221 pounds in a person who is 6' or 186 pounds in someone who is 5'6".

Studies using other definitions of overweight and obesity find a high prevalence of overweight and obesity

### KEY TERMS

**Height and weight table** assessment tool used to determine ideal or healthy weight

among Hispanics and American Indians. The prevalence of overweight and obesity in Asian Americans is lower than in the general population.

BMI is strongly associated with total body fat, and BMI levels above 25 are linked with adverse health consequences, including cardiovascular disease, hypertension, type 2 diabetes, high cholesterol, bone and joint diseases such as arthritis, and even some forms of cancer. As BMI levels rise, blood pressure increases, total cholesterol levels increase, and the HDL (good) cholesterol levels decline.

Men in the highest obesity category have more than twice the risk of hypertension and high blood cholesterol, compared with men who have BMIs in the healthy range. Women in the highest obesity category have four times the risk.

## EFFECTS OF OBESITY

**Obesity** generally is defined as an accumulation of fat (adipose tissue) beyond what is considered normal for a person's age, sex, and body type. In today's society obesity is considered a disease, not a moral failing. It occurs when energy intake exceeds the amount of energy expended over time. Only in a small minority of cases is obesity caused by such illnesses as hypothyroidism or the result of taking medications, such as steroids, that can cause weight gain.

The more a person weighs, the more blood vessels the body needs to circulate blood throughout the body. The heart takes on a heavy burden as it has to pump harder to force the blood through so many vessels. As a result, the heart grows in size and blood pressure tends to rise. Obesity also is a factor in osteoarthritis (because of the extra weight placed on the joints), gout, bone and joint diseases (including ruptured intervertebral discs), varicose veins, respiratory ailments, gallbladder disease, complications during pregnancy and delivery, and higher accidental death rate.

Obesity can alter hormone levels, affect immune function, and cause impotence in men and reproductive problems in women. Women who are 30% overweight are twice as likely to die of endometrial cancer, and those who are 40% overweight have four times the risk. Obese women also are more likely to incur cancers of the breast, cervix, ovaries, and gallbladder. Obese men are more likely to develop cancers of the rectum, colon, esophagus, bladder, pancreas, stomach, and prostate.

Obesity also can cause psychological problems. Sufferers are associated with laziness, failure, or inadequate willpower. As a result, overweight men and women blame themselves for being heavy, thus causing feelings of guilt and depression.

Scientific evidence has found an association between greater BMI and higher death rates. However, the relative risk of being heavy declines with age. Some researchers have found that data linking overweight and death are inconclusive, while other researchers have found that losing weight may be riskier than dangers posed by the extra pounds. Some researchers counter that overweight indirectly contributes to over 300,000 deaths a year (see Figure 10.4).

A poll by Shape Up America! found that 78% of overweight and obese adults have abandoned dieting as a means of reducing weight. Diets do not teach people how to eat properly. They merely restrict food intake temporarily, so when the diet ends, weight gain resumes.

## CHILDREN AND ADOLESCENTS

Adults are not the only ones fighting the battle of the bulge. In the United States, 22% of today's children and adolescents are obese, an increase of 15% since the 1970s, and 25% are overweight. Seventy percent of children who are overweight at ages 10–13 will become overweight adults.

Scientific studies have found that both boys and girls, regardless of ethnic background, had higher blood pressure, elevated total cholesterol, and higher weight and body mass index than their counterparts a decade before. Also, these studies indicated that excess abdominal fat as a child and adolescent increases the risk of fat storage later on in adult life. A major common risk factor for childhood obesity includes physical inactivity. A moderate amount of exercise activity and starting an early intervention program with good nutrition in childhood can reverse the effects of being overweight or obese in adulthood.

## GENDER

Social physique anxiety (SPA) indicates the desire to look good and has a destructive—and often disabling—effect on one's ability to function well in interactions with others and in relationships. Issues regarding appearance dominate both men and (especially) women with this anxiety disorder, as they quest for that perfect body, known as "body beautiful."

Overweight and obesity are risks for SPA, and some experts speculate that it may be a contributing factor to eating disorders. Research studies indicate that obese women complete about half a year less schooling, earn $6,710 on an average less per year, are 20% less likely to get married, and are 10% more likely to experience household poverty than those who are not overweight. Overweight men were 11% less likely to be married and had fewer adverse economic consequences than slimmer men.

Women have a lower ratio of lean body mass to fatty mass, because of bone size and mass, muscle size, and other factors, as compared with men. After sexual maturity, for all ages, men have higher metabolic rates. It is thus easier for them to burn off excess calories than it is for women. As a result of hormonal changes, pregnancy, and other factors, women face a greater chance of weight fluctuation. Men are socialized into physical activity from birth while women's roles have been more sedentary and required lower levels of caloric expenditure to complete.

The predominance of eating disorders and the consumption of diet pills are indicators of the female obsession

**FIGURE 10.4 ▶** Health Dangers of Excess Weight

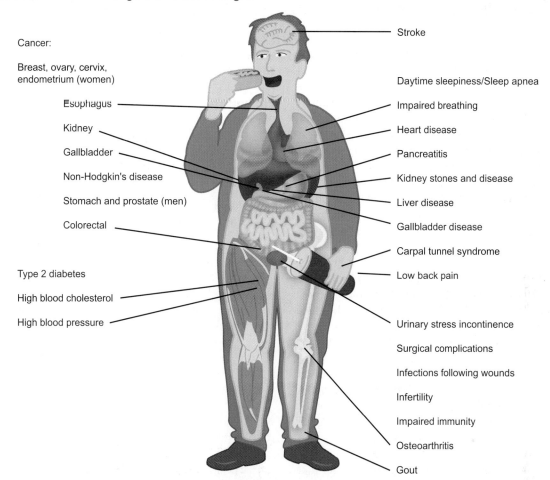

Cancer:

Breast, ovary, cervix,
endometrium (women)

Esophagus

Kidney

Gallbladder

Non-Hodgkin's disease

Stomach and prostate (men)

Colorectal

Type 2 diabetes

High blood cholesterol

High blood pressure

Stroke

Daytime sleepiness/Sleep apnea

Impaired breathing

Heart disease

Pancreatitis

Kidney stones and disease

Liver disease

Gallbladder disease

Carpal tunnel syndrome

Low back pain

Urinary stress incontinence

Surgical complications

Infections following wounds

Infertility

Impaired immunity

Osteoarthritis

Gout

with being thin. As the male image of body builders increases, so will other maladaptive responses such as eating disorders and exercise addictions.

## Body Composition and Metabolic Rate

Body composition is one of the five components of health-related fitness. The others are cardiovascular endurance, muscular flexibility, muscular strength, and muscular endurance (discussed in Chapter 11). Because diet is a major determinant of body composition, and of health-related fitness, its regulation is essential to a healthy life.

**Body composition** consists of **percent body fat** and **lean body mass.** The ratio of body fat to lean body mass, not total body weight, is what is important. Excessive fat is unhealthy because it increases the risk for chronic diseases. However, too little body fat (less than 8% for women and 3%–5% for men) can cause health problems, including muscle wasting and fatigue. In women, a low percentage of body fat (8%–13%) is associated with amenorrhea (lack of menstruation) and loss of bone mass.

Total body fat is further broken down into **essential fat** and **storage fat.** Storage fat is lost through exercise

and lean diet, but if a person loses too much storage or reserve fat, the body will resort to breaking down muscle tissue as a last effort to obtain nourishment or energy, which may be detrimental to health.

### KEY TERMS

**Obesity** a condition in which a person has an excessive amount of body fat, usually about 30% accumulation above recommended body weight according to body size

**Body composition** proportionate amounts of fat tissue and nonfat tissue in the body

**Percent body fat** adipose (fat) tissue as a percent of total body tissue

**Lean body mass** nonfat body tissue made up of muscle, bone, and organs (heart, brain, liver, kidneys)

**Essential fat** body fat needed for normal physiological functioning

**Storage fat** fat found beneath the skin and around major organs that acts as an insulator, as padding, and as a source of energy for metabolism

■ Increase the proportion of adults who are at a healthy weight.

A balance between caloric intake and caloric expenditure is necessary to maintain proper body fat content. Applying the **energy-balancing equation,** if caloric intake exceeds output, the person gains weight; when caloric output exceeds input, the person loses weight. One pound of fat equals 3,500 calories. If a person's daily caloric expenditure is 500 calories, this person should be able to lose about 1 pound of fat in one week by decreasing the daily intake of calories by 500 calories per day (500 × 7 = 3,500). Another formula to determine how many calories to consume to lose weight is to multiply your target weight (not your current weight) by 12. For example, if your target weight is 140 pounds, your recommended calories per day is 140 × 12 = 1,680. Or the calories could be expended by doing various exercises.

By consulting calorie charts for various foods and exercises, a person theoretically should be able to achieve an optimum weight by following a precisely determined formula of diet and physical activity. Unfortunately, translating the energy-balancing equation to one's life is not that simple. It relates to differences in human metabolism and other lifestyle factors such as physical activity and composition of one's diet.

Metabolism refers to how the body utilizes its fuel from nutrients (food) to carry on vital processes. The metabolic rate is the total amount of energy the body expends in a given time and, hence, the number of calories it uses, either at rest or while active.

Energy expenditure is composed of resting metabolism, digestion, and physical activity. As Figure 10.5 indicates, most of the energy (55%–75%) is required to maintain vital bodily functions including respiration, temperature regulation, and blood pressure while the body is at rest (called basal metabolic rate [BMR] or resting metabolic rate [RMR]). The energy required to digest food accounts for 5% to 15% of the daily energy expenditure, and 10% to 40% of energy is expended during physical activity.

## FACTORS CONTRIBUTING TO WEIGHT PROBLEMS

The rate of obesity is continually climbing in the United States. At the close of the 20th century, one in five American adults was considered obese. The reason for obesity is simple. If you consume more calories than you expend, you will gain weight, and if you do this throughout life, you become obese.

Research has identified a number of factors that contribute to those who gain weight and those who remain

**FIGURE 10.5** ▶ Energy-Balancing Equation

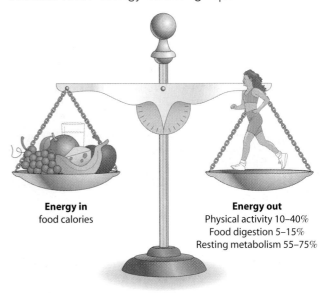

**Energy in**
food calories

**Energy out**
Physical activity 10–40%
Food digestion 5–15%
Resting metabolism 55–75%

*Note:* Energy expenditure is composed of food digestion, physical activity, and resting metabolism.
*Source:* U.S. Department of Agriculture, "The Great Nutrition Debate" (2000) (see http://www.usda.gov/cnpp). (page 286 Donatell, 8th edition).

thin. Although inherited factors undoubtedly play a role, the actual extent has not been determined. Contemporary theories that have some credibility point to factors such as body size and composition, sex, diet, age, genetics, hormones, activity level, overeating, eating pattern, culture, and psychological makeup.

**Genetic Predisposition.** You have your mother's eyes and body build and your father's smile. If you have a weight problem, did you inherit that from one or both of your parents as well? An estimated 80% of identical twins reared apart weigh almost the same as each other throughout their lives. These studies suggest that a **genetic predisposition** to weight gain exists. Genes seem to set metabolic rates—that is, how the body uses calories.

Children inherit their general body type (height, bone structure) from their parents. Body fat can be altered, but body type cannot be changed. If both parents are overweight or obese, the child has an 80% chance of being overweight; one parent is overweight or obese, 40%; and if neither parent is overweight or obese, 7%. Therefore, if obesity runs in the family, the chances of the children being obese are higher.

Genes influence body weight, size, type, and the propensity toward obesity. The pattern of fat distribution in the body (hips, waist, abdomen) is a function of heredity. Your food preferences are not inherited but for the most part are set during childhood. If you were brought up on sweets and junk foods, they probably remain an important part of your diet. If you were brought up on healthy foods, you probably include them regularly in your diet as an adult.

Two theories, which are yet to be proven on humans, connect inherited traits with body fat: setpoint theory and fat cell theory.

**Setpoint theory** stipulates that every person has a genetically determined weight range that the body works to preserve. If your set point is around 150 pounds, you will gain and lose weight within a given range of that point. The setpoint theory indicates that after losing a predetermined amount of weight, the body will sabotage additional weight loss by slowing down metabolism. Other researchers indicate that it is possible to raise set point over time by lack of exercise and gaining weight by consuming too many calories. Therefore, exercising over a long period of time and reducing caloric intake can slowly decrease one's set point. Diet is important, but exercise seems to be the most important factor in readjusting one's set point.

According to the **fat cell theory,** the amount of fat stored in the body is genetically determined by the number and size of fat cells a person has in the body. Having extra fat cells **(hyperplasia)** creates a biological pressure to keep those fat cells full. New fat cells may develop due to prolonged overeating when existing fat cells reach the limit of their fat storage capacity. Also, fat cells may swell, shrink **(hypertrophy),** and even disappear if body weight is held down for an extended period of time. Childhood-onset obesity is thought to be the result of the child's developing too many fat cells. Adult-onset obesity is thought to be the result of the adult's developing larger, not more, fat cells. Some obese people have the combined problem of large fat cells and too many fat cells. The more fat cells, the greater is the capacity to store more energy in the form of fat. Additional research is needed to determine whether these theories are relevant to obesity in humans.

In summary, heredity forms a strong foundation for obesity. Even so, family environment, parents' food consumption patterns, and exercise habits strongly influence what is built on that foundation.

**Prenatal Factors.** A child's weight may be influenced by the mother's weight gain during pregnancy. Women who gain too much weight during their pregnancy—more than 20–25—pounds are at risk for developing gestational diabetes. Mother's excess weight gain during pregnancy increases the risk of the baby being above normal birth weight. Refer to Chapter 5.

**Body Size and Composition.** Obese people have lower metabolic rates than thin people generally because thin people dissipate more calories through heat loss. The more muscle and less fat you have, the more energy your body will use even at rest. If an obese person and a person who is not obese weigh exactly the same, the obese person has a lower metabolic rate.

**Sex.** In general, males develop more muscle tissue than females. Muscle is metabolically active tissue. Therefore, men tend to have a higher metabolic rate than women, who have a larger proportion of body fat than men.

**Diet.** Diet has little effect on the resting metabolic rate, but when, what, how much, and how often you eat all have a temporary effect on metabolic rate. Constant dieting may lower the metabolic rate. After repeatedly losing and gaining weight, the body may increase its metabolic efficiency by reducing the number of calories required to maintain body functions (the setpoint theory). Each time a person diets, he or she loses weight more slowly and gains it back more quickly.

**Age.** Lean body mass decreases after age 30, at an average rate of 3% per decade for active people and 5% per decade for sedentary people. Therefore, as people age, they lose muscle mass and their metabolic rate slows down.

**Hormones.** Thyroid hormone helps to regulate metabolic rate. Therefore, certain thyroid disorders affect metabolic rate and impede the thyroid's ability to burn calories. Thyroid pills will not increase metabolic rate in healthy people except when they are taken in dangerously high amounts. Most scientific research indicates that less than 2% of the obese population have a thyroid problem and can trace their weight problems to a metabolic or hormone imbalance.

**Obesity Genes.** Recent evidence indicates the existence of a "fat gene." The Ob gene (obesity), is reported to

## KEY TERMS

**Energy-balancing equation** formula stating that when caloric input equals caloric output, an individual does not gain or lose weight

**Genetic predisposition** theory stating that inherited genes influence a person's propensities, including weight

**Setpoint theory** theory stating that individuals have a weight-regulating mechanism in the hypothalamus of the brain that controls how much one weighs

**Fat cell theory (hypertrophy** and **hyperplasia)** theory stating that the quantity of fat in the body is the result of the size and number of fat cells a person has

disrupt the body's "I've had enough to eat" signaling system and individuals may continue to eat past the point of being comfortably full. The beta-3 adrenergic-receptor gene has been identified in mice and humans. When mutated, it is thought to impede the body's ability to burn fat. The Ob gene may produce leptin, and a new leptin receptor in the brain. These studies have reported that leptin is the chemical that signals the brain when you are full and need to stop eating. Leptin and leptin receptors do not seem to work properly in obese people. It is still not clear when altering leptin levels would help in treating obesity.

Still other scientists have isolated a protein called GLP-1, which is known to slow down the passage of food through the intestines to allow the absorption of nutrients. It is speculated that leptin and GLP-1 might play complementary roles in weight control. Leptin and its receptors may regulate body weight over the long term and call on fast-acting appetite suppressants such as GLP-1 when needed.

### Physical Activity Level.

By exercising regularly and watching your weight, you can increase your overall metabolic rate. Exercise is important in long-term weight control. Exercise increases the resting metabolic rate and lean body mass (associated with higher metabolic rate). Exercise expends calories, thus raising total energy expenditure. The more energy is expended, the more calories a person can consume without gaining weight. A dramatic drop in physical activity often occurs during the college years.

### Other Factors Contributing to Weight Gain.

**Childhood Development.** Today's children eat more high-fat, high-calorie foods and they exercise less than children in the past. Fewer than half of grade schoolers participate in daily physical education classes. Many spend five hours or more a day in front of a television or computer screen.

**Socioeconomics.** The less money one makes, the more likely one is to be overweight or obese. Households earning $67,000 or more are less obese compared to those at the poverty level. Minorities are at a greater risk of being overweight or obese since one in three low-income African Americans is obese.

**Excess Calories.** At any given time, TV/radio commercials tempt us with junk foods and treats. In some cases, Americans are eating 200 to 400 calories more per day than they did several decades ago. These extra calories come from refined carbohydrates, therefore raising blood fats (triglycerides) and increasing the risk of diabetes and obesity.

**Overeating.** Research does not show that obese people eat more than people who are not obese. Both obese and nonobese people tend to underestimate their caloric intake in daily diet records, but obese people tend to underreport their intakes by 30% to 35% more than nonobese people. Binge eating, a pattern of eating in which normal food consumption is interrupted by episodes of high consumption, may account for obesity in overweight individuals who do not generally overeat.

**Oversize Portions.** As Table 10.1 indicates, the portions of packaged foods and food in many popular restaurants have increased in size drastically. Studies of appetite and satiety report that people presented with larger or oversize portions eat up to 30% more than they usually would eat.

**Eating Pattern.** Researchers have compared obese and nonobese people to discern a pattern that may account for overweight. No distinctive pattern was identified, but results of the research tend to indicate that when food tasted good, obese people ate longer. Also, researchers found that external cues such as time of day, sight of food, and elapsed time between eating episodes exist for people in every weight category, and not only the obese.

**Modernization.** Technology and the growth of industry have led to an abundance of high-calorie foods, less need for physical activity, labor-saving devices, urbanization, and a more sedentary lifestyle. People who walk to work or school tend to be less obese than those who drive. Each hour spent in a car was associated with a 6% increase in the likelihood of obesity and each half-mile walked per day reduced those odds by nearly 5%.

**Passive Entertainment.** Technology such as computers, computer games, and television are culprits in an estimated 30% of new cases of obesity. TV viewers tend to eat more while watching TV and spend less time in physical activity, which lowers metabolic rate so viewers burn fewer calories. A 15-year study of more than 3,700 African Americans and white young adults found that watching television (at least 2½ hours) and eating fast food more than twice a week triples the risk of obesity.

According to the U.S. Department of Agriculture (USDA), the food and restaurant industries spend in excess of $40 billion a year on ads designed to induce hunger. Americans—especially children, adolescents, and college students—are preoccupied with the fast-food

**TABLE 10.1 ▶** Supersized Portions

| FOOD/BEVERAGE | ORIGINAL SIZE (YEAR INTRODUCED) | TODAY (LARGEST AVAILABLE) |
|---|---|---|
| Budweiser (bottle) | 7oz. (1976) | 40 oz. |
| Nestle's Crunch | 1.6 oz. (1938) | 5 oz. |
| Soda (Coca-Cola) | 6.5 oz. (1916) | 34 oz. |
| French fries (Burger King) | 2.6 oz. (1954) | 6.9 oz. |
| Hamburger (McDonald's) (beef only) | 1.6 oz. (1955) | 8 oz. |

*Source:* "Are Growing Portion Sizes Leading to Expanding Waistlines." American Dietetic Association, www.eatright.org.

industry. Fast food is high in calories, sodium, carbohydrates, and fat; portions are large and tend to be quickly eaten, which does not allow enough time for the stomach to send the "full" signal to the brain. College students are faced with fast-food courts right on or near campus.

**Psychological Factors.** Eating tends to be a social ritual associated with enjoyment, celebration, and companionship. The all-you-can-eat buffets and endless snack machines at work, malls, schools, and college campuses present major problems to all individuals regardless of weight.

Researchers found that overweight people are no more neurotic, do not suffer more psychiatric disturbances, and have no particular personality characteristics different from those of normal-weight people. However, an increase in emotional problems among obese people may result from failed efforts to reduce weight and their concern about weight. Dieting can cause emotional disturbances such as depression, anxiety, irritability, and a preoccupation with food.

## DIETS AND DIETING

People take risks when nothing seems to work. They search continuously for a fat-burning quick fix, which often leads to extreme health risk (see Analyzing Popular Diets). Drastic dietary restriction (fasting, starvation diets), and pharmacological and surgical measures should be considered carefully and discussed with several health professionals before final decisions are made. There are only two effective ways for losing weight: consume fewer calories and increase physical activity. The following are some of the most common diet strategies and products and traps to avoid.

**The Yo-Yo Syndrome.** **Yo-yo dieting** is common when people repeatedly gain weight and then starve themselves to lose the weight, thus lowering their BMR. Once returning to eating after the weight loss, they have a BMR that is set lower, making it almost certain that they will regain the weight they just lost. Repeating the cycle of dieting and regaining, these individuals find it harder to lose weight and increasingly easy to regain the weight and they become fatter.

**Metabolic Products.** Many diet products claim to increase the metabolic rate. The popular Chinese herb ma-huang, for example, contains ephedrine, a stimulant that has been shown in some studies to raise the metabolic rate slightly. Subsequent research, however, has not shown this herb to speed the loss of fat. Caffeine is another product that has a stimulatory effect on metabolism, but it has shown little promise as a weight-loss aid. The mineral chromium also has been said to regulate carbohydrate metabolism and assist in burning fats. This claim, too, has no basis in research.

One of the newest diets is called the Zone. The metabolic pathways described by the author of *The Zone*, which supposedly connect diet, insulin-glucagon, and eicosanoids, do not exist in standard nutrition or biochemistry texts or research. However, proponents of the Zone diet stress that it is an attempt to help people eat more healthy foods and it addresses the importance of all macronutrients.

**Very Low Calorie Diets.** Very low calorie diets (VLCDs) usually are low in nutrients, which can result in a serious metabolic imbalance and even death. Usually these diets have a caloric value of 400 to 700 calories per day. On this type of diet, as much as half of the weight lost may be lean protein tissue. The heart is a muscle, so it can become weak and unable to pump enough blood through the body. When the body uses protein instead of carbohydrates and fat as a source of energy, the weight lost is in the form of water, causing faster weight loss. As much as 50% of the weight loss may be muscle, therefore making the person look flabbier. Water loss, however, results in the loss of essential vitamins and minerals. The blood pressure may drop, causing dizziness, blood sugar imbalance, cold intolerance, constipation, decreased BMR, dehydration, emotional problems, diarrhea, headaches, heart irregularity, ketosis, kidney infections and failure, loss of lean body tissue, fatigue, lightheadedness, and eventually weight gain due to the yo-yo effect. Over time, the body begins to run out of liver tissue, heart muscle, and blood, and a person may lose hair, become nauseated, and have abdominal pain. In women the menstrual cycle may become irregular. Only after depleting the available proteins from these sources does the body begin to burn fat reserves. In this process, known as ketosis, the body adapts to prolonged fasting or carbohydrate deprivation by converting body fat to ketones, which can be used to fuel some brain cells. Within about 10 days after the typical adult begins a complete fast, the body will have used many of its energy stores and death may occur.

Cutting calories slows the metabolism. A person may eat as few as 800 calories a day and still not lose weight. Once the person goes off the diet, the metabolism remains slow. The body continues to use fewer calories and the pounds come back. This illustrates the setpoint theory.

**Liquid Protein and High-Protein Diets.** Liquid diets generally consist of protein formula and water. Advocates of these high-protein diets blame the rise in obesity in the United States on excessive carbohydrate intake. One popular high-protein diet is the 40–30–30 (the Zone): 40% of total calories from carbohydrates, 30% from protein, and

## KEY TERMS

**Yo-yo dieting** losing and regaining weight again and again

**TABLE 10.2** ▶ Analyzing Popular Diets

| BOOK/PROGRAM AND AUTHOR | PREMISE OF THE DIET | HOW IT CLAIMS TO WORK | EXPERTS' OPINIONS | COMMENTS |
|---|---|---|---|---|
| *The Atkins Diet,* Robert Atkins. M.D. | Says overweight people eat too many carbohydrates. High-protein diet allows you to eat all the protein you want (meat, eggs, cheese, and more) and restricts refined sugar, milk, white rice, and whiteflour. | Restrict carbohydrates and body goes into ketosis. In ketosis, body gets energy from ketones, little carbon fragments that are the fuel created by breakdown of fat stores. You feel less hungry. | Highly controversial. Low intake of fruits and vegetables a problem. | Possible side effects: nausea, fatigue, low blood pressure, elevated uric acid/kidney problems, bad breath, constipation, fetal harm if pregnant. |
| *Dean Ornish Diet,* Dean Ornish, M.D. | Diet and exercise are important. Watch what you eat; there are foods you should eat all of the time, some of the time, and none of the time. Less than 10% of your calories should come from fat. Eat lots of little meals. | Metabolism is a result of our ancestors. We need to change old metabolic patterns. Meditation is a part of this: when your soul is fed, you have less need to overeat. | Mostly positive for highly restrictive diet and healthy lifestyle regimen. Documented studies show heart blockage reversal. Drawbacks are that it is tough to stick to this diet, and new eating patterns must be learned. Only the most committed will stick to this rigid diet. | May be tough for all but strict vegans to adhere to this plan. Eating smaller, more frequent meals may be difficult. Otherwise a good model. |
| *Eating Well for Optimum Health,* Andrew Weil. M.D. *Eating Well for Optimum Health,* (continued) | Eat less, exercise more. Take a more Eastern than Western approach. Avoid quick fixes, and set realistic goal of 1-2 pounds of weight loss per week. Balance the amount and type of food. Describes meats as "flesh foods." Minimize dairy, and take a Mediterranean dietary approach. | Keeps it simple. Criticizes high-protein diets because of rise in cholesterol and calcium depletion. Moderation is a key. | A more holistic approach to dieting than most. Considers exercise and stress as factors. | May not be sustainable for those who are used to diets high in diary or meat. Nutrition experts support this common-sense approach. The vegetarian emphasis is substantiated as healthy by numerous studies. |
| *The Pritikin Principle,* Robert Pritikin | Concern not for calories, but for density of calories. Eat more foods that are not calorie dense, such as apples and oatmeal. | Fill up on foods that have fewer catories. Large volume of fiber and water will keep you full. Emphasis on vegetables, fruits, beans, unprocessed grains; exercise strongly recommended | Weight loss will occur but frequent feelings of hunger. Weight will usually creep back. Low in fat so healthy in general, except when taken to extreme or for certain groups of people. | Strict limitations of animal products a plus. Incorporates exercise and stress management. Not an easy plan to stick to. |

30% from fat. (The American Heart Association advises that the proper balance of calories in a diet is no more than 30% of daily calories from fat, 55%–60% from complex carbohydrates, and 10%–12% from protein.) The extra protein is supposed to keep insulin levels down. Insulin is essential for processing carbohydrate in the body and also inhibits fat burning. So, in theory, less insulin should result in more fat burning.

Low-carbohydrate diets such as the Atkins Diet and the South Beach Diet advocate eliminating nearly all of the bread, pasta, sweets, and high-carbohydrate food from your diet, and eating red meat and other high-protein and high-fat foods until you are satisfied. The American Heart Assocation and the American Dietetic Association have issued warnings about low-carb diets. Many people did benefit from these diets and did not experience the harmful effects in blood cholesterol. Their LDL (bad) cholesterol and triglycerides were reduced and the HDL (good) cholesterol increased, but these benefits were only short-term. Problems associated with low-carb diets are now being recognized, especially for diabetics, because whole grains, beans, and other fiber-rich foods are not allowed in the Atkins Diet or other similar diets. Most research suggests that you should choose food with low glycemic loads and continue to reduce your total caloric intake and saturated fat intake. Most fruits, beans, vegetables, and whole grains have low glycemic loads and their sugars enter the bloodstream gradually and trigger only a moderate rise in insulin. The glycemic index is a ranking of foods according to how quickly their sugars are released into the bloodstream. (see Analyzing Popular Diets).

**TABLE 10.2** ▶ Analyzing Popular Diets (Continued)

| BOOK/PROGRAM AND AUTHOR | PREMISE OF THE DIET | HOW IT CLAIMS TO WORK | EXPERTS' OPINIONS | COMMENTS |
|---|---|---|---|---|
| The South Beach Diet, Arthur Agatston, M.D. | As with other low-carbohydrate diets, argues that carbohydrates are to blame for obesity. | Carbohydrates lead to overeating and cravings. Advocates combining small amounts of undesirable carbohydrates with vegetables and proteins. | As with other low-carbohydrate diets, research is still being conducted into effectiveness of this style of dieting. | Does not include recommendations to incorporate exercise into program, which is a key to any weight loss. Less restrictive on portion sizes than are other diets. |
| Sugar Busters, H. Leighton Steward, Morrison Bethea, M.D., Samuel Andrews MD, and Luis Balart, M.D. | Cut sugar to trim fat. Pay attention to portion size. Eliminate potatoes, corn, rice, bread, carrots, refined sugar, honey, soft drinks, and beer. | Glucose, insulin production theory: the more insulin produced, the more fat. | Most don't like this diet. When you gain weight, it doesn't matter where calories come from; it is total calorie intake that is most important. | You'll lose weight due to decreased calorie intake, but this not a good long-term strategy. |
| Weight Watchers | Eat from food groups, tally points to monitor intake. Based on weight and dietary goals. Eat what you want, but use discretion in amount. | Based on calories in, calories out. Includes exercise and social support. | Life focus rather than diet focus. Has support of most national organizations. One of the most highly recommended diets. | Works well for many people, particularly those for whom social support is important. |
| The Zone, Barry Sears, Ph.D. | Offers a wellness philosophy to develop a metabolic state in which the body works efficiently. Recommends eating different calories than you do now and a small amount of protein. Identifies favorable versus unfavourable carbohydrates. | Claims that his percentages of fat, protein, and carbohydrates are the best ratios for health. | Superiority of given ratios is unsubstantiated by research. Mixed reviews from experts: easy to follow, but don't count on results. Some recommendations (eating high-fat ice cream) are questionable. | Not a lot of do's and don'ts. Dieters may find it easy to follow. |

Source: Rebacca J. Donatelle, Health: The Basics, 6th ed. Pearson (Benjamin Cummings), 2005.

Note: In our ongoing quest to find an effective way to lose weight, Americans consider many seemingly reputable options. Are any of these diet plans really the miracles that they often claim to be? Don't count on it. Some are quite good, but others produce no long-term effects and may even be dangerous. Each year, "new and improved" versions of the same old dietary ploys surface in bookstores, where they sell millions of copies. Then there are reports of successes and dangers. And finally, professional groups jump into the fray to label these diets as ineffective or dangerous. Just when we think we've seen the last of a fad, its authors re-invent themselves and capture our interest yet again. Dr. Kelly Brownell, noted obesity researcher at Yale University, describes this pattern: "When I get calls about the latest diet fad, I imagine a trick birthday cake candle that keeps lighting up and we have to keep blowing it out over and over again." Virtually anyone can write a book making diet claims. Just because the authors have Ph.D.s or other credentials, they may not have expertise in the area that they write about. If they do have the expertise, they may base their arguments on unproven science or faulty scientific reasoning. Although health claims should only be published after solid research has proven the results repeatedly with different populations, this happens all too infrequently. Above is a summary of some of the most popular diets and the consensus opinions of the U.S. Department of Agriculture, the American Heart Association, the Center for Science in the Public Interest, and several other professional groups and individuals regarding effectiveness and safety.

In actuality, on a high-protein regimen the body will begin to burn its own fat. When the body burns fat all the time (which it does) without carbohydrates, it does not burn the fat completely. Ketones are formed and released into the bloodstream, creating a condition known as ketosis. Ketosis is the body's normal reaction to a low-carb diet, just as it would be to fasting. This theoretically should make dieting easier because it kills the appetite and may even cause nausea. Over time, though, ketosis will increase blood levels of uric acid, a risk factor for gout and kidney stones. At the same time, numerous controlled research studies show no evidence that carbohydrates, especially complex carbohydrates (starches), stimulate appetite or lead to fat storage and weight gain. Further, excessive protein intake carries potential health risks, from kidney damage to osteoporosis.

Side effects of liquid diets also can include hair loss, dry skin, gum disease, constipation, sensitivity to cold, and mood swings. Consuming inadequate amounts of carbohydrates can produce adverse effects such as diarrhea, dizziness, headaches, and weakness. And only 10%–20% of the people who have gone on a liquid diet manage to stay within 10 pounds of their target weight a year and a half after embarking on the diet.

**Over-the-Counter Diet Pills, Diet Aids, and Prescription Appetite Suppressants.** The search for the perfect quick fix to a weight problem is a $5 billion market to drug makers. Additional products such as diet sodas and low-fat foods are a big business. Among the numerous over-the-counter diet products and prescription appetite suppressants are Pondimen, Redux (known as "Fen Phen") snack

## FYI | RED-FLAG WORDS IN DIETS

| | |
|---|---|
| **Amazing** | As in "amazing breakthrough." |
| **May** | Does not mean "will." |
| **Proves** | Scientific studies gather evidence in a systematic way, but one study, taken alone, seldom proves anything. |
| **Breakthrough** | Happens only now and then—for example, the discovery of penicillin and the polio vaccine; today the word is so overworked as to be meaningless. |
| **Contributes to, is linked to, is associated with** | Does not mean "causes." |
| **Significant** | A result is "statistically significant" when the association between two factors has been found to be greater than might occur at random (this is worked out by a mathematical formula). But people often take "significant" to mean "major" or "important." |
| **Doubles the risk, triples the risk** | May or may not be meaningful. Do you know what the risk was in the first place? If the risk was 1 in a million, and you double it, that is still only 1 in 500,000. If the risk was 1 in 100 and doubles, that is a big increase. |
| **Other words** | Secret, safe, special, quick, painless, natural, instant, immediate, inexpensive, home-cure, and exciting. |

bars, pyruvate, chromium picolinate, Meridia (sibutramine), Xenical (orlistat), Wellbutrin (bupropion), ear patch, slimming soap, diet magnets, apple cider vinegar, and exercise pills in a bottle. Pondimen and Redux were found to damage heart valves and contribute to pulmonary hypertension, resulting in massive recalls and lawsuits.

Marketed as weight-loss aids are fiber diets containing oat bran, hemicellulose, corn bran, pectin, cellulose, guar gum, pectin, psyllium seed, lignin, and apple fiber. Manufacturers say these fibers swell in the stomach and absorb liquids, thereby providing a feeling of fullness. Dietary fiber in reality acts as a bulking agent in the large intestine, not in the stomach. Most of these products provide 1 to 3 grams of fiber per day, which is not close to the recommended daily intake of 20 to 35 grams.

The Food and Drug Administration (FDA) has found no data to warrant classifying any type of fiber as an aid in weight control or as an appetite suppressant. The principal caveat emptor ("let the buyer beware") was used in previous times to warn people to investigate before buying. It is still a good idea.

Appetite suppressants works by increasing the level of the brain chemical serotonin, which curbs hunger and makes those who take the drugs feel full. The drugs are intended for people who are 30% over a healthy body weight or 20% overweight with medical problems such as diabetes or high blood pressure. They are supposed to be prescribed along with an exercise program and sound diet.

Appetite suppressants known as fen-phen were taken off the market after being linked to heart valve problems. The FDA has warned users about Ephedra (ephedrine) and ma-huang, which are often combined with caffeine and cause heart attacks, strokes, and death. These suppressants may reduce weight but at a risk to mental and physical well-being. Ephedrine is a nonprescription stimulant medication that increases heart rate and blood pressure and is often found in certain cold and allergy pills and is believed to cause heart attacks, seizures, and strokes. It slightly increases metabolic rate and decreases appetite. St. John's wort is a herbal product that has some antidepressant effects. The problem with this combination is that ephedrine can result in heart attacks, strokes, and other fatal complications. Extreme caution is recommended.

Meal replacements in the form of shakes or snack bars have become popular to lose or keep off weight. If used appropriately as a replacement for, instead of a supplement to, regular meals and snacks, they can be a successful means of weight loss. Foods made with fat substitutes may have fewer grams of fat, but may not have fewer calories. Many foods are low in fat but still high in sugar and calories. Refined carbohydrates, absorbed quickly into the bloodstream, raise blood glucose levels. As glucose levels fall, your appetite increases.

Pyruvate, promoted as a metabolic stimulant, is a three-carbon intermediary in the metabolism of glucose. There is no scientific evidence that supplementing your diet with pyruvate will result in weight loss. A six-week scientific study involving fewer than 18 women found that women who were given pyruvate instead of polyglucose had less of a weight gain. Pyruvate did not result in any weight loss; it resulted in less weight gain.

Chromium picolinate has not been scientifically proven to increase metabolism and suppress appetite, therefore leading to weight loss as claimed by some weight loss companies.

Currently only two weight loss drugs are FDA approved. Meridia (sibutramine) and Xenical (orlistat) are intended only for individuals with a BMI greater than 30 or a BMI equal to or greater than 27 with risk factors such as high blood pressure that increase their risk of the disease.

Meridia slows the body's dissipation of the serotonin it produces naturally. Even though studies indicate Meridia is moderately effective in helping people shed seven to 11 pounds (or approximately 10% of their body weight) more than dieters not taking the drug, it can cause increases in blood pressure and heart rate. This drug is in the same chemical class as amphetamines and works by suppressing appetite. Blood pressure should be monitored regularly, and the person should be under a physician's care while using this drug. Side effects include insomnia, dry mouth, constipation, and headache. Many individuals taking this drug regain weight after they stop treatment.

Orlistat (Xenical) blocks fat absorption by the gut but also inhibits absorption of water and vitamins in many people, which may cause cramping and diarrhea. Its side effects include bloating, flatulence, fecal incontinence, and diarrhea, and its long-term effects are unknown at this time. This drug works by preventing gastrointestinal and pancreatic enzymes from breaking down fat for absorption by the body. Because it blocks absorption of the fat-soluble vitamins A, D, E, and K, a daily supplement is necessary. Combined with a supervised diet, orlistat has proven effective in attaining weight loss, lessening weight regain, and improving some obesity-related risk factors. Additional risks for individuals with eating disorders may result from the use of this drug.

Wellbutrin (bupropion) is an antidepressant and anti-smoking drug that has shown potential weight loss in obese people. All of these drugs should be available by prescription only. However, Xenical and Meridia are being marketed over the Internet to anyone who completes a form that is reviewed by a company doctor.

There is no scientific evidence that weight loss results from wearing a special patch behind the ear; bathing with so-called slimming soap to wash away extra fat; using diet magnets to attract fat; or wearing Get Slim Slippers, which are specially designed with no heel. Neither reflexology science nor gravity will cause a person to lose weight. Furthermore, apple cider vinegar will not remove toxins from the body or speed up metabolism. Exercise pills in a bottle may contain ephedrine, which may speed up metabolism—and result in some minimal weight loss initially—but also increase blood pressure, heart rate, and the risk of death.

Diet patches have not been proved to be effective or safe. Spirulina is a blue algae that has no documented record of success as a weight loss supplement. Glucomanan is a plant root, advertised as "The Weight Loss Secret That's Been in the Orient for over 500 Years." No scientific evidence exists to support this claim. The Federal Trade Commission is suing several marketers because of unfounded statements about magnet diet pills, which claim to flush fat out of the body.

Among the numerous over-the-counter diet aids are amino acids (L-glutamine, L-arginine) and grapefruit juice extract. The most common diet aids sold in drugstores are phenyl propanolamine hydrochloride (PPA) and fiber. PPA is similar to amphetamines (available legally only by prescription). It acts as a mild stimulant and suppresses the appetite. PPA, however, may cause dizziness, headaches, insomnia, hypertension, heart palpitations, and rapid pulse in some people. It is not approved by the FDA, which is proceeding with steps to ban the ingredient completely. As former U.S. Surgeon General C. Everett Koop said, "The best prescription is knowledge." Save your time and especially your money by avoiding these so-called miracle treatments. There is a very simple, safe, and effective strategy to losing weight: eat less and exercise more.

**Obesity Surgery.** The easy but very risky solution may lie in gastric or bariatric surgery (Figure 10.6). It is recommended only for individuals who have BMIs higher than 40 or who have BMIs of 35 along with severe health complications. The operation uses bands or staples to section off a small portion of the stomach. A small outlet, about the size of a pencil eraser, is left at the bottom of the stomach pouch. Since the outlet is small, food (a few tablespoons) stays in the pouch longer so people feel full for a longer time. Dieters cannot eat enough calories, so they lose weight. This procedure should be reserved for the morbidly obese who face imminent health risks. Complications include infections, leaking of stomach juices into the abdomen, injury to the spleen, slippage or erosion of the band, vomiting, nausea, vitamin and mineral deficiencies, and dehydration. Lifelong medical and sometimes psychological monitoring is needed for those who have this procedure. The long-term weight loss success rate is 40% to 63% of excess body weight over a three-year period and 50% to 60% after five years. Up to 25% of patients may require reoperation within five years.

Liposuction is another surgical procedure for spot reduction. It also carries risks such as infection, severe scarring, and even death. Some people regain the fat and must have multiple surgeries to repair lumpy, irregular surfaces from which the fat was removed.

**Crash Diets.** Losing even a moderate amount of weight could improve the health of millions, but crash diets are not the answer. Losing weight too quickly may result in damage to body systems. Furthermore, many dieters develop a pattern of going on diets, then abandoning them after they have lost weight. When they regain the weight, they go on yet another diet. This yo-yo dieting is risky. The weight fluctuation poses health problems and may shorten the life span.

## EATING DISORDERS

The media, fashion industry, and television commercials suggest that "thin is in, fat is out," and "zeros become heroes". For example, fashion icons such as Paris Hilton, Nicole Richie, and Victoria Beckham with their extra thin

**FIGURE 10.6A** ► Biliopancreatic Diversion

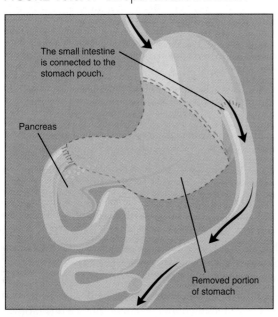

**FIGURE 10.6B** ► Restrictive Surgery

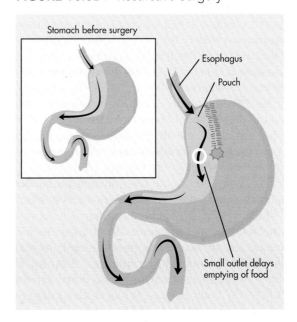

**FIGURE 10.6C** ► Gastric Binding

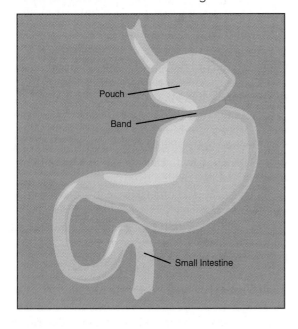

**FIGURE 10.6D** ► Vertical Banded Gastroplasty

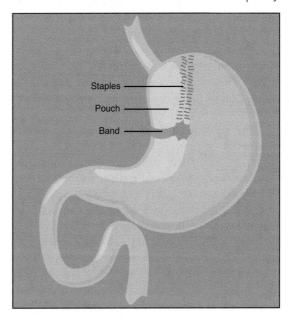

looks dominate fashion and the media, while Ashley Olsen received world-wide media attention for her diagnosed eating disorder. No underweight, super-skinny, minuscule-waisted models boasting "size zero" and even "double zero" (00) sizes can be healthy. Clothing companies such as Nicole Miller and Banana Republic, which is owned by Gap, are advertising "00" clothes on their websites. The Madrid City Council in Spain, organizer of the city's annual fashion week, imposed a ban on models with a body mass index (BMI) under 18. Many models are surviving off cocaine and cigarettes rather than risking eating. In August 2006, fashion model Luisel Ramos died of a heart attack moments after stepping off a catwalk, and industry insiders allege she suffered from anorexia. Another model, Lauren Martin, is struggling for survival after being ravaged by the same eating disorder. Adolescents, teens, and adults preoccupied with trying to mimic these fashion models and celebrities are making themselves ill.

An eating disorder is about anxiety and control and healing from trauma and food and weight are just the tools of destruction. Stringent dieting can play a key role in causing **eating disorders.** As a result of the cultural emphasis on thinness, in combination with psychological and physiological factors that are not fully understood, people with eating disorders have a perception of being too fat, which may not be the case at all. They engage in destructive eating behaviors under the veneer of weight control. These disorders are obsessive and in most cases require intensive intervention to cure. Sufferers tend to be women (5 to 10 million) from white middle-class or upper-class families in which there is undue emphasis on achievement, appearance, and body weight. However, eating disorders span social class, gender, race, and ethnic backgrounds, and are present in countries throughout the world. Limited studies of eating disorders in minority college students report that African-American female undergraduates had a slightly lower prevalence of eating disorders than whites. Asian Americans reported fewer symptoms of eating disorders but more body dissatisfaction, concerns about shape, and more intense efforts to lose weight. In addition, there is an increase of males (1 million) suffering from various forms of eating disorders. Studies suggest that eating disorders may have familial associations, such as the presence of these disorders in identical twins or in a mother or sister. Many persons have other problems, including: 50% are clinically depressed; 25% are alcoholics; and a large number have problems such as compulsive stealing, gambling, or other addictions. Possible physical components are hypothesized to be

- A predisposition to eating disorders caused by a biological factor linked to clinical depression
- Insufficient serotonin (a neurotransmitter that sends nerve messages to and from the brain)
- Malfunctioning of the hypothalamus

Psychologically and emotionally, people with eating disorders tend to share the emotional traits of low self-esteem, feelings of helplessness, depression, and perfectionism. Most eating disorders seem to develop as a way of handling stress and anxiety, using self-imposed eating behaviors to gain a sense of control.

The three forms of eating disorders—anorexia nervosa, bulimia nervosa, and binge eating—are taking a toll on the health of a growing number of people. More than 90% of those afflicted with eating disorders, according to the National Institute of Mental Health, are adolescent girls and young women. Approximately 1% of adolescent girls develop anorexia nervosa, and another 2% to 3% develop bulimia nervosa. The U.S. Department of Agriculture has estimated that 5% to 20% of college-age women are bulimic and that males account for 5% to 10% of all cases of eating disorders. Of the three eating disorders, males seem more predisposed to binge eating; one-third to one-fourth of those with binge eating disorder are male.

Anorexia and bulimia are found most often in Caucasians. Perhaps because African Americans have not subscribed as fully to the preoccupation with slimness, eating disorders are not as prevalent in that population. Socioeconomically, eating disorders seem to be more common in middle and upper-middle classes—those to whom the cultural message of slimness may have the greatest appeal.

## FYI | DSM CRITERIA FOR EATING DISORDERS

**Anorexia**
According to the DSM-IV, people who meet the criteria for anorexia nervosa experience all of the following symptoms.

- Refusal to maintain the minimum body weight for one's height and age.
- Intense fear of gaining weight even though underweight.
- Disturbed perception of one's body weight or size.
- In post-pubescent women, the absence of at least three consecutive menstrual cycles. (In some women, the loss of periods precedes any significant weight loss.)

**Bulimia**
People with bulimia experience all of the following.

- Recurrent episodes of consuming a much larger amount of food than most people would during a similar time period (this is usually about two hours) and a sense of loss of control over eating during each episode.
- Accompanying attempts to compensate for eating binges by vomiting, by abusing laxatives or other drugs, or by fasting or excessive exercise.
- Both the binge eating and purging occur at least twice a week for three months.
- A negative perception of one's shape and weight.

*Note:* Anorexia and bulimia are included in the *Diagnostic and Statistical Manual of Mental Disorders*. Binge eating is not included in DSM-IV but is a proposed entry.

Perhaps 4% of all female athletes (a field that emphasizes thinness) develop anorexia nervosa or bulimia. Tennis star and Wimbledon finalist Zina Garrison-Jackson has acknowledged her battle with bulimia, which began in 1983 following the death of her mother. Eating disorders as a whole, in males and females alike, are more prevalent in athletes perhaps because they perceive that they must sacrifice the nutritional principles governing the general population if they are to win competitive events.

The consequences of eating disorders can be severe, including death. The death rate is about one in 10, usually from starvation, cardiac arrest, or suicide. Three well-publicized deaths attributed to eating disorders are those of singer Karen Carpenter, gymnast Christy Henrich, and Boston Ballet dancer Heidi Guenther.

## KEY TERMS

**Eating disorder** severe disturbance in eating behavior; three forms are anorexia nervosa, bulimia nervosa, and binge eating

**Anorexia Nervosa.** **Anorexia nervosa** is an eating disorder in which the person does not eat enough food to maintain normal body weight. This leads to severe weight loss, malnutrition, and possibly death. Of all anorexics, 90%–95% are female, and most are in the upper teen and college-age group, although the condition has been documented in middle-aged women and in children as young as nine.

These individuals are more afraid of gaining weight or becoming fat than death from starvation. Thus, most are not even aware that they are starving themselves. Men account for only about one in 20 cases in the general population, but eating disorders among male athletes and dancers are much more common, possibly equaling the incidence of female peers. The typical anorexic eats only 50 to 100 calories a day. Often the preoccupation with weight begins with a distressing situation, such as the loss of a boyfriend or the divorce of parents. Anorexia nervosa is characterized by

- Intense fear of becoming fat, even though the person is underweight

- A distorted body image that allows the person to see oneself as overweight when the person is underweight

- Refusal to maintain body weight

- Cessation of menstrual cycle

- Failure to mature sexually or, if mature, loss of interest in sex

Figure 10.7 points out the physical characteristics of anorexia nervosa. Physiologically, the anorexic's body tries to protect itself by lowering the metabolism. As thyroid activity decreases, the hair and nails become brittle, and the skin becomes dry. Depletion of body fat causes the person to be intolerant to cold. The electrolyte imbalance can result in less bone density and heart failure. Treatment consists of medical, psychosocial, and dietary facets to initiate and sustain weight gain along with psychological techniques to resolve personal and family problems. Initially, anorexics often reduce total food intake, but eventually they restrict their intake of almost all foods and they often purge through vomiting or using laxatives. They never seem to feel thin enough and constantly identify body parts that they feel are too fat. High-risk individuals may require hospitalization and may need to be force-fed by tube to forestall death.

**Bulimia Nervosa.** Like anorexia nervosa, **bulimia nervosa** begins typically during adolescence. It is characterized by a pattern of **bingeing** followed by **purging.** For bulimics, overeating is an attempt to gain comfort and compensate for anxiety, depression, anger, or loneliness. To offset the ensuing guilt and fear of getting fat, the bulimic's solution is to purge the food consumed during the binge. A binge can last as long as eight hours with the consumption of 20,000 calories (approximately 210

## FYI | SOME CLUES TO AN EATING DISORDER

- Excessive weight loss (15%–25% below recommended weight)
- Frequent weight fluctuations (rollercoaster dieting may show up in erratic weight gains or losses)
- Unusual eating habits (taking tiny bites, moving food around on the plate)
- No longer eating meals with the family or group (making excuses such as "too busy," and so on)
- Secretive behavior, especially in eating and bathroom use
- Taking laxatives or diet pills
- Food disappearing regularly
- Overdoing exercise
- Menstrual periods stopping
- More dental cavities and gum disease (induced by malnutrition and vomiting)
- Extreme sensitivity to cold
- Distorted body image (continually saying "I'm too fat")

*Source: Facts About Eating Disorders* (Denver: Children's Hospital, 1994).

brownies), although the average binge involves about 3,400 calories (the equivalent to an entire pecan pie).

The pattern of gorging and purging eventually becomes ingrained. Bulimia is characterized by

- A feeling of lack of control during binges

- Any or some combination of self-induced vomiting, taking laxatives or diuretics, fasting, exercising excessively and strenuously, taking enemas

- Excessive concern with body shape and weight

Bulimics may retain close to normal weight and may not present obvious signs of their eating disorder because they binge and purge in private. In college they are most often discovered by friends and roommates who share bathrooms and eat with them in cafeterias. An estimated one in five women on college campuses is bulimic, and more men suffer from bulimia nervosa than from anorexia nervosa.

Eventually, bulimia can lead to serious physical problems including

- Trauma to the lining of the mouth, esophagus, and stomach

- Erosion of tooth enamel and receding gums

- Electrolyte imbalance in the bloodstream

- Fatigue and muscle cramps

- Endocrine and metabolic changes affecting the menstrual cycle

**FIGURE 10.7 ▶** Physical Symptoms of Anorexia Nervosa

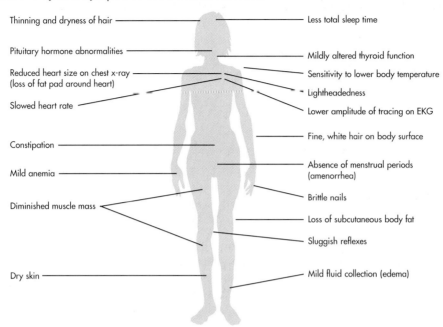

Thinning and dryness of hair

Pituitary hormone abnormalities

Reduced heart size on chest x-ray
(loss of fat pad around heart)

Slowed heart rate

Constipation

Mild anemia

Diminished muscle mass

Dry skin

Less total sleep time

Mildly altered thyroid function

Sensitivity to lower body temperature

Lightheadedness

Lower amplitude of tracing on EKG

Fine, white hair on body surface

Absence of menstrual periods
(amenorrhea)

Brittle nails

Loss of subcutaneous body fat

Sluggish reflexes

Mild fluid collection (edema)

## FYI · WHAT IS PICA?

One of the more unusual practices that survived the journey from Africa is *pica*, the practice of eating clay and other nonfood items. Clay eating was common in West Africa because it alleviated hunger and soothed the irritation caused by intestinal parasites. Clay eating also may have been part of religious rituals. Eating clay also may have added calcium, iron, and phosphorus to mineral-deficient diets.

In America clay eating was present during slavery and is still fairly common in some parts of the South and even in northern cities, especially by pregnant women. In rural areas clay is the substance of choice. In urban areas, laundry starch is often preferred, though some people eat coffee grounds, plaster, paraffin, and milk of magnesia.

Pica eating seems to be passed on from mother to daughter. Whether it is harmful is not known. It may lead to weight gain and hypertension (from the sodium in clay), and it may interfere with nutrition, blocking the absorption of vitamins and minerals and substituting for real food.

*Source: Good Health for African Americans* by Barbara Dixon: (New York: Crown Publishers, 1994), p, 25.

It can contribute to osteoporosis and heart failure. Repeated use of laxatives causes constipation. Treatment requires adherence to a structured eating plan. Anorexia nervosa and bulimia nervosa disorders sometimes overlap—that is, the same person can suffer both diseases—or one can lead to the other. Treatment appears to be more effective for bulimia than for anorexia.

**Binge Eating Disorder. Binge eating disorder (BED)** is the most recently recognized eating disorder. The binge eater often is obese, and dieters may be more susceptible to the disorder. The condition is similar to bulimia nervosa except that the person rarely purges or uses other compensatory behaviors such as misuse of laxatives or excessive exercise. It is found in about 2% of the general population.

Characteristics of binge eating include

- Rapidly consuming large amounts of food in a short time (consume more than 2,000 calories in a single binge)

## KEY TERMS

**Anorexia nervosa** an eating disorder involving extreme weight loss—at least 15% below recommended body weight

**Bulimia nervosa** an eating disorder in which a person consumes large quantities of food in a short time, followed by self-induced vomiting or taking laxatives or diuretics

**Bingeing** Consuming a large amount of food in a short time; gorging

**Purging** self-induced vomiting

**Binge eating disorder (BED)** an eating disorder characterized by consuming large quantities of food in a short time

The age-adjusted prevalence of combined overweight and obesity in racial and ethnic minorities—especially minority women—is generally higher than in whites in the United States.

- Black women (20+ years old): 65.8%
- Mexican American women (20+ years old): 65.9%
- White women (20+ years old): 49.2%

- Black men (20+ years old): 56.5%
- Mexican American men (20+ years old): 63.9%
- White men (20+ years old): 61.0%

*Note:* That studies using BMI 25 as the definition of overweight and obesity provide ethnicity-specific data only for these three racial and ethnic groups.

---

- Feeling unable to stop eating (lack of control)
- Feeling disgusted, guilty, out of control, or depressed after eating
- Eating more rapidly than other people
- Eating large amounts of food when not hungry
- Eating until an uncomfortable feeling sets in
- Eating large amounts of food when alone (compulsive eaters)
- Eating throughout the day with no planned mealtimes
- Bingeing at least twice a week for at least a six-month period

Some binge eaters develop bulimia nervosa, inducing vomiting at times or using laxatives to avoid weight gain. Others continue to binge or overeat. Treatment almost always requires professional assistance by psychologists, dietitians, and physicians who use therapeutic methods such as individual and group therapy. In some cases an antidepressant drug has been helpful. Binge eaters are usually overweight or obese. An estimated 8% to 19% of obese patients in weight loss programs are binge eaters. A behavior technique, habit reversal, is used to replace bingeing with alternative behaviors, such as checking e-mail, calling a friend, or other activities to keep one from eating. To date, binge eating disorder is still under consideration as a psychiatric disorder.

**Treatment for Eating Disorders.** There are no quick fixes or simple solutions in the treatment for eating disorders. Treatment first focuses on reducing the threat to life, and once the person is stabilized, a long-term therapy involves friends, family, and other significant people in the person's life. Therapy focuses on the medical, social, environmental, psychological, and physiological factors that have led to the problem. The person must focus on building new eating behaviors, recognizing threats, building self-confidence, and finding other ways of dealing with problems associated with life. Support groups often help the person and family to gain understanding and emotional support and learn self-development techniques designed to foster positive reactions and actions. Treatment of depression also may be a major focus.

When a person is overweight or underweight, changes are necessary for a healthier future. People can apply this knowledge to weight loss or gain by first assessing their body composition and then taking steps to produce the desired results.

The remaining variables—attitude, commitment, determination, and motivation—are psychological.

## Assessing Your Body Composition

Many different means exist of assessing body composition (ratio of lean to fat tissue). Body mass index (BMI) is the most commonly accepted measure of weight based on height. Other methods include waist circumference (WC), waist-to-hip ratio (WHR), whole body counting, girth and circumference measures, soft-tissue roentgenogram, total body electrical conductivity (TOBEC), hydrostatic weighing, skinfold measurements, and bioelectrical impedance analysis (BIA). Some techniques are highly accurate but inaccessible, whereas other techniques can be done by almost anyone but may not be as accurate.

> **VIEWPOINT** *Do you see patterns of overweight or obesity in your family? Define a risk factor for overweight or obesity that is most relevant to you. What can you do to decrease your risk?*

### BODY MASS INDEX

**Body mass index** is a mathematical formula that correlates height and weight to estimate critical fat values (see Tips for Action and Figure 10.8). A higher BMI may indicate an increased risk of developing cardiovascular disease, hypertension, adult-onset diabetes (type 2), osteoarthritis, sleep apnea, and other conditions. BMI should not be used to estimate body fat of competitive athletes and body builders, given that their BMI is high because of a relatively larger amount of muscle.

## Tips for Action Calculating Your Body Mass Index

1. Multiply your weight in pounds by 703.
2. Multiply your height in inches by itself.
3. Divide the first number by the second and round up to the nearest whole number.

For example, take a 140 lb., 5' 6" (66") person.

$$140 \times 703 = 98,420$$
$$66 \times 66 = 4,356$$
$$98,420 \div 4,356 = 22.59$$

This person's body mass index, rounded to the nearest whole number, is 23.

*Note:* The Body Mass Index Calculator (http://www.nhlbisupport.com/bmi/) and Dr. C. Everett Koop's (http://www.drkoop.com) websites instantly calculate body mass index.

**FIGURE 10.8** ▶ BMI Values Used to Assess Weight for Adults

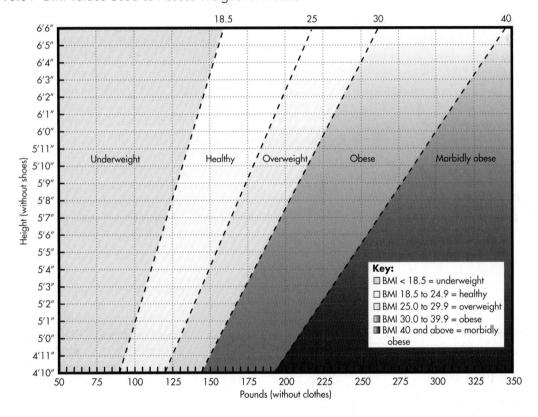

Also, BMI should not be used with pregnant or nursing women, growing children, or sedentary and frail older persons.

According to BMI, a healthy range is classified as 18.5 to 24.9. Your weight may be healthy at a higher BMI if you are muscular and have a higher lean body mass. A BMI of 25 or greater is classified as overweight, indicating an increase in the risk of disease. If your BMI is between 25 and 29.9 (23.4 for Asians), your overweight is affecting the quality of your life. You may have a higher risk of serious health problems and you will have more pains and aches, which will cause you discomfort. A BMI of 30 or greater defines obesity and indicates an increase in the risk of death. The risk of premature death increases even more so if your BMI is over 40, a sign of severe or "morbid" obesity. A BMI under 18.5 is a sign of being underweight. BMI is a useful tool to screen the general population. Similar to height and weight tables, however, it fails to differentiate fat from lean body mass or where most of the fat is located.

## KEY TERMS

**Body mass index (BMI)** technique incorporating height and weight to estimate critical fat values

## FIGURING HEALTHY BODY WEIGHT

Figure 10.9 provides a general guideline to determine your healthy body weight. Because African Americans tend to have denser bones than Caucasians, they are allotted an extra 4–6 pounds on the average. The healthy weight determined in Figure 10.10 is the basis used to calculate caloric needs using the BMR plus sex and activity factors. The BMR factor for men is higher than for women because muscle tissue is more active than fat tissue, and men generally have more muscle tissue than women do. Although age is not factored into the data presented in Figure 10.10, the younger you are, the higher your BMR will be, generally speaking. The BMR is highest during

infancy, puberty, and pregnancy, when the body is undergoing rapid changes and thus requires the most energy. After age 30, the BMR decreases by 1% or more each year, so people find that they have to work harder to take off extra pounds.

## WAIST CIRCUMFERENCE (WC)

Waist circumference (WC) is a simple measurement of the waist and is nearly as effective as more complex measures of obesity such as the body mass index to indicate risk for weight-related health problems. Studies report that stress hormones have a physiological impact on the body, and that fat accumulates around the midsection in times of tension and stress. An apple shape (widening waist) correlates with high levels of harmful blood fats (LDL cholesterol and triglycerides). Abdominal fat increases the risk of high blood pressure, high cholesterol, type 2 diabetes, and metabolic syndrome (a perilous combination of overweight, high blood pressure, and high levels of cholesterol and blood sugar). To measure your waist circumference, place a tape measure around your bare abdomen just above your hip bone. The tape should fit snug but does not compress the skin. The general guideline is that a waist measuring over 35 inches (88 cm) for women signals a serious risk. For men, the figure is approximately 40 inches (102 cm). Waist circumferences indicate the "central" abdominal area of the body. This "visceral" fat is more dangerous than "subcutaneous" fat just below the skin since it moves into the bloodstream and directly raises levels of harmful cholesterol. When men diet, they tend to lose more visceral fat located around the abdominal area,

**FIGURE 10.9** ▶ Guidelines for Determining Healthy Body Weight

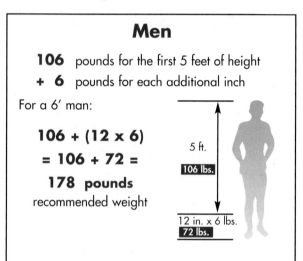

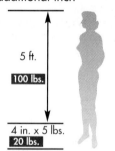

## Men

**106** pounds for the first 5 feet of height
**+ 6** pounds for each additional inch

For a 6' man:

**106 + (12 × 6)**
**= 106 + 72 =**
**178 pounds**
recommended weight

5 ft.
106 lbs.

12 in. × 6 lbs.
72 lbs.

## Women

**100** pounds for first 5 feet of height
**+ 5** pounds for each additional inch

For a 5'4" woman:

**100 + (4 × 5)**
**= 100 + 20 =**
**120 pounds**
recommended weight
± 10% to account for individual differences (small or large frame)

5 ft.
100 lbs.

4 in. × 5 lbs.
20 lbs.

### Modifications for African Americans

**Men: 110** pounds for the first 5 feet of height
**Women: 104** pounds for the first 5 feet of height

Source: *Good Health for African Americans* by Barbara M. Dixon and Josleen Wilson, copyright ©1993 by Barbara M. Dixon and Josleen Wilson. Used by permission of Crown Publisher, a division of random House, Inc.

**FIGURE 10.10** ▶ Calculation of Daily Caloric Needs

Daily caloric needs =
Weight (pounds) × BMR factor
× 24 (hours/day) × activity factor
= _____ daily caloric needs

BMR factor
Men = .45          Women = .41

| **Activity factors** | **Range** |
|---|---|
| Sedentary | 1.40 – 1.50 |
| Light activity | 1.55 – 1.65 |
| Moderate activity | 1.65 – 1.70 |
| Heavy work | 1.75 – 2.00 |

For example, how many calories a day does a male 180-pound construction worker need?

Daily caloric needs =
180 (pounds) × .45 × 24 hours × 1.75
(activity factor) = 3,402 daily calorie needs

BMR = basal metabolic rate.

therefore producing cardiovascular benefits, a decrease in triglycerides (fats circulating in the blood), and an increase in the "good" form of cholesterol, or high-density lipoprotein (HDL). Body composition varies with race and ethnicity. Asians may be more likely and African Americans less likely to accumulate visceral fat than Caucasians.

## WAIST-TO-HIP RATIO (WHR)

The **waist-to-hip ratio** or WHR is a technique that focuses on the distribution of body fat. Fat in the waist and abdomen (the apple shape) is more active metabolically and is associated with higher risk for disease and premature death than is fat in the thighs, hips, and buttocks (the pear shape). The higher the ratio of waist-to-hip measurement, the greater is the risk. More men are apples, and more women are pears. Women tend to be the pear shape because of fat stored for special purposes such as pregnancy and nursing. This fat is more difficult to lose.

To determine the waist-to-hip ratio, the waist circumference measurement is divided by the measurement of the widest circumference around the hips.

Waist-to-hip ratio = waist circumference ÷ hip circumference

For males this ratio should be less than 0.95, and for females the ratio should be less than 0.80. Higher ratios suggest a higher risk. For both men and women, a 1.0 or higher is considered "at risk" or in the danger zone and indicates health consequences such as heart disease and other illness associated with being overweight. Table 10.3 shows the risk for disease according to the waist-to-hip ratio.

## HYDROSTATIC WEIGHING

One of the most accurate methods for assessing body composition is underwater or **hydrostatic weighing.** While under water the person sits in a chair, exhales air, and bends over, feet not touching the floor. Because the density of fat is different from that of lean tissue, these masses can be estimated by measuring the amount of water displaced or by comparing the difference between the underwater and dry weighing.

This method can be intimidating, especially for those who have a fear of water. On the plus side, it covers both

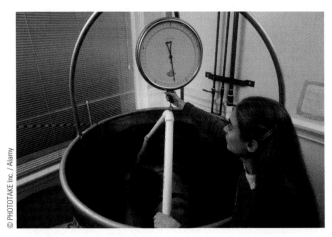

▲ Hydrostatic weighing is one technique used to assess body composition

essential and storage fat and is inexpensive compared with utilizing specialized labs and hospitals. It is inconvenient, though, and not widely available. Measurements can be affected by eating foods that create internal gas or engaging in activities that affect fluid retention or cause dehydration. Reliability depends on the individual doing the weighing and the respiration effort of the person taking the test. The standards used for assessment were developed by testing middle-aged sedentary males, so they may be inaccurate for most people.

## SKINFOLD MEASUREMENT

The **skinfold measurement** is a more convenient method to measure body composition. It indicates how much of the weight is fat and where the fat is located. A technician grasps a fold of skin at a predetermined location and measures it using an instrument called a **caliper.** The skinfold measurement assessment usually is available at colleges, universities, and health clubs. Repeated measurements are taken from several areas of the body, and the results are computed from formulas that predict body fatness from skinfold thickness. The more sites measured, the more valid is the measure of percentage of body fat.

### KEY TERMS

**Waist-to-hip ratio** waist circumference measurement divided by measurement of the widest circumference around the hips

**Hydrostatic weighing** method of determining body composition by measuring the amount of water displaced when a person exhales and sits under water

**Skinfold measurement** method of determining body composition by measuring the thickness of fat under the skin

**Caliper** instrument used to measure the thickness of fat under the skin

**TABLE 10.3 ▶** Risk for Disease According to Waist-to-Hip Ratio

| WAIST-TO-HIP RATIO | | |
| --- | --- | --- |
| MEN | WOMEN | DISEASE RISK |
| ≤0.95 | ≤0.80 | Very low |
| 0.96–0.99 | 0.81–0.84 | Low |
| ≥1.00 | ≥0.85 | High |

© PHOTOTAKE Inc. / Alamy

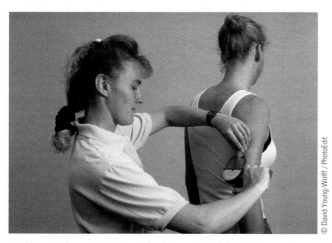

▲ *Various types of skinfold calipers used to assess skinfold thickness*

Because the distribution of body fat is not uniform, taking the measurements can be difficult. Differences in age, sex, and ethnic group can cause measurement errors, as can pinching muscles in conjunction with the skin. Because criteria have not been defined to take these differences into account, measurements always should be done by trained personnel.

## WHOLE BODY COUNTING

Another method of determining body fat measures the total amount of K-40, a naturally occurring form of potassium found primarily in lean tissue. Data are fed into a computer and results are determined.

## BIOELECTRICAL IMPEDANCE ANALYSIS

**Bioelectrical impedance analysis** involves attaching electrodes to the body in several areas, usually on the right hand and right foot. A weak, harmless electrical current is transmitted from electrode to electrode. Electrical conduction through the body favors the path of the lean tissues over the fat tissues. The easier the conductance, the leaner the person. A computer is used to calculate fat percentage from these measurements. The test results may be inaccurate if a person has used diuretic medications within the previous seven days or has exercised 12 hours before testing. This may cause water retention or affect the body's electrolyte balance. Excessive fluid during the menstrual cycle and dehydration both skew the results by showing a higher body fat.

## GIRTH AND CIRCUMFERENCE MEASURES

Diagnosticians use a measuring tape to take girth, or circumference, at various body sites. These measurements are converted into constants, and a formula is used to determine percentages of body fat. It is easy to administer but lacks accuracy.

## AIR DISPLACEMENT

**Air displacement** compares with hydrostatic weighing and takes about five minutes to measure. This technique is administered when an individual sits inside a small chamber (Bod Pod), and body volume is determined by subtracting the air volume with the person inside the chamber from air volume of the empty chamber. The amount of air in the lungs of the person is also taken into consideration when determining the body volume. Percent of body fat and body density are calculated from the obtained body volume. Because of the high cost of the equipment, the **Bod Pod** is usually not available in exercise laboratories and fitness centers. Because it is relatively new, more research is needed to determine its accuracy among various age groups, athletes, and ethnic backgrounds.

## SOFT-TISSUE ROENTGENOGRAM

Another new technique for body fat assessment involves injecting a radioactive substance into the body to penetrate lean muscle tissue so distinctions can be made between lean tissue and fat by means of imaging.

## TOTAL BODY ELECTRICAL CONDUCTIVITY

One of the newest and most expensive assessment techniques uses an electromagnetic force field to assess relative body fat. TOBEC is similar to BIA and requires expensive equipment. Furthermore, well-trained testers are essential.

Additional methods to measure body fat include imaging methods, such as computerized tomography (CT), magnetic resonance imaging (MRI), and ultrasonography, which uses high-frequency sound waves. Although all of the above methods can be useful, they can be inaccurate and unsafe unless well-trained personnel and experienced technicians administer them.

## The Role of Physical Activity

According to a Centers for Disease Control and Prevention survey, 58% of U.S. adults said that they exercise sporadically or not at all. Inactivity was prevalent among African Americans, Hispanics, low-income people, and the unemployed. Also, budget cuts are causing fewer physical education classes in schools throughout the country. To lose weight, a person has three options: diet, exercise more, or combine diet and exercise.

Researchers at Baylor College of Medicine in Houston tested more than 100 overweight men and women in each of these weight-loss methods to determine which worked best over the long term. Exercise was the winner. Physical activity is a necessary component of any weight-management program. A combination of strength-training exercises and aerobics is best. Strength training increases lean body mass, and aerobic exercise lowers the set point.

**TABLE 10.4** ▶ Walking for Weight Loss

| IF YOU WALK (MINUTES) | IF YOU CUT DAILY CALORIES BY | DAYS TO LOSE WEIGHT | | | | |
|---|---|---|---|---|---|---|
| | | 5 lb | 10 lb | 15 lb | 20 lb | 25 lb |
| 30 | 400 | 27 | 54 | 81 | 108 | 135 |
| 30 | 800 | 16 | 32 | 48 | 64 | 80 |
| 45 | 400 | 23 | 46 | 69 | 92 | 115 |
| 45 | 800 | 14 | 28 | 42 | 56 | 70 |
| 60 | 400 | 21 | 42 | 63 | 84 | 105 |
| 60 | 800 | 13 | 26 | 39 | 54 | 65 |

*Note:* The combination of walking and cutting calories results in greater weight loss than either alone.

The underlying principle is that body fat requires fewer calories to maintain itself than lean muscle tissue does. By adhering to an exercise and proper nutritional program, the desirable weight change will follow.

The safest and best way to increase metabolism is to increase physical activity (see Table 10.4). Increasing the metabolism increases the delivery of oxygen to the exercising muscles. The more capable the body is of utilizing oxygen, the more fat is expended.

People who diet without some type of exercise lose not only fat tissue but lean tissue as well. If they regain weight without exercising, the gain is mostly in the form of fat. Because fat tissue expends fewer calories to maintain itself, the person will gain weight if he or she eats the same amount of food as before. However, in studies conducted on calorie burning, persons were placed in a controlled respiratory chamber environment where calories consumed, motion, and overall activity were measured. It was found that some people are better fat burners than others. Therefore, the results may infer that some people may not produce as many of the enzymes needed to convert fat to energy. Also, results may indicate that they may not have as many blood vessels supplying fatty tissue, therefore making it harder for them to deliver fat-burning oxygen.

Some people engage in body sculpting, which is another dead-end to weight loss. A person cannot lose **cellulite** (or any fat) in specific body locations by doing localized, isolated exercises. Fat cells release fat into the blood (not the muscle), and all the muscles share the fat. **Spot-reducing** exercises, such as curl-ups for the abdominal area or side bends in an attempt to have a smaller waist, however, will tone muscles in those areas by strengthening muscle tissue under the stored body fat.

## EXERCISE INTENSITY

The proportion of fat to carbohydrate burned is greater with low-intensity exercise, such as walking. Higher-intensity exercise, such as brisk running, however, expends more total calories and the absolute number of fat calories is greater.

As you increase the intensity, that percentage shifts in favor of carbohydrate, at the expense of fat. At higher intensities, you still are expending more total fat calories. The percentage of fat versus carbohydrate may be lower, but it is based on a much higher total of expended calories.

The optimum for fat burning is high-intensity exercise. Exercise physiologist Edward Coyle, of the University of Texas, has found that a person burns significantly more fat calories per unit of time running at an easy pace than he or she does when walking.

## PASSIVE EXERCISE

Gimmicks such as vibrators, steam baths, rubber suits, body wraps, motor-driven cycles, and motor-driven rowing machines are not necessary in a successful weight management plan. They basically are a waste of time and money.

- Vibrators (tables, belts, pillows) result in negligible caloric expenditure and do not generate weight loss. They may aggravate the back and can be dangerous to pregnant women.

- Attempted weight loss by using rubber suits causes the person to sweat. Weight loss comes from the loss of body fluid, which causes unhealthy changes in

### KEY TERMS

**Bioelectrical impedance analysis (BIA)** method of determining body composition by analyzing electrical conduction through the body

**Air displacement** A relatively new technique to assess body composition by calculating the body volume from the air displaced by an individual sitting inside a small chamber

**Bod Pod** Commercial name of the equipment used to assess body composition through the air displacement technique

**Cellulite** fat that appears lumpy

**Spot-reducing** exercising to reduce fat in a specific location of the body

**Tips for Action** Want to Gain Weight?

■ Control your exercise and reduce exercising if you are doing too much.

■ Eat more calories by eating more frequently, spending more time eating, and eating high-calorie foods.

■ Eat high-calorie snacks and supplement your diet with high-calorie drinks that have a healthy balance of nutrients.

■ Eat more peanut butter, cream cheese, and cheese, and consume sandwiches with thick bread.

■ Slow down, relax, rest more, and control stress levels.

TABLE 10.5 ► MyPyramid Food Intake Pattern Calorie Levels

| | MALES | | | | FEMALES | | |
|---|---|---|---|---|---|---|---|
| ACTIVITY LEVEL | SEDENTARY* | MOD. ACTIVE* | ACTIVE* | ACTIVITY LEVEL | SEDENTARY* | MOD. ACTIVE* | ACTIVE* |
| AGE | | | | AGE | | | |
| 2 | 1000 | 1000 | 1000 | 2 | 1000 | 1000 | 1000 |
| 3 | 1000 | 1400 | 1400 | 3 | 1000 | 1200 | 1400 |
| 4 | 1200 | 1400 | 1600 | 4 | 1200 | 1400 | 1400 |
| 5 | 1200 | 1400 | 1600 | 5 | 1200 | 1400 | 1600 |
| 6 | 1400 | 1600 | 1800 | 6 | 1200 | 1400 | 1600 |
| 7 | 1400 | 1600 | 1800 | 7 | 1200 | 1600 | 1800 |
| 8 | 1400 | 1600 | 2000 | 8 | 1400 | 1600 | 1800 |
| 9 | 1600 | 1800 | 2000 | 9 | 1400 | 1600 | 1800 |
| 10 | 1600 | 1800 | 2200 | 10 | 1400 | 1800 | 2000 |
| 11 | 1800 | 2000 | 2200 | 11 | 1600 | 1800 | 2000 |
| 12 | 1800 | 2200 | 2400 | 12 | 1600 | 2000 | 2200 |
| 13 | 2000 | 2200 | 2600 | 13 | 1600 | 2000 | 2200 |
| 14 | 2000 | 2400 | 2800 | 14 | 1800 | 2000 | 2400 |
| 15 | 2200 | 2600 | 3000 | 15 | 1800 | 2000 | 2400 |
| 16 | 2400 | 2800 | 3200 | 16 | 1800 | 2000 | 2400 |
| 17 | 2400 | 2800 | 3200 | 17 | 1800 | 2000 | 2400 |
| 18 | 2400 | 2800 | 3200 | 18 | 1800 | 2000 | 2400 |
| 19–20 | 2600 | 2800 | 3000 | 19–20 | 2000 | 2200 | 2400 |
| 21–25 | 2400 | 2800 | 3000 | 21–25 | 2000 | 2200 | 2400 |
| 26–30 | 2400 | 2600 | 3000 | 26–30 | 1800 | 2000 | 2400 |
| 31–35 | 2400 | 2600 | 3000 | 31–35 | 1800 | 2000 | 2200 |
| 36–40 | 2400 | 2600 | 2800 | 36–40 | 1800 | 2000 | 2200 |
| 41–45 | 2200 | 2600 | 2800 | 41–45 | 1800 | 2000 | 2200 |
| 46–50 | 2200 | 2400 | 2800 | 46–50 | 1800 | 2000 | 2200 |
| 51–55 | 2200 | 2400 | 2800 | 51–55 | 1600 | 1800 | 2200 |
| 56–60 | 2200 | 2400 | 2600 | 56–60 | 1600 | 1800 | 2200 |
| 61–65 | 2000 | 2400 | 2600 | 61–65 | 1600 | 1800 | 2000 |
| 66–70 | 2000 | 2200 | 2600 | 66–70 | 1600 | 1800 | 2000 |
| 71–75 | 2000 | 2200 | 2600 | 71–75 | 1600 | 1800 | 2000 |
| 76 and up | 2000 | 2200 | 2400 | 76 and up | 1600 | 1800 | 2000 |

*Calorie levels are based on the Estimated Energy Requirements (EER) and activity levels from the Institute of Medicine Dietary Reference Intakes Macronutrients Report, 2002.

SEDENTARY = less than 30 minutes a day of moderate physical activity in addition to daily activities.
MOD. ACTIVE = at least 30 minutes up to 60 minutes a day of moderate physical activity in addition to daily activities.
ACTIVE = 60 or more minutes a day of moderate physical activity in addition to daily activities.

*Note:* MyPyramid assigns individuals to a calorie level based on their sex, age, and activity level.

The chart above identifies the calorie levels for males and females by age and activity level. Calorie levels are provided for each year of childhood, from 2–18 years, and for adults in 5-year increments.

*Source:* U.S. Department of Agriculture, Center for Nutrition Policy and Promotion, April, 2005.

## Tips for Action Choices in Eating

Which of the following would you choose?

### Breakfast

| Good choices | Poor choices |
|---|---|
| English muffin | Biscuits and gravy |
| Boiled egg | Cheese omelet |
| Cereal with low-fat milk | Sugared cereal with cream |
| Wheat toast, plain | Bagel and cream cheese |
| Whole-grain muffin | Chocolate muffin |
| Low-fat yogurt | Bacon or sausage |

### Lunch and Dinner

| Good choices | Poor choices |
|---|---|
| Steamed perch | Deep-fried shrimp |
| Baked chicken breast | Southern-fried chicken |
| Baked potato, plain | French fries |
| Vegetable soup | Cream soup |

| Good choices | Poor choices |
|---|---|
| Tossed salad | Cole slaw |
| Chili | BBQ ribs |
| Black-eyed peas | Ham hocks and beans |
| Bean burrito | Cheese nachos |
| Spaghetti | Hush puppies |
| Stir-fried vegetables | Egg roll |

The hidden ingredient in the poor choices is fat—in the form of butter and other dairy products, oil, and mayonnaise. Or the key may lie in the method of cooking. Methods that require fat or oil are poor choices. Better methods are roasting, baking, broiling, braising, poaching, stir-frying, steaming, and microwaving.

Some ethnic fast-food restaurants have been chastised for the high calorie counts of their items. The foods themselves usually are not the problem. The problem is in the cooking methods and add-ons.

---

water metabolism and in kidney and circulatory functions, thus increasing body temperature.

- Massage is relaxing and may improve circulation, but it will not reduce weight.

- Body wraps (wrapping the body in bandages soaked in a "special formula") may alter the body circumference temporarily, but the body will regain its shape within hours after unwrapping. Body wraps may limit circulation and can be dangerous.

- Steam baths and saunas remove fluids from the body. Rapid fluid loss can cause severe dehydration and chemical imbalance. Consuming water immediately after a sweat session will return the body to normal weight.

- Motor-driven cycles and motor-driven rowing machines are devices that do the work for the person. They may help maintain flexibility and increase circulation, but the most effective means of weight reduction is for the body, not a machine, to be active.

- Sales of body shapers (girdles) and control-top panty hose are booming. These support garments have been called "a one-minute diet" and "instant slimmers." This suggests that they are substitutes for true weight loss and not the camouflage items they really are.

> **VIEWPOINT** *The vitamin, herbal medicine, and natural remedy industries are booming. Do you believe these constitute a passing fad, or will they become staples in weight management on the path to healthier living?*

## Weight Management

The number of calories needed each day depends on gender, age, body frame size, percentage of body fat, activity level, and resting metabolic rate (the number of calories needed to sustain the body at rest). To lose or gain weight, there must be an imbalance of energy. If you consume more calories than are required to maintain your size and do not expend energy in physical activity, your body will convert the excess to fat. To gain lean muscle, you must take in more calories and exercise. For weight maintenance (balance must be met), caloric input (eating) must be equal to caloric output (daily activity) (see Table 10.5).

### WEIGHT MAINTENANCE

Weight maintenance (staying the same weight) is keeping the same composition of lean tissue and fat that is carried in the body. To remain at your constant weight, energy must be in balance; that is, energy in (eating, diet) is equal to energy out (expenditure, exercise). Thus, to remain the same weight, you must intake (eat) the number of calories expended (burned up) each day. The metabolism of older adults slows down and the activity level decreases. Therefore, you must select a variety of nutritious foods (food plan) and eat fewer calories as you age.

### WEIGHT LOSS

By following the guidelines on weight management, you will have a safe weight loss program. A safe weight loss (1/2 to 1 pound per week for women and 1–2 pounds per

---

**Tips for Action** Nonhunger Eating Cues

| | | | |
|---|---|---|---|
| Time | You are conditioned to eat at certain times, even when you are not hungry. | Situations | A study break, for example, can trigger a trip to the refrigerator. |
| Mood | Mood can be a cue to eat even when you are not hungry. This is the most common kind of nonhunger cue. | TV | TV flashes an average of eight eating cues per hour. |
| Place | Various places (such as movie theatres) can trigger a desire to eat. | Food | The smell and sight of food—vending machine, grocery store, bakery—encourage you to eat. |
| People | You eat candy or other foods because someone special gave it to you. | | |

---

week for men) for all ages and ethnic groups can be accomplished by eating less and exercising more.

To lose 1 pound of fat in a week, you must consume 3,500 fewer calories or 500 calories a day less than the maintenance number for each day in the week (seven days). To lose 2 pounds of fat in a week, you must take in 1,000 calories a day less than the maintenance number.

Overweight females who wish to lose weight should consume a minimum of 1,200 calories a day; overweight males, 1,500 calories.

## WEIGHT GAIN

Many underweight young men and women need and want to gain weight. They seem to eat everything in sight and still have a caloric deficit due to a variety of metabolic, psychological, hereditary, or other reasons. First, in order to gain weight, determine the reasons for your difficulty in gaining weight. Older adults may lose some of the senses of taste and smell that make food taste differently and be less pleasurable. Visual problems and other disabilities may make meals difficult to prepare and dental problems may make meals difficult to eat. Active individuals who engage in extreme sports that require extreme nutritional supplementation may be at risk for nutritional deficiencies.

In gaining weight, you should strive to do so in the form of lean body mass and not body fat. If one consumes more calories than used, whether the calories are from carbohydrates, proteins, or fat, weight will be gained. The food plan must be higher in calories and be nutritious, with adequate amounts of dietary protein, and the exercise program should be designed to increase muscle mass.

To increase lean body weight, an increase in caloric intake, an adequate amount of rest, and an exercise program should be effective. A safe approach is gaining about 1 pound per week after acquiring basic strength through a month of weight training. However, aerobic exercise is necessary for good health, so increased food intake (calories) should compensate for depleting calories aerobically.

To add 1 pound of body muscle in a week, you must consume 2,500 calories (this accounts for approximately 600 calories for the muscle and the extra energy needed for exercise to develop the muscle). The daily caloric excess, over the maintenance number, is about 360 calories.

Once you know what is causing a daily caloric deficit, the following steps can help you to gain extra weight.

- Eat at regularly scheduled times (whether you are hungry or not).
- Eat more. Eat more frequently, spend more time eating, eat the high-calorie foods first if you fill up fast and always start with the main course. Put extra spreads such as peanut butter, cream cheese, or cheese on your foods. Make sandwiches with extra-thick slices of bread, and add more filling. Take second helpings, and eat high-calorie snacks during the day.
- Supplement your diet. Consume high-calorie drinks that have a healthy balance of nutrients.
- Eat with people who will not analyze what you eat or who make you feel like you should eat less.
- Avoid diuretics, laxatives, and other medications that cause you to lose body fluids and nutrients.
- If you aren't exercising, exercise to increase your appetite. If you are exercising or exercising to extremes, moderate your activities until weight gain is evident.
- RELAX. Slow down, get more rest, and control stress. Try to avoid operating in high gear most of the time.

## ATTITUDE AND BEHAVIOR MODIFICATION

Eating healthier often requires a person to make fundamental changes. In contrast to dieting, which promotes the myth that long-lasting changes are brought about from the outside in, weight change should be considered from the inside out. People must correct their attitudes and habits, according to Jennifer Carney, a Denver nutritional

**Tips for Action** 10 Successful Ways to Lose Weight

**1.** Take control of your weight. Consider weight management a lifelong commitment, not a diet.

**2.** Develop your own personal plan to meet your needs. Your plan should fit you—your work schedule, priorities, personality—and should allow time for rest and relaxation.

**3.** Set realistic goals. Why do you want to lose weight? Make a commitment and set out ways to reach your goals.

**4.** Keep records in your food and exercise diary. Record what, how much, where you eat, and why you eat, and count calories. Record each exercise activity session. Make a moderate amount of exercise a priority in your daily activities.

**5.** Select nutrient-dense foods. Include natural fiber, which fills you up and speeds food through your body, cutting calorie consumption. Reduce sugar and sweeteners.

**6.** Eat several small meals throughout the day instead of eating one or two bigger meals. Do not skip meals. Eat slowly and savor each bite. Avoid seconds.

**7.** Plan snacks. Select plain popcorn, vegetables, fruit, rice cakes, and low-fat foods.

**8.** Plan for plateaus. Exercise helps to get past plateaus. Plan for success and chart your setbacks. Consider what caused the setback.

**9.** Exercise. Losing weight requires hard work and time. The more active you are, the more calories you burn.

**10.** Accept yourself. Feel good about you and why you are losing unwanted pounds. Get a friend to support, exercise, and grocery shop with you. Remember, there is no weight-loss magic, only you can make it happen.

---

consultant. She says people should find ways other than eating to nurture themselves.

Many people have to unlearn habits ingrained since childhood, such as being rewarded with sweets and being urged to "hurry up and eat" and "clean up your plate." In conflicting messages, the media promote slimness to the point of emaciation, which makes overweight people feel guilty and leads to the loss of self-esteem and to depression.

Weight management is promoted most successfully as a key to health. Individuals in weight management programs must recognize their bad habits and be motivated to lose or gain the weight. The behaviors of the person who is overeating or undereating must be modified. When the behaviors of eating fewer calories and expending more energy through exercise are attained, the outcome is a healthier person.

Behavior modification can change an individual from being inactive to active, from overeating fast food to eating nutritional foods. Half the battle of breaking bad habits lies in recognizing them. Jotting down what you eat and what your feelings are at the time you eat is a good idea. You may realize that you reach for snacks when you are bored or worried.

Weight gain usually has developed over time. Likewise, weight loss should be a slow and gradual process. Make specific lifestyle changes.

- Set realistic expectations. What you are doing is good for you. You are doing this for yourself, not to please anyone else.

- Be sure your weight management plan is medically safe.

- Include both short- and long-term goals. Break long-term goals into small, reasonable steps to get you where you want to go.

- Keep a record (chart or journal) of your weight and daily eating intake so you can measure your progress. Write down the quantity and the caloric content of the foods you eat. Pay attention to what, when, where, and why you eat.

- Make a mental note of what makes you want to eat. Anticipate problems, and plan ways to avoid them.

- Refrain from buying and stashing ice cream, cookies, soft drinks, and candy.

- Keep a variety of nutritious foods on hand.

- Never skip meals, and limit snacking after the evening meal.

- Make healthy substitutes. For instance, eat low-fat frozen yogurt instead of ice cream.

- Eat breakfast. It increases metabolism. To lose weight, consume approximately 75% of your daily calories within six hours of starting your day.

- Eat meals slowly (20–30 minutes), pausing often. Put down utensils between bites. Swallow before reloading the fork. It takes the appetite control center about 20 minutes to receive the message that you have eaten enough.

- When feeling bored or down, reach for the phone instead of food, or take a break by walking. Post a list of substitute activities you enjoy.

- Avoid stimulants, diuretics, laxatives, diet pills, and dehydration techniques (steam baths, saunas).

- Limit your alcohol intake. Alcohol may slow the body's ability to burn fat, and it favors fat storage. Alcohol is also high in calories (7 calories per gram) and may increase your appetite.

- Drink a minimum of eight 8-ounce glasses of water daily. Limit beverages such as colas and other caffeinated drinks.

- Maintain a regular aerobic exercise program. Walking after a meal will expend fat while it is still in the bloodstream and before it reaches the fat storage stage.

- Choose activities you enjoy to burn calories.

- Ask for help from others. Eat and exercise with friends and family members who offer support and encouragement. Avoid negative environments and people.

- Praise yourself, think positive, and avoid self-criticism even when you fail.

- Learn from failure. Everyone backslides. You are only human. Do not demand too much from yourself. Instead, decide how you can avoid failure so you can be successful in the future.

- Forgo diets. Tell yourself to eat nutritional foods and abstain from overeating.

- Follow the 80–20 rule: 80% of the time, make healthy food choices; 20% of the time, indulge yourself a little.

- Ban all problem foods from the home.

- Use smaller plates, bowls, and glasses. A full, small plate is psychologically more satisfying than a half-full, large plate.

- Choose a way of eating that will give you all the needed nutrients, fit your time schedule and tastes, keep you from feeling hungry and tired, and work for you for the rest of your life.

- Keep foods only in the kitchen. Remove snack foods and beverages from other rooms.

- Your reward for losing weight should be internal gratification. However, you may wish to get a new outfit, go to a movie, or something else you enjoy, when you make progress.

- Make lunch, not dinner, your main meal. Take a 10-minute walk after you eat if larger meals make you feel sluggish. At night, eat light—soup, cereal, bread, salad, or fruit.

- Eat more fresh fruits and vegetables—up to five servings a day. They also make good snacks.

- Never eat directly out of cartons, bags, or bowls. Place what you want on a plate, close the container, and put it away.

- Wait for your stomach to rumble before you eat. Stop eating before you feel full, even if there is food on your plate.

- Do not eat while watching TV, reading, driving, or studying; do not eat while standing up or walking. Eat at regular mealtimes and in designated areas (kitchen or dining room).

- Prepare foods wisely. Use less fat and refined foods. Bake, broil, and boil instead of frying. Remove all visible fat from meats. Do not use coconut oil, cocoa butter, or palm oil.

Most people go through five stages when shedding unhealthy eating habits and replacing them with healthy eating behaviors.

1. "So what?" In this stage, a person may be getting some pressure to lose weight, but he or she is resisting.

2. "I'm thinking about it." Now the person is more open to thinking, reading, and talking about changing his or her eating habits. He or she begins to consider the benefits and drawbacks.

3. "I'm ready." The person make a firm decision to change and perhaps tells family or friends about it. The change becomes a priority, and he or she starts to make a specific plan.

4. "I'm doing it." The person puts a plan into action. For example, he or she discards high-calorie foods, curtails fast-food trips, and starts to cook, using low-fat cooking methods.

5. "I did it." The person made the switch to healthier eating habits and has lost some weight. Now he or she is in for the long haul and must be careful not to backslide.

If caloric intake is more than caloric output, weight increases. If caloric intake is less than caloric output, weight decreases. Fat cannot be starved off, slept off, or melted off. No quick, easy methods or devices can help you change body weight, whether you want to gain or lose weight. Your reward for losing or gaining weight should be internal gratification. Weight management takes time, patience, and persistence. It is a lifetime adventure of setting and achieving one goal at a time.

## Summary

- The metabolic rate depends on body size and composition, gender, diet, age, genetic factors, hormones, and activity level.

- Many factors contribute to the risk for overweight or obesity. Included are genetic predisposition, set point, fat cells, body size and composition, gender, lifestyle, diet, age, hormones, physical activity level, overeating, metabolic changes, eating patterns, and psychological factors. Women are prone to have more difficulty with weight reduction.

- In general, Americans regardless of age, gender, and ethnicity are eating more, exercising less, and therefore, are gaining extra pounds.

- In the United States 22% of today's children and adolescents are obese and 25% are overweight.

- To determine healthy body weight, a person can figure basal metabolic rate and caloric needs.

- There are many different means of assessing body composition. BMI is the most commonly accepted measure of weight based on height. Other methods include waist circumference, waist-to-hip ratio, whole body counting, girth and circumference measures, soft-tissue roentgenogram, air displacement, total body electrical conductivity (TOBEC), hydrostatic weighing, skinfold measurements, and bioelectrical impedance analysis.

- Americans in general are becoming fatter, weighing an average of 12 pounds more than they did a decade ago.

- Health hazards of obesity include higher rates of cardiovascular diseases, respiratory problems, diabetes, arthritis, some cancers, and other serious conditions, as well as a shorter life span.

- The three classifications of eating disorders are anorexia nervosa, bulimia, and binge eating, all of which are most prevalent in young Caucasian women.

- To determine healthy body weight, a person can figure basal metabolic rate and caloric needs.

- Determining body composition—the proportion of fat tissue to lean body mass—is the basis for making a weight change.

- Weight-loss gimmicks include fad diets, unsupervised liquid diets, over-the-counter diet pills and aids, and passive exercise devices.

- Weight change requires not only changes in eating habits but also a regular exercise program as well as attitude and behavior modifications, foremost of which is a commitment to a lifetime weight management program.

## Personal Health Resources

ThomsonNOW  Visit the ThomsonNOW website at http://thomsonedu.com/thomsonnow for valuable resources that will:

- Help you evaluate your knowledge of the material.
- Guide you through tutorials to help you understand and apply the material.
- Allow you to take an exam-prep quiz to better prepare for class tests.

### American Obesity Association
This is the leading organization for advocacy and education on the nation's obesity epidemic. This website features statistics on overweight and obesity.

**www.obesity.org**

**Measuring Your Percentage of Body Fat.** This site features a wellness link, nutrition information, and a virtual gym. It enables you to determine your exercise efficiency by calculating your target heart rate and your body mass index.

**www.fitnesslink.com/exercise/bodyfat.shtml**

**Home Body Fat Test.** This site allows you to calculate your approximate percentage of body fat by answering three simple questions pertaining to your age, gender, and weight in pounds (or kilograms). It contains information about body composition as discussed by Covert Bailey, a fitness expert.

**www.healthcentral.com/cooltools/CT_Fitness/bodyfat1.cfm**

**BMI.** Calculate your BMI free and learn more about fitness

**www.prevention.com**

### Weight Control Network
This government site features a variety of publications on nutrition, physical activity, and weight control. There are links for research, a newsletter, statistical data, and a bibliographic collection of journal articles on aspects of weight management and obesity.

**win.niddk.nih.gov/index.htm**

**Body Composition and Somatype.** This site includes a table listing male and female percent body fat ranges, body fat myths and truths, and specific activities to help achieve proper body composition.

**www.worldguide.com/Fitness/med.html**

### National Eating Disorders Center
**www.nationaleatingdisorders.org**

This website features a comprehensive database of educational information for patients, health professionals, and students. It features referrals, advocacy, support, prevention, and professional conferences.

## It's Your Turn for Study and Review

1. What kinds of pressures affect one's personal body image? Where do these pressures come from?

2. List the risk factors for overweight and obesity. Evaluate each of them, and determine which is most important to determine if a person will be overweight or obese in later adult years.

3. Different cultures have different standards for attractiveness and body weight. Can you think of reasons that men and women in these cultures differ in why body weight is attractive and how much weight is desired?

4. Calculate your BMI using the formula provided in this chapter, and compare the results to the formulas provided by the Body Mass Index Calculator.

5. Test your percentage of body fat with skinfold calipers and one of the other methods listed in this chapter. Are the results similar?

6. What are two methods for weight reduction that offer the lowest risk and the best chance for success? Why?

7. Develop a plan to help you or a friend to maintain, lose, or gain weight. What suggestions would you provide for a safe weight maintenance, weight loss, or weight gain program?

8. What programs or services on your campus or in your community are available to help you with a weight maintenance, weight loss, or weight gain program? If in doubt, ask your instructor to find out where you can get assistance to start this lifelong journey to better health.

## Thinking about Health Issues

■ Are herbs safe and effective for weight loss?

Jennifer Sardina, "Misconceptions and Misleading Information Prevail—Less Regulation Does Not Mean Less Danger to Consumers: Dangerous Herbal Weight Loss Products," *Journal of Law and Health*, 14:1 (Spring 1999), p. 107.

1. How does the Dietary Supplement Health and Education Act of 1994 classify dietary supplements? What are the advantages and disadvantages of this classification?

2. What regulations are now being considered to further protect consumers from the dangers of herbal weight-loss products?

## Selected Bibliography

American Obesity Association, www.obesity.org.

Berkowitz, R., et al. "Behavior Therapy and Sibutramine for the Treatment of Adolescent Obesity." *Journal of the American Medical Association*, 289:14, April 9, 2003, p. 1833.

"Controlling the Global Obesity Epidemic." International Obesity Task Force (IOTF), www.iotf.org.

Delrue, M. and Michaud, J. "Fat Chance: Genetic Syndromes with Obesity." *Clinical Genetics*, 66:2, August 2004, p. 83.

Deen, D. "Metabolic Syndrome: Time for Action." *American Family Physician*, 69:2, June 15, 2004, p. 2875.

Dixon, B. *Good Health for African Americans*. New York: Crown, 1994.

Donatelle, R. J. *Health: The Basics*, 6th ed. San Francisco, CA: Pearson Education, Inc., 2005.

Floyd, P. A. and Parke, J. *Walk, Jog, Run for Wellness Everyone*, 5th ed. Winston-Salem, NC: Hunter, 2006.

Franzoi, S. and Koehler, V. "Age and Gender Differences in Body Attitudes: A Comparison of Young and Elderly Adults." *International Journal of Aging and Human Development*, 47:1, July/August 1998.

"Global Strategy on Diet, Physical Activity and Health," World Health Organization, www.who.int/dietphysical-activity/publications/facts/obesity/en/.

Hales, D. *An Invitation to Health Brief*, 4th ed. Belmont, CA: Wadsworth Publishing Co., 2006.

Health and Human Services Press Office. "Citing Dangerous Increase in Deaths, HHS Launches New Strategies against Overweight Epidemic," March 9, 2004.

Kilpatrick, M., et al. "Adolescent Weight Management and Perceptions: An Analysis of the National Longitudinal Study of Adolescent Health." *Journal of School Health*, 69:4, April 1999.

Landers, S. "Policy-makers Take Aim at Obesity Rates." *American Medical News*, www.amednews.com, July 19, 2004.

Ludwig, D. and Gortmaker, S. "Programming Obesity in Childhood." *Lancet*, 364:9430, July 17, 2004, p. 226.

Midgley, J., Matthew, G., and Celia, M. "Effect of Reduced Dietary Sodium on Blood Pressure." *Journal of the American Medical Association*, 275:20, 1996, pp. 1590–1595.

National Center for Health Statistics, www.hhs.gov.

National Heart, Lung, and Blood Institute, Communications Office. *First Federal Obesity Clinical Guidelines Released*. Bethesda, MD: NHLBI, June 17, 1998.

"Obesity in the U.S.," *AOA Fact Sheet*, American Obesity Association, www.obesity.org.

Sanders, T. A. "High- Versus Low-Fat Diets in Human Diseases." *Current Opinion of Clinical Nutrition and Metabolic Care*, 6:2, March 2003, p. 151.

"State Efforts to Control Obesity," University of Baltimore, www.ubalt.edu/experts/obesity/index.html.

Willett, W. "Reduced-Carbohydrate Diets: No Role in Weight Management?" *Annals of Internal Medicine*, 140:10, May 18, 2004, p. 836.

Willett, W. C. and Leibel, R. L. "Dietary Fat Is Not a Major Determinant of Body Fat." *American Journal of Medicine*, 113:9B, December 30, 2002, pp. 475–595.

"Your Message to Patients: Supersize, Shorter Life." *American Medical News*, www.amednews.com, February 17, 2003.

Name _____     Course _____

Date _____     Section _____

## Women

100 pounds for the first 5 feet                                    =  _____

      OR

104 pounds for the first 5 feet (African American)    =  _____

+ 5 pounds for each additional inch                         =  _____

± 10% to account for individual differences             =  _____
   (small or large frame)

## Men

106 pounds for the first 5 feet                                    =  _____

      OR

110 pounds for the first 5 feet (African American)    =  _____

+ 6 pounds for each additional inch                         =  _____

± 10% to account for individual differences             =  _____
   (small or large frame)

*Note:* To lose 1 pound of fat, subtract 500 calories per day (exercising = 250 calories and proper nutrition = 250 calories, a total of 500 calories) seven days per week for a total of 3,500 calories per week.

**Name** _____     **Course** _____

**Date** _____     **Section** _____

Weight in pounds: _____ × _____ (BMR factor)

= _____ × 24 (hrs/day) _____ = _____ × (activity factor) = _____

Daily caloric needs = _____

## BMR Factor

Men     = 0.45

Women = 0.41

| Activity factor | Range |
|---|---|
| Sedentary (sitting) | 1.40–1.50 |
| Light activity (washing dishes) | 1.55–1.65 |
| Moderate activity (mail carrier, delivery person) | 1.65–1.70 |
| Heavy work (manual laborer) | 1.75–2.00 |

*Note:* To maintain your present weight, consume the number of calories calculated above. To lose weight, consume fewer calories and increase your activity.

**Name** _____     **Course** _____

**Date** _____     **Section** _____

Calculate your waist-to-hip circumference ratio.

Waist (inches):  =  _____

Hip (inches):  =  _____

Ratio:  $\frac{\text{Waist}}{\text{Hip}}$  =  _____

Evaluate your ratio. A ratio above 0.95 for males or 0.80 for females indicates a need to reduce body fatness to lessen health risks.

**Name** _____   **Course** _____

**Date** _____   **Section** _____

Your eating pattern can show you what you eat, where you eat, why you eat, when you eat, and how you eat. Keep a record for several days of the foods you consume. Be honest. Make sure one of the days is a Saturday or Sunday and the others are weekdays.

Use the below sample as a guide.

SAMPLE:

| DAY | WHAT FOODS? How much? | WHEN? Start/Stop | WHERE? Doing what? | WHY? |
|-----|----------------------|------------------|--------------------|------|
| Sat. | Candy bar | 7:15 – 7:18 | Watching TV | Bored |

Afterward, take a look at your eating patterns. Do you have a problem area? The checklist below can assist you. Did you

|  | Yes | No |
|--|-----|-----|
| 1. Eat when you were bored? | _____ | _____ |
| 2. Eat high-calorie snack foods? | _____ | _____ |
| 3. Eat while watching TV or a movie? | _____ | _____ |
| 4. Eat fast foods more than once? | _____ | _____ |
| 5. Skip meals and then eat too much? | _____ | _____ |
| 6. Eat vegetables? | _____ | _____ |
| 7. Eat fruits? | _____ | _____ |
| 8. Drink water? | _____ | _____ |
| 9. Drink milk? | _____ | _____ |
| 10. Eat breakfast? | _____ | _____ |

If you answered "no" to questions 1–5 and "yes" to questions 6–10, good for you. If you answered "yes" to any of the first five or "no" to any of the last five, you need to make changes in your eating habits.

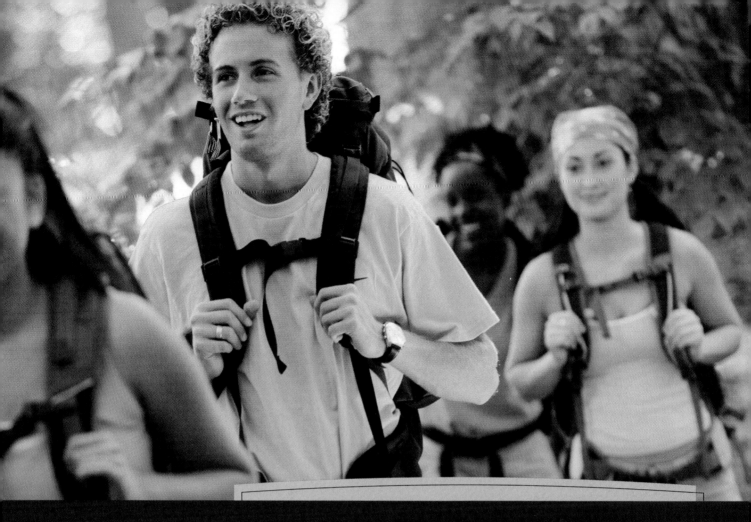

# Chapter Eleven  Physical Activity and Health

**OBJECTIVES** ■ Define physical activity and physical fitness.
■ Explain several physical and psychological benefits of fitness.
■ Explain the FITT formula and its components. ■ Explain the three
phases of an exercise session. ■ Explain the principles of overload,
progression, specificity, and reversibility. ■ Explain the PRICE injury
treatment concept. ■ List safety precautions to take when exercising.
■ Be able to design a personal fitness program.

ThomsonNOW™  Log on to ThomsonNOW at http://thomsonedu.com/
thomsonnow to access and explore self-assessments, interactive
tutorials, and practice quizzes.

© Andersen Ross/Blend Images/Jupiterimages

Many Americans may be surprised at the extent and strength of the evidence linking **physical activity** to health. Regular physical activity greatly reduces the risk of dying from coronary heart disease, the leading cause of death in the United States. In addition, physical activity is directly related to preventing disease and premature death and to maintaining a high quality of life. However, according to the Centers for Disease Control and Prevention (CDC), one in four Americans reports no physical activity at all and about half exercise occasionally but not enough. Only one in four adults meets the level of physical activity recommended by federal health officials.

The federal government promotes health for all Americans. A healthy population is a nation's greatest resource, the source of its vigor and wealth, whereas poor health drains a nation's resources and raises health care costs. The U.S. government has developed *Healthy People 2010 Objectives* (2000) and *Physical Activity and Health: A Report of the Surgeon General* (1996).

Every 10 years the U.S. Department of Health and Human Services releases a list of objectives for preventing disease and promoting health. This 10-year plan has helped instill a new sense of purpose and focus for public health and preventive medicine. Leading health indicators established by *Healthy People 2010* will be used to measure the health of the nation over the next 10 years (see Chapter 1).

In July 1994 the Office of the Surgeon General authorized the CDC to serve as lead agency in preparing the surgeon general's first report on physical activity and health. The surgeon general's report, published July 11, 1996, is a landmark review of the research on physical activity and health. It is on par with the surgeon general's historic first report on smoking and health, published in 1964, and a second one on nutrition and health, in 1988. The document on physical activity and health is a summary of more than 1,000 scientific studies from the fields of epidemiology, exercise physiology, medicine, and the behavioral sciences.

The report's key finding is that people of all ages can improve the quality of their lives through lifelong practice of moderate physical activity. A person does not have to be in training for the Boston Marathon to derive real health benefits from physical activity. A regular (preferably, daily) regimen of at least 30–45 minutes of brisk walking, bicycling, or even working around the house or yard will reduce the risks of developing coronary heart disease, hypertension, colon cancer, and diabetes. People who already are physically active will benefit even more by stepping up their activity.

Factors affecting physical activity levels include geographic location, income, gender, and education. According to the CDC, country people are less active than city people, westerners are more active than people in other regions, and men and people with higher educational levels and higher income work out more often. According to the CDC, ethnicity correlates with activity levels: 40% of Mexican Americans did not engage in any physical activity in their leisure time, compared with 35% of blacks and 18% of whites. Even when the educational levels were similar, African-American and Hispanic men and women reported less physical activity than white individuals. Watching television lowers the metabolic rate, therefore burning fewer calories, and increases obesity because viewers are inclined to snack. Adult women spend an average of 34 hours per week while men spend an average of 29 hours per week viewing television.

Physical activity declines dramatically during adolescence and the college years. These are dangerous trends for the health of American citizens. One national study of 439 undergraduates found that students spent almost 30 hours a week on sedentary behavior, mainly studying. Men reported more time in front of a computer or television but were generally more physically active than women (see Figure 11.1). Of the students reporting no physical activity, Asian, African-American, and Hispanic women reported the lowest rates of physical activity. The most physically active men are African Americans; the most physically active women are white (Figure 11.1). Lifelong activity levels are influenced by patterns set in college. Research reports that those active in college tend to be active after graduation and vice versa.

Families need to weave physical activity into the fabric of their daily lives. Health professionals need to be role models for healthy behavior and to encourage their patients to get out of their chairs and start fitness programs tailored to their individual needs. Businesses need to learn from what has worked in the past and promote worksite fitness. Community leaders need to reexamine whether enough resources have been devoted to maintenance of parks, community centers, playgrounds, and physical education. Schools and universities need to reintroduce daily, quality physical activity as a key component of a comprehensive education. And the media and entertainment industries need to use their vast creative abilities to show all Americans that physical activity is healthful and fun.

In contrast to physical activity is **physical fitness.** Physically fit people are able to meet the ordinary and the extraordinary demands of daily life effectively without being exhausted and with energy to spare for recreational activities or emergencies.

The opposite of physical fitness is a sedentary life, ironically misnamed the "good life." Contemporary society relies on cars, golf carts, elevators, remote controls, and other labor-saving devices to make life easier. Unfortunately, that is not what people need. These conveniences hasten the rate of deterioration of the body, threaten health, and shorten life. Sedentary people have twice as many health problems as active people. Exercise is essential to fitness and adds years to one's life and life

**FIGURE 11.1 ▶** Physical Activity among Ethnically Diverse College Students

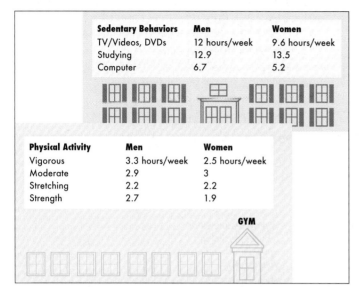

| Sedentary Behaviors | Men | Women |
|---|---|---|
| TV/Videos, DVDs | 12 hours/week | 9.6 hours/week |
| Studying | 12.9 | 13.5 |
| Computer | 6.7 | 5.2 |

| Physical Activity | Men | Women |
|---|---|---|
| Vigorous | 3.3 hours/week | 2.5 hours/week |
| Moderate | 2.9 | 3 |
| Stretching | 2.2 | 2.2 |
| Strength | 2.7 | 1.9 |

GYM

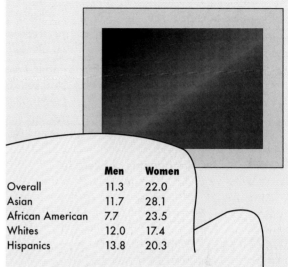

| | Men | Women |
|---|---|---|
| Overall | 11.3 | 22.0 |
| Asian | 11.7 | 28.1 |
| African American | 7.7 | 23.5 |
| Whites | 12.0 | 17.4 |
| Hispanics | 13.8 | 20.3 |

to one's years. An active person has more energy, a leaner physique, and a stronger and more flexible body.

Physical fitness can be classified into two categories: skill-related fitness and health-related fitness. Skill-related fitness, primarily the domain of athletes, is composed of agility, balance, coordination, power, reaction time, and speed. Because the emphasis of this book is on health, we are concerned with the basic components of **health-related fitness:** cardiorespiratory endurance, body composition, muscular flexibility, and muscular strength and endurance (Figure 11.2). Body composition was

**FIGURE 11.2 ▶** Health-Related Fitness Components

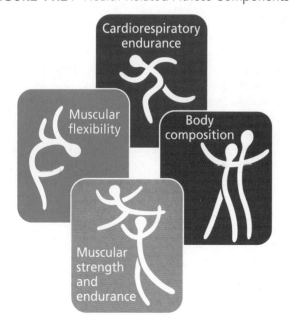

Cardiorespiratory endurance

Muscular flexibility

Body composition

Muscular strength and endurance

discussed in Chapter 10, so that information will not be repeated here.

## Benefits of Physical Activity

When asked why they exercise, most people indicate that it makes them feel better—an improved quality of life. Even modest levels of physical activity are beneficial (Figure 11.3). In contrast, a sedentary lifestyle promotes high blood pressure, coronary heart disease, ulcers, insomnia, low back pain, blood vessel disorders, atherosclerosis, strokes, obesity, cancer, and diabetes, among other conditions. The American Heart Association has established physical inactivity as a major risk factor for the development of coronary artery disease and a contributor to other risk factors including obesity, high blood pressure, and a low level of HDL (good) cholesterol. In general, diseases associated with a sedentary lifestyle are called **hypokinetic** (hypo = under, kinetic = activity) disorders.

### KEY TERMS

**Physical activity** bodily movement produced by skeletal muscles that requires an expenditure of energy and has health benefits

**Physical fitness** the general capacity to adapt and respond favorably to physical effort

**Health-related fitness** the five components are body composition, cardiovascular endurance, muscular flexibility, muscular strength, and muscular endurance

**Hypokinetic** underactive

---

HEALTHY PEOPLE 2010 Selected Physical Activity Objectives

- Improve the health, fitness, and quality of life of all Americans through the adoption and maintenance of regular, daily physical activity.
- Increase the proportion of adults who engage regularly, preferably daily, in moderate physical activity for at least 30 minutes per day.

- Enhance the cardiovascular health and quality of life of all Americans through prevention and control of risk factors and through promotion of healthy lifestyle behaviors.

---

**FIGURE 11.3 ▶** The Benefits of Exercise

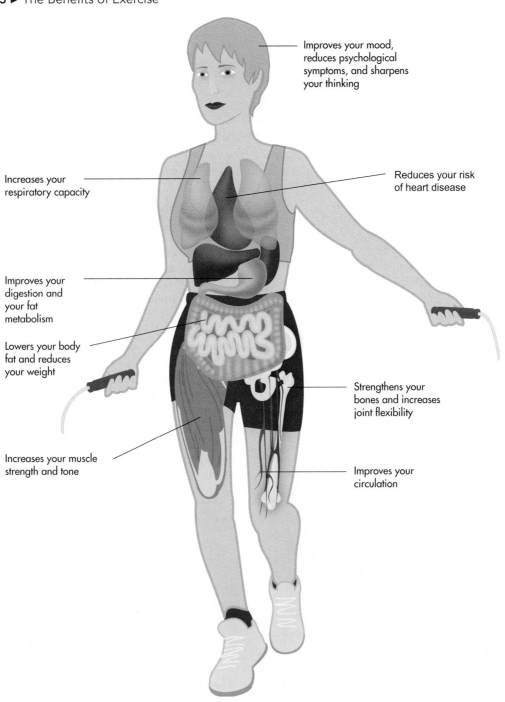

Improves your mood, reduces psychological symptoms, and sharpens your thinking

Reduces your risk of heart disease

Increases your respiratory capacity

Improves your digestion and your fat metabolism

Lowers your body fat and reduces your weight

Strengthens your bones and increases joint flexibility

Increases your muscle strength and tone

Improves your circulation

**FIGURE 11.4 ▶** Summary of FITT Components

**Lifetime Activity
Recommendations
CDC/ACSM/PCPFS**

| | **F** REQUENCY | Moderate<br>3+ Days<br>per week | Vigorous<br>5+ Days<br>per week |
|---|---|---|---|
| **I** NTENSITY 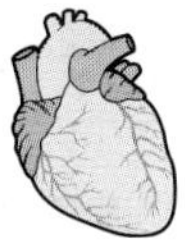 | | 50-70% of<br>Maximum<br>Heart Rate<br>(50-60% for<br>beginners)<br>3-6 METS | 70-90% of<br>Maximum<br>Heart Rate<br>(85-90% for<br>once per week<br>for athletes)<br>Over 6 METS |
| **T** IME 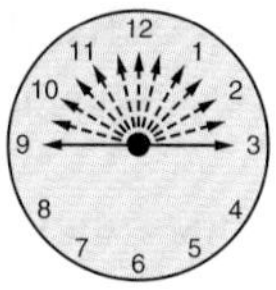 | | 30+ Minutes<br>(Continuous<br>preferred or<br>Cumulative in<br>10+ minutes<br>segments) | 20-60 Minutes<br>(Continuous<br>30-45 Minutes<br>Preferred) |
| **T** YPE 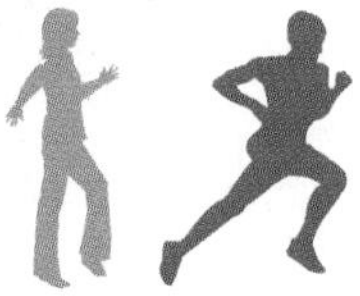 | | Moderate Activites:<br>Moderate to<br>Brisk Walking,<br>Dancing, Moderate<br>Swimming, Leisurely<br>Cycling, Leisurely<br>Skating, Mowing lawn<br>with power mower,<br>Moderate Housework | Vigorous Activities:<br>Very Brisk Walking,<br>Jogging, Running,<br>Lap Swimming,<br>Fast Cycling,<br>Fast Skating, Mowing<br>lawn with push mower,<br>Heavy Housework |

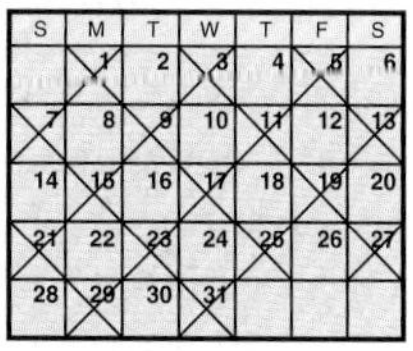

*Source:* Adapted from Patricia A. Floyd and Janet E. Parke, *Walk, Jog, Run for Wellness Everyone,* 5th ed. (Winston-Salem, NC: Hunter Textbooks, 2006).

## Training Principles

In order to improve your physical condition you must consider the principles of FITT, overload, specificity, and reversibility when working toward your fitness goals. The components of the **FITT formula,** recommended by the American College of Sports Medicine for **aerobic exercise,** are frequency, intensity, time, and type of activity.

## FREQUENCY

Frequency refers to how many days per week a person is physically active. FITT recommends a minimum of three to five days. The CDC's recommendations say daily activity is preferable. Beginners should consider, as a start, at least three nonconsecutive days at 50%–70% of maximum

heart rate, progressing to more days. Vigorous exercisers should consider rest or moderate activity one or two days per week to enable the body to recuperate and avoid injury, following at least five days of vigorous activity at 70%–90% of maximum heart rate. Individuals on a weight-loss program should exercise 45 to 60 minutes at low to moderate intensity, five to six days per week. Exercising longer increases caloric expenditure for quicker weight loss (see Summary of FITT Components, Figure 11.4).

---

### KEY TERMS

**FITT formula** frequency, intensity, time, and type of workout applied to each of the physical fitness components

**Aerobic exercise** activity that requires oxygen to produce the necessary energy to carry out the activity

## INTENSITY

Intensity refers to how hard a person must work to improve physical fitness. The terminology used is easy, moderate, and vigorous. FITT recommends that a person exercise at 50%–70% of his or her predicted **maximum heart rate.** Very low fit individuals should use 40%–50%. Some individuals may start at 60%–70% and then move into the 70%–85% zone. Individuals should calculate their target heart zone (see Self-Assessment 11.2) and maintain the heart rate in that zone throughout the workout. The heart rate should be monitored periodically during the workout and adjustments made in intensity as needed.

Intensity is measured in **METs.** One MET is equivalent to the calories expended while at rest. Two METs require twice as much energy; 3 METs require three times as much energy, and so forth. The surgeon general's report advocates moderate-intensity activity of 4–6 METs of energy expenditure, such as brisk walking, but does not discourage vigorous activity of 7 METs or higher, such as jogging or running. Moderate physical activity is roughly equivalent to physical activity that uses about 150 calories of energy per day or 1,000 calories per week. Figure 11.5 gives examples of minutes of activity required to burn 150 kcalories.

## TIME (DURATION)

FITT recommends a workout session of 20–60 minutes. Beginners and older people should start at 20 minutes and build up gradually to 30–60 minutes. The surgeon general's report recommends 30 minutes (minimum five to 10 minutes per session) on most, preferably all, days of the week (see Figure 11.4).

## TYPE OF ACTIVITY (SPECIFICITY)

The type of activity a person selects is a function of cardiorespiratory endurance, flexibility, and muscular strength and endurance. FITT recommends aerobic exercise such as walking, jogging, running, and hiking. Figure 11.4 summarizes the CDC's recommendations for each of the FITT components.

## HOW MUCH EXERCISE IS ENOUGH?

What are your goals? To improve fitness or avoid obesity? Regular physical activity is the key to success in improving fitness and avoiding overweight and/or obesity. The American College of Sports Medicine, the U.S. Surgeon General, and *Health Canada's Physical Activity Guide to Healthy Active Living* recommend a minimum of 30–60 minutes of moderate activity (walking at a speed of 3–4 miles per hour) most days of the week. Recent research reports that a minimum of 150 minutes a week of moderate-intensity exercise takes men and women out of the "low-fitness" category and lowers their risk of cardiovascular disease and diabetes, regardless of weight or body composition. Frequent, more intensive workout sessions can

**FIGURE 11.5 ▶** Minutes of Activity Required to Burn 150 Kcalories

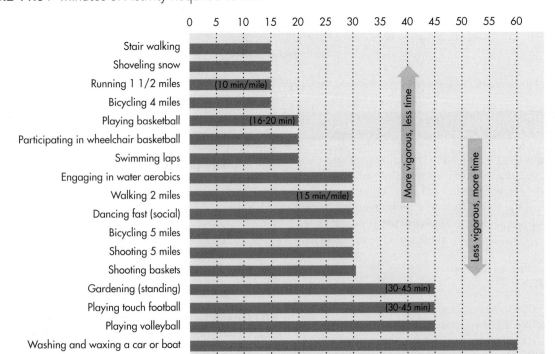

*Source:* Centers for Disease Control and Prevention, www.cdc.gov/accdphp/dnpa/physical/recommendations/adults.htm.

## Tips for Action Warm-Ups

1. Slowly stretching while concentrating on movements and flexibility exercises raises the temperature of heart and skeletal muscles.

2. The heart rate should reach about 120 beats per minute.

3. Warm-up activities help prevent injury and muscle soreness.

4. Preparation for cardiorespiratory training should include approximately two minutes of walking, jogging, or mild exercises in place.

5. Static stretching of the major muscle groups is emphasized.

6. The entire warm-up should begin slowly and gradually increase to 10 minutes of light exercise.

7. Warm-up activities should model the workout being done. For example, joggers and runners should briskly walk or jog a slow mile; swimmers should swim some laps slowly; aerobic exercisers should do a few easy rhythmic routines; golfers should stretch and do a few practice swings; tennis players should do some easy strokes and serves; and weight lifters should work on a rowing machine, treadmill, or stationary bike to loosen major muscle groups.

provide more health dividends, including improved muscular strength and endurance. Exercising longer and harder is the best way to maintain a healthy weight and lose excess pounds. According to the *2005 Dietary Guidelines for Americans*, individuals who have lost weight may need to exercise 60–90 minutes a day to keep off the pounds.

## Phases of Exercise

Each exercise session has three basic phases: the warm-up, the aerobic workout, and the cool-down. These phases apply to whichever health-related component (cardiorespiratory, flexibility, muscular strength, or endurance) is to be developed, though the specific exercises are unique to each.

### WARM-UP

The **warm-up** helps the body progress gradually from rest to exercise as blood moves more freely in the joints and increases the speed of nerve impulses to the active muscles. To help the body adjust from inactivity to exertion, start by walking briskly for about five minutes, and proceed with a five-minute general warm-up of simple stretches of the muscles that you will use often during your workout.

### AEROBIC ACTIVITY

After the warm-up, it is time for the aerobic activity workout. The key components of the aerobic activity are intensity and duration. The heart and lungs obtain their best benefits when the workout is continuous, using the large muscle groups for 30–60 minutes. When you first start exercising, you may not be able to exercise continuously

for 30 minutes without resting. As you exercise each day, you will find that you will be exercising longer without tiring.

If a person is not sweating or breathing hard or the heart rate has not increased, he or she is not exercising hard enough. People who are getting a good workout will be sweating, their heart will be beating faster, and they will be breathing harder, but they should be able to converse at the same time. Also, using your target heart rate range is necessary to make certain that you are working at the proper intensity.

### COOL-DOWN

During a vigorous workout the heart pumps blood to all of the body's muscles. These muscles contract and return the blood to the heart for reoxygenation, preventing blood from pooling in the arm and leg muscles. Ceasing activity abruptly can cause the exerciser to become faint, dizzy, and even pass out, and blood can pool in your legs. You should continue to move at a slower pace to ensure an adequate supply of blood to your heart.

Stretching plus an aerobic activity (walking or light jogging) are recommended **cool-down** activities done

### KEY TERMS

**Maximum heart rate (MHR)** the fastest heart rate obtained during all-out exercise

**METs** measurement of body's expenditure of energy

**Warm-up** the beginning phase of each workout session that helps the body progress gradually from rest to exercise

**Cool-down** the ending phase of a workout that helps the body begin to return to its resting state immediately following each exercise session. The person continues to exercise at a lower level so the body can return safely to its resting state. The cool-down phase should last about five to 10 minutes at a comfortable pace or until the heart rate generally is below 120 beats per minute. The cool-down should be longer for more intense and longer workouts.

## YOUR LIFE-TIME PLAN

Beginning an aerobic program is the most difficult phase. Often people push too hard and too fast and injure themselves, becoming discouraged and finally quitting. The three phases in an exercise plan are: beginning, progression, and maintenance.

- Beginning (approximately 4–6 weeks). Start slowly and gradually increase your workout. Monitor your heart rate and aim for 50% of your maximum heart rate. If you can't talk, you are exercising too hard.

- Progression (16–20 weeks). Slowly increase the intensity and time of your workouts. Use your target heart rate as a guide and keep a log of your workouts until you reach your goal.

- Maintenance (lifetime). Once you have reached your exercise goal of 60 minutes per day, select aerobic activities you enjoy to keep up your enthusiasm and avoid monotony. Alternate your aerobic activities and keep the pace; this is called cross-training (see section on cross training).

## Fitness Training Principles

Certain training principles are incorporated in any exercise program. These include overload, progression, specificity, retrogression, reversibility, and slow and gradual exercise.

1. **Overload.** According to the **overload principle,** to improve physical fitness, the body must be subjected gradually to more stress than it is accustomed to. The body is an adaptive mechanism. When the level of stress increases, the body will adjust and must work harder to see improvement. Overload is specific to each body part, as well as each component of fitness (cardiorespiratory, flexibility, strength, and endurance). Progressive overloading provides the benefits of exercise without the risk of injury.

2. **Progression.** The **progression principle** combines overload and adaptation. To achieve fitness, additional stress (overload) must be placed on the body once it has adapted to stress. If the overload is increased too soon before the body has had time to adapt to that stress, exhaustion or regression may result.

**FYI** FITT FORMULA FOR CARDIORESPIRATORY ENDURANCE

| | |
|---|---|
| **F** = Frequency | Three to five days per week |
| **I** = Intensity | 55%–90% maximum heart rate |
| **T** = Time | 20–60 minutes of continuous or cumulative aerobic activity |
| **T** = Type of activity | Aerobic (walking, race walking, jogging, water jogging, skipping rope, stair climbing, bench stepping, cycling, aerobic dance, soccer, skating, lap swimming) |

3. **Specificity.** The principle of **specificity of training** states that overload must be aimed specifically at the desired outcome of the fitness component. Physical exercise programs should be designed to closely match the activity with specific results in mind. For example, if you are training for strength, you must lift weights (a resistance) to get the desired results.

4. **Retrogression.** During the exercise process, the exerciser will reach plateaus when improvement stops temporarily. Performance may level off for a time before it improves again. This is the **retrogression principle.** Once the body has adjusted to the overload, performance levels will improve.

5. **Reversibility.** The principle of **reversibility** is the opposite of the overload principle. If you stop exercising, you can lose as much as 50% of your fitness improvements within two months. In other words, "use it or lose it." If your exercise schedule has to be changed, keep the intensity constant and reduce the time of your exercise in order to avoid the reversibility principle.

6. **Slow and gradual exercise.** The key to success in an exercise program is to begin slowly and be consistent. Increasing the frequency, intensity, time, and type of exercise too rapidly may invite injury. The body requires time to adjust to a sudden change in lifestyle. Training must be sensible.

## Cardiorespiratory Endurance

The single most important component of health-related physical fitness is **cardiorespiratory endurance** or aerobic exercise. The term *cardiovascular* often is used

- According to the surgeon general's report on fitness, nearly half of Americans between the ages of 12 and 21 are not vigorously active on a regular basis.
- More white and Hispanic students work out than do African-American undergraduates.
- At all ages men are more physically active than women, even on college campuses.

- According to the surgeon general's report, 25% of women are sedentary and more than 60% do not exercise regularly. According to the Centers for Disease Control and Prevention black women between the ages of 25 and 34 are more likely to gain weight than any other female group in the United States. Exercise will keep that weight down.

instead. The American College of Sports Medicine prefers to use *cardiorespiratory* because it describes the total function, including that of the lungs, more accurately.

Cardiorespiratory fitness is achieved by aerobic exercises, which improve the heart and lung functioning by boosting the body's consumption of oxygen. Aerobic means "with oxygen." Some common examples are brisk walking, jogging, running, swimming, cycling, spinning, skipping rope, rowing, aerobic dancing, step training or bench aerobics, stairclimbing, and inline skating. These generally are continuous and rhythmic, and they require the heart to beat faster to produce the oxygen necessary to perform the activity.

In contrast to aerobic exercise is **anaerobic exercise.** Anaerobic exercises are high-intensity and can be performed for only short periods. They do not develop the cardiorespiratory system. Examples of anaerobic exercise are sprinting and weight lifting. Another type of exercise that does not promote cardiorespiratory fitness is called **nonaerobic exercise.** Examples are bowling, softball, golf, and tennis.

The primary benefits of aerobic exercise are that it

- Improves the ability of the heart, lungs, and circulatory system to carry oxygen to the body's cells
- Requires the heart to pump more blood per beat, which increases its efficiency
- Slows the resting heart rate
- Improves the supply of blood to the tissues
- Decreases the resting blood pressure
- Improves the cardiorespiratory system so it works less at rest and during lower levels of exercise
- Has positive effects on blood lipids (fats)
- Helps protect a person from the effects of stress
- Improves the body's metabolism, thus providing better control of body fat
- Improves psychological and emotional well-being

Aerobic exercise also is classified in two ways.

1. **High-impact aerobics.** These exercises are not recommended for individuals with a low level of fitness.
2. **Low-impact aerobics.** These are recommended for people with low fitness levels. Examples are walking, cycling, rowing, water jogging, and swimming. Computerized and noncomputerized machines have been manufactured to simulate many of these activities— rowing machines, treadmills, stationary bicycles, and cross-country skiing machines, to name a few.

## KEY TERMS

**Overload principle** gradually subjecting the body to more stress than it is accustomed to

**Progression principle** placing additional stress on the body once it has adapted to its current stress factor

**Specificity of training** aiming overload specifically at the desired outcome of the fitness component

**Retrogression principle** leveling of performance for a period of time before performance improves again

**Reversibility** the physical effects of exercise are lost due to inactivity or disuse

**Cardiorespiratory endurance** the ability of the heart, lungs, and blood vessels to deliver blood and nutrients to the cells efficiently to meet the demands of prolonged, aerobic physical activity

**Anaerobic exercise** high-intensity activity that does not require oxygen to produce the desired energy to carry out the activity

**Nonaerobic exercise** activity that has frequent rest intervals between outlays of energy

**High-impact aerobics** aerobic exercise that has a running or jumping component

**Low-impact aerobics** activities that place minimal stress on the joints and are recommended for people with low fitness levels

---

**Tips for Action** To Prevent Injury from Low-Impact Aerobics

- Wear recommended shoes.
- Work out on resilient wood floors.
- Keep arm movements smooth and controlled.
- Use good form.
  —Abdomen tight
  —Pelvis tucked in

- —Rib cage up
- —Knees bent slightly
- Warm up beforehand, and cool down afterward.

---

## PRINCIPLES AND CONCEPTS OF AEROBIC EXERCISE

Some basic principles apply to cardiorespiratory or aerobic endurance for health-related purposes.

1. Frequency, intensity, and time should be considered in relation to the person's fitness level.

2. Low-impact activities are safer, especially for older people and for those who need to minimize strain to the joints.

3. The rate of progression usually is slower for individuals who are not fit.

4. Self-concept and motivation are important when continuing a health-fitness program for a lifetime.

The selected activity must be continuous and sufficiently strenuous to elevate the heart rate to the **proper training intensity.** *Continuous* is defined as an activity that takes three minutes or longer and marks the approximate point at which the contracting skeletal muscle shifts to aerobic metabolism to produce energy.

Before undertaking an aerobic program, a person should understand the applicable concepts, including resting, target, and recovery heart rates, and rate of perceived exertion. A physician's approval is necessary if you have any concerns regarding your state of health to safely start an exercise program.

## RESTING HEART RATE

To calculate target heart rate, you first must learn how to measure resting heart rate. **Resting heart rate** can be a good indicator of your fitness level. Slow resting heart rates tend to indicate an active lifestyle, and fast rates are associated with sedentary habits.

Resting heart rate can be determined by counting the heart rate for one minute upon waking naturally early in the morning (without an alarm.) Perhaps to get the best results, you should take your resting heart rate several days in a row and get an average.

You can take your pulse in two different ways: The **radial pulse** may be taken by placing your fingers on the thumb side of your upturned wrist below the heel of the hand. Some people have trouble counting the pulse at this site while resting but find it easy to count when exercising. The **carotid pulse** is taken by locating the carotid artery in the neck and gently tilting the head back slightly to one side. You should use the middle finger or forefinger (or both) to feel the pulse. You should not use the thumb, because it has a beat of its own. Pressure to the carotid artery should be applied lightly; a firm pressure will result in a reflex response, causing a temporary drop in heart rate.

---

**VIEWPOINT** *Do you know your resting heart rate? Target heart rate zone? Blood pressure? FITT formulas for each of the health-related components of physical fitness? Calculate your resting heart rate, maximum heart rate, and target heart rate zone. What specific actions will you take to improve your physical activity level?*

---

## TARGET HEART RATE

To determine your **target heart rate,** you must first learn to estimate your maximum heart rate (MHR). This is done by subtracting your age from 220. Cardiorespiratory development takes place when working between 50% and 85% of **heart rate reserve.** For health purposes, the 60% level allows conversation during exercise and is considered safe. Moderate is about 70%. Starting too low is better than starting too high.

The goal is to increase the intensity gradually until you can tolerate the 85% intensity. Factors including emotional stress, high humidity, and hot temperatures must be taken into account, as they may affect the heart rate response. Infections and fever elevate the body temperature, increasing the heart rate response.

Medications such as **beta-blockers** decrease the heart activity and may constrict air passages in the lungs. Any person taking prescription medications should exercise with the physician's knowledge and recommendations.

**FIGURE 11.6 ▶** Calculating Target Heart Zone Using Karvonen Formula

| Example: | Age = 20 years old |
|---|---|
| | Resting pulse = 70 |
| | MHR = maximum heart rate |
| | RHR = resting heart rate |
| | THR = target heart rate |

1. Determine maximum heart rate.

| 220 | 220 |
|---|---|
| – AGE | –20 |
| MHR | 200 |

2. Subtract resting heart rate from maximum heart rate.

| MHR | 200 |
|---|---|
| – RHR | –70 |
| number | 130 |

3. Multiply number (130) by .60, then add resting heart rate.

| | 130 |
|---|---|
| × | .60 |
| | 78 |
| + | 70 |
| Lower limit = | 148 |

4. Multiply number (130) by .80, then add resting heart rate.

| | 130 |
|---|---|
| × | .80 |
| | 104 |
| + | 70 |
| Upper limit = | 174 |

Maintain a target heart rate above 148 and below 174 beats per minute.

The best way to determine if the exercise is intense enough to condition the heart and lungs, but not too intense, is to take the pulse often during an exercise session. A heart responding normally to exercise shows a rapid increase during the first three to five minutes, followed by a steady state or plateau. Beginning exercisers should aim for the lower end of the target zone (60%) and increase gradually to 85% of the maximum heart rate. To determine your target zone according to the **Karvonen formula,** see Figure 11.6.

**Recovery Heart Rate.** **Recovery heart rate** after exercising helps determine whether the exercise demands are appropriate or excessive. As part of the cool-down, the pulse should be checked at five minutes and 10 minutes after exercising. After five minutes the pulse rate should be below 120 beats per minute, and after 10 minutes the pulse rate should be below 100 beats per minute. The closer the pulse is to your resting heart rate, the better is your condition. If it takes a long time for your pulse to recover and return to its resting level, you are unfit. Fast recovery indicates a good fitness level.

The pulse rate of most individuals decreases to fewer than 100 beats per minute during the first minute of rest; during the following two to three minutes, the pulse rate decreases at about the same rate it increased during exercise. For healthy young people, cool-down should last until the heart rate is about 120 or below. For middle-aged and older adults, the rate should be 100 or below.

## RATE OF PERCEIVED EXERTION

An alternative method of determining the intensity of exercise is the **rate of perceived exertion (RPE)** developed by Gunnar Borg. Individuals may perceive less or do more than they think they do while exercising. Therefore, associating your own inner perception of the exercise with the ratings given on the scale in Figure 11.7 is important.

Adding a 0 to each number provides a rough estimate of heartbeats per minute; therefore, an RPE range of 6 to 20 is preferred. For example, *hard* corresponds to a heart rate of 150. *Very hard* is comparable to a heart rate of 170. Generally, warm-ups and cool-downs range between 7 and 11. The typical intensity for training is 11 to 16 (110–160).

### KEY TERMS

**Proper training intensity** the intensity that gives the best cardiorespiratory development results as determined by heart rate

**Resting heart rate** heartbeats per minute while at rest

**Radial pulse** pulse taken by locating the radial artery in the wrist

**Carotid pulse** pulse taken by locating the carotid artery in the neck

**Target heart rate** the number of heartbeats desired during exercise for maximum benefit

**Heart rate reserve (HRR)** the difference between resting heart rate and maximal heart rate

**Beta-blockers** medications prescribed to control high blood pressure and heart conditions

**Karvonen formula** a method for determining if exercise is demanding enough to condition the heart and lungs by ascertaining the optimal target zone

**Recovery heart rate** heartbeats per minute after exercising

**Rate of perceived exertion (RPE)** an alternative method of determining the intensity of exercise, associated with Gunnar Borg

**FIGURE 11.7 ▶** Revised Scale for Rating of Perceived Exertion (RPE)

| | |
|---|---|
| 6 | |
| 7 | Very, very light |
| 8 | |
| 9 | Very light |
| 10 | |
| 11 | Fairly light |
| 12 | |
| 13 | Somewhat hard |
| 14 | |
| 15 | Hard |
| 16 | |
| 17 | Very hard |
| 18 | |
| 19 | Very, very hard |
| 20 | |

*Source:* Original scale from Borg, G. "Psychophysical Bases of Perceived Exertion." *Medicine and Science in Sports and Exercise*, Vol. 14, No. 5, 2003, pp. 377–381.

RPEs eliminate the problem of counting pulse rate during aerobic activities. Use RPE with caution. Perhaps for safety, exercisers should check the target zone against the RPE during the first weeks of an exercise program to ensure that they are within the proper heart rate intensity guidelines.

**Frequency and Time.** Frequency of exercise is an important variable in increasing the body's ability to use oxygen (aerobic capacity). Beyond a certain frequency and duration, exercise does not benefit the exerciser and can be risky. Dr. Kenneth Cooper, a pioneer in the field of aerobics, advises that unless you are preparing for a race, running more than 15 miles a week is not necessary for fitness. Cooper's research indicates that exercising more than five times a week triples the injury rate in amateur athletes. Further, increasing the duration of each exercise session from 30 to 45 minutes doubles the risk, unless it is done gradually over several months.

**Cross-Training. Cross-training** can provide relief from monotony and renew motivation. Some sports-medicine specialists believe that cross-training also may reduce the risk of injury by moderating the addiction to a single sport that can result in overtraining. The best method of cross-training is to pair sports that train different parts of the body: swimming with cycling, rowing with running, tennis with brisk walking. If you are cross-training for the first

time, start slowly, as you would for any physical activity program.

## ASSESSMENT OF CARDIORESPIRATORY FITNESS

Laboratory measurements (treadmill, bicycle ergometer) or field tests (distance and speed measures and step tests) can be used to determine aerobic function. The most commonly used tests for health-related purposes are the field tests used to estimate aerobic fitness level, such as step tests, distance runs, and walking tests. Distance runs (12-minute or 1–1½ mile), in which a constant speed or pace is maintained, are popular. Fast walking is recommended for unfit persons and older adults. The Rockport Fitness Walking Test provides a good measure of aerobic fitness. The goal of this test is to walk one mile as fast as possible. To make valid comparisons, the same test should be used for both pre- and post-assessments. Field test results should be considered only estimates of the person's ability.

## Flexibility

A full range of motion in a joint or group of joints is necessary to perform most active sports and daily activities without straining the muscles and developing back problems, as well as to maintain good posture. The extent of **flexibility** depends on genetics, age, gender, occupation, posture, body composition, and musculoskeletal differences. Females tend to be more flexible than males, regardless of age. Generally, flexibility improves from childhood through adolescence. Afterward, a gradual loss of joint mobility continues throughout adult life. The benefits of a flexibility program include: prevention of injuries, relaxation, relief of soreness after exercise, relief of muscle strain, improved posture, and better athletic performance. Pole/vertical gymnastic dancing, yoga, tai chi, and Pilates are examples of exercise programs that can improve flexibility.

The Pilates method is one of the fastest growing forms of exercise in the world. In the United States, this innovative system of mind-body exercise evolved from the principles of Joseph Pilates using a floor mat or equipment that transforms the way your body looks, feels, and performs. Designed for all ages and levels of physical fitness, Pilates builds strength without excess bulk, creating a toned body with slender thighs and a flat abdomen. Pilates improves core strength, agility, flexibility, and economy of motion. It can even help alleviate back pain and other chronic ailments.

Yoga is one of the six orthodox systems of Indian philosophy. In Indian thought, everything is permeated by the Supreme Universal Spirit (Paramatma or God) of which the individual human spirit (jivatma) is a part. Yoga is the disciplining of the intellect, the emotions, and

## FYI   FITT FORMULA FOR FLEXIBILITY

| **F** = Frequency | After initial daily stretching, eight weeks, two to three days per week to maintain |
| **I** = Intensity | Stretch to the point of mild discomfort |
| **T** = Time | Five times per exercise, final stretch position 10–60 seconds |
| **T** = Type of activity | Static (slow-sustained) |

the will, which enables one to achieve balance in life. Yoga, like tai chi, centers on breathing, stretching exercises, and flowing gestures. Tai chi is especially beneficial for the aged population and those with osteoarthritis, as it can alleviate joint pain and serve as a low-impact form of exercise for the entire body. Tai chi can improve flexibility, range of motion, balance, and strength. Proper technique is essential for safety. Because the range of motion is specific to body parts (trunk, shoulder, ankle), a complete stretching program should include all body parts and follow basic guidelines for improving flexibility.

Pole/vertical gymnastic dancing is a fun, sexy, and exciting way to get back into fitness or to try the latest physical fitness trend that is also the workout behind the fit and fabulous physiques of Jessica Alba, Jennifer Aniston, Kim Cattrall, Carmen Electra, Heather Graham, Daryl Hanna, Teri Hatcher, Angelina Jolie, Kylie Minogue, and Kate Moss, just to name a few. This creative new approach to improving physical fitness, core strength, and flexibility incorporates complete choreography with each class beginning with a warm-up which provides stretching but also serves to teach the fundamentals of pole skills. Practicing exercise sessions in high heels are included before moving on to pole skills.

Figure 11.8 shows the major muscle groups exercised.

## TYPES OF STRETCHING

Stretching exercises are of three types.

1. Static or slow-sustained
2. Ballistic or dynamic
3. Proprioceptive neuromuscular facilitation (PNF)

**Static** or **slow-sustained stretching** is the most frequently used and recommended stretching technique. It refers to the ability to assume and maintain an extended position at one end point in a joint's range of motion. This type of stretch should not be painful. It also has a low injury rate. Therefore, beginners and older adults in particular should use it.

The **dynamic** or **ballistic stretching** technique can be dangerous and counterproductive. It refers to moving a joint quickly and fluidly through its entire range of motion with little resistance. The bouncing movements can overstretch muscle fibers, causing the muscle to contract, not stretch. This may produce muscle soreness and injury from small tears to the soft tissue. Dynamic stretching is not recommended for the average person.

**Proprioceptive neuromuscular facilitation** requires the assistance of another person, and stretching should involve the entire body. The procedure is as follows.

1. The person assisting with the exercise provides initial force by slowly pushing in the direction of the desired stretch. The first stretch does not cover the entire range of motion.

2. The person being stretched then applies force in the opposite direction of the stretch, against the assistant, who tries to hold the initial degree of stretch as close as possible. An **isometric (static) muscle contraction** is being performed at that angle.

3. After four or five seconds of isometric contraction, the muscle being stretched is completely relaxed. The assistant then slowly increases the degree of stretch to a greater angle.

4. The isometric contraction then is repeated for another four or five seconds, following which the muscle is relaxed again. The assistant then can slowly increase the degree of stretch one more time. Steps 1 to 4 are repeated two to five more times, until the exerciser feels mild discomfort. On the last trial the final stretched position should be held for several seconds.

## KEY TERMS

**Cross-training** combining more than one activity to attain cardiorespiratory fitness and allow some muscles to rest

**Flexibility** the ability of a joint to move freely through its full range of motion

**Static** or **slow-sustained stretching** technique in which muscles are relaxed and lengthened gradually through a joint's complete range of motion and held for a short time (10–60 seconds)

**Dynamic** or **ballistic stretching** technique using rapid, bouncy, or bobbing movements to stretch muscle fibers

**Proprioceptive neuromuscular facilitation (PNF)** technique based on the contraction and relaxation of muscles

**Isometric (static) muscle contraction** muscle remains the same length and no movement occurs while a force is exerted against an immovable object

**FIGURE 11.8** ► Major Muscle Groups of the Body

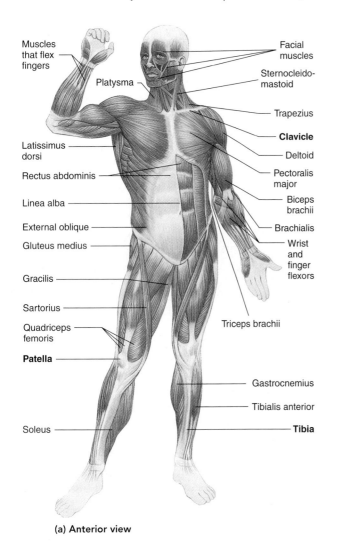

Muscles that flex fingers
Platysma
Latissimus dorsi
Rectus abdominis
Linea alba
External oblique
Gluteus medius
Gracilis
Sartorius
Quadriceps femoris
**Patella**
Soleus

Facial muscles
Sternocleido-mastoid
Trapezius
**Clavicle**
Deltoid
Pectoralis major
Biceps brachii
Brachialis
Wrist and finger flexors
Triceps brachii
Gastrocnemius
Tibialis anterior
**Tibia**

**(a) Anterior view**

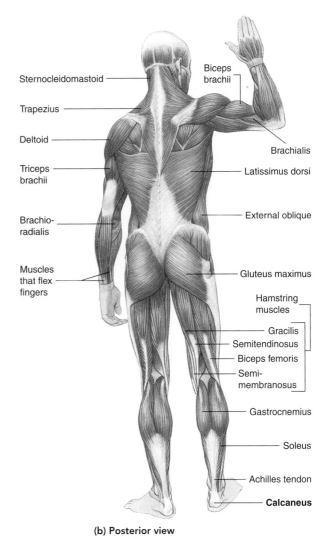

Sternocleidomastoid
Trapezius
Deltoid
Triceps brachii
Brachio-radialis
Muscles that flex fingers

Biceps brachii
Brachialis
Latissimus dorsi
External oblique
Gluteus maximus
Hamstring muscles
Gracilis
Semitendinosus
Biceps femoris
Semi-membranosus
Gastrocnemius
Soleus
Achilles tendon
**Calcaneus**

**(b) Posterior view**

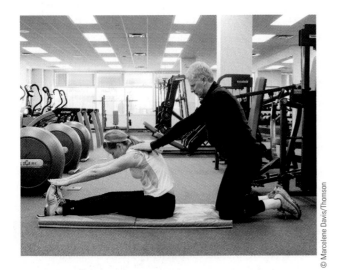

© Marcelene Davis/Thomson

▲ *The PNF stretching technique requires the assistance of another person*

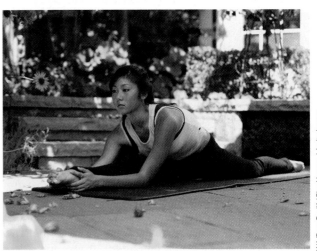

© LWA/Dann Tardif / Blend Images / Jupiterimages

▲ *Stretching should involve the entire body*

**TABLE 11.1 ▶** RX: Healthy Bones

| MODE | INTENSITY | FREQUENCY | DURATION |
|---|---|---|---|
| Weight-bearing<br><br>Endurance activities, such as tennis and jogging; activities that involve jumping; and resistance exercise such as weight lifting | Moderate to high | Weight-bearing activities, 3 to 5 times per week; resistance exercise, 2 or 3 times per week | 30 to 60 minutes |

*Source:* "Physical Activity and Bone Health." Position Stand, American College of Sports Medicine, www.acsm/msse.org.

Some researchers believe the PNF technique results in greater muscle length and therefore is more effective than the static stretch. The disadvantages of this type of stretch are that two people are needed, more time is required, the probability of injury is greater, and both persons must be knowledgeable about the procedure.

## ASSESSMENT OF FLEXIBILITY

Flexibility is specific to each muscle group. Therefore, different tests determine the range of motion in various groups of muscles. Two tests commonly used for an indication of flexibility levels are the Sit-and-Reach and the Total Body Rotation tests. The most widely known test, the Modified Sit-and-Reach, estimates hip, hamstring, and spine flexibility. An improvement over the traditional Sit-and-Reach test, arm and leg lengths are taken into consideration. When these muscle groups are tight, chronic lower back problems and injury may result. Tightness of these muscles is associated with too much sitting, an indicator of a sedentary lifestyle.

Stretching prior to testing is necessary before performing any flexibility testing. The Backsaver Sit-and-Reach test is commonly substituted for the Modified Sit-and-Reach. The Modified Sit-and-Reach is in Self-Assessment 11.4.

## Muscular Strength and Endurance

Strength is the absolute maximum weight that can be lifted, pushed, pulled, or pressed in one effort. Examples of muscular strength are pull-ups and rope climbing. Strong muscles provide greater endurance, resistance to fatigue, and power, and they help to maintain correct posture. In addition, strong muscles protect the body joints, resulting in fewer strains, sprains, and muscular difficulties such as back pain.

Age and sex differences parallel changes in muscle mass. Strength in females tends to decline after age 30, and this decline usually is the result of decreasing physical activity. Males gain strength rapidly at puberty (13–14 years) because the sex hormone testosterone stimulates muscle growth. The continuing production of testosterone contributes to strength. Women's strength may increase from strength training, but women do not develop muscle bulk as males do because they produce much smaller amounts of testosterone. Thus, the average male is stronger than the average female.

Research shows that the best way to reduce your body fat is to add muscle strengthening exercise to your workouts. Muscle tissue is your very best calorie-burning tissue, and the more you have, the more calories you burn, even when you are resting. Muscle strengthening also contributes to healthy bones (Table 11.1). Bones are more resistant to falls when muscles are stronger.

Closely related to muscular strength is **muscular endurance.** A person who is strong does not become fatigued as readily as one who is not, because less effort is required to produce repeated muscular contractions. Muscular endurance usually implies specific groups of muscles—for example, abdominal, thighs, and chest. Examples of exercises that increase endurance are abdominal curl-ups, push-ups, and sit-ups when these are repeated more than 10 times.

If muscles are not used, they will degenerate and **atrophy** (decrease in strength and size). Muscles begin to atrophy after three to four days if they are not exercised. If muscles are used regularly and vigorously, they will increase in size and improve in strength. This is termed **hypertrophy.** A weight training program consists of repetitions (reps), the single performance of an exercise, such as lifting 30 pounds at one time, and sets (number of repetitions of the same movement), such as a set of 10 push-ups.

Muscular training is highly specific, and specific muscles must be exercised to achieve certain results. A workout with weights should exercise major muscle

### KEY TERMS

**Muscular endurance** the ability of muscles to exert force or sustain a muscle contraction repeatedly for an extended period

**Atrophy** to decrease in strength or size of tissue from disuse

**Hypertrophy** an increase in size and strength of muscles that are used regularly and vigorously

## QUAD STRETCH

Grasp the foot and lift the foot to buttocks level and pull backward with opposite hand.

**Result:** Stretches quadriceps muscle.

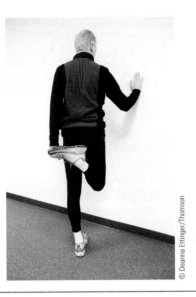

© Deanna Ettinger/Thomson

## TRUNK ROTATION AND LOWER BACK STRETCH

Sit on the floor and bend the left leg, placing the left foot on the outside of the right knee. Place the right elbow on the left knee and push against it. At the same time, try to rotate the trunk to the left (counter-clockwise). Hold the final position for a few seconds. Repeat the exercise with the other side.

**Result:** Stretches lateral side of the hip and thigh; trunk; lower back.

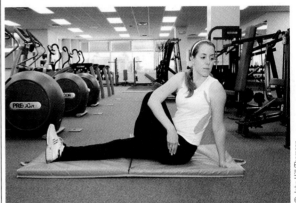

© John Hill/Thomson

## SINGLE-KNEE TO CHEST STRETCH

Lie down flat on the floor. Bend one leg at approximately 100° and gradually pull the opposite leg toward your chest. Hold the final stretch for a few seconds. Switch legs and repeat the exercise. Lower back should remain in contact with floor.

**Result:** Stretches lower back and hamstring muscles; lumbar spine ligaments.

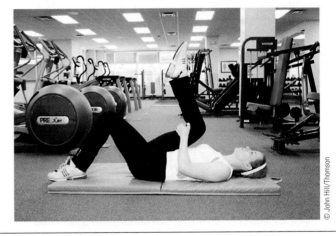

© John Hill/Thomson

## DOUBLE-KNEE TO CHEST STRETCH

Lie flat on the floor and then slowly curl up into a fetal position. Hold for a few seconds. Lower back should remain in contact with floor.

**Result:** Stretches upper and lower back and hamstring muscles; spinal ligaments.

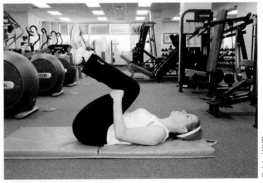

© John Hill/Thomson

## TRICEPS STRETCH

Place the right hand behind your neck. Grasp the right arm above the elbow with the left hand. Gently pull the elbow backward. Repeat the exercise with the opposite arm.

**Result:** Stretches back of upper arm (triceps muscle) and shoulder joint.

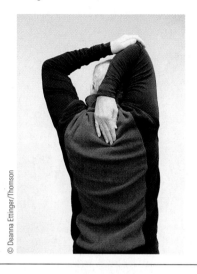

© Deanna Ettinger/Thomson

## HEEL CORD STRETCH

Stand against the wall or at the edge of a step and stretch the heel downward, alternating legs. Hold the stretched position for a few seconds.

**Result:** Stretches heel cord (Achilles tendon); gastrocnemius; soleus muscles.

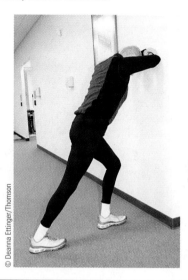

© Deanna Ettinger/Thomson

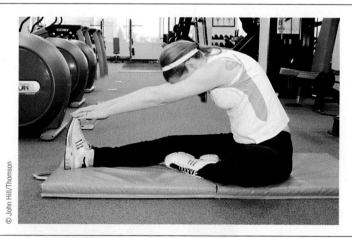

© John Hill/Thomson

## HAMSTRING STRETCH

Extend right leg. Position the left leg with knee bent, with the bottom of the foot touching the extended leg. Reach with both hands toward the ankle or foot and pull head to knee while keeping the leg straight. Hold for a few seconds. Repeat other side.

**Result:** Stretches hamstrings.

## LATERAL HEAD TILT

Slowly and gently tilt the head laterally. Repeat several times to each side.

**Result:** Stretches neck muscles and ligaments of the cervical spine.

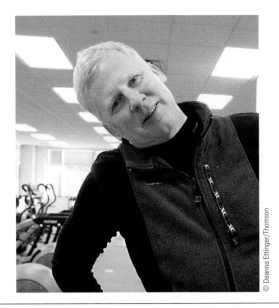

© Deanna Ettinger/Thomson

## SIDE STRETCH

Stand straight up, feet separated to shoulder width, and place your hands on your waist. Now move the upper body to one side and hold the final stretch for a few seconds. Repeat on the other side.

**Result:** Stretches muscles and ligaments in the pelvic region.

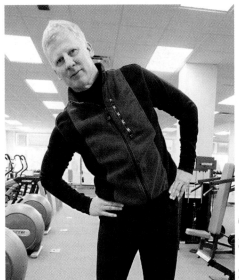

© Deanna Ettinger/Thomson

## SHOULDER HYPEREXTENSION STRETCH

Have a partner grasp your arms from behind by the wrists and push them upward slowly. Hold the final position for a few seconds.

**Result:** Stretches deltoid and pectoral muscles; ligaments of the shoulder joint.

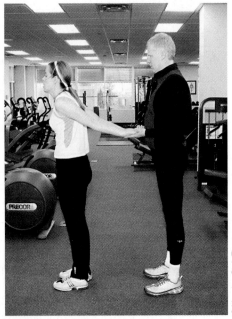

© Marcelene Davis/Thomson

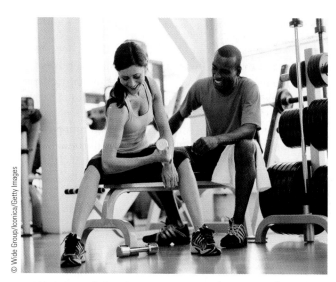

▲ *Weight training increases muscular strength and endurance*

groups: the deltoids (shoulders), pectorals (chest), triceps and biceps (back and front of upper arm), quadriceps (front thigh), hamstrings (back of thigh), gluteus maximus (buttocks), trapezius and rhomboids (back), and abdomen (Figure 11.8).

Numerous machines and freeweight routines focus on each muscle group. When the weight is raised and lowered, muscle fibers lengthen (eccentric) and shorten (concentric) during muscle contraction. The exercise routine is repeated until the muscle group is fatigued. Free (hand) weights are good for strength training, because they allow you to perform a variety of exercises that work certain muscle groups such as shoulders and legs. Machines allow only one exercise but are advantageous because they can protect you against injury, isolate specific muscles (good for rehabilitating an injury), prevent cheating when fatigue occurs, and offer varying resistance during the lifting motion.

Power Plate Acceleration training, an exercise originated from Europe, is based on vibration and increasing the gravitational force on the body. Power Plate acceleration training machines aim not just to strengthen muscles but to improve overall wellness. The equipment targets bone density loss and poor circulation, has a massage/relaxation function and targets cellulite in the thighs and buttocks. The plate at the base of the machine vibrates in three directions, back and forth, side to side and up and down. It goes in frequency, number of times per second and the plate moves up and down creating extra gravitational force in the body causing involuntary resistance in addition to whatever voluntary resistance training or stretching you are doing simultaneously. Twenty minutes of a strengthening workout on the Power Plate is equivalent to an hour or so in the weight room. Fitness trendsetters, including Chicago Bulls and Miami Dolphins, celebs Madonna, Brad Pitt and George Clooney are the latest

fitness trend users. *Medicine and Science in Sports and Exercise* and *The Journal of Sports Science* show this equipment increases muscle strength, circulation, bone density, flexibility and even testosterone and human growth hormone. Studies also show a decrease in the "bad" hormone, cortisol.

Recovery time of no less than 48 hours but not more than 96 hours between training sessions is suggested to prevent injury and overtraining. Also, atrophy occurs if more than three or four days pass without exercising the muscles. Two or three 30-minute sessions a week are sufficient for building strength and endurance. Training twice a week at greater intensity and for a longer duration can be as effective as training three times a week.

## TYPES OF MUSCULAR CONTRACTIONS

Muscles can contract or relax. As they contract or relax, skeletal muscles either pull on bones or stop pulling on bones. All exercise involves muscle pulling on bones across a joint, and this movement depends on the structure of the joint and the position of the muscle attachments.

Strength and endurance can be developed by doing three types of exercise: isotonic, isometric, and isokinetic. In **isotonic (dynamic) muscle contraction** the muscle changes length, either shortening (concentrically) or lengthening (eccentrically). Isotonic exercises are those in which a resistance is raised and then lowered, such as in weight lifting (bench press), or the resistance comes from the body's own weight (push-ups, sit-ups).

Isotonic exercise develops the most muscular strength when the resistance is high with few repetitions. Isotonic exercise equipment includes free weights; barbells (dumbbells); floor, wall, or ceiling pulleys; bars for pull-ups; and Nautilus and Universal (variable resistance) machines. Nautilus and Universal weight-training machines follow the principle of variable resistance. These machines are equipped with mechanical devices that provide different amounts of resistance, with the intent of overloading the muscle group maximally through the entire range of motion.

In isometric (static) muscle contraction, the muscle remains the same length and no movement occurs while a force is exerted against an immovable object. Squeezing a tennis ball to develop handgrip strength, pressing against doorways or walls, and pulling against ropes or towels with the arms or legs are examples of isometric exercise. Isometrics are most useful for individuals who are recovering from an injury, are bedridden, or are limited in

## KEY TERMS

**Isotonic (dynamic) muscle contraction** muscle changes in length, either shortening or lengthening

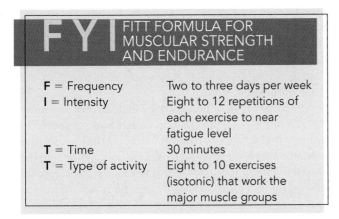

**FYI FITT FORMULA FOR MUSCULAR STRENGTH AND ENDURANCE**

| | |
|---|---|
| **F** = Frequency | Two to three days per week |
| **I** = Intensity | Eight to 12 repetitions of each exercise to near fatigue level |
| **T** = Time | 30 minutes |
| **T** = Type of activity | Eight to 10 exercises (isotonic) that work the major muscle groups |

movements for reasons other than cardiorespiratory disease.

**Isokinetic (constant speed contraction) exercises** are isotonic concentric activities utilizing constant resistance machines that regulate movement velocity and resistance to overload muscles throughout the entire range of motion. Isokinetic exercises are most effective in strengthening specific muscle groups. The machines are more expensive than traditional weight-training equipment and are found principally in hospitals and commercial fitness clubs.

## ASSESSMENT OF MUSCULAR STRENGTH AND ENDURANCE

Strength and endurance are specific to the angle of the joint at which movement occurs. Therefore, when assessing muscular endurance and strength, the **specificity principle** is important.

The most widely accepted tests include the abdominal crunches and exercises involving the upper arm and shoulder (modified pull-up, pull-up, push-up, flexed arm hang) and the hip and thigh (distance jump or sprint). Abdominal crunches are done with heels 12 to 18 inches from the buttocks. Pull-ups use different muscle groups when the palms are facing inward (easier to do) than when palms are facing outward.

## VALSALVA EFFECT

Increased pressure from the **Valsalva effect** decreases the return of blood to the heart, which in turn raises the blood pressure and slows the heart rate. In addition, tissues may be ruptured, especially in the abdominal region (hernias) and in the eyes when pathology is already present (such as glaucoma). A torn or detached retina of the eye may result when holding the breath. This tendency is not good, and exercisers have to guard against it. The rule of breathing during resistance exercise is exhale while exerting force (push or lift), inhale when muscles are relaxed. Never hold your breath, since oxygen flow helps prevent muscle fatigue and injury.

## ANABOLIC STEROIDS

**Anabolic steroids** stimulate the development of bone, muscle, skin, and hair growth, as well as emotional responses. Competitive athletes looking for an extra edge and young men and women attempting to transform their bodies sometimes use black-market and quack steroid products.

Many performance-enhancing drugs come from underground laboratories or foreign countries and often are not even steroids. Some athletes and body builders are using alternatives to steroids, including human growth hormone (HGH) and gamma hydroxybutyrate (GHB). Both substances are dangerous. HGH is an injectable form of the hormone that produces normal growth, causing a risk of hepatitis or HIV infection from tainted needles as well as other medical problems. GHB, naturally found in the central nervous system, may cause short-term coma, vomiting, sudden sleepiness, dizziness, headache, nausea, and seizures. Anabolic steroids are dangerous, with serious side effects, as shown in Table 11.2. Olympian Ben Johnson was stripped of his gold medal when tests showed he had taken anabolic steroids.

## ERGOGENIC AIDS

Ergogenic aids are dietary supplements that boost energy and strength and enhance athletic performance. Teenage

**TABLE 11.2** ▶ Side Effects of Anabolic Steroids

| MEN | WOMEN | BOTH MEN AND WOMEN |
|---|---|---|
| Prominent breasts | Deeper voice | Severe acne |
| Baldness | Enlarged clitoris | High blood pressure |
| Shrinking of the testicles | Increased facial | Decreased immune function |
| Infertility | and body hair | Liver abnormalities and tumors |
| | Hair loss | Increased harmful low-density lipoprotein (LDL) and decreased |
| | Changes in | beneficial high-density lipoprotein (HDL) cholesterol |
| | menstrual cycle | Aggressive behaviors, rage, or violence |
| | | Psychiatric disorders, such as depression |

boys and men in their twenties use these aids the most. Some of these well-known ergogenic aids include the following.

- **Androstenedione ("andro") and dehydro-epiandrosterone (DHEA).** These are weak male hormones produced in the adrenal glands of men and women. Both are broken down into testosterone. These drugs are taken to stimulate muscle growth and aid in weight control. They are promoted as food supplements and are sold in health-food stores and supermarkets. Studies show they are of little value in improving athletic performance. Since baseball player Mark McGwire admitted to using this supplement, many young people began using it. Androstenedione has not been proven to be safe or effective.

- **Caffeine.** Caffeine stimulates the nervous system and increases fat levels in the blood. This natural plant species may improve endurance but does not seem to enhance short-term maximal exercise capacity. Caffeine is addictive, increases insomnia, and may cause abnormal heart rhythms.

- **Carbohydrate beverages.** Beverages are used immediately following exercise to help people recover from intense training. Beverages are used to speed the replenishment of liver and muscle glycogen. Other substances like these are vitamin C,

inosine, beta-hydroxy-beta-methylbutyrate (HMB), and N-acetyl-L-cysteine (NAC). There is not enough positive research to support the claim that they are useful.

- **Creatine.** Creatine is an amino acid made by the body and stored predominantly in skeletal muscle. It serves as a reservoir to replenish adenosine triphosphate (ATP), a substance involved in energy production. Other functions in the body remain unknown. People taking creatine have been reported to experience muscle cramping, dehydration, and diarrhea, as well as a few cases of kidney dysfunction. There is no evidence so far that creatine may damage internal organs.

- **Energy bars.** These performance-boosting proteins, amino acids, and antioxidants come in numerous flavors. Some energy bars are high in carbohydrates and protein but less appealing, while others are sweet and tasty, containing as many as 300 calories and 6 grams of fat (see Figure 11.9).

- **Gamma butyrolactone (GLB).** Gamma butyrolactone (GBL) is marketed on the Internet and in gyms as a muscle builder and performance enhancer. It is used to treat narcolepsy, a disabling sleep disorder. The Food and Drug Administration in 1999 warned consumers to avoid products containing GBL because it was associated with at least 55 reports of adverse health effects, including one death and 19 incidents in which users became comatose.

- **Glycerol.** Sport-drink manufacturers are testing formulas using glycerol, a natural element derived from fats, which may lower heart rate and limit exhaustion in marathon events. Glycerol-induced hyperhydration (holding too much water in the blood) can have negative effects on the body.

- **Insulin-like growth factor.** Insulin-like growth factor (IGF-1) is produced by the pituitary gland and is stimulated by growth hormone. It speeds delivery of amino acids and sugar into cells, helps build bone

---

## HEEL RAISE

From a standing position with feet flat on the floor, raise and lower your body weight by moving at the ankle joint only (for added resistance, have someone else hold your shoulders down as you perform the exercise).

**Result:** Develops gastrocnemius muscles.

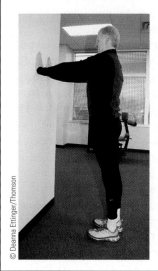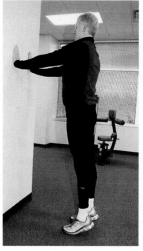

© Deanna Ettinger/Thomson

---

### KEY TERMS

**Isokinetic (constant speed contraction) exercises** isotonic concentric activities utilizing constant resistance machines that regulate movement and resistance to overload muscles

**Specificity principle** holds that exercise must target the muscles identified for development

**Valsalva effect** an increase in pressure in the abdomen and chest that results from holding one's breath during exercise (as in straining to lift a heavy object)

**Anabolic steroids** synthetic derivatives of the male hormone testosterone

**FIGURE 11.9 ▶** Which Snack Boosts Energy Most?

| Snack | Energy bar | Candy bar | Orange (1 medium) |
|---|---|---|---|
| Calories | 220 | 280 | 65 |
| Fat (grams) | 5 | 14 | .1 |
| Vitamin A* | 100% | 0% | 0% |
| Vitamin C* | 100% | 0% | More than 100% |
| Vitamin E* | 100% | 0% | 0% |

*Percentage of the Daily Values for women aged 25 to 50.
Note: Fresh fruit provides a no-fat pick-me-up. Energy bars and candy bars can be high in calories and fat, but at least the energy bars provide nutrients.

*Source:* Diane Hales, *An Invitation to Health,* 9th ed. (Belmont, CA: Wadsworth, 2001), p. 141.

and cartilage, and stimulates protein and glycogen synthesis. The immediate effects of taking IGF-1 remain unclear, but in the long term, it is known to promote cancer.

■ **Insulin.** Insulin supplementation is dangerous because it can cause insulin shock (low blood sugar), which can lead to unconsciousness and death. Insulin is used in the body to help control carbohydrate, fat, and protein metabolism. People take insulin injections to promote muscle hypertrophy.

■ **Metabolic-optimizing meals.** These substances are used by athletes as well as active people. Studies suggest that these meals may increase the hormone concentrations for the development of fitness, but the effects on muscle growth and performance are questionable.

■ **Sodium bicarbonate.** This well-known substance, more commonly known as baking soda, is believed to delay fatigue by neutralizing lactic acid in the muscles, therefore enhancing performance briefly. One must use a large amount to get any benefits, and the side effects include diarrhea.

## Conditions and Clothing for Physical Activity

People exercise in all kinds of conditions and settings, from tropical islands and ski resorts to the outdoor basketball court at the community center. Life-sustaining processes require a fairly constant internal temperature, and deviations to either extreme can cause problems. Exercise is most difficult in hot and humid weather because the excess heat generated in the body is more difficult to dispel. The optimum temperature range for exercising is below 70°F when the humidity is below 45%. The higher the humidity, the lower the temperature must be for safe activity. Conversely, the lower the humidity, the higher the temperature can be.

The type of clothing worn during exercise is critical to optimum performance and benefit. Exercisers should dress appropriately for the environment and the specific workout. In general, the clothes worn should enable free movement and be comfortable and safe.

Exercise during a moderate workout raises the body temperature, which can make the body feel that the surrounding temperature is 20°F warmer than the actual temperature. Therefore, when exercising on a 40°F day, you should dress for a 60°F day. Dressing in several layers of loose-fitting, thin clothing is best, as the layers insulate and trap heat generated by the workout. This also allows the person to remove a layer of clothing at a time as body heat increases.

In warm weather minimum clothing should be worn. It should be loose, airy, light in color, and lightweight, and it should not restrict movement when exercising. It also should be constructed to draw (wick) moisture away from the skin to the surface, providing more efficient evaporation and cooling of the body.

During wet, icy, cool, and snowy weather, a wind-resistant fabric or wool may be used as an outer layer. A wool-blend fabric (such as wool and polypropylene) is recommended. Materials worn should allow moisture to escape from the body. A visor or cap may be necessary to keep water out of the face.

Acrylic socks are most absorbent and prevent blisters and foot irritation. They dry more quickly than cotton and wick moisture away from the skin, preventing blistering and chafing. Socks with extra cushioning at the toes, balls of the feet, and heel areas may be more expensive, but these features reduce friction better than regular socks do.

During warm weather a light-colored straw-type hat or visor will allow air to circulate around the head and protect the eyes and forehead from sun rays. During cold weather 40% of the body's heat can be lost if the head is left uncovered. A wool or synthetic cap or hood will help to hold in body heat.

Mittens keep the fingers together, so the surface area from which to lose heat is smaller than that afforded by gloves. Inner liners made of polypropylene or other materials are recommended to draw moisture from the skin.

Shoes are perhaps the most important piece of equipment for any exercise. Properly fitting shoes are essential to avoid injuries (Achilles tendon strain, blisters, heel bruises). In selecting the correct shoe, body type, degree of pronation or supination (if any), the activity itself, and

## Tips for Action When Selecting Shoes

- Choose shoes according to your specific activity.

- Be sure the shoes have good stability, motion control, durability, and fit.

- Get fitted for shoes in the middle of the day when your feet have expanded and may be one-half size larger. (Also, each foot may be a different size.)

- To allow the feet to breathe, choose shoes with nylon or mesh uppers (cooler).

- Buy shoes at a reputable shoe store where the salespeople are knowledgeable. Expect to pay more for a good shoe.

- Break in new shoes slowly. Examine your shoes closely after six months or so, as that is the point at which many shoes begin to lose their cushioning. Replace your shoes when they wear out.

- For special conditions (unusual foot width; rigid, high arch; flat feet; obesity; pronation; toe shape), ask an expert to assist you. An evaluation from a podiatrist may be necessary.

- Ask to test-drive the shoes on a noncarpeted surface to help you determine the amount of comfort and cushion of the shoes.

*Source:* Adapted from Patricia A. Floyd and Janet E. Parke, *Walk, Jog, Run for Wellness Everyone*, 5th ed. Winston-Salem, NC: Hunter Textbooks, 2006. Photo courtesy of Nike, Inc.

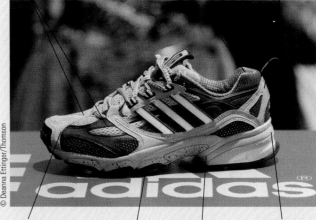

UPPER
Should consist of breathable material such as nylon mesh

COLLAR
Consists of soft material that wraps around and protects the Achilles tendon

HEEL COUNTER
Rigid cup that surrounds and stabilizes the heel

© Deanna Ettinger/Thomson

TOE BOX
Should be wide and tall enough to provide room for the toes to spread comfortably

OUTSOLE
Made of durable solid rubber or carbon rubber; protects the midsole and provides traction

MIDSOLE
Absorbs most of the shock to the heel strike upon push-off. Loses its shock-absorbing ability at approximately 500 miles of use

EXTERNAL STABILIZER
Supports the base of the heel counter for extra stability

---

surfaces should be considered. Walking shoes, court shoes (tennis or basketball), and shoes for aerobics have different characteristics and should be purchased for that specific exercise program. The average exercise shoe loses half its shock-absorbing ability (located at midsole and therefore not visible) and arch support after about 300 miles of running or 300 hours of aerobic classes. The life of the shoe is shorter for overweight people. The average exerciser should purchase a new pair about every six months.

Additional attire to consider when exercising may be an athletic bra, or for men, compression shorts (a cross between skin-tight bike shorts and a girdle). Compression shorts vary in their amount of compression and usually are worn under shorts. They cause less friction and chafing than jockstraps. Other aids may be workout watches, reflective materials (to be used at night), heart rate monitors, and sunglasses.

Wearing rubberized suits during hot weather is dangerous. They do not allow body moisture to evaporate and may cause heat-related injuries.

## Exercise-Related Injuries and Conditions

The benefits of exercise outweigh the risks of injury. Even when activities are planned carefully, though, injuries do happen. Usually they are not serious or permanent. Most injuries occur simply because people take unnecessary risks when exercising. If an injury does not receive the proper attention, it can escalate into a serious problem, sometimes to the point of permanent damage. If you experience pain during a workout, stop. Your body is telling you something is amiss.

Half or more of all new exercisers suffer exercise-related injuries during the first six months of their program. The injuries often result from anatomical problems. Few individuals have perfect body alignment. Other injuries result from training errors, improper shoes, and environmental conditions. Surfaces such as asphalt, concrete, and Astroturf can pose problems, as they absorb and hold heat. Grass softens the impact and reduces

## Tips for Action Specific Guidelines for Hot- and Cold-Weather Exercise

**In hot, humid weather**

■ Drink 12 to 20 ounces of fluid such as Gatorade 15 to 30 minutes before exercising. Water stimulates the production of urine, leaving less liquid for sweating.

■ Drink 6 to 8 ounces every 15 minutes during exercise.

■ Avoid alcoholic and caffeinated beverages as these stimulate the production of urine.

■ If need be, modify your exercise program by

— Working out during cooler times of day

— Choosing a cooler place to exercise

— Slowing your pace and shortening the duration of exercise

— Wearing light, porous clothing

**In cold weather**

■ Dress in layers to trap air warmed by the body, which provides an insulating effect.

■ Adequately protect exposed areas—fingers, nose, ears, facial skin, toes—and

— Wear mittens, not gloves

— Wear thick socks

— Wear a stocking cap that also covers the ears

**In very cold weather**

— Wear a ski mask or scarf that covers the mouth so you will be breathing moist air

— Consider polypropylene underwear plus wool outer garments

---

stress on the body. Holes, cracks in pavement, gravel, and slippery spots are potentially dangerous. Prevention is more important than any physician or self-treatment.

## HEAT-RELATED CONCERNS

Hot, humid weather raises caution signals. Prolonged exposure to hot temperatures coupled with high relative humidity can result in heat cramps, heat exhaustion, or heat stroke.

**Heat cramps,** the least severe of the heat-related health concerns, nevertheless are extremely painful. Heat cramps result from tightness of the muscles, fatigue, or dehydration, leading to imbalance of electrolytes (sodium, calcium, potassium), which are essential to muscle contraction. When heat cramps occur, the arteries temporarily decrease the blood flow to the muscles.

Proper stretching before exercising, drinking plenty of water, and consuming sufficient electrolytes—sodium (salting food), calcium (milk or cheese), and potassium (bananas)—may prevent heat cramps. People should avoid exercising during the hottest part of the day (11 a.m.–4 p.m.). The temperature usually is highest at about 4 p.m. When heat cramps occur, massaging the affected area sometimes helps.

**Heat exhaustion** results from depletion and inadequate replacement of fluids, which is caused by heavy sweating during vigorous exercise in a warm, humid place. It is not a serious threat to life. Symptoms include cold or clammy skin, dilated pupils, profuse sweating, mildly elevated temperature, headache, dizziness, rapid and weak pulse, nausea and vomiting, and hyperventilation. Immediate treatment of heat exhaustion requires relocating the person to a cooler place, loosening clothing, having the person drink large quantities of cool water, and apply-

ing cold packs to the skin or immersing the person in cold water as soon as possible.

**Heat stroke,** the most severe of the heat-related disorders, is a life-threatening emergency. The temperature control system that produces sweat to cool the body stops working. Symptoms include relatively dry skin, serious disorientation, constricted pupils, very high body temperatures (105°F or higher), sudden collapse, and loss of consciousness.

If the body temperature is lowered to normal within 45 minutes, the possibility of death from heat stroke can be reduced significantly. Treatment includes cooling the person rapidly by immersing the person in cool water or wrapping wet sheets and ice packs around the entire body, especially the head, torso, and joints. Fanning the person and giving him or her plenty of cold liquids is helpful. The affected person should be taken immediately to a hospital or an emergency treatment facility.

## COLD-RELATED CONCERNS

When exercising in cold weather, conserving heat is a major concern. **Wind chill** is a contributing factor. The wind chill index is given in Figure 11.10. Cold-related injuries include frostbite, hypothermia, and hyperthermia.

**Frostbite** is a common injury caused by overexposure to cold temperatures. When blood flow is restricted, ice crystals form in body tissues on the feet, hands, ears, nose, cheeks, and chin. The frozen body parts should be immersed in warm, not hot, water, and then covered loosely or bandaged. The affected area should not be rubbed or massaged. Medical attention should be sought immediately. Amputation is the most extreme treatment when tissue has been destroyed irretrievably.

**FIGURE 11.10 ▶** Wind Chill Index

| Wind speed (mph) | What the thermometer reads (°F) | | | | | | | | | | | |
|---|---|---|---|---|---|---|---|---|---|---|---|---|
| | 50 | 40 | 30 | 20 | 10 | 0 | -10 | -20 | -30 | -40 | -50 | -60 |
| | What it equals in its effect on exposed flesh | | | | | | | | | | | |
| Calm | 50 | 40 | 30 | 20 | 10 | 0 | -10 | -20 | -30 | -40 | -50 | -60 |
| 5 | 48 | 37 | 27 | 16 | 6 | -5 | -15 | -26 | -36 | -47 | -57 | -68 |
| 10 | 40 | 28 | 16 | 4 | -9 | -21 | -33 | -46 | -58 | -70 | -83 | -95 |
| 15 | 36 | 22 | 9 | -5 | -18 | -36 | -45 | -58 | -72 | -85 | -99 | -112 |
| 20 | 32 | 18 | 4 | -10 | -25 | -39 | -53 | -67 | -82 | -96 | -110 | -124 |
| 25 | 30 | 16 | 0 | -15 | -29 | -44 | -59 | -74 | -88 | -104 | -118 | -133 |
| 30 | 28 | 13 | -2 | -18 | -33 | -48 | -63 | -79 | -94 | -109 | -125 | -140 |
| 35 | 27 | 11 | -4 | -20 | -35 | -49 | -67 | -82 | -98 | -113 | -129 | -145 |
| 40 | 26 | 10 | -6 | -21 | -37 | -53 | -69 | -85 | -100 | -116 | -132 | -148 |

Little danger if property clothed    Danger of freezing exposed flesh    Great danger of freezing exposed flesh

*Wind speeds greater than 40 mph have little additional effect.

*Source:* B. J. Sharkey, *Physiology of Fitness* (Champaign, IL: Human Kinetics Books, 1990). Reprinted by permission.

**Hypothermia** usually occurs in damp, windy conditions and temperatures in the 50°F to 60°F ranges. The body's temperature drops below 95°F, and heat is lost faster than it can be produced. Symptoms include shivering, followed by loss of coordination and difficulty speaking. When the shivering stops, the muscles stiffen and the person becomes unconscious. Treatment includes warming the body slowly, placing dry clothing on the person immediately, and not giving anything to eat or drink unless the person is fully conscious. Medical attention should be sought immediately.

**Hyperthermia** can occur when a person is wearing too much clothing. To prevent this overheating, the exerciser should dress in several layers of light clothing and remove clothing as the body temperature increases.

## PRICES CONCEPT FOR TREATMENT OF INJURY

The standard recommended treatment for acute injuries is

P = Protect
R = Rest
I = Ice application
C = Compression
E = Elevation

The purpose of **PRICE** is to minimize injury and its risks. An injury may require one or more of the following treatments.

1. **P = Protect, stabilize, and support.** Protect the injured part as much as possible to prevent further injury. Maintain support on the injured part until all indications of the injury are gone. The use of a brace, sling, splint, cane, crutches, air cast, tape, or strap still allows the person to be active. Supports or splints are available from medical supply companies and pharmaceutical agencies

2. **R = Rest.** If you experience pain, stop immediately. Listen to your body. Resting a few days will help stop

### KEY TERMS

**Heat cramps** muscle spasms in the arms, legs, or abdomen as a result of overexercise in warm weather

**Heat exhaustion** fatigued condition resulting from depletion and inadequate fluid replacement during heavy exercise

**Heat stroke** an emergency condition resulting from overexercise in hot weather

**Wind chill** real temperature as affected by wind so as to feel colder and increase the effects on the body

**Frostbite** a skin condition caused by overexposure to cold temperatures

**Hypothermia** a condition in which body temperature drops below 95°F and loses its ability to produce heat because heat is lost faster than it can be produced

**Hyperthermia** abnormally high body temperature

**PRICE** recommended treatment for acute injuries: protect, rest, ice application, compression, and elevation

excess bleeding and pain, and it will promote healing of damaged tissues without complications. "Train, don't strain; if stressed, get rest." Unless indicated by a physician, absolute rest should not exceed 48 hours because muscles may become weak, joints may stiffen, and scar tissue may form around the injured part.

3. **I = Ice.** Icing is the most effective, safest, and cheapest form of treatment. Ice (icebag, cold whirlpool) acts as a local anesthetic by reducing the impulses of pain receptors, blood flow, muscle spasms, and inflammation (though inflammation is a part of the healing process, and too much icing can impede healing). Ice helps to limit tissue damage and hasten the healing process.

Apply ice compresses for 10 to 20 minutes, and then reapply every two waking hours for the next 48 to 72 hours. Once the skin is numb, stop icing. Be sure not to exceed the 20-minute limit, as longer than that may damage skin and nerves. Packs that remain flexible when frozen, such as a gel pack, two plastic bags of ice, or even a bag of frozen peas, can provide more cooling because they mold to the body. Self-freezing chemical packs or refreezable packs may be colder than regular ice. Chemicals in the packs can burn if they are allowed to be in direct contact with the skin.

People who are hypersensitive to cold or have a circulatory problem should not use ice. Never place an unwrapped ice pack over the elbow or the outside of the knee, because it may cause nerve damage (nerves are near the surface).

4. **C = Compression.** Pressure reduces swelling and blood flow to the injured part. Use an Ace-type elastic bandage or wet wrap for compression (not so tight that circulation is cut off).

5. **E = Elevation.** Combine elevation of the affected part with icing and compression. Elevation reduces internal bleeding and pooling of blood in the injured part. Elevate the injury above heart level to reduce swelling and eliminate pain caused by blood rushing to the injured part. After 48 hours, if swelling is gone, apply warmth or gentle heat, which speeds healing. Apply cold to sore areas after a workout to prevent inflammation and swelling.

PRICE is not a substitute for seeing a doctor in case of a serious injury or an injury that does not respond to self-treatment in 24 hours. PRICE does not include heat treatment (which is indicated for some injuries).

## HEAT TREATMENT

Heat stimulates blood flow and may increase inflammation. Therefore, it should be applied with caution. Only after the swelling has subsided (in approximately two to three days) should a person apply heat. At that point the increased blood flow caused by heating promotes healing.

## FYI EXERCISE AND NUTRITION

During heavy exercise, glycogen is broken down into glucose, which then becomes available to the muscles for energy production. Glucose provides about 6% more energy per unit of oxygen consumed than fat does. Heavy and prolonged exercise over several days depletes glycogen faster than the body can replace it through nutritive intake.

Therefore, athletes and people with similar physical demands are advised to switch to a carbohydrate-rich diet to restore glycogen levels. People who exercise less than an hour a day need not worry, as the regular recommended diet is sufficient to restore glycogen stores.

Following an exhaustive workout, eating a combination of carbohydrates and protein (tuna sandwich) within 30 minutes of exercise seems to speed up glycogen storage at an even faster rate. Protein intake increases insulin activity, thus enhancing glycogen replenishment. A 70% carbohydrate intake then should be maintained throughout the rest of the day.

Heat also helps to relax muscles, prevent spasms, reduce joint stiffness, and relieve pain.

Before using heat on an injury, a physician should be consulted to determine whether to use dry heat (heating pad or heating lamp) or moist heat (hot bath, hot water bottle, heat pack, whirlpool). Those who have heart conditions or a fever should avoid hot baths and whirlpools. If infection or loss of sensation is present, heat should not be applied.

Warm (not hot) heat should be applied for 20 to 30 minutes, two to three times a day. Using warm heat five to 10 minutes before exercising reduces stiffness. A hot water bottle, heating pad, or hot pack that does not have a cover can be wrapped in a towel. If the nature of the injury is in doubt, medical evaluation should be sought immediately. If the area becomes inflamed or painful after heating an injury, self-treatment should be stopped immediately.

## Exercise for People with Special Needs

Exercise is just as important to those individuals with disabilities as for anyone else. Approximately 54 million Americans have significant chronic disabilities due to, for example, illness, chronic pain (arthritis), injury, and birth defects. The Americans with Disabilities Act has ensured individuals with disabilities access to public health clubs and recreational facilities. Activities including adaptive horseback riding, swimming, fishing, golf, and skiing are offered for people of all ages and types of disabilities. Also there are wheelchair versions of tennis, hockey, billiards, and basketball as well as sports for those with mental retardation and visual and hearing impairments.

In 1988 Jamie Goldman lost both legs below the knee from frostbite. She wears carbon fiber artificial legs and runs competitively. She was in the advertisement promoting the 2000 Olympic and Paralympic Games. No matter what your level of ability or special need, exercise can be an integral part of your life. Call your local YMCA/YWCA, community center, health club, or independent living center if you have a special need and wish to begin an exercise, sport, or recreational program.

Equally important is physical education, and/or physical activities appropriate for students with special needs. All students regardless of their ability level should be involved in a daily physical education/physical activity program that is developmentally appropriate for their age and ability level. Individual differences affect social acceptance and inclusion. The attitudes, knowledge, and skills of adapted physical education and/or physical activity must be infused into all regular education classes. Schools and teachers must assume their responsibility for active, healthy lifestyles for all children. Regular and adapted physical education teachers can work together to meet the individual needs of all students in order to achieve a healthier lifestyle.

## Exercise for Older Adults

Retiring from your job does not mean that you are retiring from life. You never get too old to get in shape. Even though research proves exercise to be beneficial to the older person, many are not active. Research shows that by the age of 75, about one in three men and one in two women engage in no physical activity. Older adults should always consult a physician before engaging in a new physical activity program.

The American College of Sports Medicine now encourages older people to engage in a full range of physical activities, including aerobic conditioning, flexibility exercises, and strength training. Gerontologists describe exercise as "the closest thing to an anti-aging pill." Exercise slows down the changes that are associated with aging: increased body weight and fat, decreased work capacity, loss of lean muscle tissue, increased brittle bones, back problems, less mobility of joints, and more depression. Aerobic exercise helps to lower the risk of heart disease and stroke, and it also helps the older person retain the strength and mobility needed to be independent. Flexibility activities reduce the risks of sprains, injuries, and strains. Yoga, tai chi, and Pilates are beneficial exercise methods for older adults. Strength activities build stronger muscles, improve balance, increase bone

mass, provide greater mobility, and improve mood and feelings of well-being. Specific guidelines that apply to older adults include the following.

- Drink plenty of water, avoid exercising in hot or cold climates, and wear warm clothes to prevent heat loss in cold environments.
- Warm up slowly. Increase intensity and duration gradually. Do static stretching to prevent soft tissue pain.
- Cool down slowly until heart rate is below 100 before stopping.
- Include resistance, endurance, and flexibility types of activities.

## Backache

Backache is one of the most prevalent physical health problems in America today. It is the second-leading reason people go to doctors (after the common cold). Only rarely does a back problem have a serious cause or prognosis, but it debilitates huge numbers of people. About 75% consist of chronic low back pain. Much of the backache problem is caused by physical inactivity, poor postural habits and body mechanics, and overweight.

Research recommends surgical intervention only as a last resort. It is suggested that about nine of 10 people who have lower back problems will recover on their own within a month. Research reports have not found a scientific basis for spinal traction or acupuncture. Some formerly recommended treatments, such as bed rest, have been found to weaken muscles or bones. Instead, the experts advise that people with lower back pain do low-stress exercises such as walking, swimming, and biking and that they take aspirin (or acetaminophen) for pain. Spinal manipulation (chiropractic) also was found to be helpful.

Some recommendations to prevent back pain are as follows.

- Regular exercise
- Comfortable, low-heeled shoes
- Work surfaces placed at comfortable heights
- A chair with good back support
- Lifting objects close to the body
- Resting feet on a low stool when sitting a long time
- Placing a pillow or rolled-up towel behind the small of the back when driving long distances

### SAFETY GUIDELINES

- Avoid busy streets as much as possible when you are outdoors exercising (walking, jogging, running, cycling). Exercising on major streets is the most dangerous. The peak traffic hours between 4:00 and 6:00 p.m. are the most hazardous. Obey all traffic regulations. Cars always have the right-of-way.

■ Wear light-colored clothing; use reflective gear when exercising at night.

■ Be alert to objects thrown from vehicles.

■ Walkers, joggers, and runners: Face the traffic. Cyclists: Ride with the traffic, keeping to the right of the road.

■ Limit exercising in areas of severe smog, as pollutants (ozone and nitrogen oxides) may be damaging to the lungs.

■ Dress appropriate to the weather.

■ Use headphones only on trails and paths, not streets.

■ Exercise with friends, especially at night.

■ Tell friends and family your exercise destination and approximate time you plan to return.

■ Stick to your predicted arrival time.

■ Carry identification. Tuck a small business card into your exercise attire, or wear an identification bracelet. Carry the name of a person to contact in case of emergency. Females may want to consider carrying a protective warning device such as a whistle.

The following guidelines pertain to cyclists.

■ Check your cycle every time before you ride.

■ Use proper hand signals for turning and stopping.

■ Stop and look both ways to make sure sidewalks or streets are clear before you enter.

■ Walk your bicycle across busy streets at corners or crosswalks.

■ When cycling at night, use proper headlights and red taillight or reflector.

■ Keep your hands on the handlebars, and never show off.

■ Do not hitch rides or accept passengers.

■ Never tailgate or ride too closely to cars or trucks.

## Fitness Products and Facilities

Being an informed consumer will help a person distinguish between valid information and health fraud. Books, magazine articles, and other nonadvertised printed materials are available to help people select products and facilities.

### FITNESS EQUIPMENT

Good equipment enhances the enjoyment and decreases the risk of injury from exercise. It will not make you fit unless you find the motivation to use it.

Active equipment improves fitness because the exerciser has to provide the muscle and aerobic power to perform the activity. Active exercise devices include stair climbers, stationary cycles, treadmills, weight machines, and ski machines. In contrast, passive equipment does not work for you and, therefore, is a waste of time and money.

Passive equipment includes steam and sauna baths, rubberized suits (also dangerous because they do not permit sweating), hot tubs, vibrators (tables, pillows, belts), and motor-driven cycles.

Guidelines for selecting fitness equipment include the following.

1. Investigate the equipment before purchasing it. Seek advice from knowledgeable personnel in local colleges or universities, community wellness centers, and YMCAs, as well as sports instructors and coaches. Ask questions and shop around for the best buys.

2. Make sure the equipment is safe, is in good working order, and fits properly.

3. Test-drive equipment before you buy it. Does it provide a good workout? Select equipment according to your physical and lifestyle needs.

4. Do not be in a hurry. Give yourself a cooling-off period so you will not buy on impulse.

5. Buy quality equipment, or wait until you can afford it. Check the length of warranty. Look for warranties of one or two years or more.

6. Buy according to your needs, and buy equipment you will continue to use. Will the equipment fit into your lifestyle and exercise space? Can it be stored easily?

**VIEWPOINT** *Many people have personal trainers. Thus far, anyone can be a personal trainer. Although some organizations issue certificates of competency, no licensing body governs this relatively new specialty. Do you believe personal trainers should be required to have a license to practice?*

### HEALTH AND FITNESS CLUBS

Most people who join a health or fitness club do not go regularly or quit within six months. Still, clubs may provide motivation and expert advice on better ways to exercise. Before joining one of these facilities, a person should consider the following.

1. **Location and hours of operation.** The facility should be within 15 minutes of you and open at convenient hours.

**FIGURE 11.11** ► Physical Activity Pyramid for Adults

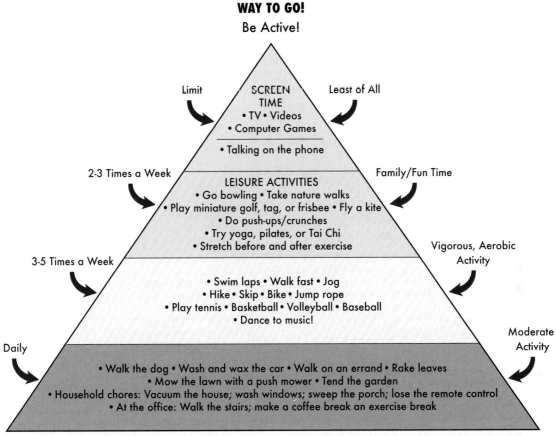

To create and sustain well-being, accumulate a minimum of 30–35 minutes daily of moderate physical activity

2. **Individual concerns.** Are you allowed, before signing the contract, to discuss your physical limitations, risk factors, and individual problems? Does the facility recommend that you consult with your doctor before beginning an exercise program?

3. **Stress test.** If you have any doubts regarding your present state of health, consult your physician, who may recommend an exercise stress test.

4. **Facility and equipment.** Is the facility in good order, clean, and well ventilated? Is it overcrowded (waiting lines)? Does the club have programs such as aerobics classes and enough cardiorespiratory fitness equipment, such as treadmills, stair-climbing machines, stationary bicycles, running track, swimming pool, and rowing machines? Does it include devices for strength and flexibility development? Is the equipment maintained properly and in good condition? What type of floor is used for aerobic workouts—suspended wood floor, high-density matting, carpet over cushioning? Beware of aerobic floors made of tile, linoleum, or cement.

5. **Qualified and certified personnel.** What type of in-house training does the club require of its instructors?

Law does not mandate certification, but it should be considered. Exercisers may find that working with a trained professional makes exercise enjoyable, prevents injury, and provides motivation. Are warm-up and cool-down periods included? Ask to observe instructors and classes, and talk with club members. Do the instructors address the participants' various ability levels? Do they give personalized attention and move around? Is safety stressed? Are they certified in CPR (cardiopulmonary resuscitation) and first aid? If not, look elsewhere.

6. **Membership.** Does membership include lockers, showers, towels, classes, or will you have to pay extra for these amenities? Select a no-contract plan if possible. If not, choose a short-term contract before you commit to join for a year or more. Read the contract carefully. Many clubs go out of business, and some change ownership often. Get all agreements in writing. "Pay as you go" is the best plan.

7. **People.** Are the participants older or younger than you are? Are they in better or worse shape? Perhaps you will enjoy the exercise program more if you feel compatible with the people who exercise with you.

**FIGURE 11.12** ▶ Activity Pyramid for People Over 60

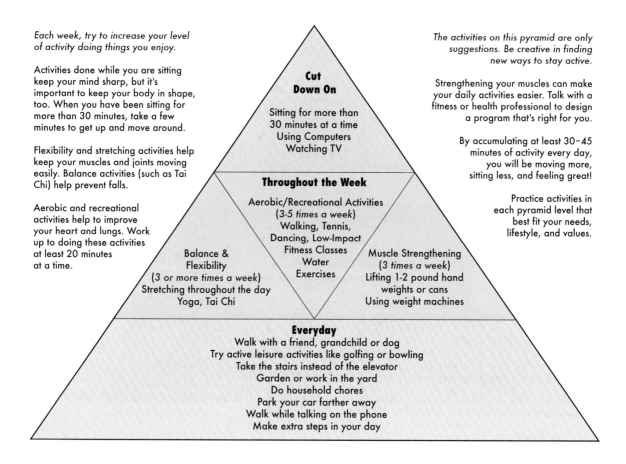

**Activity Pyramid for People Over 60**

*Each week, try to increase your level of activity doing things you enjoy.*

*Activities done while you are sitting keep your mind sharp, but it's important to keep your body in shape, too. When you have been sitting for more than 30 minutes, take a few minutes to get up and move around.*

*Flexibility and stretching activities help keep your muscles and joints moving easily. Balance activities (such as Tai Chi) help prevent falls.*

*Aerobic and recreational activities help to improve your heart and lungs. Work up to doing these activities at least 20 minutes at a time.*

**Cut Down On**
Sitting for more than 30 minutes at a time
Using Computers
Watching TV

**Throughout the Week**
Aerobic/Recreational Activities
(*3-5 times a week*)
Walking, Tennis, Dancing, Low-Impact Fitness Classes
Water Exercises

**Balance & Flexibility**
(*3 or more times a week*)
Stretching throughout the day
Yoga, Tai Chi

**Muscle Strengthening**
(*3 times a week*)
Lifting 1-2 pound hand weights or cans
Using weight machines

**Everyday**
Walk with a friend, grandchild or dog
Try active leisure activities like golfing or bowling
Take the stairs instead of the elevator
Garden or work in the yard
Do household chores
Park your car farther away
Walk while talking on the phone
Make extra steps in your day

*The activities on this pyramid are only suggestions. Be creative in finding new ways to stay active.*

*Strengthening your muscles can make your daily activities easier. Talk with a fitness or health professional to design a program that's right for you.*

*By accumulating at least 30–45 minutes of activity every day, you will be moving more, sitting less, and feeling great!*

*Practice activities in each pyramid level that best fit your needs, lifestyle, and values.*

8. **Visit.** Visit the club at the time of day you plan to use it. How many people are using the facility when you plan to exercise?

9. **Drugs.** Is it a drug hangout? Is steroid and other drug use apparent?

10. **Check it out.** Call the Better Business Bureau to see if complaints have been filed.

## Health and Physical Activity Prescription

Personal health is unique to the individual. No single physical activity program is suitable for all people. Your wellness prescription should consist of your own interests, objectives, time, and schedule. The physical activity pyramids as shown in Figure 11.11 and Figure 11.12 are handy references for the following guidelines to help you in planning your health and physical activity prescription.

1. **Goals and objectives.** What is my purpose for this program? My short-term (days, weeks) and long-term (months, years) goals? Objectives? Are these attainable and realistic? Make certain that you enjoy your exercise activity.

2. **Medical readiness.** Am I ready for this physical activity program? Do I have any health risk factors? Have I consulted with my physician if indicated?

3. **Attire.** Am I ready to exercise in hot or cold weather? Do I have comfortable clothing and shoes?

4. **Present level of health and fitness.** What is my health and fitness status? Have I had a preevaluation as to my current status on health-related components of physical fitness?

5. **Written plan.** Do I have a method for maintaining a written record of my daily and weekly physical activity program? Write "jogging" or "weights," for example, on a calendar. Stick with the plan.

**Tips for Action** At the Fitness Starting Line

■ Select one or more activities you enjoy. Books, videos, and magazines are available to help you learn about various activities.

■ Set a time and schedule. Among your day's activities, make exercise a top priority.

■ Make a personal contract stating a realistic goal and your commitment to reach it. Include the beginning date, clear description of what you want to accomplish, ways to measure your progress, and the date you expect to accomplish your goal. Start by writing down your major goal, and then list smaller objectives to accomplish it.

■ Do not overdo it. Overexertion can cause soreness and fatigue, which might discourage you.

■ Seek support. Network with family, friends, a partner, a group, and ask them to join you. Make exercise a social event. Talk with people and discover the strategies that worked for them. Borrow from their experience.

■ Listen to music. Music enhances your training and helps the time pass quickly.

■ Do not feel guilty or blame yourself when you slip in your exercise program. Deal with your reasons and move on.

■ Seek assistance when you need it. Controlling counterproductive behaviors such as alcohol and drug abuse,

overeating, and cigarette smoking may require outside help. Programs such as Weight Watchers, Alcoholics Anonymous, Smoke Enders, and services provided by health departments and counseling centers are just a few of the community resources available.

■ Get plenty of rest and sleep.

■ Make exercise a daily choice. Once you have started, do not stop. See yourself as a capable person in charge of your health and well-being. Notice how much better you look and feel.

■ Participate in team sports—volleyball, softball, basketball, bowling.

■ Park the car a few blocks away from where you are going, and then walk the rest of the way.

■ Always take stairs instead of elevators.

■ Walk the dog at a brisk pace.

■ Mow the lawn and work in the yard.

■ Vary your routine to prevent monotony and boredom.

■ Keep a record of your progress, and reward yourself when you show improvement.

■ Be patient.

■ Have fun and enjoy your new lifestyle.

6. **Time and convenience.** Do I have a set daily and weekly time to devote to my physical activity program? Always try to exercise at the same time of day. For example, before breakfast or before dinner. How far do I have to go to exercise? Get someone to exercise with you. Are the equipment and facilities convenient?

7. **Components.** Does my physical activity prescription include warm-up, activity session, cool-down, overload principle, principle of progression, principle of specificity, being active, and safety? Does it adhere to the FITT formula for cardiorespiratory endurance, muscular flexibility, and muscular strength and endurance?

8. **Nutrition.** How am I doing with basic nutrients? Do I need more vitamins, minerals, and water? Does my diet provide sufficient complex carbohydrates (grains, fruits, and vegetables) and some protein? Have I cut down fat intake to less than 30% of total dietary calories? Remember not to skip breakfast, because it gets your metabolism going. Water is essential to an exercise program.

9. **Drugs.** Am I drug-free (including tobacco)? If not, do I plan to become drug-free?

10. **Stress management activities.** Do I take time for myself? What relaxation techniques do I use?

11. **Flexibility.** Do I need to add, modify, or adjust my current physical activity program?

12. **Enjoyment and motivation.** Am I enjoying and happy with the results of my physical activity program? Do I look forward to being active?

13. **Cost.** Can I afford to purchase the necessary equipment? Pay the fees for a fitness or health club? Can I find other means to exercise with little or no cost involved?

14. **Rewards.** How am I going to reward myself after achieving short-term goals? Long-term goals? Savor the moment while you are walking, jogging, lifting weights, cycling, and so on at the beginning of a fresh new day or after a stressful day. Enjoy the pure pleasure of waking up each morning and living the moment.

## Summary

- The surgeon general's report on physical activity and health provides a landmark review of the research on physical activity and health.

- Exercise has both physical and psychological benefits including reduced risk for many diseases, plus more energy and vitality.

- The FITT formula is an acronym for **f**requency, **i**ntensity, **t**ime, and **t**ype of activity. It applies to each of the physical fitness components.

- The health-related physical fitness components are body composition, cardiorespiratory endurance, muscular flexibility, and muscular strength and endurance.

- Phases of exercise include the warm-up, the workout, and the cool-down.

- Principles of fitness training include the overload principle, progression principle, and specificity of training.

- The purpose of aerobic exercise is to increase your heart rate to higher levels and thus increase cardiorespiratory fitness.

- The three types of stretching are static or slow-sustained, dynamic or ballistic, and proprioceptive neuromuscular facilitation (PNF).

- Types of muscular contractions are isotonic (dynamic) and isometric (static).

- A shortcut to building muscle is the use of steroids and ergogenic aids. Long-term side effects are not known.

- Clothing should be comfortable and allow the person to move freely. Proper shoes are particularly important.

- Heat-related concerns include muscle cramps, heat exhaustion, and heat stroke.

- The most common cold-weather concerns are frostbite and hypothermia.

- The PRICE treatment for injury consists of protect, rest, ice, compression, and elevation. In addition, heat treatment sometimes is indicated.

- Prevention is the best treatment. Common sense heads the list of safety precautions.

## Personal Health Resources

**ThomsonNOW** Visit the ThomsonNOW website at http://thomsonedu.com/thomsonnow for valuable resources that will:

- Help you evaluate your knowledge of the material.

- Guide you through tutorials to help you understand and apply the material.

- Allow you to take an exam-prep quiz to better prepare for class tests.

American Council on Exercise. This site features information for the general public as well as for certified fitness trainers. Information such as Fit Facts information sheets, whole-body exercise workouts, daily fitness tips, newsletters, and information on ACE certification.

**www.acefitness.org**

National Center for Chronic Disease Prevention and Health Promotion: Physical Activity and Health. This website is sponsored by the CDC and features a report from the U.S. Surgeon General. Two important CDC reports, the national physical activity initiative and the link between physical activity and health are available for download.

**www.cdc.gov/nccdphp/sgr/sgr.htm**

Your Personalized Health Portrait. Complete this confidential health questionnaire to determine your personal lifestyle score. Also included is a list of screening tests and immunizations to discuss with your doctor.

**www.thriveonline.com/cgi-bin/hmi/healthportrait.cgi**

Customized Five-Step Fitness Test. This site includes information on five physical fitness tests, with illustrations and easy step-by-step directions. You will enter your exercise data online for the appropriate test. Test items include Sit-and-Reach test (flexibility), walking test for one mile (cardiovascular fitness), upper-body strength (push-ups), abdominal strength (curls), and body fat (using an online calculator).

**www.phys.com/fitness/analysis/fittest**

Check Your Physical Activity and Heart IQ. This site, sponsored by the National Heart, Lung, and Blood Institute, provides a true-false quiz to allow you to assess what you know about how physical activity affects your heart. The answers provided will uncover exercise myths and give you information on ways to improve your heart health.

**www.nhlbi.nih.gov/health/public/heart/
obesity/pa_iq_ab.htm**

Choosing Exercise for Health. This site describes the health benefits of regular exercise.

**www.physsportsmed.com/issues/jul-96/wooten.htm**

Shape Up America Fitness Assessment. A battery of physical fitness assessments, including activity level, flexibility, strength, and an aerobic fitness test, is provided. Enter your age, height, weight, and gender and take the screening test to assess your physical readiness for physical activity. The final results in each of these areas will be based on the personal data entered.

**www.shapeup.org/fitness/ass/fset2.htm**

Create Your Personal Contract to Healthy Behavior Change. This site includes information on establishing your goals in writing to become a healthier you. Also, it provides you with the opportunity to print your personal contract and have a friend sign it for validation.

**www.thriveonline.com/seasonal/new_year/ resolutions/contract.html**

Healthy People 2010. This site provides a list of national goals for improving the health of all Americans by the year 2010.

**www.health.gov/healthypeople**

American Council of Exercise Cardiovascular Fitness Facts. This site features information about a variety of cardiovascular forms of exercise, including walking, running, jumping rope, spinning, swimming, cross-training, and interval training.

**www.acefitness.org/fitfacts_list.cfm#1**

Improving Cardiovascular Health in African Americans. This document from the National Heart, Lung, and Blood Institute provides information on the value of cardiovascular exercise to improving health.

**www.nhlbi.nih.gov/health/public/heart/other/ chdblack/energize.htm**

2005 Dietary Guidelines Advisory Committee. Report of the Dietary Guidelines Advisory Committee on the Dietary Guidelines for Americans, 2005. Washington, DC: Health and Human Services and U.S. Department of Agriculture, 2004, **www.health.gov/dietaryguidelines/dga2005/report.**

## It's Your Turn for Study and Review

1. Which one of the health-related fitness components do you do well? Which one do you need to improve? What types of activities will help you to improve your fitness level?

2. Calculate your maximum heart rate. What is your intensity level, for example, 60% or 80% of your maximum heart rate? Is it easy or hard for you to exercise at the 60% level? Eighty percent level?

3. Why do you need good flexibility? What specific actions can you take to improve your flexibility?

4. Why do you need good muscular strength and muscular endurance? What specific actions can you take to improve your muscular strength and muscular endurance? How would you measure your improvement?

5. Does your college or university have facilities for you to exercise? Does your community have facilities for you to exercise? What types of equipment are located in these facilities? What hours are available in those facilities?

6. List five to eight of the most important steps that you think will help you put together a successful personal fitness program. Consider your interests, your current fitness level, cost, convenience, time, and any special health concerns that you may have.

7. Make a list of your favorite physical activities that may increase your cardiorespiratory fitness, flexibility, muscular strength, and muscular endurance. Choose five that you would like to do regularly. Make a schedule, setting aside a regular time to exercise. Make a regular appointment with a friend to exercise with you. Then enjoy the experience to a healthier you.

8. How often should you exercise? Every day? Once a week? Three or four times per week? Where can you get advice about exercise?

9. A person is concerned about his or her safety when exercising alone. What actions can this person take to make sure that he or she is safe and can enjoy an exercise session? Where can this person exercise?

10. Are exercise and nutrition related? Is one more important than the other? If so, which one?

## Thinking about Health Issues

Do ergogenic aids enhance performance and are they safe?
Dee Murphy, "What You Should Know about Creatine," *Current Health 2: A Weekly Reader Publication*, 26:6 (February 2000), p. 13.

1. What are natural sources of creatine in the body?

2. Physiologically, how does creatine enhance physical performance? What types of exercises are not enhanced by creatine ingestion?

3. What are the major adverse effects of creatine supplementation? What questions should you ask before considering taking any supplement?

## Selected Bibliography

American College of Sports Medicine. "ACSM Position Stand: The Recommended Quantity and Quality of Exercise for Developing and Maintaining Cardiorespiratory and Muscular Fitness, and Flexibility in Healthy Adults." *Medicine and Science in Sports and Exercise*, 30:6, 1998, pp. 975–991.

American College of Sports Medicine. *Guidelines for Exercise Testing and Prescription*, 6th ed. Baltimore, MD: Lippincott Williams and Wilkins, 2000.

"Biology Shows Women and Men Are Different." *Mayo Clinic Women's Healthsource*, September 2002.

Birch, B. B. "Make It Routine: The 10 Best Stretches." *Runner's World*, 2001, pp. 52–56.

Blair, S. N., et al. "The Evolution of Physical Activity Recommendations: How Much Is Enough?" *American Journal of Clinical Nutrition,* 79:5, May 2004, p. 913S.

Blair, S. and Church, T. "The Fitness, Obesity, and Health Equation." *Journal of the American Medical Association,* 292:10, September 8, 2004, p. 1232.

Borg, G. "Psychophysical Bases of Perceived Exertion." *Medicine and Science in Sports and Exercise,* 14, 1982, pp. 377–381.

Branch, J. D., et al. "Moderate Intensity Exercise Training Improves Cardiorespiratory Fitness in Women." *Journal of Women's Health and Gender-Based Medicine,* 9:1, 2000, pp. 65–73.

Brant, J. "Drink This." *Runner's World,* 2001, pp. 42–44.

Buckworth, J. and Nigg, C. "Physical Activity, Exercise, and Sedentary Behavior in College Students." *Journal of American College Health,* 53:1, July–August 2004, p. 28.

Carter, M. J. "Moving beyond the Surgeon General's Report: An HPERD Challenge." *Journal of Physical Education, Recreation, and Dance,* 70:2, 1999.

Centers for Disease Control and Prevention. "Heat-Related Mortality—United States, 1997." *Morbidity and Mortality Weekly Report,* 47:23, 1998, pp. 473–476.

College of Family Physicians of Canada, www.cfpc.ca.

Daley, M. J. Spinks, W. L. "Exercise, Mobility, and Aging." *Sports Medicine,* 29:1, 2000, pp. 1–12.

Donatelle, R. J. *Health: The Basics,* 6th ed. Needham Heights, MA: Allyn and Bacon, 2005.

Dunn, A., et al. "Comparison of Lifestyle and Structured Interventions to Increase Physical Activity and Cardiorespiratory Fitness." *Journal of the American Medical Association,* 281:4, 1999.

Fahey, T., Insel, P. M., and Roth, W. T. *Fit and Well: Core Concepts and Labs in Physical Fitness and Wellness,* 4th ed. Mountain View, CA: Mayfield Publishing Company, 2001.

Feldman, E. "Creatine: A Dietary Supplement and Ergogenic Aid." *Nutrition Reviews,* 57:2, 1999.

Floyd, P. A. and Parke, J. E. *Walk, Jog, Run for Wellness Everyone,* 5th ed. Winston-Salem, NC: Hunter Textbooks, 2006.

Galloway, M. T. and Jokl, P. "Aging Successfully: The Importance of Physical Activity in Maintaining Health and Function." *Journal of the American Academy of Orthopedic Surgeons,* 8:1, pp. 37–44.

Hales, D. *An Invitation to Health,* 12th ed. Belmont, CA: Wadsworth, 2007.

Hass, C. J., et al. "Single versus Multiple Sets in Long-Term Recreational Weightlifters." *Medicine and Science in Sports and Exercise,* 32:1, 2000, pp. 235–242.

Hoeger, W. W. K. and Hoeger, S. A. *Principles and Labs for Physical Fitness,* 3rd ed. Belmont, CA: Wadsworth, 2002.

Hu, F., et al. "Television Watching and Other Sedentary Behaviors in Relation to Risk of Obesity and Type 2 Diabetes Mellitus in Women." *Journal of the American Medical Association,* 289:14, April 9, 2003, p. 1785.

Hu, F. B., et al. "Physical Activity and Risk of Stroke in Women." *Journal of the American Medical Association,* 283, 2000, pp. 2961–2967.

MacIntosh, D. "Getting the Facts on Physical Activity." *Canadian Family Physician,* 49, January 2003, p. 23.

Martin, D. R. "Athletic Shoes: Finding a Good Match." *Physician and Sports Medicine* 25:9, 1997, pp. 138–144.

Metzl, J. D. "Strength Training and Nutritional Supplement Use in Adolescents." *Current Opinion in Pediatrics,* 11, 1999, pp. 292–296.

National Institute on Aging. *Exercise: A Guide from the National Institute on Aging.* Gaithersburg, MD: NIA Information Center, 1998.

Nies, M., Vollman, A. and Cook, M. T. "African-American Women's Experience with Physical Activity in Their Daily Lives." *Public Health and Nursing,* 16, 1999, pp. 23–31.

Noonan, T. J. "Muscle Strain Injury: Diagnosis and Treatment." *Journal of the American Academy of Orthopedic Surgeons,* 7, 1999, pp. 262–269.

Novy, D. M., et al. "Physical Performance: Differences in Men and Women with and without Low Back Pain." *Archives of Physical Medicine and Rehabilitation* 80, 1999, pp. 195–298.

Patel, A. T. and Ogle, A. A. "Diagnosis and Management of Acute Low Back Pain." *American Family Physician,* 61:6, 2000, pp. 1779–1786, 1789–1790.

"Physical Activity and Health: Adults." A Report of the Surgeon General, President's Council on Physical Fitness and Sports, www.cdc.gov.

Pollock, M. L., et al. "Resistance Exercise in Individuals with and without Cardiovascular Disease." *Circulation,* 101, 2000, pp. 828–833.

"Poor Fitness in Young Adults Associated with Later Cardiovascular Problems." *FDA Consumer,* 38:1, January–February 2004, p. 7.

Rose, V. "CDC Report on Physical Inactivity." *American Family Physician,* 59:6, 1999.

Sachtleben, T., et al. "Serum Lipoprotein Patterns in Long-Term Anabolic Steroid Users." *Research Quarterly for Exercise and Sport,* 68:1, 1997.

Sallis, J., et al. "Evaluation of a University Course to Promote Physical Activity: Project GRAD (Graduate Ready for Activity Daily)." *Research Quarterly for Exercise and Sport,* 70:1, 1999.

Shepherd, R. J. "Exercise and Training in Women. Part 1: Influence of Gender on Exercise and Training Responses." *Canadian Journal of Applied Physiology* 25:1, 2000, pp. 19–34.

Shepherd, R. J. "How Much Physical Activity Is Needed for Good Health?" *International Journal of Sports Medicine* 20, 1999, pp. 23–27.

Suminski, R., et al. "Physical Activity among Ethnically Diverse College Students." *Journal of American College Health*, 51, September 2002, p. 75.

"Surgeon General's Report on Physical Activity and Health." *Physical Activity and Fitness Research Digest*, 2:6, 1996.

Terjung, R. L., et al. "American College of Sports Medicine Roundtable: The Physiological and Health Effects of Oral Creatine Supplementation." *Medicine and Science in Sports and Exercise*, 32:3, 2000, pp. 706 717.

U.S. Department of Health and Human Services. *Healthy People 2010 Objectives*, Draft for Public Comment. Washington, DC: Public Health Service, 1998.

U.S. Department of Health and Human Services. *Physical Activity and Health: A Report of the Surgeon General*. Atlanta, GA: U.S. Department of Health and Human Services, 1996.

Volek, J. S. Update: "What We Now Know about Creatine." *ACSM's Health and Fitness Journal* 3:3, 1999 pp. 27–33.

Waldron, M. "Fitness Equipment: Are These Your Symptoms?" *Runner's World*, 1994, p. 30.

Witvrouw, E., et al. "Stretching and Injury Prevention: An Obscure Relationship." *Sports Medicine*. 34:7, 2004, p. 443.

Name _____     Date _____

Course _____     Section _____

What would be the two most important benefits of physical activity for you? Be specific.

1. _____.

2. _____.

Did you know you can get a moderate amount of physical activity by just brisk walking, gardening, or raking leaves preferably most, if not all, days of the week? You do not have to do vigorous exercises such as jogging or running.

Check the activities that apply to you that interfere with your physical activity program.

| | |
|---|---|
| _____ Too tired to exercise | _____ Too old to exercise |
| _____ The weather is too bad | _____ Exercise is boring |
| _____ Exercise makes me sweat | _____ No convenient place |
| _____ Do not enjoy exercise | _____ Too overweight |
| _____ No safe place to exercise | _____ Cannot stick with it |
| _____ No one to exercise with me | _____ Do not like to fail |
| _____ Do not have the time | _____ It is too late to get in shape |
| _____ No exercise equipment at home | |

People can select activities that they enjoy and that fit into their daily lives. What are the two main reasons that keep you from being physically active?

1. _____.

2. _____.

Good news: You can do something about the reasons you are not physically active. You can change your behavior toward physical activity starting today.

How can you change your behavior(s) that keep you from being physically active?

1. _____.

2. _____.

*The first step in being physically active is to begin today—right now. Are you ready?*

**Name** _____     **Date** _____

**Course** _____     **Section** _____

Determine your target heart zone for aerobic exercise for your selected range by using the procedure below. During an aerobic workout, attempt to keep your heart rate within your target heart zone. First, find your resting heart rate (RHR) by taking your pulse for one minute after waking from a night's sleep or a nap, without the assistance of an alarm and without getting up from the prone position. Next, find your maximum heart rate (MHR) by subtracting your age from 220. Now apply the rest of the formula below to determine the lower and upper limits of your training heart zone.

**1.** Determine your MHR.

$$
\begin{array}{cc}
220 & 220 \\
\underline{-\ \text{your age}} & \underline{-} \\
\text{Maximum heart rate} & \text{MHR} = \underline{\hspace{2cm}}
\end{array}
$$

Your maximum heart rate is _____ beats per minute (RHR)

**2.** Subtract resting heart rate (RHR) from maximum heart rate (MHR).

$$
\begin{array}{c}
\text{MHR} \\
\underline{-\ \text{RHR} \qquad\qquad\qquad -} \\
\end{array}
$$

**3.** Multiply the above number by .60 (60%), then add resting heart rate (RHR).

$$
\begin{array}{l}
\text{Number} \\
\underline{\times \qquad .60} \\
\underline{+ \qquad \text{RHR}} \\
\end{array}
$$

Lower limit = _____

**4.** Multiply number by .80 (80%), then add resting heart rate (RHR).

$$
\begin{array}{l}
\text{Number} \\
\underline{\times \qquad .80} \\
\underline{+ \qquad \text{RHR}} \\
\end{array}
$$

Upper limit = _____

Maintain a target heart rate     above _____ beats per minute

below _____ beats per minute

**Name** _____     **Date** _____

**Course** _____     **Section** _____

Count your heart rate (pulse) at two locations: the carotid artery (side of neck) and the radial artery (wrist).

1. Practice locating both your carotid and radial artery heartbeats, or pulses. Count your pulses as soon as possible after exercising.

2. Count your pulse at both the carotid (neck) and radial (wrist) locations. Use a watch or clock to count for 10, 15, or 30 seconds. To establish your heart rate in beats per minute, multiply the 10-second count by 6, the 15-second count by 4, or the 30-second count by 2.

3. Count the pulse of a partner using both the carotid and radial locations.

4. Record the results in the spaces below.

**Carotid pulse count**

|  | Self<br>Heart rate/min. | Partner<br>Heart rate/min. |
|---|---|---|
| _____ 10 seconds × 6    = | _____ | _____ |
| _____ 15 seconds × 4    = | _____ | _____ |
| _____ 30 seconds × 2    = | _____ | _____ |

**Radial pulse count**

|  | Self<br>Heart rate/min. | Partner<br>Heart rate/min. |
|---|---|---|
| _____ 10 seconds × 6    = | _____ | _____ |
| _____ 15 seconds × 4    = | _____ | _____ |
| _____ 30 seconds × 2    = | _____ | _____ |

Which method do you prefer when counting your heart rate? Why?

Name _____     Date _____

Course _____     Section _____

### Before you begin

Precede an exercise program with a medical exam if you have any of the following risk factors.

- Elevated blood pressure or cholesterol                                                                       _____

- Cigarette smoking                                                                                                          _____

- Family history of coronary disease in parents or siblings before age 55; any heart, lung, or metabolic disease, such as diabetes                                                                                                          _____

- Man over 40 years of age                                                                                               _____

- Woman over 50 years of age                                                                                          _____

## FLEXIBILITY

## MODIFIED SIT-AND-REACH

### The Test

To perform this test, you need a yardstick on a 12″ box or the Acuflex I Sit-and-Reach Flexibility Tester.

Warm up and remove your shoes prior to the test. Sit on the floor with legs straight out and hips, back, and head against the wall. An assistant now places the box against the bottom of your feet. Put one hand on top of the other and reach forward as far as possible leaving the head and back touching the wall. At this point, the assistant places the yardstick on top of the box and slides the stick along the top of the box until it touches the person's fingers. The yardstick now is held firmly in place. Gradually reach forward, releasing head and back from the wall, stretching as far as possible on the yardstick and holding the final position two seconds. Repeat and average the two scores.

### The Results

Men in their 20s with good flexibility should be able to reach 15 inches; in their 30s, 14 inches; in their 40s, 13.5 inches; and in their 50s, 11.5 inches. Women in their 20s should be able to reach 16 inches; in their 30s, 15.5 inches; in their 40s, 14.5 inches; and in their 50s, 12.5 inches.

### The Future

Add some stretching to your daily routine. Stretch your muscles only after they are warm.

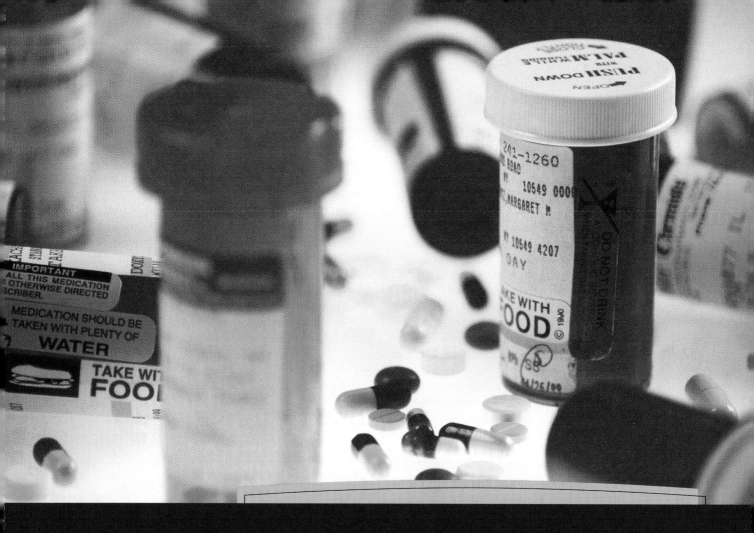

# Chapter Twelve Psychoactive Drugs and Medications

**OBJECTIVES** ■ Cite reasons people give for taking drugs. ■ Describe the narcotics and their effects. ■ Describe the depressants and their effects. ■ Identify the stimulants and their effects. ■ Describe the forms and effects of marijuana. ■ Describe the effects of anabolic steroids. ■ Identify the properties of inhalants. ■ Outline various drug treatment options. ■ Discuss the use and misuse of over-the-counter drugs.

ThomsonNOW™ Log on to ThomsonNOW at http://thomsonedu.com/ thomsonnow to access and explore self-assessments, interactive tutorials, and practice quizzes.

Americans are bombarded with drugs and information relating to drugs (psychoactive substances) on a daily basis. New pharmaceuticals are introduced often, in order to treat or cure specific health conditions and diseases. Illicit substances are extremely common. Voluminous information is presented on drug use, misuse, and abuse; who is taking drugs; what drugs are being taken; when and where the drugs are being used; how the drugs are taken, and how much.

Drugs, often called **psychoactive substances,** are any agent—natural or artificial—that has the ability to alter the normal functions and structure of the body. This includes altering mood, perception, or behavior. Whether drugs are effective or ineffective depends upon their function, purpose, and how they are used, misused, or abused. Some drugs play a major role in the treatment of medical and psychological conditions. Prescription drugs and over-the-counter (OTC) medications are capable of curing diseases, easing pain, calming fears, alleviating anxiety and frustration, relieving sleeplessness, and treating many health problems. Medications can be effective when they are used properly, but some can be addictive and dangerous when misused. More than 6.3 million Americans reported current use of prescription drugs for nonmedical purposes in 2004. Even when monitored carefully, some drugs can cause adverse reactions, **iatrogenic (medically induced) illnesses,** and death. Persons who misuse or abuse a psychoactive drug, legal or illegal, may develop a tolerance for the drug as well as **physiological** and **psychological dependence.**

Improved drug technology and the availability of prescribed and OTC medications have dramatically improved the health status of millions. In addition, as medications improve health, life expectancy is extended. On the other hand, many commonly abused drugs have caused tremendous human suffering and death.

The psychoactive substances and medications discussed in this chapter are the narcotics (opium, morphine, heroin, codeine), the depressants (barbiturates, quaaludes, tranquilizers), the stimulants (cocaine/crack, amphetamines, methamphetamines, caffeine), the hallucinogens (LSD, PCP), cannabis (marijuana and hashish), and inhalants. Over-the-counter medications will be discussed also. Tobacco and alcohol, the topics of Chapter 13, are also psychoactive substances.

**Drug abuse** and **drug misuse** cause deleterious effects on the health and well-being of millions of people daily. The damaging effects that can be caused by misuse and abuse of drugs—whether prescribed, OTC, or illicit (illegal)—may include the following.

- Drug dependency
- Physical and mental dysfunctioning
- Disruption of family units
- Criminal and destructive behavior
- Premature and accidental death
- Disruption of career goals and aspirations
- Incarceration

Figure 12.1 shows some of the factors associated with drug (including alcohol) use.

**FIGURE 12.1** ▶ The Social Influences of Psychoactive Drugs

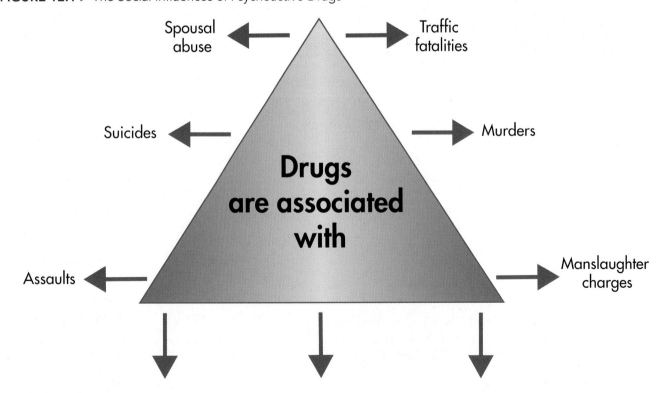

Spousal abuse · Traffic fatalities · Suicides · Murders · **Drugs are associated with** · Assaults · Manslaughter charges

**FIGURE 12.2 ▶** Past Month Illicit Drug Use among Persons Aged 12 and Older, by Race or Ethnicity, 2003 and 2004 Annual Averages

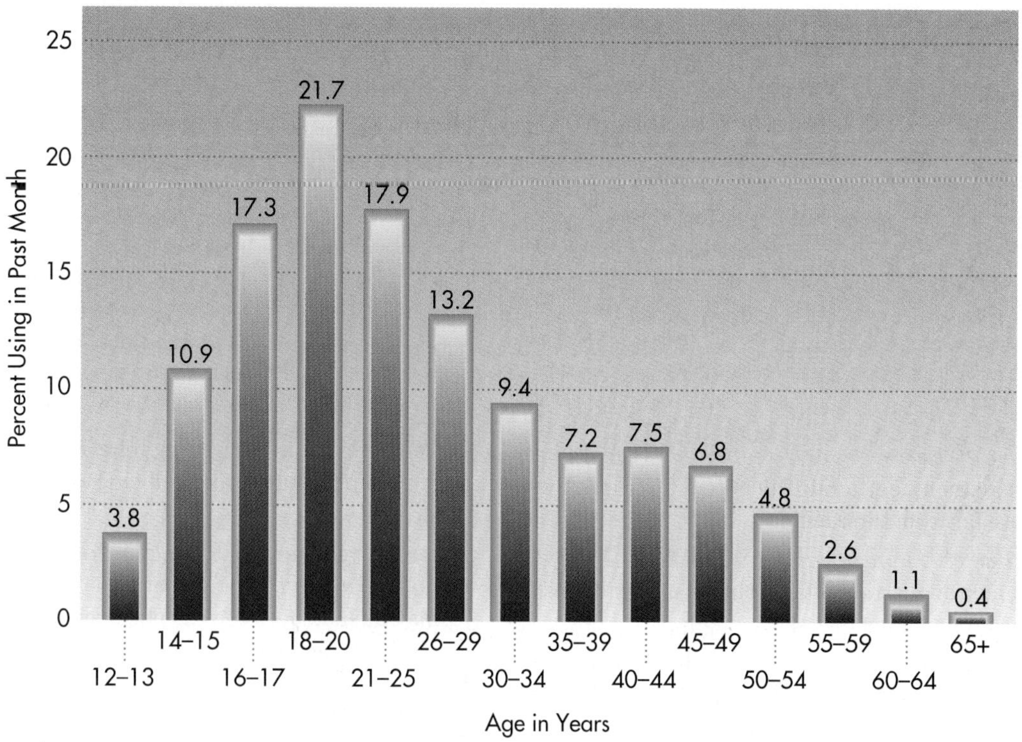

*Source:* Substance Abuse and Mental Health Services Administration; National Household Survey on Drug Abuse, 2003 and 2004.

## Prevalence

Although drug use has declined in the past three years, there are still approximately 14 million Americans who are drug users. One in five adult women, versus one in three men, abuses or becomes addicted to alcohol or other drugs during a lifetime. NIDA's 2004 Monitoring the Future survey of 8th, 10th, and 12th graders found that 5% of 12th graders reported abusing OxyContin in the past year, and 9.3% reported abusing Vicodin, making Vicodin one of the most commonly abused prescription drugs in this population. Abuse of inhalants has increased two years in a row and now stands at 17.3%.

According to the 2004 National Survey on Drug Use and Health, rates of current use of illicit drugs were highest for the young adult age group (18 to 25) at 19.4%, with 16.1% using marijuana, 2.1% using cocaine, 1.5% using hallucinogens, and 6.1% using prescription-type drugs nonmedically.

## A Reason for Drugs?

People give various reasons for using drugs. Whatever reason given, users should be knowledgeable about any chemical substance taken into the body, and how it may alter the structure and functioning of the body. Drugs are easy to take, most methods entail little effort, and they provide the means to escape from a problem in a matter of seconds (a quick fix). Other reasons may include the following.

- *Curiosity.* Especially among young people, experimentation comes naturally. When drugs are readily available, it is easy for them to follow their inclination to explore new experiences.

**KEY TERMS**

**Psychoactive substance** any agent that has the ability to alter mood, perception, or behavior

**Iatrogenic illness** medically induced sickness caused by adverse reactions to drugs

**Physiological dependence** a biochemical need to repeat administration of a substance; addiction

**Psychological dependence** a state in which individuals crave drugs to satisfy some personality or emotional need

**Drug abuse** the use of a chemical substance that results in physical, mental, emotional, or social impairment

**Drug misuse** the occasionally inappropriate or unintentional use of a medication

- *Pleasure and escape from boredom.* Many feel that drugs make them feel good. The potential destructive effects are far from their mind.

- *Peer influence.* Among teens in particular, peer pressure often is an overriding factor in what they choose to do, including taking drugs.

- *Spiritual purposes.* Throughout history people have used drugs in religious ceremonies and rituals. For example, the Native American Church incorporates peyote into its spiritual practices. Another example is illustrated by the Hindus' use of bhang, derived from the marijuana plant, during festivals, marriages, and family celebrations.

- *Self-discovery.* Drugs may be used to fill a void in one's life and as a search for meaning that the family structure formerly filled.

- *Social interaction.* Some drugs facilitate interchange among people in groups or one-to-one. Particularly for shy people, drugs may be especially attractive in this regard.

- *Rebellion.* Another hallmark of youth, taking drugs may be a way of flaunting authority.

## Drug Routes of Administration

Routes of administration are ways or methods in which drugs are introduced into the bloodstream and central nervous system. Common routes of administration are as follows.

1. **Inhalation.** Introduction of a vapor or gas into the respiratory tract via the nose and mouth or a powder through the nose. Sniffing vapors from drugs is one example of inhalation.

2. **Injection.** Introduction of drugs into the body subcutaneously (just below the surface of the skin), intramuscularly (into large muscles), or intravenously (directly into the vein). Injecting drugs directly into the vein is the most rapid route for introducing drugs into the bloodstream.

3. **Oral ingestion.** Introduction of the drug into the body through the mouth or oral cavity. These routes may include between the cheek and gum (buccal surface) and under the tongue (sublingual). A drug such as LSD, when utilized via these routes, is introduced rapidly into the bloodstream via the capillaries.

4. **Topical application and implantation.** Introduction of drugs through mucous membranes such as eyes, skin, gums, anus, and genitalia.

Whatever the route of administration, the blood system distributes the dosage of the drug to all parts of the body. This can be a positively healthy distribution if the drug is used therapeutically or a negatively damaging distribution if the drug is used abusively, illegally, or for purposes not intended. Some drugs remain in the system for several hours, and other drugs or their effects may remain for several years. Drugs vary in potency ranging from a chemical as mild as an aspirin to one as powerful as methamphetamines, heroin, crack, or LSD. When more than one drug is used at the same time, the combined interaction of these drugs is called **synergism.** Multiple substance abuse, also known as polydrug abuse and dual addiction, is especially dangerous because different substances may interact with each other to produce unexpected dangerous or life-threatening results.

## Drugs and How They Affect the Brain

The brain sends and receives messages via a network of nerve cells, or **neurons,** depicted in Figure 12.3. To receive information, each neuron has branches, called **dendrites,** and on these branches are **receptors** that receive the messages. The cell body on each neuron decides

- Reduce drug-related deaths.
- Reduce drug-related injuries.
- Reduce drug-induced deaths.
- Reduce intentional injuries resulting from alcohol and illicit drug-related violence.

- Reduce the cost of lost productivity in the workplace due to alcohol and drug use.

**FIGURE 12.3 ▶** Physiological Effects of Psychoactive Drugs on the Brain

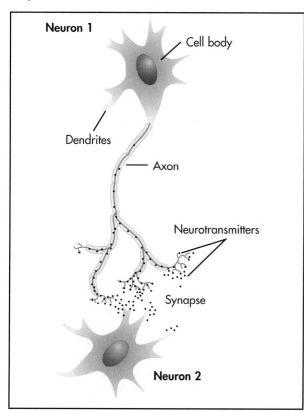

the nerve cell cannot send or receive a message. The entire nervous system depends on these neurotransmitters and receptors.

Psychoactive drugs disrupt the way messages are sent to and from the brain. Some drugs slow down or completely shut down message transmission. Other drugs speed the number of messages so much that the brain cannot make sense of them. Sometimes this is a good thing. For example, certain drugs stop pain by blocking the pain messages going from the painful area into the brain. Sometimes, though, changing the brain through psychoactive drugs is harmful. By unlocking the pleasure center, the drugs may start the person on the road to **addiction.** If the person is physically addicted to a drug and discontinues it, various **withdrawal** symptoms occur. These may consist of flulike symptoms, diarrhea, abdominal pain, delirium tremens (DTs), hallucinations, paranoia, and sometimes death, depending on the substance. In addition are the psychological symptoms of withdrawal.

### KEY TERMS

**Synergism** the combined action of two or more drugs that is greater than the effects of any drug taken alone

**Neurons** nerve cells

**Dendrites** branches of neurons that convey impulses to the cell body

**Receptors** components of a neuron that combine with the neurotransmitter to receive messages from another neuron

**Axon** a long cable connected to the neuron, receiving information from the cell body, relaying it to another neuron

**Synapse** a gap between each neuron that requires a special chemical to send messages across

**Neurotransmitters** chemicals that send messages across a synapse from the axon of a nerve cell to another nerve cell

**Addiction** a state of biochemical or psychological dependence produced by habitual drug taking

**Withdrawal** physical and psychological symptoms that occur when an individual who is addicted to a drug discontinues its use

if the information is important and, if so, sends it to another neuron. To send information, each neuron has a long cable called an **axon,** which acts like a telephone wire, receiving the message from the cell body and sending it to the receptors on the dendrites of another neuron. In this way, messages are passed from neuron to neuron throughout the nervous system. Between each neuron and the next one is a gap called a **synapse,** which requires special chemicals to get a message across the gap. These chemicals, called **neurotransmitters,** take the message from the axon of one nerve cell and send it to the receptors of another nerve cell. A neurotransmitter is like a key, and a receptor is like a lock. When the key fits, the nerve cell is turned on and sends the message. If it does not fit,

## Narcotics

A **narcotic** is a drug that induces stupor and insensibility. The term is used particularly for morphine and other opium derivatives. **Opiates** are obtained from the juice of the opium poppy, *Papaver somniferum.* **Opioids** are synthetic narcotics.

Narcotic drugs induce sleep, relieve acute pain, and are used to treat coughs, diarrhea, and various other illnesses. They are divided into four categories.

1. Natural opiates, including opium, morphine, and codeine
2. Semisynthetic opiates, including heroin, **Dilaudid,** and Percodan
3. Synthetic narcotics, including Demerol, methadone, and Darvon
4. **Endorphins** and **enkephalins,** which are naturally occurring narcotics in the body

### OPIUM

**Opium** is a drug that is obtained from the resin derived from the unripe seed pods of the opium poppy plant. It is known as the mother drug because it is the base compound for all of the natural narcotics. Opium has been a major trade commodity for centuries. During the 19th century, the smuggling of opium to China from India, particularly by the British, was the cause of the opium wars. It was during this time, which the Chinese termed the "century of shame," that Britain seized Hong Kong. Ancient Egyptian physicians used opium nearly 6,500 years ago to kill pain. When the opiates were found to sedate, relieve anxiety, create **euphoria,** and provide an escape from reality, people began to use opium recreationally.

Opium, called by street names *big O, black stuff, block, gum,* and *hop,* is usually smoked, though sometimes it is swallowed. However it enters the body, it has the potential to relieve pain, and produce euphoria, drowsiness, stupor, sleep, coma, and death. With repeated use the person may develop a strong **tolerance** and physical dependency. The first U.S. law banning opium use was passed in 1875 in San Francisco, where smoking opiates was prohibited in opium houses or dens. Opium has been taken off the market in the United States.

### MORPHINE

**Morphine,** the principal active agent in opium, is a powerful painkiller. Commercial and street names for morphine are *M, Miss Emma, monkey,* and *white stuff.* It acts directly on the central nervous system (CNS) to relieve pain. It is 10 times stronger than opium and therefore exerts rapid depressing effects on the brain receptors

that control analgesic (painkilling) action. In addition, it causes euphoria and sedation. It is used legally to relieve pain after surgery and is used in cases of trauma, cancer, and tooth extractions. It is used as an adjunct to general anesthesia and epidural anesthesia. Additionally, morphine is administered for palliative care, severe coughs, and diarrhea associated with AIDS. Morphine can be highly addictive, and tolerance and physical and psychological dependence develop quickly.

When some 400,000 injured Civil War soldiers became addicted to morphine, they suffered from what came to be known as the soldier's disease. Because it was such a useful drug, however, morphine continued to be prescribed for everything from headaches to skull fractures. Patent medicines containing morphine were readily available, and cough medicine containing morphine was even given to infants. Illicit morphine is produced mostly in powder form and also as tablets, cubes, and capsules. It may cause light sensitivity, euphoria, drowsiness, nausea, vomiting, and decreased respiration, to the point of death. When morphine is injected using nonsterile techniques, pathogens introduced into the bloodstream can cause HIV infection, abscesses, cellulitis, liver disease, and other problems.

### HEROIN

**Heroin** (often called *brown sugar, dope, H, horse, junk, skag, skunk, smack, white horse*) is processed from morphine and usually appears as a white or brown powder. In its purest form heroin is a white powder with an extremely bitter taste. When sold illegally, it is almost always diluted or cut with other substances, such as sugar or starch. Heroin is usually liquefied and injected intramuscularly (muscling), just under the skin (skin popping), or intravenously (mainlining). It also is snorted (sniffed/tooted) or smoked—methods that are becoming increasingly popular because they do not require a needle for injection.

Like other narcotic drugs, heroin affects the nerve cells of the brain and spine, dulling pain and clouding the senses. Heroin use produces immediate euphoria (a rush) accompanied by a warm flushing of the skin, dry mouth, constricted pupils, lowered sex drive, drowsiness, and loss of appetite. The euphoria from heroin may last three to eight hours. Following the initial euphoria, the user goes "on the nod," an alternately wakeful and drowsy state.

Users tend to become addicted within two weeks of consistent use. Many develop a tolerance to the drug over time, with stronger and more frequent cravings. Withdrawal symptoms occur eight to 24 hours after the last dose (fix). Sometimes serious, these may include watery eyes, runny nose, nausea and vomiting, diarrhea, chills, excruciating cramps in the abdomen and legs, and tremors. Symptoms associated with heroin withdrawal get progressively worse for approximately three to four days. The person becomes more irritable and experiences episodes of severe sneezing and coryza (inflammation of nasal passage coupled with profuse nasal discharge). Chronic users may experience collapsed veins, infection of the heart lining and valves, abscesses, cellulitis, and liver disease. Various types of pneumonia may result, due to the poor health of the user and respiratory problems caused by heroin use.

Pregnant women who have drugged their embryo or fetus or both with heroin will likely cause the infant to suffer withdrawal symptoms shortly after birth, called the **neonatal abstinence syndrome (NAS).** Newborns with NAS are highly sensitive to noise, are irritable, have poor coordination, sneeze and yawn excessively, and have uncoordinated sucking and swallowing reflexes. Research using ultrasound measurements raises questions about the rate of brain growth in fetuses exposed to narcotics. The head circumference tends to be slightly smaller than usual. Even though the head size catches up to that of nonexposed babies within six months or so, possible long-term effects of prenatal harm to the brain remain a concern.

AIDS is now the fourth leading cause of death in women of childbearing age in the United States, most of which is attributable to the woman's use of contaminated needles in conjunction with her drug use or having sex with an HIV-infected injectable drug user.

HIV infection and AIDS are especially prevalent among African-American injectable drug users. African Americans are twice as likely as Caucasians to have used drugs intravenously. While representing about 12% of the U.S. population, African-Americans account for 27% of all people with AIDS, and of those cases, 44% reported injecting an illicit substance prior to the AIDS diagnosis, according to the Centers for Disease Control and Prevention (CDC). In addition, African-Americans account for 31% of deaths from heroin and morphine.

The CDC reported that more than 48,700 Hispanics had developed AIDS, and almost half (48%) of these cases involved injectable drug use. Of the Hispanics using drugs intravenously, 74% never used bleach or alcohol to clean their needles before injecting.

The National Institutes of Health (NIH) convened a Consensus Panel on Effective Medical Treatment of Heroin Addiction that concluded that heroin addiction can be treated with medications and behavior therapies to include methadone maintenance treatment, substance abuse counseling, psychosocial therapies, and other supportive services to enhance retention.

## CODEINE

**Codeine** is a natural alkaloid derivative of opium; most codeine used in the United States is synthesized from morphine. Medically, it is used as a cough suppressant, a mild painkiller in combination with other drugs such as acetaminophen and cough medicines, and for the control of diarrhea. Codeine is less potent than morphine since only about 10% of the codeine is converted in the body. It is a widely abused prescription drug (Empirin with codeine, Fiorinal with codeine, Robitussin A-C, Tylenol with codeine) with the potential for physical dependence. However, it has a correspondingly lower risk of dependence than morphine.

Codeine is regulated by the Controlled Substance Act. It is a Schedule II controlled substance for pain-relief products containing codeine alone. When it is paired with aspirin or acetaminophen (paracetamol) it is listed as a Schedule III controlled substance.

## OTHER NARCOTICS

A synthetic opiate, OxyContin **(Percodan),** is a prescription pain reliever that is causing major problems among recreational users. Although it is prescribed to relieve pain due to injuries, bursitis, dislocations, fractures, neuralgia, arthritis, and lower back and cancer pain, the pharmacological effects make it a desirable substitute for heroin. OxyContin is a tablet that should be swallowed whole; however, abusers often chew the tablets or crush

### KEY TERMS

**Narcotic** a drug that induces stupor and insensibility; in legal terms, any addictive drug subject to illegal use

**Opiates** drugs obtained from the juice of the opium poppy

**Opioids** synthetic narcotics

**Dilaudid** derived from morphine, legitimately used as cough suppressant and as analgesic for treating severe pain

**Endorphins** and **enkephalins** naturally occurring narcotics in the body, produced by the immune system

**Opium** base compound for all natural narcotics

**Euphoria** a heightened sense of well-being associated with drug use

**Tolerance** condition in which an individual must increase drug dosage to experience the same effects over time

**Morphine** main alkaloid found in opium; used medically to kill pain and sedate

**Heroin** narcotic drug derived from morphine that is 35 times stronger than morphine

**Neonatal abstinence syndrome (NAS)** set of withdrawal symptoms occurring shortly after birth in newborns who have been exposed to heroin in utero

**Codeine** a natural derivative of opium used as a cough suppressant or mild painkiller

**Percodan** a cough-suppressing and analgesic medication

the tablets and snort the powder. Because it is water soluble, crushed tablets can be dissolved in water and the solution injected. OxyContin has a high abuse potential and people who take the drug repeatedly can develop a tolerance or resistance to the drugs' effects. Many deaths have resulted specifically from the abuse of OxyContin.

Other chemically constructed and often prescribed opioids are meperidine **(Demerol),** pentazocine (Talwin), **methadone** (Dolophine), and propoxyphene (Darvon). These substances work similarly to the major natural narcotics. Their differences are presented in potency, duration, and effectiveness.

Another opiate-like drug is **Special K** (ketamine hydrochloride). Special K, known as psychedelic heroin, is smoked or snorted and may cause amnesia, impaired motor movement, and fatal respiratory problems.

# Depressants

**Depressants,** informally called downers, are drugs that inhibit neural activity and slow physical and mental functions. They do this by decreasing awareness and incoming stimuli to the brain cells and spinal cord. Depressants cause drowsiness, relax muscles, and, if taken in excessive quantities, can even cause death.

## SEDATIVE-HYPNOTICS

**Barbiturates.** In the early 1900s, two German chemists derived a substance from barbituric acid that had a calming and relaxing effect and could put a person to sleep. Since then, scientists have developed more than 2,500 **barbiturates,** 15 or so of which are still in use to treat conditions such as anxiety, insomnia, epilepsy, and peptic ulcers. Many uses, however, are illegal. The commercial barbiturates are Amytal, Nembutal, Seconal, and Phenobarbital. Street names are *barbs, reds, red birds, phennies, tooies, yellows,* and *yellow jackets.*

Today, barbiturates are prescribed most often as sleeping pills. However, barbiturates produce a less than ideal sleep that is accompanied by fewer rapid eye movements (REMs) and fewer dreams than normal sleep. Doctors also prescribe barbiturates to relieve anxiety, tension, and irritability.

Abusers quickly develop a tolerance to the drug and typically take 20 times the amount recommended by the medical profession. Heroin addicts often resort to barbiturates if they cannot obtain the narcotic. Overdose is a real danger. Effects include cold, clammy skin; a weak, rapid pulse; and difficulty breathing. The usual treatment is to pump the stomach and administer CPR if necessary. Otherwise the person may lapse into a coma and die.

Barbiturates become even more dangerous when they are combined with other depressants such as alcohol.

This speeds the absorption of barbiturates into the bloodstream and adds to the drug's physically depressing effects on the body.

Withdrawal symptoms are similar to those from alcohol: anxiety and agitation, loss of appetite, nausea and vomiting, sweating, rapid heartbeat, tremors, and cramping. These symptoms peak during the second or third day or longer after discontinued use. The person may go into convulsions and become delirious. Some people have hallucinations. The withdrawal symptoms that follow excessive, prolonged, heavy barbiturate use may be more serious than those of any other drug. Withdrawal symptoms caused by using barbiturates are difficult to treat and create true medical emergencies.

**Chloral hydrate.** Chloral hydrate is a depressant with hypnotic (sleep-inducing) properties. Taken as syrups or gelatin capsules, it becomes effective in approximate 30 minutes to an hour. Though rarely used medically, some medical professionals consider it a drug of choice for sedation of children having dental and various other medical procedures. The "Mickey Finn" ("knockout drop") made famous in the cinema was a combination of chloral hydrate and alcohol. Abuse of chloral hydrate can cause severe respiratory depression, low blood pressure, liver damage, confusion, seizures, shortness of breath, irregular heartbeat, staggering, and weakness. Severe respiratory depression reduces the sensitivity of respiratory centers, resulting in a depression in breathing. This could be fatal.

**Methaqualone.** Another form of depressant is methaqualone (Quaalude, Sopor, Parest), a nonbarbiturate sedative-hypnotic. It is also a painkiller. Methaqualone is known on the street as *ludes, mandrex, quad,* and *quay.* **Quaalude** is the most familiar trade name. This drug is used often interchangeably with barbiturates, as it has similar effects and was believed to be nonaddictive—a supposition that has proved to be false. Quaaludes have high potential for both physical and psychological dependence. High doses may cause headaches, drowsiness, depression, unusual excitement, fever, irritability, poor judgment, dizziness, abdominal cramping, major motor convulsions, insomnia, and possible coma and death. Although they are no longer marketed in the United States, large amounts of illicit Quaaludes are imported for black-market sale.

**Benzodiazepines.** In the 1940s the American Medical Association began to search for a substitute for barbiturates (thrill pills), and the pharmaceutical companies developed a new class of drugs known as benzodiazepines or **tranquilizers.** These antianxiety drugs depress the central nervous system but have milder effects than the other classes. The most popular benzodiazepines are Ativan, Halcion, Valium, Xanax, and Librium. They are known on the street as *candy, downers, sleeping pills,* and *tranks.*

Used medically as anticonvulsants and muscle relaxants, they reduce tension, irritability, and stress and sometimes are prescribed to manage panic disorders.

Although benzodiazepines are milder than the other forms, they may have serious side effects and toxic reactions, including confusion, depression, poor judgment, respiratory depression and arrest, muscular incoordination, nausea, lethargy, skin rashes, and constipation. They may alter the sex drive, cause menstrual irregularities, and produce blood cell abnormalities. Benzodiazepines have the potential to cause physical and psychological dependence.

A person quickly develops a tolerance to benzodiazepines. Used in conjunction with alcohol, barbiturates, opiates, or other depressant drugs, the outcome can be life-threatening. Drug overdose is common.

The typical abuser is Caucasian, female, and 20–40 years old. Taking three or four tablets of Valium a day for about six weeks is enough to cause addiction. Addicts frequently take the tablets with alcohol or marijuana to ensure a high. Withdrawal symptoms last about seven to 10 days. The withdrawal is like that from the barbiturates.

A relatively new benzodiazepine is **Rohypnol** (flunitrazepam). It is swallowed or snorted and is known on the street as *forget-me pill, Mexican Valium, R2, Roche, roofies, roofinol, rope,* and *rophies.* This drug is prescribed as an effective sleep medication in other countries. Manifestations of Rohypnol use include impaired judgment, slurred speech, difficulty walking, irritability, angry outbursts with little provocation, and personality changes. Some people become more aggressive and, after the effects wear off, do not remember what happened while they were under the influence of the drug.

It commonly is referred to as the rape drug. Unscrupulous men have used Rohypnol to secretly spike soft drinks and alcoholic beverages of females and other males, then raped them while they were in a sedated state. If a woman suspects that she has been sexually assaulted while under the influence of Rohypnol, a urine test is available to help prove that she has been drugged. This drug test for women is free of charge (from Hoffman-La Roche, manufacturer of the drug) to law enforcement officials, rape crisis

centers, and hospital emergency rooms investigating cases of assault.

A pattern of Rohypnol use can result in tolerance and physical dependence. Like other benzodiazepines, withdrawal symptoms may include insomnia, anxiety, tremor, elevated blood pressure, and grand mal seizures.

**GHB and GHB Analogs.** Gamma-hydroxybutyric acid (GHB), known as *G, Liquid X, scoop,* and *grievous bodily harm,* is a synthetic depressant. In July of 2002, GHB was approved for treatment for an extremely rare form of a sleep disorder (narcolepsy). Prior to that time the FDA banned the depressant because it proved to be extremely dangerous, causing vomiting, respiratory problems, seizures, amnesia, comas, and death. GHB and its analogs, gamma-butyrolactone (GBL) and 1,4-butanediol (BD) are considered rape drugs because they are easily mixed with water and other liquids. With these prepared mixtures, the victim's senses of smell and taste are severely altered. The victim is unaware that the otherwise salty/soapy tasting substance is present. These drugs are difficult to trace because they quickly leave the body and may be impossible or difficult to detect in medical settings.

GHB has surpassed Rohypnol (flunitrazepam) as the most common substance used in drug-facilitated sexual assault. GHB can mentally and physically paralyze an individual, and its effects, when coupled with alcohol, are intensified. In response to the use of drugs in sexual assaults, Congress in 1996 passed the Drug-Induced Rape Prevention and Punishment Act to combat drug-facilitated crimes of violence, including sexual assaults. This act

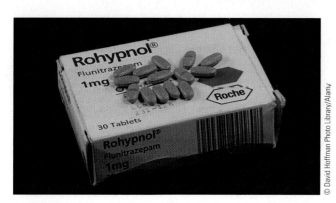
▲ *Rohypnol*

**KEY TERMS**

**Demerol** short-acting synthetic narcotic used as an analgesic or a painkiller; usually injected

**Methadone** a synthetic narcotic used as a heroin substitute

**Special K** or ketamine hydrochloride; an opiate-like drug that impairs motor movements and respiration when smoked or snorted.

**Depressants** a classification of drugs that inhibit neural activity and slow physical and mental functions; downers

**Barbiturates** sedative-hypnotic substances that depress the central nervous system

**Quaaludes** a depressant often used interchangeably with barbiturates; high potential for physical and psychological dependence

**Tranquilizers** psychoactive drugs that depress the central nervous system but have milder effects than the other depressants

**Rohypnol** a benzodiazepine that sedates a person and makes him or her vulnerable to assault; "rape drug"

imposes harsh penalties for distribution of a controlled substance to an individual without the individual's knowledge and consent with the intent to commit a crime of violence and rape.

## Stimulants

### COCAINE/CRACK

**Cocaine** is a white powder that comes from the dried leaves of several species of *Erythroxyl coca* or coca plant native to the Andes Mountains of South America (see Figure 12.4). The leaves of the coca plant are stripped and mixed with an organic solvent, which forms a coca paste. The paste is synthesized into cocaine hydrochloride, the white crystalline powder known by users as *coke, white lady, blow, toot, snow, base, flake, bump, Charlie,* and *nose candy.*

Cocaine is a stimulant that enters the body in a matter of seconds or minutes, depending upon the route of administration. Cocaine often is inhaled (snorted or tooted). It

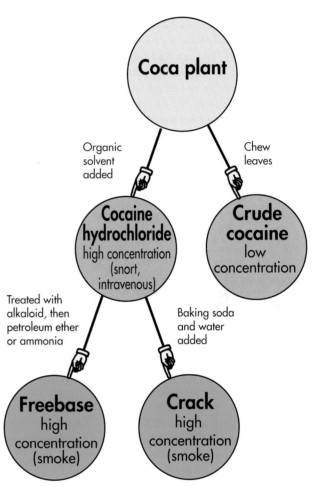

**FIGURE 12.4 ▶** Forms of Cocaine

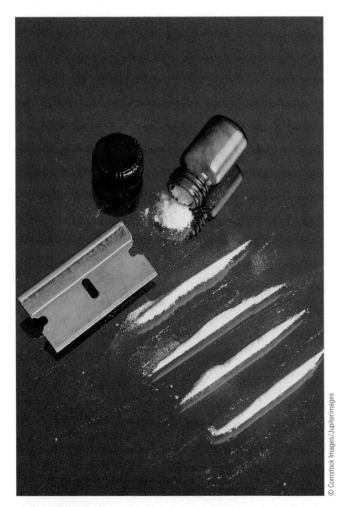

▲ *Powdered cocaine*

© Comstock Images/Jupiterimages

also can be injected intravenously alone or mixed with heroin; the latter is called speedballing. The user will experience an intense rush or feeling of power, energy, and alertness. With cocaine use the sense of euphoria lasts only a few minutes, after which the user crashes. To relieve the resulting depression (dysphoria), the person takes another dose of the drug. And so the cycle continues. Chronic use of cocaine has a number of adverse effects on the body.

The heart beats faster and abnormally. Cocaine can constrict the blood vessels and cause angina, irregular heart rhythm (ventricular fibrillation), and heart attacks.

- It causes the heart to beat too fast (tachycardia), which can cause it to stop functioning.

- It can raise blood pressure, and may cause arterial constriction in the brain, leading to a brain attack (stroke).

- With repeated use over time it can cause long-term psychological effects such as restlessness, excitability, anxiety, insomnia, irritability, mood swings, paranoia, and depression.

- The mucous membrane in the nasal passages dries and deteriorates. Cilia (the hairlike projections that protect the nasal lining) are destroyed, producing nasal discomfort, hemorrhaging, and perforation of the nasal septum (the cartilage that separates the nostrils).

- Crack users may have severe chest congestion and a chronic cough in which they expel black phlegm.

Chronic, long-term cocaine use can result in the inability of men to retain an erection for orgasm and ejaculation and the inability of females to reach orgasm. Cocaine-addicted women are four times as likely as drug-free women to experience premature separation of the placenta from the uterus, which causes hemorrhaging and threatens the lives of both mother and fetus. Cocaine also can precipitate miscarriage or premature delivery by promoting uterine contractions. Maternal cocaine use endangers the fetus by constricting arteries leading to the uterus, which in turn diminishes blood supply and, hence, oxygen to the fetus. For statistics on drug use by pregnant women, see Figures 12.5 and 12.6.

Cocaine that is smoked has been converted into freebase by treating the cocaine powder with an alkaloid and then with petroleum ether or ammonia. The more popular

**FIGURE 12.5 ▶** Past Month Illicit Drug Use among Pregnant Women Aged 15 to 44, by Race or Ethnicity, 2003 and 2004 Annual Averages

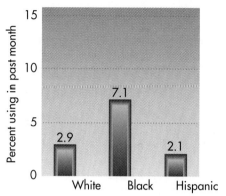

*Source:* Substance Abuse and Mental Health Services Administration, National Household Survey on Drug Abuse, 2003 and 2004.

**FIGURE 12.6 ▶** Past Month Illicit Drug Use among Pregnant Women, by Age, 2003 and 2004 Annual Averages

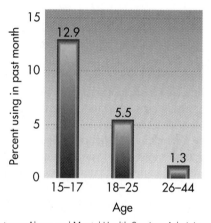

*Source:* Substance Abuse and Mental Health Services Administration, National Household Survey on Drug Abuse, 2003 and 2004.

cocaine freebase method is to mix cocaine hydrochloride with baking soda and water. A base forms and is dried into small pieces called rocks or **crack.** When a piece of rock cocaine is heated in a glass pipe, cocaine vapors are produced and inhaled. Space-basing refers to smoking crack mixed with phencyclidine (PCP or angel dust).

Crack can cause serious problems in pregnant females. The embryos and fetuses robbed of oxygen and nutrients are called crack babies after they are born. Crack babies

## KEY TERMS

**Cocaine** powerful stimulant derived from the coca plant

**Crack** small pieces or rocks formed from a dried mix of cocaine hydrochloride, baking soda, and water

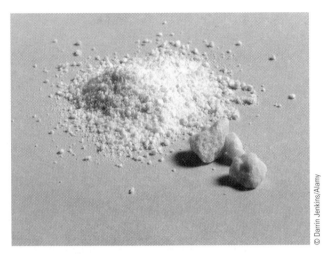

▲ *Crack*

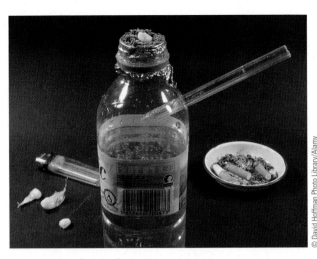

▲ *Homemade crack pipe*

exhibit various characteristics, including prematurity, irritability, neurological disorders, and strokes. They bond poorly, have difficulty sucking, and experience short, irregular periods of restless sleep.

Because crack makes the user more aggressive, dangerous, and paranoid, cocaine and crack are allied closely with drug-related crimes, including homicides and shootouts among gang members and organized crime groups. Unfortunately, children often are enlisted to work in the crack distribution network. They are being lured into gangs and into the streets as lookouts (to alert crack dealers when police are nearby), to run (transport drugs between dealers), and to deal (sell crack).

The key to cocaine's addiction is **dopamine,** a neurotransmitter that controls pleasure sensations. Cocaine causes the release of more dopamine but also blocks reuptake from the brain. As a result, neurons make less and less of it, and gradually the user tries larger and more frequent doses of cocaine to recapture the feeling of pleasure.

According to the National Institute on Drug Abuse, the number of illegal users of cocaine exceeds 1.6 million. In addition, 2.7% of the general U.S. population has tried cocaine during their lifetime. Adults aged 18 to 25, particularly men, have the highest rates of cocaine use.

The active ingredient in cocaine was first isolated in the mid-19th century. Famed psychoanalyst Sigmund Freud partook of cocaine and advocated its use to treat a variety of ills, including asthma, digestive upset, and morphine addiction. He suggested that it might be used as an **aphrodisiac.** Freud participated in the events leading to the discovery of the one valid medical use of cocaine: as a local anesthetic. It still is used as a local anesthetic in throat, nose, eye, and ear surgery. Novocaine and Xylocaine are cocaine synthetics.

Another user was William Halstead, often called the father of American surgery and one of the four founders of the Johns Hopkins Medical School. Halstead's experiments with cocaine led to an intense addiction that threat-

ened his career. Like other scientists at that time who used themselves as guinea pigs, Halstead injected himself often with cocaine and as a result developed a dependence on the drug. He finally was able to overcome his dependence and resume his illustrious work. History shows, however, that he turned to morphine to subdue the cocaine addiction and remained addicted the rest of his life.

In the past, ground coca leaves were sold as tonics. Coca-Cola took half of its name from the cocaine in it. When the dangers of the drug became obvious, cocaine was removed from the beverage just before the Pure Food and Drug Act was passed in 1907. The federal government erroneously classified cocaine as a narcotic and outlawed its use with passage of the Harrison Narcotic Act in 1914. This law made cocaine available only by medical prescription, although that did not put an end to its illicit use.

A new study funded by the National Institutes of Health (NIH) suggests that a common over-the-counter herbal supplement, *N*-acetylcysteine (NAC), can reduce the cravings associated with chronic cocaine use. This research, released at the American College of Neuropsychopharmacology's (ACNP) annual conference, is among the first to identify NAC as a potential agent to modulate the effects of cocaine addiction. There is also evidence in animal models of addiction to suggest that this chemical works similarly in the treatment of heroin addiction, and possibly alcoholism. In clinical trials, when modafinil (in daily doses of four 100-mg pills) is administered, the cocaine addict is able to abstain for three weeks. The long, continuous abstinence on modafinil is a strong and encouraging signal that this medication can help patients avoid relapse during the critical first weeks of treatment.

## AMPHETAMINES

**Amphetamines** are groups of synthetic amines that stimulate the body's own epinephrine (adrenaline hormone) and norepinephrine (neurotransmitter hormone). They affect the portion of the brain that controls breathing, heart rhythm, blood pressure, and metabolic rate. Amphetamines act directly on the central nervous system by inducing feelings of well-being, exhilaration, wakefulness, confidence, excitement, increased mental alertness, and talkativeness. They are known as *bennies, black beauties, crosses, hearts, LA turnaround, speed, truck drivers,* and *uppers.*

These drugs have a number of medicinal uses. The original (and current) use of amphetamines was for the treatment of narcolepsy, a sleep disorder. Later, amphetamines became a component of nasal inhalants, as well as an agent to counteract fatigue and enhance alertness. Because they were found to curb the appetite, they were marketed with weight-loss programs. They still are used for short-term treatment and management of obesity and weight control. Amphetamines are administered to individuals who have attention deficit disorder (ADD), a condition characterized by extreme motor restlessness, poor attention span, and impulsivity. Appropriate doses also can enhance physical performance.

Amphetamine use became widespread during the 1920s, eroding the popularity of cocaine. Amphetamines produced a similar high and their effects lasted longer. More important, they were cheap and easy to obtain.

As with the other wonder drugs, the downside to amphetamines became apparent. Drivers who took amphetamines (pep pills) to stay awake ended up having more accidents when the pills' effects wore off suddenly. Students who took the pills to stay up all night cramming for exams displayed bizarre behavior. Executives who used the pills to stay alert discovered that their judgment and decision-making ability were impaired.

The same problems are present with amphetamines today, particularly when they are not controlled. Additional effects of amphetamines include elevated body temperature, dry mouth, irritability, slurred speech, repetitive movements, nausea, vomiting, blurred vision, aggressive behavior, and insomnia. Most users take amphetamines in capsules, also called uppers, bennies, dexies, jolly beans, and copilots.

## METHAMPHETAMINES

**Methamphetamine** (*meth, speed, crystal, chalk, ice, glass, quartz, bantu, crank*) is one of the most dangerous and deadliest drugs criss-crossing the United States. It is a synthetic stimulant made from available ingredients and the cold medication pseudoephedrine. Some other common ingredients used for meth are red phosphorus, battery acid, lye, and antifreeze. Methamphetamines are swallowed, inhaled, smoked, or injected into the vein.

Probably the most dangerous form of methamphetamine is ice, which is smoked in a glass pipe or injected. It looks like a lumpy crystal of ice (hence the nickname *crystal*). It first brings on intense euphoria, which may be followed by nausea and vomiting. Over time it is associated

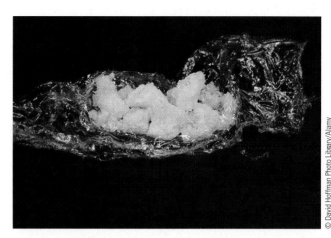

▲ *"Ice" (methamphetamine)*

© David Hoffman Photo Library/Alamy

with aggressive and violent behavior, paranoia and psychosis, weight loss, kidney and lung failure, cardiovascular disorders, and possible death. Many first-time users become addicted instantly. The high can last as long as 24 hours in a regular user and as long as seven days in a novice user. When deprived of the drug, regular users feel strong cravings for it. Withdrawal symptoms cover a wide range and can include depression, cramps, sleepiness, apathy, irritability, mental confusion, and hallucinations.

Women use meth to lose weight. An extremely major concern is meth mouth. After short periods of use (sometimes just a month), a perfectly healthy set of teeth can turn grayish-brown, twist and begin to fall out, and take on a texture like ripened fruit rather than hard enamel. Meth dries out saliva and causes users to grind their teeth, resulting in decay and rot. The urban gay community has seen an increase in AIDS because meth makes many users feel hypersexual and uninhibited. This has meant a sharp increase in unsafe sex. People of all sexual orientations are taking part in "speed sex" (using speed and having sex all weekend).

Mothers who ingest ice during pregnancy can damage their unborn babies. These infants, called ice babies, have tremors and may cry up to 24 hours nonstop. They tend to

---

## KEY TERMS

**Dopamine** brain chemical that controls pleasure sensations; the key to cocaine's addiction

**Aphrodisiac** a substance that stimulates sexual desire

**Amphetamines** a group of synthetic amines affecting portions of the brain that control breathing, heart rhythm, blood pressure, and metabolic rate

**Methamphetamines** powerful stimulants that induce intense euphoria; one form is ice

avoid any type of closeness, bonding, or contact with other people.

The Substance Abuse and Mental Health Services Administration (SAMSHA) shows that meth treatment admissions for young people have recently increased fourfold.

> **VIEWPOINT** *Methamphetamine laboratories are springing up all across America. These labs are found in homes, hotel rooms, and other public places. They are extremely dangerous (fires, explosions, toxic fumes) due to explosive chemicals used to make the meth. What do you think can be done to stop this serious and dangerous problem?*

## METHYLPHENIDATE (RITALIN) AND OTHER STIMULANTS

A group of drugs, Ritalin, Metadate CD, Concerta, and Adderall are mild central nervous system stimulants that are prescribed to treat attention deficit/hyperactivity disorder (ADHD). ADHD sufferers manifest three distinct symptoms: impulsiveness, inattention, and hyperactivity.

Due to its stimulant properties, methylphenidate **(Ritalin)** has become increasingly popular as a recreational drug. Known on the street as *Vitamin R, JIF, Skippy, the smart drug, MPH,* and *R-Ball,* Ritalin is snorted or injected. It has effects similar to, but more potent than, caffeine and less potent than amphetamines. It has a notably calming and focusing effect on persons with ADHD, especially children. Ritalin works by activating the brain stem arousal system and cortex.

When abused, methylphenidate can have the following adverse effects: dizziness, change in heart rate and blood pressure, abdominal pain, weight loss, drug dependence, appetite suppression, wakefulness, euphoria, and severe depression upon withdrawal. Higher doses of the drug will cause convulsions, irregular heartbeat and respirations, anxiety, hallucinations, and fever. Abusers take the tablets either orally or crushed and snorted. Some abusers dissolve the tablets in water and inject the mixture. This method of usage can be very dangerous because insoluble fillers in these tablets can block small blood vessels.

## CAFFEINE

**Caffeine,** one of the world's most widely used drugs, has been ingested by humans for centuries. It is an alkaloid substance found in beverages such as coffee, tea, cola, and other soft drinks, as well as in chocolate, prescriptions, and over-the-counter medications. The average American drinks about 34 gallons of soda and 28 gallons of coffee each year.

Among the 63 natural sources from which caffeine is extracted are seeds of *Coffea arabica* (coffee); roasted leaves of the *Camellia sinensis,* which is an evergreen shrub (tea); the West African kola or guru nut; and the Brazilian soapberry plant. Table 12.1 shows the amounts of caffeine in various items.

Caffeine levels peak in the body within an hour of consumption, and more than half of the caffeine is metabolized (broken down, becoming inactive) in three to seven hours. As a stimulant, caffeine produces a feeling of well-being and alertness. It is a diuretic, so too much of it will deplete the body's water content. The effects of caffeine are hard to study because the response varies from person to person. Some people are caffeine-sensitive and should not consume it at all. Generally, however, the effects of lower doses may include the following.

- Increased muscle capacity
- Stimulation of learning
- Heightened intellectual processes
- Improvement in certain motor skills
- Faster heartbeat
- Relaxed bronchial muscles
- Increased output of urine
- Increased basal metabolic rate (BMR)
- Increased blood levels of glucose and lipids (fats)
- Stimulation of the respiratory center

**TABLE 12.1 ▶** Caffeine Content of Selected Items

| PRODUCT | AMOUNT | AVERAGE CAFFEINE (mg) |
|---|---|---|
| Coffee | | |
| Drip | 6 oz. | 137 |
| Brewed | 6 oz. | 117 |
| Instant | 6 oz. | 60–117 |
| Decaffeinated | 6 oz. | 3 |
| Cola | 12 oz. | 30–45 |
| Chocolate | | |
| Cake | 1 slice | 25 |
| Baking chocolate | 1 oz. | 25 |
| Milk chocolate | 1 oz. | 6 |
| Chocolate milk | 8 oz. | 5 |
| Hot cocoa | 6 oz. | 5 |
| Tea | | |
| Five-minute steep | 6 oz. | 50 |
| Decaffeinated | 6 oz. | 1 |
| Instant | 6 oz. | 33 |
| Medications | | |
| Pain relief | Standard dose | 41 |
| Diuretics | Standard dose | 167 |
| Alertness | Standard dose | 150 |
| Diet | Standard dose | 168 |
| Cold or Allergy | Standard dose | 27 |

Higher doses of caffeine have the following potential effects.

- Constricted blood vessels in the brain (usually associated with hypertensive headaches)
- Irregular heartbeat
- Extreme nervousness
- Flushed appearance
- Muscle twitching or tremor
- Irritability
- Tinnitus (ringing in the ears)
- Insomnia

Rarely does anyone die of a caffeine overdose. To overdose, a person would have to drink more than 80 cups of coffee in a short time.

No consensus has been reached as to whether caffeine is addictive. Although it has been consumed throughout history, evidence has not proven any dangers in moderate consumption for most people. Nevertheless, the scientific community often has investigated linkages between caffeine and heart disease, cancer of the pancreas, and, in women, problems associated with reproduction, aggravated premenstrual syndrome (PMS), fibrocystic breast disease, and calcium depletion and bone loss. In 1985 the National Institute of Mental Health reported that caffeine can cause panic attacks in some people. These attacks are characterized by irrational feelings of anxiety, accompanied by heart palpitations, shortness of breath, sweating, and mental confusion.

Conflicting studies about the risks of consuming caffeine during pregnancy have been published. Researchers discourage consumption of more than 300 milligrams (two to three cups of coffee) per day, and even lower levels may not be safe. The potential risk to the fetus posed by caffeine is small but real. To be safe, pregnant women should avoid caffeine altogether or keep their intake to a minimum.

## Cannabis

**Marijuana** is a mind-altering drug that is the product of shredded leaves, flowering tops, stems, and seeds of the hemp plants *Cannabis sativa*, *Cannabis indica*, and *Cannabis ruderalis*. The plants are dried and sometimes rolled into paper and called a *joint*, *reefer*, or *nail*. It is smoked in a pipe, or a water pipe (*bong*). Marijuana also is eaten in foods such as brownies, cakes, and cookies or brewed in teas. Other popular uses include stuffing it in cigar leaves (blunts) and adding cocaine (primo). Sometimes blunts contain PCP (angel dust) or crack cocaine. Some common names for marijuana are *weed*, *chronic*, *pot*, *grass*, *joint*, *cannabis*, *Mary Jane*, *hashish*, and *blunt*. "B.C. Bud" is a form of marijuana cultivated by growers in British Columbia and considered highly desirable for its potency by U.S. consumers.

Although there are more than 400 chemicals in marijuana, the mind-altering and primary psychoactive ingredient is THC (delta-9-tetrahydrocannabinol). Potency of marijuana depends on the type of plant, the soil, the weather, and fertilization.

Marijuana is the most widely used illegal drug in the United States (Figure 12.7).

Marijuana affects users in different ways. Some become ebullient, gaining an exaggerated sense of well-being and a feeling of self-confidence. Others become reflective and quiet. Marijuana usually enhances social interaction and bestows what many users refer to as

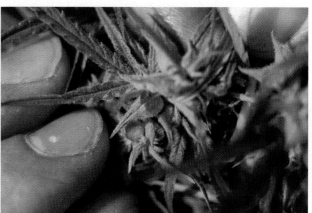

▲ *Colas—Buds of the marijuana plant*

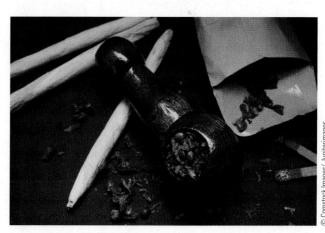

▲ *Marijuana cigarettes and pipe*

### KEY TERMS

**Ritalin** a central nervous system stimulant prescribed for attention deficit/hyperactivity disorder (ADHD)

**Caffeine** mild stimulant found in coffee, tea, chocolate, and medications

**Marijuana** the drug derived from the cannabis plant, *Cannabis sativa*, that contains THC, an ingredient that causes mild euphoria when inhaled or eaten

**FIGURE 12.7** ▶ Frequency of Marijuana Use among Past Year Users Aged 12 and Older, 2003 and 2004

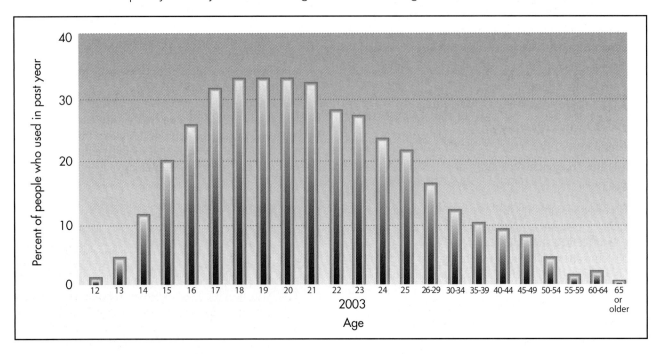

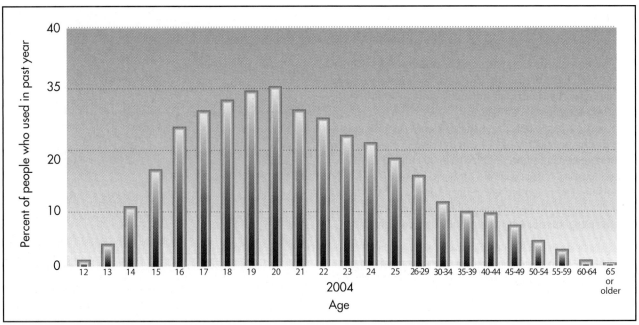

*Source:* Substance Abuse and Mental Health Services Administration, National Household Survey on Drug Abuse, 2003 and 2004.

"mellowing out"—a dreamy sense or state. The user may have more intense and vivid sensory perceptions of sight, taste, hearing, and smell. The sense of time is distorted. Thoughts may become fragmented, and moods vary from calm to argumentative and violent.

The most immediate physical changes are faster heartbeat and pulse rate, reddening of the eyes, and a dry mouth and throat. Acute panic anxiety reaction, or fear of losing control, is a common serious reaction. Symptoms usally subside within a few hours of use. The long-term

effects are more sobering. These include loss of motor coordination, difficulty concentrating, and trouble learning new facts and remembering old ones. Memory lapses are common. People often describe regular users as slow and dull. Among the most severe physical problems is permanent damage to the reproductive organs, including sterility in males. Also, heavy marijuana use by pregnant women is associated with low birthweight and possible abnormalities in children born to them. In short, evidence continues to accumulate that long-term marijuana use has a

According to the Federal Bureau of Investigation's *Uniform Crime Reports,* a total of 1,005,385 arrests were made for drug abuse violations during 1999. The majority of those arrested for drug violations were white (63.6%), followed by African Americans (35.2%), Asian or Pacific Islanders (0.7%), and American Indians or Alaska Natives (0.5%). In addition, the U.S. Sentencing Commission reported in that same year that a total of 22,499 federal defendants were charged with a drug offense. A quarter of these defendants were white (25%), nearly one-third were black (31%), and the majority were Hispanic (42%). The most common drug for white and Hispanic defendants was marijuana; for black defendants, crack cocaine.

**FIGURE 12.8 ▶** Types of Illicit Drug Used by Aged 12 and Older, 2003 and 2004

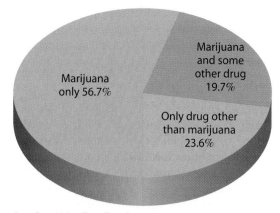

*Note:* Based on 14.0 million illicit drug users.
*Source:* Substance Abuse and Mental Health Services Administration, National Household Survey on Drug Abuse, 2003 and 2004.

over 16% of auto accident fatalities. The drug is involved in 20% of all traffic accidents. In one study, marijuana was detected in the blood of 37% of young adults killed in auto accidents.

THC, the active ingredient in marijuana, is absorbed in most body organ tissues (especially fat tissue). Before the body rids itself of THC, it is chemically transformed into metabolites. These THC metabolites can remain in the urine for a week or so after smoking.

> **VIEWPOINT** *Marijuana's therapeutic value has been utilized in the treatment of nausea and vomiting associated with cancer chemotherapy, glaucoma, asthma, and other conditions. Should the physician of patients suffering from these health problems make the ultimate decision about utilizing marijuana for treatment?*
> **What is your opinion?**

harmful effect on the heart, lungs, brain, and reproductive system. Marijuana smoke contains cancer-causing agents. Long-term cannabis smoking has been associated with cellular changes in the lungs (metaplasia) that are considered precancerous.

Medicinally, marijuana has proven to be effective in reducing nausea caused by chemotherapy, improving the appetites of AIDS patients, and reducing intraocular pressure in persons with glaucoma. Medicinal use is illegal and those using the drug as medicine risk arrest and imprisonment.

Marijuana increases the appetite (the munchies), which is a pitfall for overweight people who are trying to manage their weight. Finally, the combined effects of marijuana and alcohol are greater than when either substance is used alone.

Effects of marijuana are not limited to the person using it. Intoxication by marijuana alone is responsible for

## Hashish and Hashish Oil

Hashish is concentrated delta-9-tetrahydrocannabinol (THC), which is the resin from the *Cannabis indica* plant. Once collected, hashish is prepared into various forms such as balls, flat sheets, and squares. This is usually added to marijuana or cigarettes (*joint, biff,* or *spliff*) and smoked. It is also added to cookies or other foods and ingested. It is used for its relaxing and mind altering effects. The THC in hashish available in America can range from 2% to 7% and as high as 20%.

Hashish oil is produced by using a solvent to extract cannabinoids from plant material. Hash oil is more concentrated than hash and may have a percentage of THC ranging from 15% to 70%. The dangers of both are the same as those of marijuana. Other forms of hash are *Hard hash, Soft hash, Honey Oil, Soap Bar,* and *Kief.*

# Hallucinogens or Psychedelics

**Hallucinogens** are a group of mind-altering drugs that affect the brain and nervous system, bringing about changes in thought, self-awareness, emotion, and sensation. The synonymous term is *psychedelic,* which means "revealing to the mind." These drugs create a distorted perception of reality, irrational thinking patterns, and modified states of consciousness. The most pronounced effect may be sensory: sounds become louder, colors brighter, smells stronger.

True to their name, these drugs produce hallucinations. This happens because hallucinogenic drugs cause the blood vessels in the brain to constrict, limiting the amount of blood that reaches the brain and thus depriving it of its normal amount of oxygen. Some hallucinations are pleasant. Others are "bad trips" or bummers. Occasionally a user gets a panic reaction. Impurities in street drugs may alter or exacerbate the effects.

Because of the nature of hallucinations, users have been known to jump out of windows and walk in front of cars. Another common reaction is Hallucinogen Persisting Perception Disorder or HPPD **(flashback),** a recurrence of the trip, which can happen unexpectedly during drug-free periods. Long-term reactions from using hallucinogens include recurrent anxiety, depression, and mental disturbance or psychosis.

Some of the most common hallucinogens are described briefly below and summarized in Table 12.2.

**TABLE 12.2** ▶ Summary of Hallucinogens

| DRUGS | COMMON RX NAMES | STREET NAMES |
|---|---|---|
| Lysergic acid | LSD | Acid, blotter, boomers, cubes, microdot, yellow sunshine |
| Phencyclidine | PCP | Angel dust, boat, hog, love boat, peace pill |
| Methylenedioxy-methamphetamine | MDMA | Adam, ecstasy, Eve, X, lover's speed, peace, STP, XTC, clarity drug, M&M |
| Dimethoxymeth-amphetamine | STP | Serenity, peace |
| Dimethyl-tryptamine | DMT | Businessman's trip |
| Peyote cactus | Mescaline | Mesc, buttons, cactus, peyote |
| Psilocybe | Psilocybin | Magic mushrooms, sacred mushrooms, purple passion, shrooms |
| Mushrooms | | Magic mushrooms, 'shrooms |

## MESCALINE AND PEYOTE

In modern times **mescaline,** or peyote, derived from the **peyote** cactus (*Lophophora williamsii*), is still part of religious ceremonies of American Indians of the southwestern United States. The crown of the cactus has buttons that are cut, dried, and chewed or soaked in water to produce a potent liquid. Mescaline users experience vivid color imagery, distortions in the perception of time, and enhanced senses. Problems associated with the use of this drug can range from visual hallucinations to mental illness.

## LSD

**LSD** (lysergic acid diethylamide) is a colorless, odorless, tasteless liquid that is a major drug in the hallucinogen class. It is manufactured from lysergic acid, found in the ergot fungus *Claviceps purpures*, which grows on rye and other grains, or it can be made synthetically. LSD is sold under at least 80 street names, which include *acid, cid, blotter, trips,* and *doses.* It is the most potent hallucinogen known to humans. For many years a drop of LSD was placed on a sugar cube and taken by mouth. Today it appears more often as a tablet or soaked into heavy blotter paper, which is divided into small decorated squares, with each square representing a dose. It is licked off of the squares or placed under the tongue for absorption. It can be found in other forms such as powder or crystal, liquid, and gelatin squares. LSD takes effect in 30 to 90 minutes. The effects continue for 12 hours or more.

Physical reactions include dilation of the pupils, higher body temperature, increased heart rate and blood pressure, loss of appetite, sleeplessness, tremors, and dry mouth. Some people may experience nausea, aching body, tingling, and sweating. If taken in large doses, the drug produces delusions and visual hallucinations. The user's sense of time and self changes. Sensations can "cross over," giving the user the feeling of seeing sounds and hearing colors. LSD users refer to their use as a *trip.* A bad trip is an acute adverse reaction, which is long and begins to clear after 12 to 14 hours. Many LSD users experience flashbacks (recurrence of certain aspects of a person's experience, without the user having taken the drug again), often suddenly and without warning. LSD users may manifest long-lasting psychoses, such as schizophrenia or severe depression.

Research with animals indicates that LSD may cause genetic damage, manifested in children born to users.

## PSYCHEDELIC MUSHROOMS

**Psilocybin** (a psychedelic alkaloid) is present in more than 80 hallucinogenic species of fungi such as *Psilocybe cubensis* and *Psilocybe semilanceata*. These are commonly called *magic mushrooms, Liberty Caps,* or *shrooms.* Magic mushrooms are eaten (fresh or dried), taken as a powder in

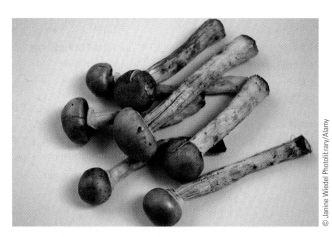

▲ *Psilocybin mushroom*

capsule, brewed in teas, and mixed and eaten with foods. If taken in low doses, it makes the user relaxed, euphoric, and will cause the user to laugh a lot. Higher doses intensify colors, diminish concentration, distort perceptions of time and space, and produce hallucinations. The high usually lasts from four to 10 hours. Users may experience "bad trips," causing anxiety, panic, and confusion. Recurring episodes of HPPD can occur days, weeks, or even months after previous use. Little is known about the long-term effects of mushrooms, with no serious problems with dependency reported. Shrooms are illegal. Possession can result in extended prison terms.

# Dissociative Anesthetics

## PCP

**PCP,** or phencyclidine hydrochloride, is an anesthetic that blocks nerve receptors from pain and temperature without producing numbness. It was first synthesized in 1959 as an intravenous surgical anesthetic. Its harmful side effects of confusion, delirium, intense anxiety, and depression quickly became apparent. For these reasons it was discontinued for use with humans in 1967. However, it is illegally manufactured in labs and sold as tablets, capsules, or colored powder. It is known as *angel dust, ozone, boat, peace pill, tranq, wack, hog, killer weed,* and *rocket fuel.* PCP can be snorted, smoked, or eaten.

PCP became a popular drug in the mid-1960s because of its low cost and ready availability. Taken in small doses, it induces feelings of euphoria. Moderate doses cause blurred vision, slurred speech, sleepiness, violence, heavy sweating, and rapid breathing. Higher doses cause intoxication accompanied by mental confusion, violence, hallucinations, and trouble speaking. Still higher dosages can produce symptoms of serious mental illness. A massive overdose will result in coma and death. Most PCP deaths stem from mental confusion. Abusers have drowned in shallow pools because they did not think to stand up or died in fires because they could not feel the flames or could not figure out how to escape.

One of the most serious consequences is the loss of inhibitions and ensuing threat of harm to others. PCP can cause extreme, unpredictable rages. Numerous gruesome murders have been committed by people under the influence of PCP. Many PCP users are brought to emergency rooms because of overdose or because of the drug's unpleasant psychological effects. In a hospital or detention setting, people high on PCP often become violent or suicidal.

## KETAMINE

Ketamine is a dissociative anesthetic used for humans and in veterinary procedures. Ketamine is produced as a powder or liquid that can be injected, prepared in drinks, or mixed with smokable substances and smoked. The effects of ketamine are similar to PCP (physical) and LSD (visuals). Low doses can produce colorful images and experiences known as *K-land.* Higher doses produce an "out-of-body" or "near death" experience called *K-Hole.* Ketamine use can cause psychedelic effects, numbess, muscle weakness, loss of coodination, slurred speech, violent and aggressive behavior, blank stares, and exaggerated feeling of strength. Additionally, its dangerous effects may include vomiting and convulsions, brain death due to oxygen starvation, and death.

The effects of each experience with ketamine could last up to 48 hours. Effects in chronic users who stop taking the drug may take up to two years to wear off completely and can include recurrent flashbacks. Physical and/or psychological dependence can occur from long-term use.

---

### KEY TERMS

**Hallucinogens** a group of mind-altering drugs that affect the brain and nervous system

**Psychedelic** literally, "revealing to the mind"

**Flashback** recurrence of a drug trip

**Mescaline** hallucinogen derived from peyote cactus

**Peyote** a type of cactus that yields mescaline

**LSD** lysergic acid diethylamide-24; a psychedelic drug that produces distorted reality

**Psilocybin** primary psychoactive agent in psychedelic mushrooms

**PCP** an anesthetic that blocks nerve receptors from pain and temperature without producing numbness; angel dust

**TABLE 12.3** ▶ Summary of Drugs, by Category

| DRUG | OTHER NAMES | APPEARANCE | ROUTE OF ADMINISTRATION |
|---|---|---|---|
| **NARCOTICS (OPIOIDS AND MORPHINE DERIVATIVES)** | | | |
| Opium | Paregoric, Dover's powder, parepectolin | Dark brown chunks, powder | Smoked, eaten, injected |
| Morphine | Pectoral syrup | White crystals, hypodermic tablets, injectable solutions | Taken orally, injected, smoked |
| Heroin | Smack, horse, stuff, junk, black tar, big H, downtown | White to dark-brown powder or tarlike substance | Injected, smoked, inhaled |
| Codeine | Empirin compound with codeine, Tylenol with codeine, codeine in cough medicine | Dark liquid varying in thickness, capsules, tablets | Taken orally, injected |
| **DEPRESSANTS** | | | |
| Barbiturates | Downers, barbs, blue devils, red devils, yellow jacket, yellows, Nembutal, Tuinals, Seconal, Amytal | Red, yellow, blue, or red and blue capsules | Taken orally |
| Chloral hydrate | | Soft capsules, syrup | Taken orally |
| Methaqualone | Quaaludes, ludes, sopors | Tablets | Taken orally |
| Benzodiazepines | Valium, Librium, Miltown, Serax, Equanil, and Tranxene | Tablets or capsules | Taken orally |
| **DISSOCIATIVE ANESTHETICS** | | | |
| Ketamine | Cat valium, k, special k, powder, vitamin k | | Injected, snorted, smoked |
| PCP and analogs | Phencyclidine, angel dust, boat, hog, love boat, peace pill | | Injected, swallowed, smoked |
| **STIMULANTS** | | | |
| Cocaine | Coke, snow, nose candy, flake, blow, big C, snowbirds, white lady, ready rock | White crystalline powder | Inhaled, injected |
| Crack cocaine | Crack, rock, freebase | White to tan pellets or crystalline rocks that look like soap | Smoked |
| Amphetamines | Speed, uppers, black beauties, pep pills, copilots, hearts, benzedrine, dexedrine, footballs | Capsules, pills, tablets | Taken orally, injected, inhaled |
| Methamphetamines | Crank, crystal meth, crystal methedrine, speed | White powder, pills, rock that resembles a block of paraffin | Taken orally, injected, inhaled |
| Caffeine | | Ingredient in coffee, soda, chocolate, and other food items | Taken orally |
| **CANNABIS** | | | |
| Marijuana | Pot, reefer, grass, weed, bo, primo, joint, bud, chronic | Like dried parsley, with stems or seeds; rolled into cigarettes | Smoked or eaten |

# Inhalants

**Inhalants** are chemicals containing volatile solvents that produce mind-altering vapors that are sniffed, snorted, or huffed (holding an inhalant-soaked rag in the mouth). "Bagging" is commonly used—sniffing or inhaling fumes from substances sprayed or placed into plastic or paper bags. The user gets an immediate rush or high. For many years the most popular inhalant was the glue used in making model airplanes. Today, inhalants used more often are solvents (paint thinner, nail polish remover, degreaser, dry cleaning fluid, gasoline, glue), gases (butane, propane, whipped cream dispensers, aerosol propellants, medical anesthetic gases), and nitrites (isoamyl, isobutyl, cyclohexyl). These are referred to as *laughing gas, poppers,*

**TABLE 12.3** ▶ Summary of Drugs, by Category *(Continued)*

| DRUG | OTHER NAMES | APPEARANCE | ROUTE OF ADMINISTRATION |
|---|---|---|---|
| **CANNABIS (CONT.)** | | | |
| Tetrahydro-cannabinol | THC | Liquid, tablets | Taken orally |
| Hashish | Hash | Brown or black cakes or balls | Smoked or eaten |
| Hashish oil | Hash oil | Concentrated syrup liquid varying in color from clear to black | Smoked—mixed with tobacco |
| **HALLUCINOGENS** | | | |
| Phencyclidine | PCP, hog, angel dust, loveboat, lovely, killer weed, rocket fuel, peace pill | Liquid, white crystalline powder, pills, capsules | Taken orally, injected, smoked (sprayed on joints or cigarettes) |
| Lysergic acid diethylamide | LSD, acid, white lightning, blue heaven, sugar cubes | Colored tablets, blotter paper, clear liquid, thin squares of gelatin | Taken orally, licked off paper, gelatin and liquid can be put in the eyes |
| Mescaline and peyote | Mesc, buttons, cactus | Hard, brown discs, tablets, capsules | Discs—chewed, swallowed, or smoked; tablets and capsules—taken orally |
| Psilocybin | Magic mushrooms, 'shrooms | Fresh or dried mushrooms | Chewed or swallowed |
| **INHALANTS** | | | |
| Nitrous oxide | Laughing gas, whippets | Small 8-gram metal cylinder sold with a balloon or pipe, propellant for whipped cream in aerosol spray can | Vapors inhaled |
| Amyl nitrite | Poppers, snappers | Clear yellowish liquid in ampules | Vapors inhaled |
| Butyl nitrite | Rush, bolt, bullet, locker room, climax | In small bottles | Vapors inhaled |
| Chlorohydrocarbons | Aerosol sprays, cleaning fluids | Aerosol paint cans | Vapors inhaled |
| Hydrocarbons | Solvents | Cans of aerosol propellants, gasoline, glue, paint thinner | Vapors inhaled |
| **DESIGNER DRUGS** | | | |
| Analog of fentanyl (narcotic) | Synthetic heroin, China white | White powder | Inhaled, injected |
| Analog of meperi-dine (narcotic) | MPTP (new heroin), MPPP, synthetic heroin | White powder | Inhaled, injected |
| Analog of amphetamines or methamphetamines (hallucinogens) | MDMA (ecstasy, XTC, Adam, essence), MDM, STP, PMA, 2, 5-DMA, TMA, DOM, DOB, EVE | White powder, tablets, or capsules | Taken orally, injected, or inhaled |
| Analog of phen-cyclidine (PCP) | PCPy, PCE | White powder | Taken orally, injected, or smoked |

*snappers*, *bold*, *rush*, and *whippets*. Almost any substance that is volatile (evaporates quickly) and can be inhaled will produce some effect.

The chemical fumes from inhalants act as depressants on the central nervous system. Inhalants will produce a quick feeling of being drunk followed by dizziness, staggering, sleepiness, and confusion. Low doses produce giddiness, excitement, and silliness. Higher doses render the user less inhibited and out of control.

Many of the effects are similar to those of alcohol. These include loss of inhibition, headache, nausea or vomiting, slurred speech, loss of motor coordination, wheezing/unconsciousness, cramps, weight loss, muscle weakness,

---

**KEY TERMS**

**Inhalants** drugs that produce vapors that cause psychoactive effects when inhaled or sniffed

damage to cardiovascular and nervous system, and death. Unlike alcohol, however, these effects last only about one-half hour.

Effects of inhaling over time include gastroenteritis, depressed muscle tone, lead poisoning, damage to the liver and kidneys, nervous system dysfunction, and bone marrow disorders. Chronic use of solvents such as gasoline can lead to leukemia. Inhaling chemicals also decreases the appetite, which often is related directly to nutritional deficiencies.

Inhalants decrease oxygen to the brain, causing about one-half of chronic sniffers to suffer brain damage, which may be irreversible depending on which substance is sniffed. A few gases, such as methylene chloride (found in spray paint, for example), are extremely dangerous, and sudden deaths have followed first-time use. The oxygen level of the blood drops suddenly, producing an irregular heartbeat and heart failure. Inhaling a solvent in a plastic bag has caused some deaths by suffocation.

Inhalants are not believed to produce physical dependence. Their use, however, is associated with negative effects such as school failure. Users also tend to drink alcohol as they get older, followed by the abuse of sedatives and other illegal drugs.

Nitrous oxide, also known as *laughing gas*, is a colorless, odorless gas used medically as an anesthetic. It is a central nervous system depressant that is absorbed through the lungs, which distribute it rapidly throughout the body. Nitrous oxide causes health problems, accidents, and death. Long-term exposure may result in anemia and nerve degeneration, producing painful sensations in the arms and legs, an unsteady gait, irritability, loss of balance, and intellectual deterioration. Death from suffocation can occur. Breathing the gas without sufficient oxygen can produce asphyxiation. Many will abuse the drug using "whippets" (whipped cream dispensers) at parties, concerts, sporting events, and even at work in restaurants.

## Anabolic-Androgenic Steroids

**Anabolic-androgenic steroid** (*juice, roids*) is a synthetic version of the male hormone testosterone. Normally, testosterone has two specific effects upon male development.

1. An androgenic effect refers to increased masculine characteristics—an increase in facial hair, growth of male sex organs and glands, and deepening of the voice.

2. An anabolic effect refers to muscle building—increased muscular strength and size, increase in size of internal organs, better protein breakdown, and increased calcium in the bones.

Anabolic steroids are available legally only by prescription, to treat conditions that occur when the body

**TABLE 12.4 ▶** Primary Substances of Abuse Reported by Racial and Ethnic Groups, Percent of Admissions to Substance Abuse Treatment, 2004

| RACE OR ETHNICITY | TOTAL ADMISSIONS (THOUSANDS) | ALCOHOL ONLY | PRIMARY SUBSTANCE AT ADMISSION | | | | |
|---|---|---|---|---|---|---|---|
| | | | ALCOHOL AND OTHER DRUG | HEROIN | SMOKED COCAINE | NON-SMOKED COCAINE | OTHER DRUGS* |
| Total** | 1,875 | 22.2 | 18.0% | 14.2% | 9.9% | 3.8% | 31.9 |
| White (non-Hispanic) | 1,11 | 26.1 | 18.1 | 11.9 | 6.2 | 3.3 | 34.4 |
| Black (non-Hispanic) | 419 | 12.2 | 19.7 | 14.9 | 23.3 | 4.9 | 25.0 |
| Hispanic origin | 238 | 20.3 | 14.3 | 25.5 | 5.2 | 4.7 | 30.0 |
| Mexican | 96 | 26.9 | 11.5 | 14.8 | 4.2 | 4.1 | 38.5 |
| Puerto Rican | 73 | 9.9 | 16.8 | 46.3 | 5.7 | 5.2 | 16.1 |
| Cuban | 6 | 18.0 | 13.0 | 15.6 | 14.9 | 10.1 | 28.4 |
| Other/not specified | 63 | 22.5 | 15.8 | 19.1 | 5.2 | 4.7 | 32.7 |
| Other | 82 | 26.0 | 18.3 | 8.8 | 5.2 | 2.9 | |
| Alaska Native | 2 | 21.8 | 18.8 | 22.5 | 7.3 | 2.7 | 26.9 |
| American Indian | 36 | 34.8 | 24.3 | 4.0 | 3.6 | 1.9 | 31.4 |
| Asian/Pacific Islander | 16 | 20.8 | 12.5 | 6.7 | 5.2 | 2.4 | 52.4 |
| Other | 34 | 19.6 | 14.7 | 14.0 | 6.7 | 4.3 | 40.7 |

* Other drugs include marijuana, amphetamines and other stimulants, opiates other than heroin, tranquilizers, sedatives, PCP and other hallucinogens, and inhalants.
** Total includes admissions with unknown race and ethnicity.
*Source:* Substance Abuse and Mental Health Services Administration, Office of Applied Studies, 1998; and National Admissions to Substance Abuse Treatment Services, Treatment Episode Data Set (TEDS) 1994–2004. Rockville, MD, Table 3.2. TEDS collects data on admissions to substance abuse treatment providers that receive public funds.

produces abnormally low amounts of testosterone, such as delayed puberty and some types of impotence. They are also prescribed to treat body wasting in patients with AIDS and other diseases that result in loss of lean muscle mass.

Anabolic-androgenic steroids have been designed by drug companies to have a stronger anabolic effect than normal production of testosterone. After a few months of injecting or taking the steroids orally, the muscles are larger and stronger. Many steroid users report that the use of this drug improves their physical performance, as well as their appearance.

Steroids usually are taken in cycles of several weeks or months. After this period of use, the user gives the body a break and discontinues use for a few weeks before starting the cycle again. Steroids often are abused further through a practice known as *stacking*, which means the user may take more than one steroid at a time (for example, both injectable and oral forms).

Steroid use can cause serious side effects. When the synthetic hormone is used, it diminishes the normal production of testosterone in males. Steroid use causes bloody cysts in the liver (peliosis hepatitis), kidney disease, shrinking testicles, sterility, impotence, breast enlargement in males, male pattern baldness, hypertension, heart disease, and a change in blood lipids. Use of steroids is associated with increased risks of disorders in the reproductive and immune systems. Female anabolic steroid users may experience muscle growth, masculinization, cessation of the menstrual cycle, male pattern baldness, decreased breast size, deepened voice, enlargement of the clitoris, sterility, fluid retention, and growth of facial hair. For adolescents, growth is halted prematurely through premature skeletal maturation and accelerated puberty changes. This means that adolescents risk remaining short for the remainder of their lives if they take anabolic steroids before the typical adolescent growth spurt.

Steroids may affect the user psychologically as well. Many have reported sharp increases in aggressive behavior known as *roid rage*, personality changes, and more self-confidence. Physically, the user is able to work harder during training and increase the effort put forth during competition. After discontinuing anabolic steroids, the user may experience depression, stress, undue anxiety, irritability, and suicidal tendencies.

## Designer Drugs (China White, MDMA)

A classification of psychoactive substances is called **designer drugs.** These are **structural analogs,** or drugs that mimic the psychoactive reactions of controlled drugs. They are produced in clandestine laboratories and sold on the black market. Use of designer drugs is increasing.

The best known designer drug is **China white.** Initially promoted as a safe alternative to heroin, China

white turned out to be a thousand times more potent. Many cases of fatal overdoses have been reported.

Another category is MDA, which combines methamphetamine and mescaline analogs. On the street it is known as the love drug, because it makes people more sociable. It, too, can be fatal.

**Ecstasy,** or **MDMA** (*Adam, Bean, E, M. Roll, XTC*), is a stimulant that is chemically similar to both methamphetamine and mescaline. It has hallucinogenic/psychedelic effects that can last between four to six hours. It may be a mood elevator, or it may cause panic, anxiety, paranoia, pounding and racing heart (rapid heart rate), dry mouth, large pupils, involuntary twitching (in both the face and body), cramps, churning in the stomach, and shaking. Feeling hot and sticky is very common. Giggling uncontrollably, talking excessively, itchy and puffy eyes with blurred vision, grinding of teeth, and clenching both fists and jaws are all common reactions. Rave party attendees who ingest MDMA are at risk for dehydration, hyperthermia, and heart and kidney failure. These risks are coupled with the drug's stimulant effect and dancing for long periods of time in hot, crowded conditions. This combination has caused fatalities.

An overdose is life-threatening. In the 1980s, states began to regulate the manufacture of drug analogs. Still, the underground manufacture continues, and new designer drugs emerge. For an analysis of the long-term effects of ecstasy on memory, see Figure 12.9.

## Over-the-Counter Drugs

There are over 300,000 over-the-counter products on the market at any given time. These drugs can be purchased without a prescription. Over-the-counter, or OTC, drugs are self-prescribed, self-administered, and usually used without a physician's knowledge or supervision. Many OTC products are capable of alleviating various symptoms, disorders, and diseases—and also capable of producing ill effects, dependency, and, in some cases, addiction.

### KEY TERMS

**Anabolic-androgenic steroid** a synthesized version of the male hormone testosterone

**Designer drugs** manufactured drugs that mimic the effects of other drugs

**Structural analog** a designer drug that mimics the effects of another drug

**China white** a designer drug with more potent effects than heroin

**Ecstasy** or **MDMA** a hallucinogen with amphetamine-like properties

**FIGURE 12.9** ▶ Long-term Effects of MDMA Use on Memory

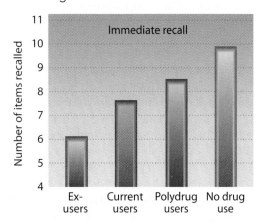

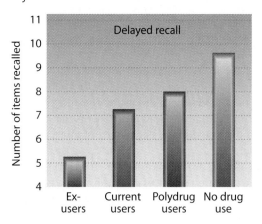

Two serious potential hazards are improper self-diagnosis and overmedication. Also, drugs can interact unfavorably with other medications, substances in the diet, and with one's own body chemistry. When self-prescribing, a person should follow the directions printed on the product, inquire about the product from the pharmacist, or read the *Physician's Desk Reference for Nonprescription Drugs* to be completely informed about the medication.

Consumers are continually bombarded with new OTC products along with the established ones. The **Food and Drug Administration (FDA)** is the federal regulatory agency charged with establishing criteria for all drugs and reviewing active ingredients in all of the following 26 classes of OTC drugs.

1. Analgesics
2. Antacids
3. Antidiarrheal products
4. Antiemetics
5. Allergy treatment products
6. Antimicrobial products
7. Antiperspirants
8. Antirheumatic products

9. Antitussives
10. Bronchodilators and antiasthmatic products
11. Cold remedies
12. Contraceptive products
13. Dandruff products
14. Dentifrices and dental products
15. Emetics
16. Hematinics
17. Hemorrhoidal products
18. Laxatives
19. Miscellaneous internal products
20. Miscellaneous dermatologic products for external use
21. Ophthalmic products
22. Oral hygiene aids
23. Sedatives and sleep aids
24. Stimulants
25. Sunburn prevention and treatment products
26. Vitamin and mineral products

For consumer protection, the FDA requires that all OTC medications be packaged with a tamper-proof seal and that the package include information about active ingredients, strength, amount of medication in the container, appropriate dose, indications for use, side effects, warnings, and expiration date.

All essential information for OTC drugs is to be placed in the same order on medicine labels, in a more readable and understandable format.

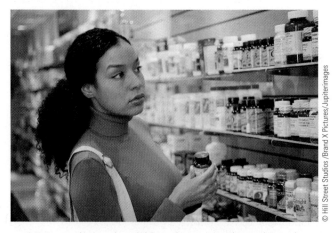

▲ *OTC products should be chosen and used wisely*

## Drug Addiction/Drug Treatment

Over 6 million Americans need drug addiction treatment. The vast majority will never get the treatment or any intervention for this serious abuse problem.

**Tips for Action** For Safe Use of Over-the-Counter Drugs

■ Do not take more than is recommended.

■ Do not take the medicine longer than is recommended.

■ Do not use medications that have expired.

■ Do not give medications to children under age 12 unless the label lists a recommended dose for children.

■ Do not continue taking the medication if the symptoms persist or get worse.

■ Do not combine medications.

Drug addiction surfaced as a social problem in the United States after the Civil War, when wounded veterans came home hooked on morphine they had received to relieve pain. With the invention of the hypodermic needle came the legal—and illegal—intravenous use of drugs. American homemakers became addicted to various prescription drugs. By the beginning of the 20th century, the public was raising questions about the misuse of drugs.

In the 1930s the federal government opened the first two drug treatment hospitals, in Lexington, Kentucky, and in Fort Worth, Texas. In the 1950s Riverside Hospital in New York City opened the first drug treatment facility designed especially for juvenile addicts. Synanon was founded on the West Coast in 1958. Programs and facilities began to multiply in the 1970s, in response to the increasing abuse of drugs by middle-class youth, a rise in the crime rate resulting from drug use, and the return of many addicted soldiers from Vietnam.

In approaching the practicalities of treatment, drugs differ in how widespread their use is and how addictive the various drugs are. Table 12.5 summarizes the effects of various drugs on the body.

The treatment programs available in the United States today are outlined briefly below. No one best method exists. Some work better with some forms of addiction. The goal is to find the treatment plan that works best for each individual. Regardless of the type of addiction, the key to success is personal motivation, backed by an ongoing support system.

## TREATMENT MODALITIES

Most drug experts view chemical dependence as a medical condition, just as diabetes or heart disease. In most cases the first step in traditional treatment and rehabilitation of psychoactive drug abuse is **detoxification.** In most cases, medications and vitamins are administered to assist in withdrawal. Detoxification utilizes three basic steps.

1. Get the person completely off drugs as quickly as possible.

2. Relieve both the physical and psychological distress of the withdrawal process.

3. Achieve and maintain abstinence—a drug-free life.

Detoxification usually requires cold-turkey withdrawal instead of gradually tapering off. Tranquilizers and other drugs usually are prescribed to reduce anxiety and tension. Most people in these detox programs are treated on an outpatient basis, and the treatment usually lasts about three weeks. Long-term results are not encouraging. One study found that the average addict is back on drugs in about eight days after treatment. Detoxification works best if it is part of a treatment program that includes counseling and psychotherapy.

## NONDRUG THERAPIES

Counseling and psychotherapy are part of most drug abuse treatment programs, whether outpatient treatment or inpatient treatment. These programs usually are based on behavior modification principles. The costlier programs are residential (hospital models), and others are administered on an outpatient basis. The programs are tailored to deal with emotional problems that triggered the drug abuse initially. Group therapy and drug education are stressed in most inpatient programs. Again, the results are mixed and not entirely promising.

## THERAPEUTIC COMMUNITIES

Independent **therapeutic communities** have shown some success in turning around the lives of addicts. Staffed largely by former addicts and graduates of the program, they stress a self-help approach. Encounter group sessions and confrontational therapy techniques based on peer pressure are part of the program. Treatment can last

### KEY TERMS

**Food and Drug Administration (FDA)** the regulatory agency charged with establishing criteria for all drugs and reviewing active ingredients in all over-the-counter drugs

**Detoxification** ridding the body of poisons or the effects of poisons

**Therapeutic communities** self-help group homes programmed to assist addicts in remaining drug-free

**TABLE 12.5** ▶ Effects of Selected Drugs on the Body

| | NARCOTICS | COCAINE AND CRACK | AMPHETAMINES |
|---|---|---|---|
| **Type of drug** | ■ Poppy derivatives (opium, codeine, morphine, heroin) and synthetics (Demerol, methadone, Dilaudid, Percodan)<br>■ Smoked, eaten, or injected<br>■ Ancient painkillers used medicinally<br>■ Deaden pain, produce euphoria and drowsiness | ■ Derived from South American coca bush (still chewed in Andes to offset fatigue)<br>■ Cocaine hydrochloride is white powder (coke, C, flake, snow)<br>■ Crack is mixture of cocaine and baking soda<br>■ Used until 1920 in many medicines<br>■ Stimulant action—like amphetamine, but now legally classed as a narcotic | ■ Synthetically produced; amphetamine (speed), dextroamphetamine (Dexedrine), methylamphetamine or ice, methylphenidate (Ritalin)<br>■ Used as pills, inhaled, or injected (speed)<br>■ Central nervous system (CNS) stimulants that resemble action of adrenaline (natural body hormone) |
| **Short-term effects (after a single dose)** | ■ Briefly stimulate, then depress higher brain centers<br>■ Give quick pleasure surge (for few minutes), then stupor (which mutes hunger, pain, sex drive)<br>■ Taken by mouth, effects slower, no initial pleasure surge<br>■ Pupils tiny, body warm, limbs heavy<br>■ Mouth dry, skin itchy<br>■ Users may nod off, alternately awake or asleep, oblivious to surroundings | ■ Short-acting, powerful CNS stimulant; also a local anesthetic<br>■ Effects vary depending on whether drug is snorted (inhaled); injected; put in mouth, rectum, or vagina; or smoked (as crack)<br>■ Transient euphoria and increased energy<br>■ Loss of appetite<br>■ Rise in heart rate and breathing<br>■ Dilated pupils<br>■ Agitated, restless, talkative<br>■ Brief rise in sex drive | ■ Nervous system briefly stimulated<br>■ Reduces appetite<br>■ Increases energy, offsets fatigue<br>■ Talkative, restless, more alert<br>■ Faster breathing<br>■ Rise in heart rate and blood pressure (with risk of burst blood vessels and heart failure)<br>■ Temperature raised, mouth dry, skin sweaty<br>■ Pupils dilated<br>■ Alleviates stuffy nose (original medicinal use) |
| **With larger doses and longer use** | ■ Extremities heavy<br>■ Permanent drowsiness<br>■ Pupils become pinpoints<br>■ Skin cold, moist, bluish<br>■ Progressively slower breathing<br>■ Depressed breathing<br>■ Dangers increase with alcohol intake | ■ Permanently stuffy nose (if snorted) and risk of perforated nasal septum<br>■ Brief euphoric effect followed by crash—depression<br>■ Anesthetic effect can depress brain function<br>■ Bizarre, erratic, perhaps violent actions<br>■ Paranoid psychosis (disappears if drug is discontinued)<br>■ Sensation of crawling under the skin<br>■ Convulsions, disturbed heart action, death | ■ Bizarre behavior, talkative, restless, tremors, excitability<br>■ Sense of power, superiority, aggression<br>■ Illusions and hallucinations<br>■ Some users become paranoid, suspicious, panicky, violent<br>■ Elevated blood pressure<br>■ Insomnia |
| **Long-term effects** | ■ Constipation<br>■ Moodiness<br>■ Risk of endocarditis (heart infection) and other infections (AIDS) from needle-sharing<br>■ Hormone upsets (menstrual irregularities)<br>■ Liver damage<br>■ Damaged offspring<br>■ Strong dependence | ■ Weight loss, malnutrition<br>■ Destroyed nose tissues (if sniffed)<br>■ Restlessness, mood swings, insomnia, extreme excitability, suspiciousness and paranoia, delusions ("psychosis")<br>■ Depression<br>■ Impotence<br>■ Risk of heart attacks<br>■ Strong psychological dependence | ■ Malnutrition, emaciation (owing to appetite loss)<br>■ Anxiety states<br>■ Amphetamine-psychosis (with schizophrenia-like hallucinations)<br>■ Kidney damage<br>■ Susceptibility to infection<br>■ Sleep disorders<br>■ Psychological dependence |
| **Withdrawal symptoms** | ■ Striking withdrawal effects (four to five hours after last dose), sweating, anxiety, diarrhea, gooseflesh, shivering, tremors | ■ Little or no withdrawal sickness; sleepiness<br>■ Extreme exhaustion<br>■ Possibly cocaine blues (depression) | ■ Long sleep, chills<br>■ Ravenous hunger<br>■ Depression |

**TABLE 12.5** ▸ *Effects of Selected Drugs on the Body (Continued)*

| HALLUCINOGENS | CANNABIS | INHALANTS | CAFFEINE |
|---|---|---|---|
| ■ Derived from mushrooms (psilocybin) or cactus (mescaline) or synthetically—for example, lysergic acid (LSD) or acid and phencyclidine (PCP)<br>■ Structures resemble catecholamines—normal brain neurotransmitters<br>■ Hallucinogens can distort reality and produce severe delusions | ■ Derived from *Cannabis sativa*; preparations vary in potency; hash most potent, marijuana least<br>■ Smoked in joints or chewed (sometimes with food)<br>■ Medicinally used for epilepsy, glaucoma, against nausea | ■ Volatile organic hydrocarbons from petroleum and natural gas (for example, gasoline, toluene, hexane, chloroform, carbon tetrachloride, nail polish remover or acetone, lighter fluid, paint thinners, cleaning fluid, airplane cement, plastic glue)<br>■ Hallucinogenic effects | ■ Derived from tea, coffee beans, kola nuts, chocolate<br>■ Used in many medicines (for example, painkillers, cold and cough, pain remedies, antihistamines)<br>■ Average cup of coffee contains 60–75 mg caffeine, colas about 35 mg (per 250 mL)<br>■ CNS stimulant |
| ■ Unpredictable effects—at first like amphetamine<br>■ Excitation, arousal<br>■ Temperature raised<br>■ Altered sense of smell, shape, size, color, distance<br>■ Exhilaration, mind expansion, or anxiety—depending on user<br>■ Rapid pulse, dilated pupils, blank stare<br>■ Exaggerated power sense with possibly violent behavior<br>■ Later—dramatic perceptual distortions<br>■ Occasionally convulsions | ■ Produces dreamlike euphoria, laughter, relaxation<br>■ Alters sense of space, time<br>■ Increases heart rate<br>■ Reddens eyes<br>■ Dreamy, stoned look<br>■ At later stages, users are quiet, reflective, sleepy<br>■ Combined with alcohol, increased effects, distorted behavior<br>■ Impairs short-term memory, thinking, and ability to drive car or perform complex tasks | ■ Exhilaration, light-headedness, excitability, disorientation<br>■ Confusion, slurred speech, dizziness<br>■ Distorted perception<br>■ Visual and auditory hallucinations<br>■ Impaired muscular control<br>■ Possible nausea, increased saliva, sneezing<br>■ Dampened reflexes<br>■ Recklessness, feelings of power, invincibility | ■ Stimulates brain, speeds nerve-cell transmission<br>■ Elevates mood and alertness<br>■ Stimulates mental activity<br>■ Speeds up breathing, metabolism<br>■ Enhances mental performance<br>■ Postpones fatigue<br>■ Shortens sleep<br>■ Increases urine output<br>■ Raises blood fats<br>■ Increases stomach acidity<br>■ Decreases appetite |
| ■ Anxiety, panic attacks, paranoid delusions, occasionally psychosis (like schizophrenia)<br>■ Injury or accidents because of drug-induced delusions or distance misjudgment<br>■ Increased risk of fetal abnormalities<br>■ Tolerance develops rapidly but also disappears fast with renewed drug sensitivity<br>■ With PCP, high fever, muscle spasm, erratic behavior, psychosis lasting weeks or more | ■ Slowed digestive (gastrointestinal) activity<br>■ Time misjudgment<br>■ Sharpened or distorted sense of color, sound<br>■ Thinking slow and confused<br>■ Apathy, loss of motivation or drive<br>■ Large doses can produce severe confusion, panic attacks<br>■ Hallucinations (even psychosis) | ■ Drowsiness and possible unconsciousness<br>■ Severe disorientation<br>■ Risks increase with fume concentration<br>■ Irregular heartbeat, heart action disturbed<br>■ Large doses may cause heart failure (especially with spot removers or airplane cement) | ■ Nervousness, hand tremors<br>■ Delayed sleep onset, reduces depth of sleep, insomnia<br>■ Abnormally rapid heartbeat<br>■ Jitteriness<br>■ Mild delirium possible<br>■ Convulsions (rare)<br>■ Suspected cancer-causing agent |
| ■ Long-term medical effects not known<br>■ May include muscle tenseness, flashbacks—brief, spontaneous recurrence of prior LSD (hallucinogenic) experiences<br>■ Prolonged, profound depression<br>■ Panic attacks<br>■ No physical dependence | ■ Loss of drive, reduced energy<br>■ Regular heavy use increases risk of<br>—bronchitis, lung cancer<br>—reduced sex hormones<br>—impaired learning<br>—memory loss<br>—possible decrease in immunity<br>■ Psychological dependence | ■ Pallor, thirst, nose, eye, mouth sores<br>■ Irritability, hostility, forgetfulness<br>■ May damage liver, kidney, and brain<br>■ Nosebleeds, impaired blood cell formation<br>■ Depression, weight loss<br>■ Other drugs compound damage<br>■ Dependence possible | ■ Raised blood cholesterol level<br>■ Risk of stomach ulcers<br>■ Suspected cancer-inducing agent<br>■ Possible damage to unborn baby<br>■ Regular coffee use (more than five cups daily) can lead to dependence |
| ■ Few withdrawal effects, possible flashbacks, anxiety | ■ Withdrawal symptoms mild—insomnia, anxiety, irritability | ■ Restlessness, anxiety, irritability, headaches<br>■ Stomach upsets<br>■ Delirium (rare) | ■ Severe headache<br>■ Irritability<br>■ Tiredness |

*Source:* Adapted with permission from *Health News*, a publication of the University of Toronto Faculty of Medicine. Subscriptions and back issues can be obtained by writing 109 Vanderhoof Ave., Suite 205, Toronto, Ontario MAG 2H7 or by calling (416) 978-5411.

from three months to two years. The average duration of treatment is less than six months, but those who have gone through treatment continue to be considered members of the therapeutic community.

## SELF-HELP GROUPS

Many addicts participate in **self-help groups** with others who have similar experiences and thus can offer personal support. Examples are Narcotics Anonymous (NA), Substance Anonymous (SA), and Cocaine Anonymous (CA). These groups are based on the 12-step program developed by the founders of Alcoholics Anonymous (AA), the premier self-help group.

Participation in these self-help groups is voluntary. Members are there because they want to be—which points toward greater success. At the meetings, people talk about their past experiences with drugs as well as their fears and hopes. Listening to others and exchanging accounts seem to help relieve the compulsions. Because the commonality is drug abuse, these groups tend to be multiracial.

## PRIVATE MEDICAL PROFESSIONALS

Physicians who specialize in addictions and withdrawal treatments are certified by the American Society of Addiction Medicine or the American Academy of Psychiatrists in Alcoholism and Addiction. In conjunction with their therapy, they highly recommend self-help support programs.

Some psychologists treat drug addiction. They emphasize the psychological aspects of anger, depression, anxiety, and other feelings that underlie the addiction. They, too, should be trained in this area of specialty. In choosing the professional to see, the person should always look for someone who puts the addiction issue first.

Other treatment facilities available are outpatient rehabilitation, mental health centers, inpatient rehabilitation, hospital inpatient, and emergency rooms.

## Summary

- Psychoactive drugs affect normal brain function and alter the mood and behavior of an individual.
- Psychoactive drugs include narcotics, depressants, stimulants, inhalants, and hallucinogens or psychedelics.
- Over-the-counter drugs (OTCs) fall into 26 different drug categories and have the potential for misuse and abuse.
- Drug addictions are treated through medication and by nondrug therapies such as therapeutic communities, self-help groups, and private physicians.

## Personal Health Resources

ThomsonNOW  Visit the ThomsonNOW website at http://thomsonedu.com/thomsonnow for valuable resources that will:

- Help you evaluate your knowledge of the material.
- Guide you through tutorials to help you understand and apply the material.
- Allow you to take an exam-prep quiz to better prepare for class tests.

American Council for Drug Education. This organization provides information on the effects of drug usage and offers treatment referrals through its hotline. 212-595-5810

**www.acde.org**

Hazelden Foundation. A foundation that distributes educational materials and self-help literature on quitting alcohol, tobacco, and drugs. 1-800-257-7810

**www.hazelden.com**

American Cancer Society. The site offers literature on smoking and referrals to local chapters. 1-800-227-2345 400-816-7800

**www.cancer.org**

National Clearinghouse for Alcohol and Drug Information. This group provides information on all psychoactive substances. 1-800-729-6686 TDD: 800 487-4889

**www.NCADI.SAMHSA.gov**

Substance Abuse and Mental Health Archive. Data have been compiled from government drug abuse and mental health surveys administered from 1970 to the present. Includes keyword site search option. 888-741-7242

**www.icpsr.umich.edu/SAMHDA**

Substance Abuse & Mental Health Services Administration (SAMHSA). This agency supplies data on national survey on drug use.

**www.samhsa.gov**

The Drug Information Conference. The Center for Substance Abuse Research site offers information on drug use, including health effects, fact sheets, and related drug topics. 301-403-8329

**www.info.com/conferences**

The National Institute on Drug Abuse. This governmental site offers voluminous materials/research on all components of drugs.

**www.nida.nih.gov**

*Medical News Today.* A compilation and reporting on latest medical research.

**www.medicalnewstoday.com/printerfriendlynews. php?newsid=34933**

**Executive Office of the President**
**Office of National Drug Control Policy**
The site is a drug policy information clearinghouse with fact sheets on various drugs.

**www.whitehousedrugpolicy.gov/publications/factsht**

## It's Your Turn for Study and Review

1. With the increase in cases of HIV/AIDS, hepatitis, human papillomavirus (HPV), and syphilis, which can be spread via injectable drug use, should the government provide heroin addicts with sterile needles?

2. Millions of Americans consume caffeine daily in coffee, tea, cola, chocolate, and various medications. Briefly discuss the effects of caffeine.

3. List and discuss 10 reasons why people use drugs.

4. Should marijuana be legalized? Discuss fully and factually your decision.

5. What factors influence drug dependence?

6. What are some treatment options for drug dependence?

## Selected Bibliography

Ambramovitz, M. "The Knockout Punch of Date Rape Drugs." *Current Health*, March 2001, pp. 18–21.

Avorn, J. "Are Your Pills Safe? Why Dangerous Medicine Gets Past FDA." *AARP The Magazine*, March/April 2006, pp. 49–51.

Bandell, B. "Crystal Meth Wave Spreads across Florida." *South Florida Business Journal*, May 10, 2006.

Barr, Naomi. "Pill Alerts." *O The Oprah Magazine*, March 2007, p. 174.

Basler, B. "Generic Drugs Stuck in the Pipeline." *AARP Bulletin*, 47:5, May 2006, p.11.

Bernstein, J., et al. "Brief Motivational Intervention at a Clinic Visit Reduces Cocaine and Heroin Use." *Drug and Alcohol Dependence*, 77:1, 2005, pp. 49–59.

Boschert, S. "Chest Pain in Young May Mean Cocaine Use." *Family Practice*, 33:6, March 2003, p. 16.

Buchert, R., et al. "A Voxel-Based PET Investigation of the Long-Term Effects of 'Ecstasy' Consumption on Brain Serotonin Transporters." *American Journal of Psychiatry*, 161, July 2004, p. 1181.

"Caffeine," National Institute on Drug Abuse, www.nida.nih.gov. 2006.

Centers for Disease Control and Prevention. *Youth Risk Behavior Surveillance—United States, 1999.* Atlanta, GA: CDC, June 2000.

"Cocaine," National Institute on Drug Abuse, www.nida.nih.gov. 2006.

Cowley, G. "Can Marijuana Be Medicine?" *Newsweek*, February 3, 1997, p. 22.

Dackis, C. A., et al. "A Double-Blind, Placebo Controlled Trial of Modafinil for Cocaine Dependence." *Neuropsychopharmacology* 30:1, 2005, pp. 205–211.

Dager, S., et al. "Human Brain Metabolic Response to Caffeine and the Effects of Tolerance." *American Journal of Psychiatry*, 156:2, February 1999, pp. 229–236.

Dreher, N. "Cramming on Ritalin." *Current Health*, September 2001, pp. 21–23.

Drug Abuse Warning Network. The DAWN Report: Club Drugs. October 2002.

Emanuel, E. J. "Drug Addiction." *The New Republic*, July 2006, pp. 9–12.

Federal Bureau of Investigation. *Crime in the United States 1999: Uniform Crime Reports.* Washington, DC: U.S. Government Printing Office, October 2000.

Fischmann, J. and Melton, M. "Drug Bazaar." *U.S. News and World Report*, June 21, 1999, pp. 58–62.

Galanter, M. and Kleber, H. D., eds. *The American Psychiatric Textbook of Substance Abuse Treatment.* Washington, DC: APA Press, 1999.

George, Liame. "A New Kind of Senior Moment." *Maclean's*, January 29, 2007, p. 41.

Goldberg, R. *Drugs across the Spectrum.* Belmont, CA: Wadsworth/Thomson Learning, 2000.

Goozner, M. "FDA Woes: Why Protecting Our Medicine Is So Complicated." *AARP Bulletin*, 47:5, May, 2006.

Hatem, M. B. "CEWG: 25 Years Tracking Emerging Drug Abuse Problems." *NIDA Notes*, 16:4, October 2001, pp. 11–13.

"Heroin." National Institute on Drug Abuse, www.nida.nih.gov. 2006.

Ingram, S. "Smart Drugs: Brain Builders or Bad Medicine." *Current Health*, January 2001, pp. 14–15.

Jaffe, H. and Chip, A. "Got Any Smart Pills?" *Washingtonian*, 41:4, January 2006, pp. 41–47.

**KEY TERMS**

**Self-help groups** addicts participating with others who have similar experiences and can offer personal support

Jardin, R. "Does Ritalin Really Add Up?' *NEA Today*, 17:7, April 1999, p. 24.

Julien, R. M. *A Primer of Drug Action*, 10th ed. New York: Worth, 2005.

Kirchheimer, Sid. "Move Your Pills." *AARP The Magazine*, January/ February 2007, p. 41.

Kowalski, K. "Stimulants: Fast Track to Disaster." *Current Health*, February 2001, pp. 6–12.

Leshner, A. "Using Science to Counter the Spread of Ecstasy Abuse." *NIDA Notes*, 16:5, December 2001, p. 3.

Mandavilli, A. "FDA Warning: Over-the-Counter Medicines Risky." *Discover*, 27:1, January 2006, p. 51.

"Marijuana." National Institute on Drug Abuse, www.nida.nih.gov. 2006.

Meadows, M. "Prescription Drug Use and Abuse." *FDA Consumers*, 13:5, September/October 2001, p. 19.

Monroe, J. "OTCs—Check Out the Labels." *Current Health*, November 21, 2001, p. 12.

Monroe, J. "Antibiotic vs. the Superbugs." *Current Health*, October 2001, pp. 24–26.

Murphy, D. "Why Diet Drugs Can Be Diet Dangers." *Current Health*, December 2000, pp. 18–21.

Nestler, E. "Historical Review: Molecular and Cellular Mechanisms of Opiate and Cocaine Addiction." *Trends in Pharmacological Sciences*, 25:4, April 2004, p. 210.

Nordenberg, T. "The Death of the Party: All the Rave, GHB's Hazards Go Unheeded." *FDA Consumer*, 34:2, March/April 2000, pp. 14–17.

O'Malley, P. M., Johnston, L. D., and Backman, J. F. "Alcohol Use among Adolescents." *Alcohol Health and Research World*, 22:2, June 1998, pp. 887–892.

Perkins, H. W., et al. "Misconceptions for the Frequency of Alcohol and Other Drug Use on College Campuses." *Journal of American College Health*, 47:6, May 1999, pp. 253–258.

Powledge, T. "Addiction and the Brain." *Bioscience*, 49:7, July 1999, pp. 513–519.

*Project Lead: High Expectation about Multiple Substance Abuse*. Washington, DC: Links Foundation, 1987.

Ragavan, C. "Cracking Down on Ecstasy." *U.S. News and World Report*, February 5, 2001, pp. 14–15.

Scheller, M. "Inhalants: Don't Let Them Take Your Breath Away." *Current Health*, September 2000, pp. 16–19.

Stephenson, J. "Cannabis Consequences." *Journal of the American Medical Association*, 291:23, June 16, 2004, p. 2809.

Stocker, S. "Cocaine Pleasurable Effects May Involve Multiple Chemical Sites." *NIDA Notes*, 14:2, September 1999, p. 7.

Substance Abuse and Mental Health Services Administration, *Mid-Year 2000 Preliminary Emergency Department Data from the Drug Abuse Warning Network*. Rockville, MD: SAMHSA, January 2001.

Substance Abuse and Mental Health Services Administration. *Summary Findings from the 1999 National Household Survey on Drug Abuse*. Rockville, MD: SAMHSA, August 2000.

Thomas, C. L., ed. *Taber's Cyclopedic Medical Dictionary*. Philadelphia: F. A. Davis Company, 2001.

Torpy, J. "Opioid Abuse." *Journal of the American Medical Association*, 291:10, September 15, 2004, p. 1213.

United Nations Office on Drugs and Crime. *2004 World Drug Report*. Vienna, Austria.

*USA Today*. Your Health, "Drug Addiction, Substance Abuse and Methamphetamine Treatment." 134:2725, October 2005.

U.S. Department of Education. *Growing Up Drug Free*. Washington, DC: U.S. Government Printing Office.

U.S. Department of Health and Human Services. *Youth Risk Behavior Survey*. Atlanta, GA: Centers for Disease Control and Prevention, 1999.

U.S. Department of Health and Human Services. *Driving after Drug or Alcohol Use: Findings from the 1996 National Household Survey on Drug Abuse*. Rockville, MD: Substance Abuse and Mental Health Services Administration, 1998.

U.S. Department of Health and Human Services. *Drug Abuse and Addiction Research: 25 Years of Discovery to Advance the Health of the Public*, Sixth Triennial Report to Congress. Washington, DC: U.S. Government Printing Office, 1999.

U.S. Office of National Drug Control Policy. *Heroin Fact Sheet*. Washington, DC: The White House, 2007.

U.S. Sentencing Commission. *1999 Sourcebook of Federal Sentencing Statistics*. 2000. Inter-University Consortium for Political and Social Research at the University of Michigan (ICPSR) www.ICPSR.umich.edu/NACSD.

Vincent, Isobel. "Where The Drug Lords Are Kings." *Maclean's*, January 29, 2007, pp. 23–24.

Zalavitz, M. "Should I Drop My Antidepressant?" *Psychology Today*, April 2006, p. 59.

Name _____    Date_____

Course _____    Section_____

Differentiate the psychoactive substances listed below in terms of category, source, and primary route of administration.

| Substance | Category | Source | Route of Administration |
|---|---|---|---|
| Barbiturates | | | |
| Benzodiazepines | | | |
| Caffeine | | | |
| Crack or cocaine | | | |
| Heroin | | | |
| Marijuana | | | |
| Mescaline | | | |
| Methamphetamine (ice) | | | |
| Morphine | | | |
| Psilocybin | | | |

**Name** _____   **Date**_____

**Course**_____   **Section**_____

The following questions were written by recovering addicts in Narcotics Anonymous.

|  | Yes | No |
|---|:---:|:---:|
| 1. Do you ever use alone? | ☐ | ☐ |
| 2. Have you ever substituted one drug for another, thinking that one particular drug was the problem? | ☐ | ☐ |
| 3. Have you ever manipulated or lied to a doctor to obtain prescription drugs? | ☐ | ☐ |
| 4. Have you ever stolen drugs or stolen to obtain drugs? | ☐ | ☐ |
| 5. Do you regularly use a drug when you wake up or when you go to bed? | ☐ | ☐ |
| 6. Have you ever taken one drug to overcome the effects of another? | ☐ | ☐ |
| 7. Do you avoid people or places that do not approve of your using drugs? | ☐ | ☐ |
| 8. Have you ever used a drug without knowing what it was or what it would do to you? | ☐ | ☐ |
| 9. Has your job or school performance ever suffered from the effects of your drug use? | ☐ | ☐ |
| 10. Have you ever been arrested as a result of using drugs? | ☐ | ☐ |
| 11. Have you ever lied about what or how much you use? | ☐ | ☐ |
| 12. Do you put the purchase of drugs ahead of your financial responsibilities? | ☐ | ☐ |
| 13. Have you ever tried to stop or control your using? | ☐ | ☐ |
| 14. Have you ever been in a jail, hospital, or drug rehabilitation center because of your using? | ☐ | ☐ |
| 15. Does using interfere with your sleeping or eating? | ☐ | ☐ |
| 16. Does the thought of running out of drugs terrify you? | ☐ | ☐ |
| 17. Do you feel it is impossible for you to live without drugs? | ☐ | ☐ |
| 18. Do you ever question your own sanity? | ☐ | ☐ |
| 19. Is your drug use making life at home unhappy? | ☐ | ☐ |
| 20. Have you ever thought you could not fit in or have a good time without using drugs? | ☐ | ☐ |
| 21. Have you ever felt defensive, guilty, or ashamed about your using? | ☐ | ☐ |
| 22. Do you think much about drugs? | ☐ | ☐ |
| 23. Have you had irrational or indefinable fears? | ☐ | ☐ |
| 24. Has using affected your sexual relationships? | ☐ | ☐ |
| 25. Have you ever taken drugs you did not prefer? | ☐ | ☐ |
| 26. Have you ever used drugs because of emotional pain or stress? | ☐ | ☐ |

**27.** Have you ever overdosed on any drugs? ☐ ☐

**28.** Do you continue to use despite negative consequences? ☐ ☐

**29.** Do you think you might have a drug problem? ☐ ☐

Are you an addict? This is a question only you can answer. Members of Narcotics Anonymous found that they all answered different numbers of these questions "yes." The actual number of "yes" responses is not as important as how you feel inside and how addiction has affected your life. If you are an addict, you must first admit that you have a problem with drugs before any progress can be made toward recovery.

*Source:* From *Am I An Addict?* Copyright© 1983, 1988 Narcotics Anonymous World Services. All rights reserved. Reprinted by permission.

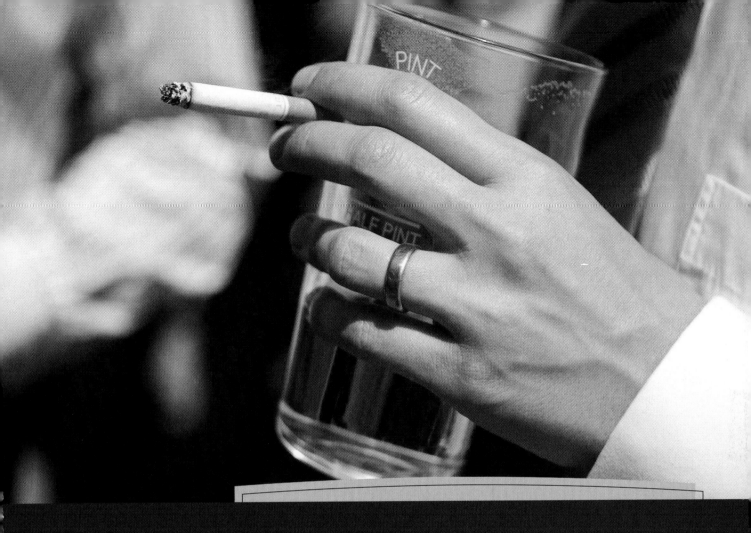

© PSL Images/Alamy

# Chapter Thirteen
# Alcohol and Tobacco

**OBJECTIVES** ■ Discuss the prevalence of drinking and binge drinking. ■ Define alcoholism and identify alcohol-related disorders. ■ Describe the societal effects of drinking alcohol. ■ Identify the physical effects of drinking alcohol. ■ Identify the types of alcoholic beverages and define "proof." ■ Cite the legal limit for blood alcohol content when driving in your state. ■ Trace the history of and trends in tobacco use. ■ Identify the physical effects of tobacco. ■ Identify the groups most likely to use tobacco. ■ Identify the effects of secondhand smoke.

ThomsonNOW™  Log on to ThomsonNOW at http://thomsonedu.com/thomsonnow to access and explore self-assessments, interactive tutorials, and practice quizzes.

When one looks at the drug problem in this country, it is notable that the two that have the largest negative impact and result in the most deaths—alcohol and tobacco—are both legal. Alcohol and tobacco, both mind-altering substances, can wreak havoc on a college community in terms of death, injury, assault, sexual abuse, unsafe sex, academic problems, serious health problems (now and later), abuse, and dependence.

Binge drinking has reached epidemic proportions on college campuses throughout the country. Alcohol can provide some beneficial effects when consumed in moderation. Its misuse, however, can have adverse physiological, social, and relational impacts. Tobacco causes many life-threatening diseases, including oral and throat cancer, lung cancer, colon cancer, emphysema, and heart disease. Tobacco, either smoked or smokeless, has no redeeming value. Its hold on people stems from its addictive properties.

The rate of tobacco smoking in U.S. society at large has been declining, although its use is rising in certain demographic groups, primarily teens. In this chapter we discuss alcohol and tobacco to include their psychological and social effects.

## Alcohol Use

Alcohol use is socially accepted and therefore, it is often used in most gatherings. Beer, wine, and distilled spirits are consumed by all economic levels of people. Wine often accompanies meals and is used to flavor certain foods. Alcoholic beverages are consumed during social gatherings to make the user feel relaxed, more convivial, and to escape from day-to-day pressures. Wine is part of sacred rites in some religious communions and ceremonies. Alcoholic beverages are used socially to celebrate occasions such as weddings, births, graduations, anniversaries, family reunions, political, and sporting events. Alcohol slows or depresses the central nervous system and reduces inhibitions in some people, allowing them to be more expressive and explorative. Except for

the brief period of Prohibition in the United States (1917–1932), alcohol has been socially acceptable and legal.

Most Americans continue to desire the effects produced after consuming the beverage **ethyl alcohol,** also known as ethanol or grain alcohol. The major types of alcoholic beverages are as follows.

1. **Distilled spirits.** Also known as hard liquor, these are made by distilling brewed or fermented grains. They contain 40%–50% alcohol by volume. Distilled liquor includes gin, scotch, whiskey, rum, vodka, and various liqueurs. The alcohol content of distilled beverages is expressed in terms of **proof,** which is equal to twice the percent of alcohol. One degree of proof, then, equals one-half of 1% of alcohol. For example if a beverage is 86 proof, the product contains 43% alcohol by volume.

2. **Wine.** Wine is made by fermenting grapes and other fruits. Table wine contains 9% to 14% alcohol by volume and often is served with food. Dessert wine or fortified wine has distilled alcohol added and contains 18% to 21% alcohol by volume. Fortified wines include sherry, port, and Madeira. Fortified wines are popular with young drinkers because they have a kick.

3. **Beer and ale.** These are made by controlled fermentation of cereal grains and malt. Hops are added to give these drinks a distinctive flavor. Lager beer contains 3% to 4% alcohol; malt liquor, 4% to 5%; and high-powered beer such as ale, porter, and stout, 6% to 7%.

Figure 13.1 gives the percentage alcohol content in selected beverages.

### PREVALENCE

Approximately 121 million Americans aged 12 and older use alcohol in some form or another. An estimated 55 million are binge drinkers and 16.7 million are heavy drinkers. Approximately 70% of adults in the United

**FIGURE 13.1** ▶ Percentage Alcohol Content in Various Beverages

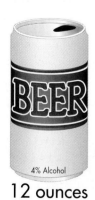
12 ounces

≠

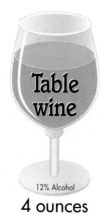
4 ounces

≠

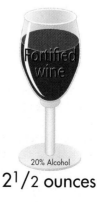
2¹/2 ounces

≠

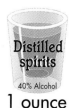
1 ounce

States are regular drinkers. More than 7.5% of the population ages 18 and older—over 13.8 million Americans—have problems with drinking, including over 9 million people who are alcoholic. Although two-thirds of the population drink, 10% of all drinkers (those who drink heavily) drink half of all alcohol consumed.

Alcohol abuse causes over 100,000 deaths in the United States and Canada each year. African Americans have higher rates of abstinence than whites, yet drink heavier on one given occasion, and have higher rates of medical problems such as cirrhosis (in some geographic areas), hypertension, homicides, cancer of the esophagus, and death. African Americans have higher rates of mortality from alcoholic cirrhosis than either whites or Asian Americans. The latter have the lowest rates of drinking, alcohol abuse, and death from alcohol-related causes. Hispanic males have high rates of alcoholism and high rates of cirrhosis.

For American Indians, alcohol abuse is a factor in five leading causes of death: motor vehicle crashes, alcoholism, cirrhosis, suicide, and homicide. The stereotype of the drunken Indian that has persisted since colonial times is pervasive. American Indian men are three times more likely than American Indian women to be heavy drinkers.

Alcohol abuse patterns differ. Some drink every day to get drunk, and some drink excessively occasionally. Whatever the pattern, when alcohol dependency develops, it can become very difficult to stop.

## GENETIC INFLUENCES

Certain ethnic minorities may have genetic traits that either predispose them to or protect them from becoming alcoholic. The differences may relate to variants of the genes for enzymes involved in alcohol metabolism by the liver. One enzyme found in Japanese, for example, has been associated with faster elimination of alcohol from the body, as compared with whites. Table 13.1 points out some of the specific risk factors by ethnic group.

Acculturation also plays a large role in drinking patterns among various ethnic groups. For example, studies of Asian Americans suggest that, as they become assimilated into the American culture, their drinking rates increase and eventually conform to those of the U.S. population as a whole.

## BLOOD ALCOHOL CONCENTRATION

The rate at which alcohol enters the bloodstream is the key factor in **blood alcohol concentration (BAC)** or **blood alcohol level (BAL).** Once the alcohol is absorbed and enters the bloodstream, it is distributed uniformly throughout the body, extending to all body fluids and tissues. The brain has a large blood supply; therefore, it absorbs alcohol quickly. If a woman is pregnant and

**TABLE 13.1 ▶** Alcohol-Related Health Risks in Minority Groups

| ETHNIC GROUP | RISK FACTORS FROM ALCOHOL ABUSE |
|---|---|
| African Americans | High risk for cirrhosis of the liver, heart diseases, nutritional deficiencies, neurological disorders, and cancer of the tongue, mouth, esophagus, and larynx; extremely high accident and homicide rates |
| American Indians | Among some tribes, very high mortality rates; cirrhosis of the liver, suicide, homicide, cancers, and emotional and neurological disorders |
| Asian Americans | Low rates and risks of drinking-related health problems; research indicates that about half carry a gene that affects metabolism in the liver, causing a buildup of a toxic metabolite, manifested by the flushing response of the face, sweating, and nausea |
| Hispanics | High risk for liver disorders and diseases, neurological disorders caused by nutritional deficiency, cancer of the tongue, mouth, esophagus, and larynx |

is drinking alcohol, it is distributed within the fetal circulation.

Ninety-five percent of alcohol in the blood has to be metabolized, converted to carbon dioxide and water, so it can be removed from the body. Recent research indicates that as much as 30% of alcohol consumed by nonalcoholic males may be metabolized in the stomach. The liver is capable of metabolizing approximately 0.25–0.3 ounces of liquor per hour. The additional 5% of alcohol, which is not metabolized and therefore is unchanged, is excreted via urination, perspiration, and respiration.

In all states a person 21 and over is considered legally intoxicated if the BAC measures 0.08%–0.10%. According to the 1996 National Highway System Act, "any individual under age 21 with a blood-alcohol concentration of 0.02% or greater when driving a motor vehicle is deemed driving while intoxicated." BAC is measured scientifically with a **breathalyzer** or by testing blood or urine samples.

### KEY TERMS

**Ethyl alcohol** colorless liquid and central nervous system depressant made by the process of fermentation and found in alcoholic beverages

**Proof** amount of alcohol in a beverage, expressed as twice the percent of alcohol

**Blood alcohol concentration (BAC)** or **blood alcohol level (BAL)** ratio of alcohol measured in the blood to total blood volume; expressed as a decimal

**Breathalyzer** device used to measure blood alcohol

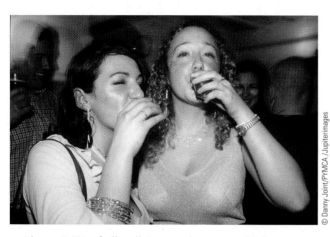

▲ *About 84% of all college students are drinkers*

When the BAC reaches 0.02%, an individual may feel mild relaxing effects from alcohol. Typically, more definite impairment begins when the BAC ranges between 0.03% and just under 0.10%. These effects include impairment of mental function/judgment. In addition, voluntary muscle control decreases, causing some difficulty when performing fine-motor skills.

As the BAC increases, alcohol causes the central nervous system to alter behavioral and physical body function. The changes can include diminished psychomotor performance and severe depression of areas responsible for motor control in the brain. The results are disorientation, slurred speech, visual and hearing difficulty, confusion, poor coordination, poor judgment, abnormal eye movements, unsteady gait, and euphoria.

When alcohol is consumed more rapidly than the liver can metabolize it, the BAC rises. The alcohol impairs brain functions, causing **intoxication.** Physical and behavioral dysfunctioning also result from intoxication. Other complications can include depressed reflexes, anesthesia, unconsciousness/stupor, and coma. A BAC of 0.50% to 0.60% may lead to death by **alcohol poisoning.** Approximately 1,500 students die each year from alcohol poisoning. When excessive amounts of alcohol depress certain involuntary muscle reactions, death is imminent. Table 13.2 summarizes the effects of alcohol related to the BAC.

## DRINKING AND DRIVING

Alcohol is involved in approximately 48% of all traffic fatalities (the leading cause of accidental death). Alcohol-related motor vehicle accidents, the most frequently committed crime, can result in serious personal injury, property damage, and economic cost. Blood alcohol levels of 0.10% or more are found in over 31% of all boating fatalities. Twenty-three percent of 16- to 20-year-old drivers fatally injured in crashes had BACs of 0.10% or more. One in 10 Americans aged 12 and older drives under the influence of alcohol at least once during a 12-month period. Drinking drivers are lethal weapons on the road. They have visual impairment, poor judgment, impaired coordination, and unrealistic sensations of speed and perception. As the blood alcohol content rises, the danger and risk of being involved in an alcohol-related motor vehicle accident increase (see Table 13.3).

To curtail this carnage on the roads, some states have taken various precautionary measures, including identifying repeat offenders, confiscating drivers' licenses and license plates, immobilizing vehicles, strongly publicizing the dangers of drinking and driving, utilizing prevention

**TABLE 13.2 ▶** Effects of Alcohol Related to Blood Alcohol Concentration

| BLOOD ALCOHOL CONCENTRATION | EFFECTS |
| --- | --- |
| 0.01 | Mild, if any; slight changes in feeling, mood elevation |
| 0.03 | Feelings of relaxation and exhilaration; slight impairment of mental function |
| 0.08 | Diminished inhibitions, difficulty performing motor skills, impaired judgment, impaired visual and hearing acuity |
| 0.10 | Typically, little or no judgment and poor condition |
| 0.12 | Difficulty performing gross motor skills, impaired vision, definite impairment of mental function |
| 0.15 | Major impairment of physical and mental functions, erratic and irresponsible behavior, distorted judgment, feeling of euphoria, difficulty responding to stimuli |
| 0.20 | Confusion, decreased inhibitions, inability to move without assistance, inability to maintain upright position; may fall asleep |
| 0.30 | Severe mental confusion, difficulty in comprehension and perception, difficulty responding to stimuli, extreme distortion of sensibility; produces sleep in most people |
| 0.40 | Nearly complete anesthesia, severely depressed reflexes, possible unconsciousness or coma |
| 0.50 | Unconsciousness or deep coma; possibly death |
| 0.60 | Total depression of nerves that control heart and breathing centers; death |

## Tips for Action If You Choose to Drink

■ Refrain from the use of alcoholic beverages, if you are not 21.

■ Do not drink and drive. For most people two drinks in one hour can raise blood alcohol level to 0.08%, which is the tolerance level for driving under the influence in most states.

■ Choose a designated driver (who will not drink) before drinking begins.

■ Offer alternative beverages for those who will not be drinking alcohol, when you are hosting.

■ Do not participate in drinking contests. Blood alcohol can rise to lethal levels (0.40%+) and produce alcohol poisoning and possible death.

■ Accept the definition of heavy drinking as five or more drinks once or twice each weekend. If your drinking pattern is suspect, you may have a drinking problem.

■ Recognize the warning signs of alcohol abuse.

**FIGURE 13.2 ▶** Intoxicated Drivers in Fatal Crashes by Age Group, 1990–2000

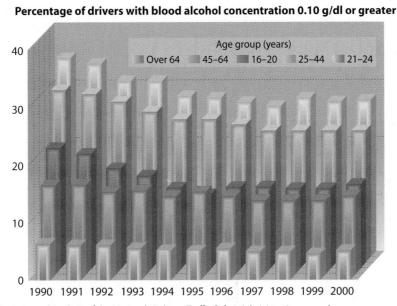

**Percentage of drivers with blood alcohol concentration 0.10 g/dl or greater**

*Source:* National Center for Statistics and Analysis of the National Highway Traffic Safety Administration www.nhtsa.gov.

methods, and incarcerating the offenders. In addition, many states are passing harsher laws and incorporating larger fines when individuals drive under the influence of alcohol. Percentages of intoxicated drivers in fatal crashes are presented in Figure 13.2.

## SOCIETAL EFFECTS OF DRINKING ALCOHOL

Abuse of alcohol continues to be a major societal problem. Use of alcohol can lead to problems in the family, and can contribute to irresponsible and dangerous sexual encounters such as pregnancy, HIV/AIDS infection, human papillomavirus (HPV), and other sexually transmitted diseases. Alcohol is a contributing factor in all of the following.

■ Motor vehicle crash injuries and deaths

■ Accidents

■ Violence

■ Fighting, assaults, abuse, homicides

■ Absenteeism from work and school

### KEY TERMS

**Intoxication** temporary state of mental confusion when alcohol content is consumed more rapidly than the body can metabolize it

**Alcohol poisoning** death attributed to BAC at 0.50% and above

**TABLE 13.3** ▶ Traffic Fatalities by State and Highest Blood Alcohol Concentration in the Crash, 2005

| STATE | TOTAL FATALITIES | NO ALCOHOL (BAC = 0.00 g/dl) | | LOW ALCOHOL (BAC = 0.01–0.09 g/dl) | | HIGH ALCOHOL (BAC = 0.10 g/dl) | | ANY ALCOHOL (BAC = 0.01 g/dl) | |
|---|---|---|---|---|---|---|---|---|---|
| | | NUMBER | PERCENT | NUMBER | PERCENT | NUMBER | PERCENT | NUMBER | PERCENT |
| Alabama | 995 | 596 | 60 | 74 | 7 | 326 | 33 | 399 | 40 |
| Alaska | 103 | 50 | 48 | 9 | 9 | 44 | 43 | 53 | 52 |
| Arizona | 1,036 | 580 | 56 | 102 | 10 | 354 | 34 | 456 | 44 |
| Arkansas | 652 | 452 | 69 | 61 | 9 | 139 | 21 | 200 | 31 |
| California | 3,753 | 2,352 | 63 | 340 | 9 | 1,061 | 28 | 1,401 | 37 |
| Colorado | 681 | 425 | 62 | 58 | 8 | 198 | 29 | 256 | 38 |
| Connecticut | 342 | 184 | 54 | 40 | 12 | 119 | 35 | 158 | 46 |
| Delaware | 123 | 63 | 51 | 11 | 9 | 49 | 40 | 60 | 49 |
| DC | 49 | 30 | 61 | 5 | 10 | 14 | 29 | 19 | 39 |
| Florida | 2,999 | 1,808 | 60 | 261 | 9 | 930 | 31 | 1,191 | 40 |
| Georgia | 1,541 | 971 | 63 | 132 | 9 | 438 | 28 | 570 | 37 |
| Hawaii | 131 | 77 | 59 | 17 | 13 | 37 | 28 | 54 | 41 |
| Idaho | 276 | 162 | 59 | 33 | 12 | 81 | 29 | 114 | 41 |
| Illinois | 1,418 | 804 | 57 | 126 | 9 | 489 | 34 | 614 | 43 |
| Indiana | 875 | 605 | 69 | 56 | 6 | 214 | 24 | 270 | 31 |
| Iowa | 445 | 321 | 72 | 24 | 6 | 100 | 22 | 124 | 28 |
| Kansas | 461 | 307 | 67 | 36 | 8 | 118 | 26 | 154 | 33 |
| Kentucky | 820 | 564 | 69 | 53 | 6 | 203 | 25 | 256 | 31 |
| Louisiana | 937 | 490 | 52 | 95 | 10 | 352 | 38 | 447 | 48 |
| Maine | 169 | 118 | 70 | 13 | 7 | 38 | 22 | 51 | 30 |
| Maryland | 588 | 363 | 62 | 64 | 11 | 161 | 27 | 225 | 38 |
| Massachusetts | 433 | 215 | 50 | 65 | 15 | 153 | 35 | 218 | 50 |
| Michigan | 1,382 | 876 | 63 | 109 | 8 | 397 | 29 | 506 | 37 |
| Minnesota | 625 | 370 | 59 | 48 | 8 | 207 | 33 | 255 | 41 |
| Mississippi | 949 | 570 | 60 | 89 | 9 | 289 | 30 | 379 | 40 |
| Missouri | 1,157 | 646 | 56 | 124 | 11 | 387 | 33 | 511 | 44 |
| Montana | 237 | 127 | 54 | 18 | 8 | 92 | 39 | 110 | 46 |
| Nebraska | 276 | 173 | 63 | 33 | 12 | 70 | 25 | 103 | 37 |
| Nevada | 323 | 178 | 55 | 32 | 10 | 112 | 35 | 145 | 45 |
| New Hampshire | 126 | 77 | 61 | 9 | 7 | 40 | 31 | 49 | 39 |
| New Jersey | 731 | 412 | 56 | 88 | 12 | 231 | 32 | 319 | 44 |
| New Mexico | 430 | 225 | 52 | 46 | 11 | 159 | 37 | 205 | 48 |
| New York | 1,458 | 1,039 | 71 | 126 | 9 | 293 | 20 | 419 | 29 |
| North Carolina | 1,472 | 949 | 64 | 103 | 7 | 419 | 28 | 523 | 36 |
| North Dakota | 86 | 45 | 52 | 5 | 6 | 36 | 42 | 41 | 48 |
| Ohio | 1,351 | 835 | 62 | 105 | 8 | 411 | 30 | 516 | 38 |
| Oklahoma | 652 | 431 | 66 | 53 | 8 | 169 | 26 | 221 | 34 |
| Oregon | 451 | 263 | 58 | 56 | 12 | 132 | 29 | 188 | 42 |
| Pennsylvania | 1,520 | 902 | 59 | 107 | 7 | 511 | 34 | 618 | 41 |
| Rhode Island | 80 | 39 | 49 | 10 | 12 | 31 | 38 | 41 | 51 |
| South Carolina | 1,065 | 643 | 60 | 94 | 9 | 329 | 31 | 422 | 40 |
| South Dakota | 173 | 92 | 53 | 15 | 9 | 66 | 38 | 81 | 47 |
| Tennessee | 1,306 | 795 | 61 | 112 | 9 | 399 | 31 | 511 | 39 |
| Texas | 3,769 | 1,871 | 50 | 448 | 12 | 1,450 | 38 | 1,898 | 50 |
| Utah | 373 | 284 | 76 | 21 | 6 | 68 | 18 | 89 | 24 |
| Vermont | 79 | 48 | 61 | 4 | 5 | 27 | 34 | 31 | 39 |
| Virginia | 930 | 589 | 63 | 85 | 9 | 257 | 28 | 341 | 37 |
| Washington | 632 | 357 | 56 | 59 | 9 | 217 | 34 | 275 | 44 |
| West Virginia | 410 | 235 | 57 | 26 | 6 | 149 | 36 | 175 | 43 |
| Wisconsin | 799 | 454 | 57 | 57 | 7 | 288 | 36 | 345 | 43 |
| Wyoming | 152 | 107 | 70 | 6 | 4 | 40 | 26 | 45 | 30 |
| **U.S. total** | **41,821** | **25,168** | **60** | **3,761** | **9** | **12,892** | **31** | **16,653** | **40** |
| Puerto Rico | 566 | 289 | 51 | 73 | 13 | 203 | 36 | 277 | 49 |

*Note:* Percentages are calculated from unrounded data. Totals may not equal sum of components due to independent rounding. BAC = blood alcohol concentration.

*Source:* National Center for Statistics and Analysis of the National Highway Traffic Safety Administration www.nhtsa.gov.

- Dissension and disharmony in the community and workplace
- Decreased productivity
- Job loss, discharge, and wage garnishment
- Skyrocketing benefit costs (insurance)

Figure 13.3 shows the percentages of various societal problems that are alcohol-related. An estimated 25% of all people admitted to general hospitals have drinking problems. Moderate to heavy alcohol consumption is a major risk factor in injury and trauma. Ten percent of all deaths in the United States are linked to alcohol, including those caused by illness, accidents, and homicide.

Alcohol use is associated closely with violent crimes. When people are under the influence of alcohol, their reasoning and judgment are impaired, so they more often resort to aggressive behavior and violence. In about half of all homicides and serious assaults, and a high percentage of sex-related crimes, robberies, and domestic violence incidents, alcohol is found in the offender, the victim, or both.

Alcohol is used all too often to anesthetize the thinking processes—to try to block out pain, fears, unpleasant thoughts, and feelings of inadequacy, loneliness, and low self-esteem. In addition, people may use alcohol as a crutch to escape problems associated with the family, job, and social relationships.

Alcohol can have detrimental psychological consequences by altering feelings, perceptions, and moods. Many drinkers do not realize that alcohol is a depressant. Individuals with low self-esteem may turn unpleasant feelings and anger toward themselves. Alcohol often is a factor in suicide attempts, vandalism, police involvement, and property damage.

In recent years, alcohol has been the drug of choice of high school and college students. Both groups are showing an increase in **binge drinking** (five or more drinks in a row for men and four or more in a row for women). Binge drinkers tend to be white males under 25 years of age, college students, "party animals," members of Greek organizations, and athletes. The consequences of excessive drinking affect virtually every college campus, college community, and college student. Other statistics on college binge drinking are given in Table 13.4. Today's college student, on the average, spends more money on alcohol than on books. Drinking alcohol is a factor in about 28% of college dropouts. Of the approximately 12.5 million college students in the United States, an estimated 4% will die from alcohol-related causes.

## PHYSICAL EFFECTS OF DRINKING ALCOHOL

Alcohol is not a nutrient. It is not digested. However, it is partially broken down in the stomach. The alcohol consumed is absorbed into the bloodstream quickly through the stomach wall and small intestine. Absorption is influenced by several factors such as the concentration of alcohol in the beverage, quantity consumed, rate of consumption, amount of food in the stomach, carbonation of the beverage or mixer, age, sex, and body weight.

The larger the body, the lower the concentration of alcohol in the blood will be. Individuals with more body weight have more body fluid, which disperses the alcohol consumed in a larger volume of blood. Therefore, they will not become intoxicated as rapidly as individuals who weigh less and consume the same amount of alcohol at the same rate. Figure 13.4 shows the BAC related to body weight.

Women and men respond differently to alcohol. Women have smaller quantities of the enzymes in the

**FIGURE 13.3 ▶** Societal Effects of Alcohol Abuse

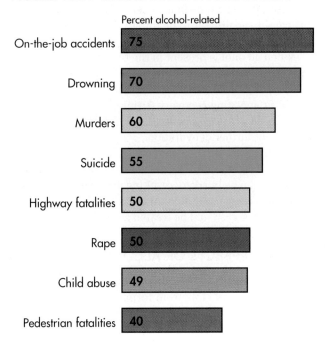

Percent alcohol-related

| | |
|---|---|
| On-the-job accidents | 75 |
| Drowning | 70 |
| Murders | 60 |
| Suicide | 55 |
| Highway fatalities | 50 |
| Rape | 50 |
| Child abuse | 49 |
| Pedestrian fatalities | 40 |

**TABLE 13.4 ▶** Binge Drinking by College Students

| DRINKING ACTIVITY | MEN | WOMEN |
|---|---|---|
| Drank on 10 or more occasions in the past 30 days | 24% | 13% |
| Usually binges when drinks | 43 | 38 |
| Drinks to get drunk | 44 | 35 |
| Was drunk three or more times in the past month | 28 | 19 |

*Source:* The National Alcohol Study conducted by Harvard University, School of Public Health, 1999.

### KEY TERMS

**Binge drinking** consuming five or more drinks consecutively for men and four consecutively for women

**FIGURE 13.4 ▶** Blood Alcohol Concentration Related to Body Weight

| Number of drinks | Body weight | | | | | | | |
|---|---|---|---|---|---|---|---|---|
| | 100–119 | 120–139 | 140–159 | 160–179 | 180–199 | 200–219 | 220–239 | 240 > |
| 10 | .38 | .31 | .27 | .23 | .21 | .19 | .17 | .16 |
| 9 | .34 | .28 | .24 | .21 | .19 | .17 | .15 | .14 |
| 8 | .30 | .25 | .21 | .19 | .17 | .15 | .14 | .13 |
| 7 | .26 | .22 | .19 | .16 | .15 | .13 | .12 | .11 |
| 6 | .23 | .19 | .16 | .14 | .13 | .11 | .10 | .09 |
| 5 | .19 | .16 | .13 | .12 | .11 | .09 | .09 | .08 |
| 4 | .15 | .12 | .11 | .09 | .08 | .08 | .07 | .06 |
| 3 | .11 | .09 | .08 | .07 | .06 | .06 | .05 | .05 |
| 2 | .08 | .06 | .05 | .05 | .04 | .04 | .03 | .03 |
| 1 | .04 | .03 | .03 | .02 | .02 | .02 | .02 | .02 |

Blood alcohol concentration

▮ Reasonably safe      ▯ Unsafe      ▮ Illegal in all states

stomach tissue that aid in breaking down alcohol. This translates to women's absorbing 30% more alcohol into their bloodstream than men. This is a main reason for a higher incidence of liver damage among women drinkers than men drinkers. Alcohol also interferes with the absorption of some major nutrients and minerals, especially calcium, in women. As menopausal and older women start to lose calcium, this loss causes bones to become brittle and thin (osteoporosis). In addition, women taking oral contraceptives remain inebriated longer. Their bodies metabolize alcohol more slowly than women who are not on the pill.

In males, metabolism of alcohol by the liver produces a chemical substance that speeds destruction of testosterone. Sex problems such as erectile dysfunction (ED) and testicle atrophy are common in heavy drinkers.

In addition, absorption may be influenced by body chemistry, emotions, and individual tolerance. When the liver becomes more efficient in metabolizing alcohol, because of repeated consumption, the body becomes more tolerant. As more alcohol is consumed and metabolized, more alcohol is needed to get the desired effect (buzz) one received initially.

**The Hangover.** For some people a **hangover** follows excessive drinking. It clearly signals to the drinker the unpleasant side effects associated with overindulging. Symptoms vary from one person to another. They include a throbbing headache, slurred speech, gastritis, nausea, vomiting, poor circulation, dizziness, thirst, irritability, fatigue, and mental depression. Alcohol acts as a **diuretic,** speeding the elimination of fluid from the body. This causes the drinker to be thirsty and dehydrated after drinking excessively.

When alcohol is present in the bloodstream, recovering from a hangover takes time. Showering, taking aspirin, and drinking coffee or more alcoholic beverages will not aid in speeding recovery. Drinking plenty of water, however, can restore needed body fluids more quickly and prevent further dehydration.

Passing out after excessive consumption can be extremely dangerous. If a person vomits while unconscious, the airway can be blocked, resulting in death. Obstruction of the air passage and alcohol intoxication are medical emergencies and should be treated as such.

## CHRONIC EFFECTS OF ALCOHOL USE

Because alcohol thins the blood, moderate drinking may help prevent blood clots from forming. A member of the American Medical Association opined via radio that 31,000 more people would die yearly in the United States

## FYI | MIXING ALCOHOL AND MEDICINES

Sometimes alcohol increases the effects and the risks of a medicine to potentially dangerous levels. About 100 prescription medicines can produce unwanted effects when mixed with alcohol.

| Analgesic pain medication | Effects |
| --- | --- |
| ■ Salicylates (aspirin) | Stomach and |
| ■ Ibuprofen (Advil, Motrin) | intestinal bleeding, bleeding ulcers |

| Antidiabetic agents | |
| --- | --- |
| ■ Chlorpropamide (Diabinese) | Altered control of blood sugar, |
| ■ Tolbutamide (Orinase) | most often hypoglycemia |
| ■ Insulin | |

| Barbiturates | |
| --- | --- |
| ■ Secobarbital (Seconal) | Greater sedative effect, drowsiness, |
| ■ Phenobarbital (Barbita) | confusion |
| ■ Pentobarbital (Nembutal) | |

| Benzodiazepines | |
| --- | --- |
| ■ Alprazolam (Xanax) | Greater sedative effect, impaired |
| ■ Diazepam (Valium) | motor |
| ■ Triazolam (Halcion) | coordination (such as driving ability) |

| Monoamine oxidase (MAO) inhibitors | |
| --- | --- |
| ■ Isocarboxazid (Marplan) | Certain alcoholic beverages contain |
| ■ Phenelzine (Nardil) | tyramine, which can cause severe |
| ■ Tranylcypromine (Parnate) | high blood pressure; may be fatal |

*Source:* Adapted from National Council on Patient Information and Education, 666 Eleventh St. N.W., Suite 810, Washington, DC.

on alcohol. As drinking opportunities are presented, drinking episodes occur more frequently and periods of intoxication lengthen. Excessive drinking may cause the drinker not to be able to recall what happened the day before or recall events in which the drinker was physically present. This is called a **blackout,** or temporary amnesia. The person rationalizes drinking behavior, physical problems, destruction of peer and family relationships, and encounters with law enforcement personnel.

The following are signals that drinking has become excessive and that the person may be an alcoholic.

- **Secret drinking.** Alcoholics sneak drinks so other people will not know how much they are drinking.
- **Guilt feelings about drinking.** Alcoholics realize they have lost control over drinking and start to rationalize drinking behavior, feel remorseful, and avoid any discussion about alcohol.
- **Gulping the first few drinks.** Alcoholics want a quick buzz, so they quickly gulp down the first drinks. They want the effects as soon as possible.
- **Periods of total abstinence.** Occasionally alcoholics go "on the wagon." They do not drink for some time. This reassures them that they can take it or leave it. Most will resume drinking.
- **Hiding bottles.** Alcoholics want to be certain they will not run out of alcohol.
- **Neglecting proper nutrition.** Alcoholics do not eat properly. They have little interest in food because alcohol is a substantial portion of their dietary intake.
- **Effects on family and friends.** In some cases family and friends become embarrassed because of the alcoholic's behavior. Family members may change their socialization patterns.
- **Decrease in sexual drive.** Alcohol is a depressant drug, so it represses sexual drive and sexual activity along with other functions.

As alcohol consumption becomes more excessive, the individual develops a drug dependency, losing control over drinking. Chronic alcohol consumption lowers resistance

### KEY TERMS

**Hangover** effects associated with consuming excessive amounts of alcohol

**Diuretic** any drug that speeds up elimination of salts and water from kidneys and other body organs

**Alcoholism** chronic, progressive condition of dependence on alcohol characterized by consumption above social and controllable limits

**Blackout** inability to remember recent events when drinking

of cardiovascular disease if Americans would become teetotalers. Many studies have found that people who drink moderately reduce their risk of dying from heart disease by about 40%.

**Alcoholism** is apparent when consumption of alcoholic beverages is no longer merely social or controllable. Its use exceeds social norms and results in inappropriate drinking patterns. The user becomes physically dependent

to disease; damages the liver, the cardiovascular system, and the central nervous system; and causes severe nutritional deficiencies that lead to further problems. Prolonged heavy drinking is also linked to increased risks of cancer of the bladder, mouth, stomach, and esophagus.

Figure 13.5 illustrates parts of the body affected by long-term alcohol use. Eleven of the more common alcohol-related disorders are listed below.

1. **Malnutrition** occurs when prolonged consumption of alcohol depresses the appetite and attacks the mucosa in the stomach. Heavy drinkers often do not obtain the needed calories. Without needed nutrients the alcohol depresses protein synthesis, interferes with the transfer of glucose into energy, increases mineral loss, and increases fatty acids.

2. **Alcoholic pellagra** is caused by a deficiency of protein and niacin. Symptoms of alcoholic pellagra are gastrointestinal disorders, mental and nervous disturbances, inflammation of the skin (dermatitis), and diarrhea.

3. Alcohol affects the heart and blood vessels by increasing the heart rate and constricting the arterial blood flow to the heart. Prolonged, excessive drinking can weaken the heart and contribute to cardiomyopathy, a disease of the heart muscle. In addition, excessive drinking can cause abnormal heart rhythms and heart failure. Alcoholics also tend to have higher blood pressure, which can lead to stroke (brain attack).

4. Alcohol causes blood vessels in the kidneys to dilate. This in turn produces an increase in urine output. An acute effect is dehydration. Prolonged and excessive use of alcohol can cause irreversible damage to the kidneys.

5. Combined cigarette smoking and alcohol drinking enhance the development of cancers of the oral cavity, larynx, esophagus, and pancreas.

6. The following liver disorders and diseases are common in heavy drinkers.

   a. **Hepatotoxic trauma,** commonly termed "fatty liver" (90%–100% of heavy drinkers show evidence of fatty liver), is reversible if the person stops drinking.

   b. **Alcoholic hepatitis,** a chronic inflammation of the liver tissue, develops in 10%–35% of heavy drinkers. Alcoholic hepatitis is often fatal.

**FIGURE 13.5 ▶** Effects of Alcohol Use

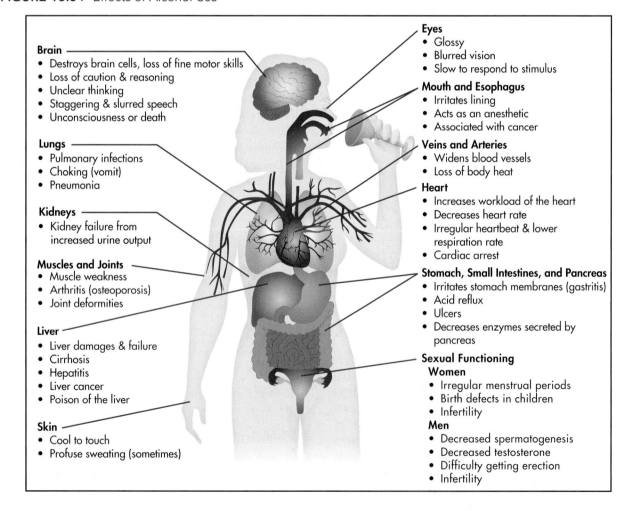

■ Reduce death and injuries caused by alcohol- and drug-related motor vehicle crashes.

■ Increase the age and proportion of adolescents who remain alcohol- and drug-free.

■ Reduce the proportion of persons engaging in binge drinking of alcohol beverages.

■ Reduce average annual alcohol consumption.

■ Reduce the proportion of adults who exceed guidelines.

---

**c. Alcoholic cirrhosis** occurs in 10%–20% of heavy drinkers and is characterized by scarring, shriveling, and hardening of the liver tissue. The scar tissue replaces functioning liver cells and blocks the flow of blood to cells that are still alive. This impairs liver functioning and the metabolism of alcohol.

7. Chronic alcohol consumption affects the central nervous system mainly because prolonged drinking depresses the appetite. When drinkers do not take in needed nutrients, they are predisposed to several neurological conditions.

   **a. Wernicke's disease** is caused by a thiamine deficiency. Symptoms include rapid, involuntary oscillation of the eyeballs and double vision, severe decrease in mental functioning, and lack of muscular coordination.

   **b. Polyneuritis** is another condition caused by thiamine deficiency. It is characterized by inflammation of several peripheral and central nerves, which causes the drinker to become weak and have tingling sensations.

   **c. Korsakoff's syndrome** is caused by a deficiency of B-complex vitamins, specifically $B_{12}$ and thiamine. Symptoms of this type of psychosis include severe amnesia, loss of contact with reality, and personality alterations. The person is apathetic and has difficulty walking.

   **d. Alcoholic hallucinosis** is a mental disorder characterized by seeing images (pink elephants, snakes, spiders), mood disturbances, and alcohol-related depression.

8. Chronic alcohol use alters the hormones that regulate the pituitary, hypothalamus, and the gonads (ovaries and testes). This can cause men to have lower levels of testosterone, shrinking testicles, loss of facial hair, low sex drive, erectile dysfunction, and infertility. Women may encounter menstrual disturbances, atrophying ovaries, and infertility.

9. A small amount of ethyl alcohol stimulates stomach activity. Alcohol can irritate the mouth, throat, esoph-

agus, stomach, small intestines, and pancreas. Two common gastrointestinal disorders in alcoholics are **gastritis** and **gastric ulcers.**

10. Fetal Alcohol Spectrum Disorders (FASD). FASD is an umbrella term describing the range of effects that can occur in and individual whose mother drank alcohol during pregnancy. These effects may include physical, mental, behavioral, and/or learning disabilities with possible lifelong implications. FASD refers to conditons such as **fetal alcohol syndrome (FAS),**

---

### KEY TERMS

**Malnutrition** effects on body due to prolonged deficiency of necessary nutrients

**Alcoholic pellagra** condition caused by deficiency of protein and niacin due to prolonged alcohol consumption

**Hepatotoxic trauma** disease of the liver caused by alcoholism; commonly called fatty liver

**Alcoholic hepatitis** chronic inflammation of the liver tissue caused by alcohol drinking

**Alcoholic cirrhosis** scarring, shriveling, and hardening of liver tissue resulting from chronic alcohol consumption

**Wernicke's disease** syndrome caused by thiamine deficiency resulting from excessive alcohol

**Polyneuritis** inflammation of several peripheral and central nerves caused by thiamine deficiency attributable to alcoholism

**Korsakoff's syndrome** psychosis caused by deficiency of B vitamins resulting from alcoholism

**Alcoholic hallucinosis** mental disorder characterized by mental disorientation and mood disturbance

**Gastritis** chronic inflammation of the stomach lining that is common in alcoholics

**Gastric ulcers** chronic inflammation of the lower end of the esophagus and the stomach

**Fetal alcohol syndrome (FAS)** group of physical and behavioral defects in a newborn caused by the mother's alcohol use during pregnancy

**fetal alcohol effects (FAE),** alcohol-related neurodevelopmental disorder (ARND), and alcohol-related birth defects (ARBD). Each year, as many as 40,000 babies are born with FASD, costing the nation about $4 billion.

11. Alcoholics are 21 times more likely than nonalcoholics to receive a diagnosis of antisocial personality disorder. The rates are four and six times higher for schizophrenia and mania, respectively. Between 35% and 50% of alcoholics have panic disorders. In addition, alcoholism often is associated with bulimia, depression, and overuse of other drugs, including sedatives, hallucinogens, stimulants, and marijuana.

## ALCOHOL ABUSE DISORDERS

Data presented by the Agency for Healthcare Research and Quality indicates that U.S. community hospitals treated nearly 210,000 patients for alcohol abuse disorders in 2003 at a cost of about $2 billion. In addition, more than 1 million patients admitted for other reasons also had diagnoses of alcohol abuse and approximately 3% of all hospital stays had some mention of the problem.

Overall, 65% of all hospital admissions due primarily to alcohol abuse disorders also involved a substance abuse disorder; 34.4% involved mood disorders such as depression or bipolar disorder; 11.5% included alcohol-related liver disease; and 8.7% included anxiety disorders.

These and additional data were drawn from hospitals that comprise 90% of all discharges in the United States.

## TREATMENT, INTERVENTION, AND PREVENTION PROGRAMS

An estimated 18 million American adults currently have problems as a result of alcohol overconsumption and approximately 610,000 seek some type of treatment yearly. The success of any treatment approach depends upon the alcohol-dependent person and his or her goal of total abstinence. The alcoholic must desire and be willing to stop drinking. He or she must take the first step. Treatment may consist of detoxification, drug therapy, psychotherapy, nutrient supplements, and ongoing maintenance.

- *Detoxification.* In most cases the first step in treatment and rehabilitation of alcoholism is detoxification, a process of removing toxic substances from the body. During this period certain drugs are given to prevent the patient from having convulsions. In addition, vitamins are administered to increase the appetite, and the person is given a highly nutritious diet so the body organs will receive proper nutrients and start to heal from damage that may have occurred during the drinking period.

- *Drug therapy.* Several drugs have been used in treating alcoholism. Once the patient has been detoxed,

tranquilizers are given for several weeks to decrease symptoms associated with agitation, anxiety, and tremors. Naltrexone is a drug that works by blocking the craving for alcohol and also the pleasure derived from drinking alcohol. It blocks opioid receptors in the brain, eliminating the feel-good effects. In clinical trials naltrexone combined with behavior modification enabled as many as three-fourths of alcoholics to avoid a relapse. However, naltrexone has a serious drawback: alcoholics must remember to take it every day. Now there is new hope. Vivitrol (naltrexone) is an extended-release injection that is administered once-monthly and cuts heavy drinking by up to 48%. It was approved by the FDA in April 2006. In aversion therapy the prescription drug disulfiram (Antabuse) is administered. This drug blocks the metabolism of acetaldehyde. If the patient takes Antabuse and drinks alcohol, the combination causes extremely unpleasant reactions such as breathing difficulty, intense headache, nausea, vomiting, and pounding heart.

- *Psychotherapy.* Psychotherapy is as individualized as the personality. It can be effective for some alcoholics by helping the person discover or uncover an underlying conflict that is contributing to or has precipitated the drinking behavior. Most psychotherapists include the family in therapy, as successful treatment may depend upon understanding and support from family members.

- *Nutrient supplements.* Some supplements that may be helpful in the treatment of alcoholism are vitamin A, vitamin $B_1$, vitamin $B_2$, vitamin $B_6$, vitamin $B_{12}$, choline, folic acid, niacin, pangamic acid, pantothenic acid, vitamin C, vitamin E, vitamin K, vitamin D, iron, magnesium, chromium, zinc, unsaturated fatty acids, manganese, and glutamine. Uses of nutrient supplements should be monitored by a healthcare provider.

## ORGANIZATIONS DEALING WITH ALCOHOLISM

Alcoholics Anonymous (AA) is a well-organized, long-established, supportive fellowship of alcohol-dependent people. Their sole purpose is to get sober and remain sober. Members decide to turn over their lives and will to a power greater than themselves. They have to desire to stop drinking, admit they are unable to stop drinking and need help, and be honest with themselves. AA has at least 19,000 affiliated groups and more than 35,000 members across the United States.

Al-Anon and Alateen are organizations that help families cope with alcohol-dependent family members. Al-Anon is for mates and other relatives. The family members are encouraged and supported by other families. They learn that they are not alone. Alateen is a supportive organization for teenagers of alcoholic parents.

Additional organizations that are helpful and supportive include the Salvation Army, Women for Sobriety, the national Institute on Alcohol Abuse and Alcoholism, university organizations, and the National Council on Alcoholism. Work-based and church-based programs are available.

# Tobacco Use

**Tobacco** is a plant, *Nicotiana tabacum* or *Nicotiana rustica*, grown in the United States and other countries. Although the Native Americans harvested and used tobacco years before introducing it to European explorers, Jean Nicot of France is credited with popularizing tobacco uses in 1559. Nicot tested tobacco on people and reported that it cured migraine headaches, other persistent headaches, and colds. His reports and the number of aristocrats praising and using the drug in France caused its use to spread rapidly. By 1565 the plant had been named nicotiana, with the active ingredient isolated and called nicotine in 1828.

The leaves of the tobacco plant are dried and processed into cigarettes, cigars, and pipe tobacco for smoking. Strips of leaves are processed to make chewing tobacco, and the leaf is pulverized into a fine powder to make snuff. Cigarette smoking is the most popular use of tobacco.

**Clove cigarettes** are used by teenagers and young adults. Although some people assume that these cigarettes are made entirely of cloves, they contain about 40% cloves and about 60% tobacco. Their levels of tar, nicotine, and carbon monoxide are even higher than regular cigarettes. The active ingredient in cloves, **eugenol** (oral anesthetic), has a numbing effect in the back of the throat that enables users to inhale the smoke more deeply.

Another cigarette, which has been popular in India for centuries, is being used by teens and young adults in the United States. **Bidis**, skinny, sweet-flavored clove look-alikes sold in various flavors, are prepared with unprocessed tobacco and are more potent than regular cigarettes. A bidi's smoke differs from regular cigarette smoke in that it contains more potent amounts of nicotine, tar, carbon monoxide, and other toxic substances and gases. Bidis are used more by young African-Americans and Hispanics than whites.

> **VIEWPOINT** *Approximately one-half of smokers believe that smoking helps to control weight. A common belief among smokers is that smoking cessation may cause weight gain. Oftentimes this will deter smokers from making attempts to stop. Research has shown that the average weight gain with cessation of smoking is eight pounds. Which is less hazardous to your health, an eight-pound weight gain or smoking?*
> **What is your opinion?**

Tobacco product manufacturers are claiming to produce safer cigarettes/cigarette products—Eclipse and Accord—with fewer chemicals and carcinogens and reduced secondhand smoke. Other such products are being developed. Not smoking is the healthiest alternative.

Strong pressure is placed on individuals, especially through the media, to smoke and to use tobacco products. Tobacco companies spend more than $2 billion each year to promote their products. Many of the tobacco companies produce ads displaying beautiful, handsome, well-dressed, athletic models. In truth, physical attractiveness is far removed from the realities of smoking and its effects.

## WHY PEOPLE USE TOBACCO

Reasons for using tobacco vary widely. Some reasons include genetics, familial influence, weight control, stress (coping response), low self-esteem, and social influence. Persons who are less educated are more likely to smoke. The initial experimentation often is associated with peer influence. Many young tobacco users admit their reasons include the need to be accepted, the idea of looking and feeling mature, and acting out a tough, iconoclastic, rebellious role.

The American Cancer Society conducted a survey of smokers, which indicated that nine of 10 smokers would like to quit. Smokers quickly find out that quitting is difficult, even if he or she has smoked a short time. A major reason for continuing to use tobacco is dependency and addiction to the nicotine that is found in all tobacco products. For whatever reason a person uses tobacco, it is hazardous to the health of the user, nonusers, and the environment.

## PREVALENCE OF SMOKING

The Centers for Disease Control (CDC) has reported that an estimated 46.5 million adults in the United States smoke cigarettes, even though this single behavior will

### KEY TERMS

**Fetal alcohol effects (FAE)** aberrant behavior patterns in newborns resulting from the mother's alcohol consumption during pregnancy

**Tobacco** plant (*Nicotiana tobacun* or *Nicotiana rustica*) with leaves that are dried and processed for smoking

**Clove cigarettes** cigarettes containing about 40% cloves, with a numbing ingredient, eugenol

**Eugenol** (oral anesthetic), has a numbing effect in the back of the throat that enables users to inhale the smoke more deeply

**Bidis** skinny, sweet-flavored clove look-alikes sold in various flavors, prepared with unprocessed tobacco, and more potent than regular cigarettes

result in death or disability for half of all regular users. Cigarette smoking is responsible for more than 400,000 deaths each year, or one in every five deaths. Additionally, if current patterns of smoking continue, over 5 million people currently younger than 18 will die prematurely from tobacco-related diseases. Coupled with this enormous health toll is the $75 billion in medical expenditures and another $80 billion in indirect costs.

Smokers worldwide spend over $85 to $100 billion annually to buy 4 trillion cigarettes. Over 70,000 Americans were current users of a tobacco product in 2004. Fifty-nine million smoked cigarettes, 137 million smoked cigars, 7.2 million used smokeless tobacco, and 1.8 million smoked tobacco in pipes. (See Figures 13.6 and 13.7.) Thirty-five million Americans age 12 or older met the criteria for nicotine dependence.

In 2004, among persons age 25 and older, 31.4% of whites, 27.3% of blacks, 33.8% American Indians or Alaska Natives, and 23.3% of Hispanics reported that they had used a tobacco product in the past month. Native Americans have a 38% rate of tobacco use, followed by African-American males with 32%. White college students tend to use tobacco more than African Americans, Asian Americans, and Hispanics. Hispanic and Asian American women continue to have the lowest rates of smoking. For survey data on cigarette use by race or ethnicity. See Figure 13.8.

## ADOLESCENT SMOKERS

Adolescent smokers do not understand the power of nicotine. However, they start smoking for various

**FIGURE 13.6** ▶ Past Month Cigarette Use by Age, 2003 and 2004

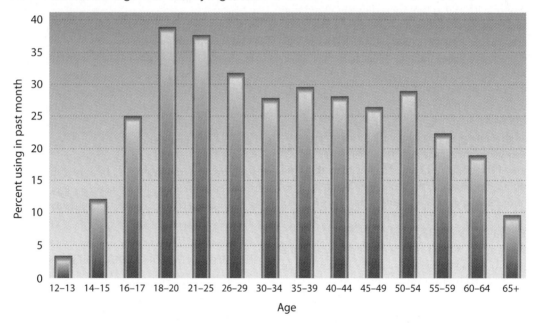

*Source:* Substance Abuse and Mental Health Services Administration, National Household Survey on Drug Abuse, 2003 and 2004.

**FIGURE 13.7** ▶ Past Month Tobacco Use among Persons Age 12 and Older, 2002 and 2003

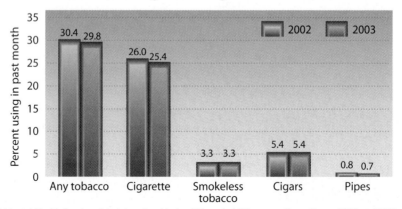

*Source:* Substance Abuse and Mental Health Services Administration, National Household Survey on Drug Abuse, 2003 and 2004.

**FIGURE 13.8** ▶ Past Month Cigarette Use Among Persons Aged 12 and Older, by Race or Ethnicity, 2003 and 2004 Annual Average

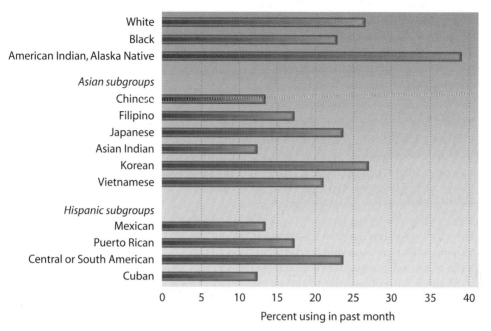

*Source:* Substance Abuse and Mental Health Services Administration, National Household Survey on Drug Abuse, 2003 and 2004.

reasons—stress, acceptance, boredom, depression, loneliness, unmet emotional needs, and fun. The longer they smoke, the more serious the smoking problem becomes. Smoking is especially harmful to the health of developing adolescents. According to Dr. Diane Gold of the Harvard University School of Public Health, smoking as few as five cigarettes per day can reduce lung function growth in both boys and girls. Males aged 12 and older are slightly more likely to smoke cigarettes than females. Adolescent smoking rates differ between whites and African Americans. By the late 1990s smoking rates among white teens were more than triple those of African-American teens. In recent years, smoking has increased among African-American male teens, but African-American female teens continue to have lower smoking rates than white female teens.

## SMOKELESS TOBACCO

Smokeless tobacco use is rising, especially in young males. Using snuff is called "dipping" because the user places a pinch of moist powdered or shredded tobacco between the gums and lower jaw/lip. Then the tobacco juice is extracted, and the user spits it out and dips again. Chewing tobacco contains forms of loose tobacco leaves. The user tears a wad off and places it in the cheek. After chewing, the used wad (quid) is discarded, and the cycle continues.

Many users believe smokeless tobacco is safer than cigarettes. Actually, the former is at least as dangerous,

because this powdered form releases more of its chemicals in the mouth. Further, it is extremely addictive, as the amount of nicotine in a dip is about two to three times that in a cigarette. Smokeless tobacco also releases cancer-causing tobacco-specific nitrosamines. The smokeless tobacco user often experiences tissue changes in the mouth, or **leukoplakia** (whitening, thickening, and hardening of the tissue), which is a precancerous lesion. Long-term snuff users have 50% greater risk of developing oral cancer than nonusers because of the nicotine. Each year doctors see 30,000 new cases of oral cancer in the United States.

An estimated 22 million people use chewing tobacco or snuff in the United States, of whom 20% to 40% are adolescent males. One in five high school males uses spit tobacco (12.2% for non-Hispanic whites, 2.2% for non-Hispanic African Americans, and 5.1% for Hispanics), more than half of whom began using it before they were 12 years old.

## CIGARS AND PIPES

Some people smoke cigars or pipes, often in the mistaken belief that these forms are safer than cigarette smoking.

**KEY TERMS**

**Leukoplakia** condition in which tissue in the oral cavity turns white, thickens, and hardens; a common effect of smokeless tobacco

## FYI FACTS ABOUT TOBACCO USE

- Men (28%) are more likely to smoke than women (23%).
- American Indians have the highest smoking rate of any ethnic group (39%).
- Men age 25 and older who dropped out of high school have the highest smoking rate of any group (42%).
- A third of all high school freshmen smoke.
- Smoking by African-American boys has doubled since 1991.

Cigar smoking, in particular, has seen a resurgence recently. In both cigar and pipe smoking, nicotine is absorbed through the gums and lining of the mouth. If the user inhales, the smoke is more damaging to the lungs than cigarette smoke, causing higher rates of cardiovascular and respiratory diseases than cigarette smoke. In either case, cigar and pipe users have increased risks for cancers of the mouth, lip, throat, and esophagus.

**VIEWPOINT** *A number of retired major league baseball players are banding together to convey the message to U.S. youth that spit tobacco is harmful. Former St. Louis Cardinals catcher Joe Garagiola says he feels particularly motivated because "baseball has become identified with scratching and spitting." Baseball Hall of Fame member Hank Aaron says, "Kids see athletes using this stuff. That can have a devastating effect on young people."* **What is your opinion? Do you feel that some athletes who publicly use smokeless tobacco are conveying a negative message to youth?**

## COMPONENTS OF TOBACCO

**Nicotine.** Tobacco contains more than 4,000 elements or compounds and toxic substances. Forty-three of these substances cause cancer. Figure 13.9 shows the proportional amounts of chemicals in smoke. The one that makes it addictive is **nicotine.** Nicotine is thought to be among the most addictive of all substances. Nicotine addiction has both physical and psychological aspects. Initially it acts as a stimulant, giving the user a brief kick. It can increase the heart rate by up to 25 beats per minute. The first cigarette of the day can raise the heart rate by 10 to 20 beats per minute and blood pressure by five to 10 points as the blood vessels constrict. In addition, nicotine decreases HDL (good) cholesterol levels, steps up the

**FIGURE 13.9 ▶** Composition of Cigarette Smoke

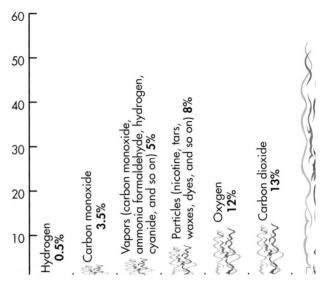

release of glycogen by the liver, slightly deadens the taste buds and the sense of smell, causes halitosis (bad breath), weakens tooth enamel, and causes dry throat and hoarseness. It paralyzes cilia (tiny hairs in the bronchial tubes), preventing them from sweeping out the bacteria and dust and dirt particles from the lungs, and thereby lowering immunity to diseases.

Nicotine causes irritation and inflammation of the walls of cardiac arteries, which eventually produces scar tissue. As the arterial lining becomes thicker, less blood travels to the heart. This can cause the blood flow to become blocked, causing a heart attack.

Withdrawal from nicotine has physical symptoms, including headaches, muscle aches, cramps, nausea, and visual disturbances. Physical withdrawal takes about a week while nicotine is being flushed from the body via the kidneys. The first three or four days are most difficult.

The psychological component of nicotine addiction is more difficult to pin down but equally problematic. Psychological withdrawal can last years, although the first two or three months are most critical. Tobacco seems to have dual stimulating and antianxiety or tranquilizing properties. For example, while intense anxiety is the most prevalent symptom of withdrawal, sleepiness also is common. These seemingly contradictory properties of nicotine compound the difficulty of psychological withdrawal.

**Gases and Vapors.** Among the more than 4,000 elements, compounds, and toxic chemicals in cigarette smoke are the gases nitrogen, carbon monoxide, carbon dioxide, acetone, vinyl chloride, hydrogen cyanide, formaldehyde, and ammonia. **Carbon monoxide,** an extremely poisonous gas in tobacco smoke, is the same gas that is emitted from auto exhausts. When the smoker inhales carbon monoxide, it combines with the hemoglobin of red blood cells. This reduces the red blood cells' capacity to carry oxygen to major organs such as the brain and heart. Carbon monoxide also decreases visual acuity, more specifically at night.

**FIGURE 13.10** ▶ Health Effects of Smoking Cigarettes

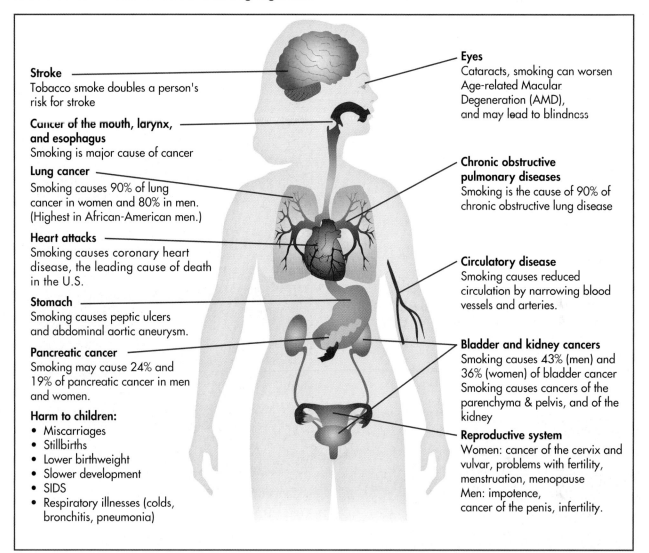

**Stroke**
Tobacco smoke doubles a person's risk for stroke

**Cancer of the mouth, larynx, and esophagus**
Smoking is major cause of cancer

**Lung cancer**
Smoking causes 90% of lung cancer in women and 80% in men. (Highest in African-American men.)

**Heart attacks**
Smoking causes coronary heart disease, the leading cause of death in the U.S.

**Stomach**
Smoking causes peptic ulcers and abdominal aortic aneurysm.

**Pancreatic cancer**
Smoking may cause 24% and 19% of pancreatic cancer in men and women.

**Harm to children:**
• Miscarriages
• Stillbirths
• Lower birthweight
• Slower development
• SIDS
• Respiratory illnesses (colds, bronchitis, pneumonia)

**Eyes**
Cataracts, smoking can worsen Age-related Macular Degeneration (AMD), and may lead to blindness

**Chronic obstructive pulmonary diseases**
Smoking is the cause of 90% of chronic obstructive lung disease

**Circulatory disease**
Smoking causes reduced circulation by narrowing blood vessels and arteries.

**Bladder and kidney cancers**
Smoking causes 43% (men) and 36% (women) of bladder cancer Smoking causes cancers of the parenchyma & pelvis, and of the kidney

**Reproductive system**
Women: cancer of the cervix and vulvar, problems with fertility, menstruation, menopause
Men: impotence, cancer of the penis, infertility.

**Tobacco Tar.** Tobacco **tar** is composed of particles that form a yellowish-brown sticky residue on hands, ashtrays, and lungs. When smokers inhale, these particles remain in the lungs. Among the carcinogenic (cancer-causing) substances in tar are **nitrosamines,** pyrenes, chrysenes, phenols, and cresols. Tar contributes to cancers of the lung, oral cavity, and others.

When smokers inhale tar into the lungs, carcinogenic components are dispersed into the bloodstream. In smokeless tobacco, carcinogens in the tar and nicotine are absorbed through the mucous membrane lining of the mouth or digestive system and passed to the bloodstream.

## ADVERSE EFFECTS OF TOBACCO

Tobacco use is responsible for more than 400,000 adult deaths in the United States each year. This is more than the number of Americans who died in World War II, and more than those who die from AIDS, multiple sclerosis, diabetes, accidents, gunshot wounds, and breast and prostate cancers combined. Medical costs related to smoking total approximately $50 billion per year. Smoking accounts for 87% of all deaths from lung cancer and 30% of all deaths from cancer. It is the cause of 40% of preventable deaths and 30% of all adult early deaths. Since 1965, female deaths have been rising due to increased smoking. The health effects of smoking are depicted in Figure 13.10.

### KEY TERMS

**Nicotine** addictive chemical component found in tobacco

**Carbon monoxide** extremely poisonous gas in tobacco smoke

**Tar** yellowish-brown sticky residue in tobacco that causes cancer

**Nitrosamines** cancer-causing substances that are found in tobacco

The facts are clear.

■ Cigarette smoking is a major cause of cancers of the lung, larynx, oral cavity, and esophagus and a contributing cause in cancers of the bladder, pancreas, and kidney.

■ Smoking increases the risk of lung cancer more than 10-fold.

■ Lung cancer risk increases steadily with the number of cigarettes smoked per day. In those who smoke 40 or more cigarettes a day (two or more packs), the rate of lung cancer is 12–25 times the rate for nonsmokers.

■ The risk of lung cancer is less in people who quit smoking, and the risk decreases as the number of years since quitting increases.

■ Smoking has made lung cancer the No. 1 cancer killer of American women.

■ More than 80% of the current smokers started before age 21.

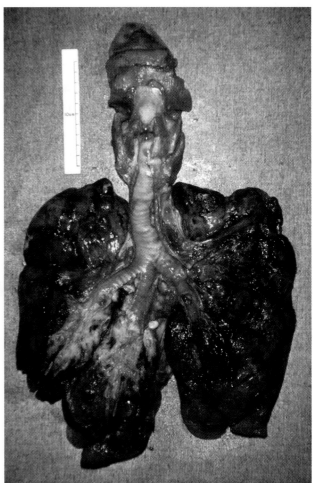

© Medical-on-Line / Alamy

▲ *Cancer of the lung is a frequent result of cigarette smoking*

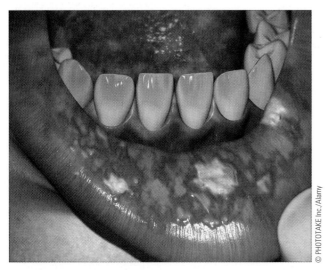

© PHOTOTAKE Inc./Alamy

▲ *Smokeless tobacco was the cause of this squamous cell carcinoma on the lower lip*

Tobacco destroys the lungs, weakens the heart, deadens the esophagus, and damages the kidneys, eyes, bladder, and uterus, according to Dr. Robert Schrier, chairman of medicine at the University of Colorado Health Sciences Center. It may be responsible for 14% of all leukemia and 80% of all laryngeal cancers.

The National Center for Environmental Health reports that smoking may inhibit sexual function. Smokers are more likely than nonsmokers to be impotent.

Smoking may clog the blood vessels in the penis just as it clogs vessels in the rest of the body. The good news is that the impotence may cease after the smoker quits smoking.

According to the American Council on Science and Health, the bone mineral content of women smokers is about 15%–30% less than that of nonsmokers. For men smokers, bone mineral content is about 10%–20% less than that of nonsmokers. This is one reason smoking is a major risk factor for osteoporosis.

**Cancers.** Smoking is the major cause of lung cancer in women and men in the United States. The incidence of lung cancer is closely associated with the length of time one has smoked, the number of cigarettes smoked each day, the accumulation of tar in the lungs, and the amount of gases, tar, and other chemicals that have been inhaled.

African Americans have long been shown to have a 50% higher incidence than do Caucasians of lung cancer and death from the disease. Initial data seem to indicate that African Americans have less capacity to detoxify NNk,

## Tips for Action For Nonsmokers Who Do Not Like Smoke

You can maintain a nonsmoke environment congenially in the following ways.

■ Do not preach, attempt to humiliate, or embarrass the smoker.

■ Do not relate your opinions about smoking. Leave it at the fact that smoke bothers you.

■ If you have a physical ailment that is aggravated by smoking, mention it directly.

■ Be sensitive to the smoker's need to smoke. Consider your own reaction if someone were to ask you to quit something you enjoy or feel compelled to do (overeating, drinking too much, and so on).

■ Be good-natured about asking someone not to smoke in your presence.

■ Thank the smoker for being considerate about your request.

*Source: HealthGUIDE,* St. Joseph Medical Center, 700 Broadway, Fort Wayne, IN 46802.

---

one of the most important tobacco-related carcinogens linked to lung cancer. Though African-American men smoke fewer cigarettes a day, they tend to be more affected by the tar and nicotine.

Cancer ravages the lungs with a vast number of wildly multiplying cells. Most often it begins with constant irritation of the bronchial lining. Because of this irritation, the cilia, which filter the air, disappear from the lining of the bronchi. Although extra mucus is secreted to substitute for the cilia and trap pollutants, this mucus itself becomes a problem. It remains trapped until finally forced out of the lung by a smoker's cough.

**TABLE 13.5 ▶** Some Methods to Quit Smoking

| METHOD | WHAT IT IS | HOW IT WORKS |
|---|---|---|
| Cold turkey | Abrupt and total smoking cessation | Willpower; initial nicotine withdrawal takes about three to four days, but symptoms can persist for weeks |
| Nicotine gum | Chiclet-sized nicotine-laced chewing gum marketed by SmithKline Beecham under the name Nicorette | Aids in cold-turkey quitting by replacing some of the nicotine smoking provides |
| Nicotine Nasal Spray | Prescription product | Delivers nicotine to nasal membranes and bloodstream |
| Nicotine inhaler | Prescription product | Delivers nicotine into mouth and bloodstream |
| Nicotine patch | Adhesive pad about 2" square | Applied to a quitter's upper arm or torso for 18 to 24 hours daily over a number of weeks; a continuous supply of nicotine is absorbed into the bloodstream |
| Breathe Free Plan | Sponsored by The Seventh-Day Adventists Four week plan | Clean living: no smoking, alcohol, coffee, tea, regular exercise, and balanced/healthy diet |
| Smokeless® | Seven or eight one-hour or 90-minute group sessions over four weeks | Uses behavioral techniques to teach stop-smoking, stress and weight management |
| Freedom From Smoking® | American Lung Association's not-for-profit program: eight one-hour to two-hour group classes over seven weeks | Motivational lectures, tips on quitting, buddies |
| Freshstart® | American Cancer Society's not-for-profit program: four one-hour group sessions over a two-week period | By third session smokers quit; lectures cover stopping strategies, stress and weight control, relapse prevention |
| How to Quit | Sponsored by American Medical Association, this new self-help kit contains instructional video and booklets as well as relaxation and support tapes | Over a four-week period helps smoker prepare, quit, develop stress-management techniques, work on relapse prevention |

## Tips for Action To Help Curb the Craving

The following are different ways smokers can retrain themselves to live without cigarettes. Any one of several of these methods in combination might be helpful to you.

- Do not smoke after you get a craving for a cigarette until three minutes have passed. During those three minutes, change your thinking or activity.

- Do not store up cigarettes. Never buy a carton. Wait until one pack is finished before you buy another.

- Never carry cigarettes around with you at home or at work. Keep your cigarettes as far from you as possible. Leave them with someone or lock them up.

- Never carry matches or a lighter with you.

- Put away your ashtrays or fill them with objects so they cannot be used for ashes.

- Change your brand of cigarettes weekly so you are always smoking a brand of lower tar and nicotine content than the week before.

- Always ask yourself, "Do I need this cigarette, or is it just a reflex?"

- Each day try to put off lighting your first cigarette.

- Decide arbitrarily that you will smoke only on even- or odd-numbered hours of the clock.

- Keep your hands occupied. Try playing a musical instrument, knitting, or fiddling with hand puzzles.

- Take a shower. You cannot smoke in the shower.

- Brush your teeth frequently to get rid of the tobacco taste and stains.

- If you have a sudden craving for a cigarette, take 10 deep breaths, holding the last breath while you strike a match. Exhale slowly, blowing out the match. Pretend the match was a cigarette by crushing it out in an ashtray. Now immediately get busy on some work or activity.

- Smoke only half a cigarette.

- Get out of your old habits. Seek new activities or perform old activities in a new way. Do not rely on the old ways of solving problems. Do things differently.

- If you are a stay-home "kitchen smoker" in the morning, volunteer your services to schools or nonprofit organizations to get yourself out of the house.

- Stock up on light reading materials, crossword puzzles, and vacation brochures that you can read during your coffee breaks.

- Frequent places where you cannot smoke, such as libraries, buses, theatres, swimming pools, department stores—or just go to bed.

- Give yourself time to think and get fit by walking a half hour each day. If you have a dog, take it for a walk with you.

*Source:* American Cancer Society, Texas Division. Used by permission.

---

If the smoker quits before cancerous lesions are present, the bronchial lining will return to normal. If the smoker does not quit and cancerous lesions are present, the abnormal cell growth will spread, blocking the bronchi and invading the lung tissue. In the latter stages of lung cancer, abnormal cells break away from the lungs and are carried by the lymphatic system to other vital organs, where new cancers begin (metastasis).

Danger signs of oral cancer include change in the voice, a lump in the neck, a growth in the mouth, blood in the saliva, and trouble swallowing. Any hoarseness or voice problem that lasts more than two weeks warrants a trip to the doctor.

Smokeless tobacco (chewing tobacco and snuff) and pipe and cigar smoking are linked to high rates of cancer of the oral cavity (mouth, lips, gums, cheeks, throat), esophagus, and pharynx. In addition, smokeless tobacco can irritate the gums, causing gingivitis and, eventually, tooth loss.

**Cardiovascular Diseases.** Tobacco smokers have high rates of coronary heart disease, pulmonary emphysema, and chronic bronchitis. Emphysema, once a relatively rare disease, now is common in smokers. Emphysema destroys the elasticity of the alveoli (air sacs) of the lung. It greatly reduces the smoker's ability to inhale and exhale properly, and the smoker is chronically short of breath. The tissue affected by emphysema never can be repaired or replaced. The disease progresses slowly but steadily and turns its victims into respiratory cripples. People with emphysema spend years gasping for breath. Many die because of an overworked heart.

Chronic bronchitis is an inflammation of the bronchial tubes. When the lining of the bronchial tubes becomes irritated, it secretes excessive mucus, causing bronchial congestion. This congestion produces chronic coughing and makes breathing extremely difficult. Chronic bronchitis and emphysema are included in the discussion of respiratory disorders in Chapter 7.

Surgeon General David Satcher stated, "When calling attention to public health problems, we must not use the word 'epidemic.' But there is no better word to describe the 600-percent increase since 1950 in women's death rates for lung cancer, a disease primarily caused by cigarette smoking. Clearly, smoking-related diseases among women is a full-blown epidemic."

In 2001 alone, lung cancer killed 68,000 U.S. women. That is one in every four cancer deaths among women, and about 27,000 more deaths than from breast cancer (41,000). In 1999 approximately 165,000 women died prematurely from smoking-related diseases: cancer and heart disease. In addition, women who smoke face unique health effects related to pregnancy.

Women are physically affected by alcohol more seriously than men. Women tend to get drunk faster than men, and they stay drunk longer than men. The absorption rate is much higher in women than in men mainly due to women having less of alcohol dehydrogenase, an enzyme that breaks down alcohol in the lining of the stomach. When women consume the same quantity of alcohol as men, women will retain a higher concentration of alcohol in the blood. In addition, the use of oral contraceptives and hormonal level changes during the menstrual cycle can slow the rate that the liver metabolizes alcohol.

Females who are heavy drinkers tend to suffer from hepatitis (alcohol-related), cirrhosis of the liver, peptic ulcers, high blood pressure, and anemia more quickly than men who consume more than they do. Females who are heavy drinkers are 40% more likely to have breast cancer than their nonsmoking contemporaries. They are more likely to be battered, sexually assaulted, and are twice as likely to die than males in the same group as a result of accidents, victimization, and suicide.

African-American women may be at even higher risk of alcohol-related health problems than Caucasian women. African-American women who drink heavily are about seven times more likely to have a child with fetal alcohol syndrome than heavy-drinking white women.

*Source: Devon Jersild, "Female Trouble: When Happy Hour Goes Sour," Health, January/February 2002, pp. 114–118, 148.*

**Smoking and Bone Health.** Osteoporosis is a condition in which bones weaken and are more likely to fracture. Fractures from osteoporosis can result in pain, disability, and sometimes death. Osteoporosis is a major health threat for an estimated 44 million Americans, 68% of whom are women. Recent studies have shown a direct relationship between tobacco use and decreased bone density. The longer one smokes and the more cigarettes smoked, the greater the risk of fractures. Exposure to secondhand smoke during youth and early adulthood may increase the risk of developing low bone mass.

**Smoking and the Embryo/Fetus.** Smoking during pregnancy can jeopardize the embryo/fetus's long-term physical growth and intellectual development. Women who smoke during pregnancy have high rates of low-birth-weight infants, premature deliveries, spontaneous abortions (miscarriages), bleeding during pregnancy, death of the embryo (stillbirth), and children who die during infancy. Each cigarette a mother smokes during the third trimester (when 70%–75% of growth occurs) causes a 1-ounce drop in birthweight. A very small decrease in the baby's birthweight can cause health problems later on. Women who use oral contraceptives (the pill) and smoke are at higher risk for stroke, heart attack, and problems associated with the circulatory system. Smoking can affect a woman's reproductive health. In addition, women smokers have higher rates of cervical cancer.

**Environmental Tobacco Smoke or Secondhand Smoke.** A 2006 report of the Surgeon General, *The Health Consequences of Involuntary Exposure to Tobacco Smoke*, clearly outlines and updates the evidence of the harmful effects of involuntary exposure to tobacco smoke.

Secondhand smoke, also known as environmental tobacco smoke (ETS), is a mixture of the smoke given off by the burning end of tobacco products (sidestream smoke) and the mainstream smoke exhaled by smokers. People are exposed to secondhand smoke at home, in the workplace, and in other public places such as bars, restaurants, and recreation venues. The ETS from cigars and cigarettes contains many of the same toxins and irritants (such as carbon monoxide, nicotine, hydrogen cyanide, and ammonia) as well as a number of known carcinogens (such as benzene, nitrosamines, vinyl chloride, arsenic, and hydrocarbons). Because cigars contain greater amounts of tobacco than cigarettes, they produce greater amounts of ETS. Secondhand smoke is harmful and hazardous to the health of the general public. A known carcinogen (cancer-causing agent), ETS causes

---

## Tips for Action After You Have Quit Smoking . . .

■ Do not skip meals (smokers often skip meals because they get an adrenaline rush from cigarettes that takes the place of eating).

■ Eat less more often. Snack on low-calorie vegetables and fruits.

■ Drink six to eight glasses of water a day.

■ Cut back on caffeine and alcohol, as both are often associated with smoking.

■ Plan exercise into your daily routine. Run up the stairs. Do some yard work.

■ Soak in the bathtub at the end of the day. This is a great relaxer.

■ Do not use weight gain as an excuse to resume smoking. You must be 90 pounds overweight to rival the cardiovascular risk of smoking a pack of cigarettes a day.

■ Chew gum.

■ Visit your dentist and get your teeth cleaned to get rid of the tobacco stains.

---

lung cancer and coronary heart disease in nonsmoking adults. Fortunately, exposures of adults are declining as smoking becomes increasingly restricted in workplaces and public places. Unfortunately, children continue to be exposed in their homes by the smoking parents and other adults. This exposure increases the risk of serious respiratory problems in children, such as bronchitis, pneumonia, greater numbers and severity of asthma attacks, lower respiratory tract infections, chronic coughs, and reduced lung functioning. Secondhand smoke also increases the risk for middle ear infections. Parents' cigarette smoke also lowers HDL (good) cholesterol in children with high cholesterol levels (about 2.9 million U.S. children). These children subsequently have a greater risk for heart disease. Infants are three times more likely to die from sudden infant death syndrome (SIDS) if their mothers smoke during and after pregnancy. Among children younger than 18 years of age, an estimated 22% are exposed to secondhand smoke in their homes, with estimates ranging from 11.7% in Utah to 34.2% in Kentucky.

### HOW TO QUIT

The dependence on nicotine—physical, psychological, or both—has a strong hold on tobacco users. Of those who try to quit, only about 8% succeed the first time. Many have been smoking since their teen years, to the point where it becomes an ingrained pattern. Some fear quitting because they believe they will gain weight. Although the metabolism does slow somewhat, ex-smokers in a 117,000-woman classic study conducted by the Nurses' Health Study weighed an average of only three to six pounds more after two nonsmoking years than those who continued to smoke.

Consider the following benefits.

■ Among former smokers, the decline in risk of death, compared with continuing smokers, begins shortly after quitting and continues at least 10 to 15 years.

■ Stopping smoking reduces the risks for cancers of the oral cavity and the esophagus by 50% as early as five years after cessation. Further reduction of risk occurs over time.

■ The risk for cervical cancer is substantially lower among former smokers than continuing smokers, even in the first few years after cessation.

■ The excess risk of heart disease caused by smoking is reduced by about one-half after one year of quitting smoking and then declines gradually.

■ After quitting smoking, the risk of stroke eventually returns to the level of the "never smoker." In some studies this has occurred within five years, and in others as long as 15 years.

■ For those without overt chronic obstructive lung disease, smoking cessation improves pulmonary function about 5% within a few months after quitting.

■ Pregnant smokers who stop smoking at any time up to the 30th week of gestation have infants with higher birthweights than do women who smoke throughout pregnancy. Quitting in the first three to four months of pregnancy and abstaining throughout the remainder of pregnancy protects the fetus from the adverse effects of smoking.

■ Smokers with gastric or duodenal ulcers who stop smoking heal more rapidly.

■ Smokers who increase the amount of time they exercise by 30 minutes a week while trying to quit are 30% more likely to be successful than those who don't exercise as reported by the Brown Medical School.

A majority of smokers have begun to understand seriously the health dangers of smoking to themselves, others, and the environment, and have begun to quit smoking on their own. However, many products and programs have been offered as aids to quit smoking. Some of

- Reduce tobacco use by adults.
- Reduce tobacco use by adolescents.
- Increase smoking cessation during pregnancy.
- Reduce the proportion of nonsmokers exposed to environmental tobacco smoke.

- Eliminate laws that preempt stronger tobacco control laws.
- Increase the average federal and state tax on tobacco products.

these are summarized in Table 13.5. Studies generally have shown that none of these aids is as effective as unaided individual effort. Nevertheless, some are helped with these products and services.

The **nicotine patch** now is available over-the-counter (OTC). This rectangular pad, usually affixed to the arm, delivers a steady amount of nicotine through the skin over a 24-hour period. Each day a new patch containing increasingly less nicotine is self-applied. The rationale is that the patch gradually reduces the addictive craving for nicotine through lower doses. Meanwhile, the person is not taking in all of the carcinogenic substances contained in tobacco smoke. After three months the craving for nicotine presumably will be reduced to the point where the person can be tobacco-free. The nicotine patch is recommended for use within a comprehensive program that addresses the psychological aspects of smoking as well.

Nicotine chewing gum delivers a consistent, low level of the drug, which helps reduce cravings and other withdrawal symptoms in smokers trying to quit. It also has few side effects and a very low potential for abuse.

One of the newest smoking cessation products is the nicotine inhaler. Small amounts of nicotine are inhaled from small tubes similar to other nasal inhalers. The rate of success in quitting is higher than comparison groups using placebo inhalers.

Several drugs for treating nicotine addiction include bupropion (Zyban) and varenicline (Chantix) tablets. Chantix is a partial nicotinic receptor agonist indicated as an aid to smoking cessation. Chantix works by providing some nicotine effects to ease the withdrawal symptoms and by blocking the effects of nicotine from cigarettes if smoking is resumed. It was approved by the FDA in May 2006.

Antianxiety drugs have been given to smokers. These relieve the irritability and tension of people who are trying to quit.

Nondrug methods have been used, too. One is an aversive technique in which smokers engage in rapid smoking until they exceed their tolerance level and become ill. The point is to make smoking unpleasant. This technique is known as negative reinforcement. Another aversive measure is to administer mild electric shock while a person is smoking. This has been found to produce only short-term benefits at best.

Along with its many other applications, behavior modification has been used in an attempt to get people to quit smoking. People are taught to avoid or deal with situations in which smokers are tempted to smoke. Many behavior modification programs include support groups or a buddy system for the person to turn to when the urge to smoke strikes. Finally, hypnosis is a successful means of teaching some people not to smoke—especially those who are highly motivated to quit.

About a third of the people who quit smoking subsequently resume smoking. Most people who have stopped for good, however, have made more than one previous attempt to stop. This should motivate smokers to keep trying even though they may not be successful until making several attempts.

Various cessation resources are available such as: Smokefree.gov, Pathways to Freedom: Winning the Fight against Tobacco (African Americans), A Breath of Fresh Air: Independence from Smoking (women), and Kick the Smoking Habit (Latino families).

## Summary

- Ethyl alcohol is an integral part of America's dietary, social, and sometimes spiritual lifestyles. It is a depressant psychoactive substance (distilled and fermented) that can enhance or devastate occasions.

- Alcohol is capable of causing a physiological addiction.

- A substantial number of the population drink alcohol. Over 60% of adults aged 18 and older report having consumed 12 or more alcoholic drinks in a given year.

- Although moderate drinking may be beneficial to health, overconsumption of alcohol has contributed to problems in relationships, high accident rates, increased violence, decreased productivity, and other societal problems.

## KEY TERMS

**Nicotine patch** pad worn on the arm that delivers a steady amount of nicotine through the skin as an aid to quitting

- Of all deaths in the United States, over 10% are linked to alcohol, including deaths caused by illness, accidents, and homicides.

- Binge drinking among college students has assumed epidemic proportions.

- Absorption of alcohol in the bloodstream depends on variables such as blood alcohol concentration, quantity consumed, rate of consumption, amount of food in the stomach, age, sex, and body weight.

- Alcohol damages the liver and developing embryos and fetuses, and causes some cancers, gastrointestinal disorders, and hormonal deficiencies, as well as psychiatric and psychological problems.

- Cigarette smoking is the single most preventable cause of disease and death in the United States.

- Over one in six deaths per day (more than 1,000 a day) is attributed to tobacco use.

- Smoking cigarettes kills approximately 400,000 adults each year.

- Tobacco contains some 4,000 gases and tars. Overwhelming evidence indicates that nicotine found in tobacco is extremely addictive.

- Tobacco is a major contributor to lung and other cancers, emphysema, chronic bronchitis, and many other diseases.

- Secondhand smoke can produce harmful effects to the lungs of those who live with smokers and those who are around smokers.

## Personal Health Resources

**ThomsonNOW**  Visit the ThomsonNOW website at http://thomsonedu.com/thomsonnow for valuable resources that will:

- Help you evaluate your knowledge of the material.

- Guide you through tutorials to help you understand and apply the material.

- Allow you to take an exam-prep quiz to better prepare for class tests.

American Cancer Society. This site presents information about smoking, statistics on smoking populations, quitting smoking, environmental smoke, and health issues related to smoking.

**www.cdc.gov/tobacco**

American Lung Association. This site contains information on all smoking populations, smoking and pregnancy and birth, secondhand smoke, and various other topics pertaining to tobacco.

**www.lungusa.org/tobacco/index.html**

Centers for Disease Control and Prevention, Office on Smoking and Health. This site contains information on smoking and pregnancy and childbirth, smoking and targeted populations, tobacco control, tobacco-related statistics and data, and other tobacco-related resources.

**www.cdc.gov/tobacco**

Hospitalizations for Alcohol Abuse Disorders, 2003. This agency compiles data from 90% of all hospital discharges in the United States.

**www.hcup-us.ahrq.gov/reports/statbriefs/sb4. jsp-34k-cached**

MADD. This site offers helpful information on talking to teens about the dangers of drunk driving. It presents national campaigns to eliminate drunk driving and underage drinking.

**www.madd.org**

National Highway Traffic Safety Administration. This site provides national statistics on national highway traffic data.

**www.nhtsa.dot.gov**

National Institute on Alcohol Abuse and Alcoholism. This site provides statistics and publications on alcohol and alcohol-related topics.

**www.niaaa**

The College Alcohol Study. This site presents study findings on Harvard University's ongoing alcohol surveys of 15,000 students at 140 colleges in 40 states.

**www.hsph.harvard.edu/cas/test/**

Tobacco.org. This site provides information on tobacco and all tobacco-related subjects.

**www.tobacco.org**

## It's Your Turn for Study and Review

1. What are some factors that influence the ways in which a drinker responds to alcohol consumption?

2. Describe the effects of alcohol on the various body systems.

3. How is a person's blood alcohol concentration (BAC) or blood alcohol level (BAL) determined?

4. What are the most common reasons that people drink?

5. Describe some reasons for tobacco use.

6. What are the major components of tobacco and how do they affect the body?

7. How does secondhand smoke pose a risk for nonsmokers?

## Thinking about Health Issues

Smoking and weight loss—safe assumption or deadly decision?
Catherine A. Tomeo and others, "Weight Concerns, Weight Control Behaviors, and Smoking Initiation." *Pediatrics*, 104:4 (October 1999); p. 918.

1. Based on the transtheoretical model of change that has been used to study adult smoking cessation, what are the four stages of adolescent smoking initiation?

2. What are two reasons that could explain the relationship between smoking rates among females and weight concerns?

3. What are the risk factors for smoking contemplation and for smoking experimentation among young women and men?

## Selected Bibliography

"Alcohol and Minorities." *Alcohol Alert.* Rockville, MD: U.S. Department of Health and Human Services, January 1998.

"Another Shot for Alcoholics." *Prevention News and Trends*, 57:9, September 2005, p. 57.

Boyle, R. G., et al. "Use of Smokeless Tobacco by Young Females." *Addictive Behavior*, 23:2, March/April 1998, pp. 171–178.

Brink, S. "Your Brain on Alcohol." *U.S. News and World Report*, May 7, 2001, pp. 50–57.

Centers for Disease Control and Prevention. "Alcohol-Attributable Deaths and Years of Potential Life Lost—United States, 2001." *Morbidity and Mortality Weekly Report* 53, 2004, pp. 866–70.

Centers for Disease Control and Prevention. *National Report on Human Exposure to Environmental Chemicals.* Atlanta, GA: CDC, Human Services, March 2001.

Cohn, Jessica. "Spitting Image." *Current Health* 2, February 2007, pp. 26–27, Vol. 33, No. 6.

Curry, A. "In the Mood for a Smoke: Teen Life Can Be a Drag." *U.S. News and World Report*, October 16, 2000, p. 60.

"Drinking and Driving: Factors Influencing Accident Risk." *Congressional Digest*, 77, 1998, pp. 164–165.

Emanuel, E. J. "Drug Addiction." *The New Republic*, July 2006, pp. 9–12.

Fairchild, A. and Colgrove, J. "Out of the Ashes: The Life, Death, and Rebirth of the 'Safer' Cigarette in the United States." *American Journal of Public Health* 94, 2004, pp. 192–205.

Friscolanti, Michael. "Rare Species of Teenager." *Maclean's* January 15, 2007, Vol. 120, No. 1, p. 46.

Gaffney, E., et al. "How I Quit Smoking." *Glamour*, 104:1, January 2006, pp. 56, 58–59.

Gorman, M. O. "How to Catch It Early—Nonsmokers? Don't Overlook the Warning Signs." *Prevention*, December 2001, p. 43.

"How to Handle a Hangover." *Harvard Health Letter*, 31:3, p. 3, January 2006.

"Huff, Don't Puff." *Prevention News and Trends*, 57:11, November 2005, p. 54.

Jersild, D. "Female Trouble: When Happy Hour Goes Sour." *Health*, January/February 2002, pp. 114–118, 148.

Johnson, J. G., et al. "The Association between Cigarette Smoking and Anxiety Disorders during Adolescence and Early Adulthood." *Journal of the American Medical Association*, 284, November 8, 2000, pp. 2348–2351.

Kandel, D. and Chen, K. "Extent of Smoking and Nicotine Dependence in the United States." *Nicotine and Tobacco Research*, 2:3, 2000, pp. 263–274.

Kowalski, K. "Debunking Myths about Alcohol." *Current Health*, 2001, pp. 18–21.

Lamburg, L. "Patients Need More Help to Stop Smoking," *JAMA* 292, 2004, p. 1286.

Lieber, C. S. "Hepatic and Other Medical Disorders of Alcoholism: From Pathogenesis to Treatment." *Journal of Studies of Alcohol*, 59:1, January 1998, pp. 9–25.

McGinnis, M. "Smoke Alert." *Prevention*, 58:5, May 2006, p. 155.

McKnight, E. and McKnight, W. L. "Women and Alcohol." University of Florida, Brain Institute, December 17, 2001.

MacNeil, J. S. "Don't Drink and Smoke: Two Vices' Bad Synergy." *U.S. News and World Report*, June 26, 2000, p. 63.

Orr, T. B. "Help Blow the Smoke Away." *Current Health*, November 2000, pp. 25–27.

Patterson, F. "Cigarette Smoking Practices among American College Students: Review and Future Directions." *Journal of American College Health*, 52:5, March/April 2004, p. 203.

Paulos, L. "Deadly Overdose." *Seventeen*, 65:3, March 2006, p. 173–175.

Russel, R. "Bright Lights, Big Waistline." *Prevention*, 57:10, October 2005, pp. 125–126, 128, 130.

Substance Abuse and Mental Health Services Administration. *National Household Survey on Drug Abuse: Population Estimates 1998.* Rockville, MD: U.S. Department of Health and Human Services, 1999.

*Surgeon General's Report: Women and Smoking 2001.* Atlanta, GA: Centers for Disease Control and Prevention, Office on Smoking and Health, 2001.

Task Force on Community Preventive Services. "Recommendations Regarding Interventions to Reduce Tobaccco Use and Exposure to Environmental Tobacco Smoke." *American Journal of Preventive Medicine*, 20:2 (Supplement), 2001, pp. 10–15.

USA Today-Your Health, "Drug Addiction, Substance Abuse and Methamphetamine Treatment." 134:2725, October 2005.

U.S. Department of Health and Human Services. *Eighth Special Report to the U.S. Congress on Alcohol and Health.* Washington, DC: U.S. Government Printing Office, 2000.

U.S. Department of Health and Human Services. *Healthy People 2010*, 2nd ed. Washington, DC: HHS, 2000.

U.S. Department of Health and Human Services. *Reducing Tobacco Use: A Report of the Surgeon General.* Atlanta, GA: Centers for Disease Control and Prevention, 2000.

Volkow, N. D. "Drug Addiction: Free Will, Brain Disease or Both." Vital Speeches of the Day, June 2006, pp. 505–508.

Wallich, P. "The Kegbot Is Watching." *Popular Science,* December 2005, pp. 111–112.

White, N. "Love with a Twist." *Oprah Magazine*, April 2006, pp. 169–170, 172–173.

Zickler, P. "Adolescents, Women, and Whites More Vulnerable than Others to Becoming Nicotine Dependent." *NIDA Notes* Research Findings, 16:2, May 2001, pp. 1–2.

Zickler, P. "Study Points to Acetaldehyde-Nicotine Combination in Adolescent Addiction." *NIDA Notes*, 20:3, October 2005.

Name _____ Date _____

Course _____ Section _____

| | Always | Frequently | Occasionally | Seldom | Never |
|---|---|---|---|---|---|
| 1. I smoke cigarettes to keep myself from slowing down. | 5 | 4 | 3 | 2 | 1 |
| 2. Handling a cigarette is part of the enjoyment of smoking it. | 5 | 4 | 3 | 2 | 1 |
| 3. Smoking cigarettes is pleasant and relaxing. | 5 | 4 | 3 | 2 | 1 |
| 4. I light up a cigarette when I feel angry about something. | 5 | 4 | 3 | 2 | 1 |
| 5. When I have run out of cigarettes, I find it almost unbearable until I can get them. | 5 | 4 | 3 | 2 | 1 |
| 6. I smoke cigarettes automatically without even being aware of it. | 5 | 4 | 3 | 2 | 1 |
| 7. I smoke cigarettes to stimulate me, to perk myself up. | 5 | 4 | 3 | 2 | |
| 8. Part of the enjoyment of smoking a cigarette comes from the steps I take to light up. | 5 | 4 | 3 | 2 | 1 |
| 9. I find cigarettes pleasurable. | 5 | 4 | 3 | 2 | 1 |
| 10. When I feel uncomfortable or upset about something, I light up a cigarette. | 5 | 4 | 3 | 2 | 1 |
| 11. I am very much aware of the fact when I am not smoking a cigarette. | 5 | 4 | 3 | 2 | 1 |
| 12. I light up a cigarette without realizing I still have one burning in the ashtray. | 5 | 4 | 3 | 2 | 1 |
| 13. I smoke cigarettes to give me a lift. | 5 | 4 | 3 | 2 | 1 |
| 14. When I smoke a cigarette, part of the enjoyment is watching the smoke as I exhale it. | 5 | 4 | 3 | 2 | 1 |
| 15. I want a cigarette most when I am comfortable and relaxed. | 5 | 4 | 3 | 2 | 1 |
| 16. When I feel blue or want to take my mind off cares and worries, I smoke cigarettes. | 5 | 4 | 3 | 2 | 1 |
| 17. I get a real gnawing hunger for a cigarette when I have not smoked for a while. | 5 | 4 | 3 | 2 | 1 |
| 18. I have found a cigarette in my mouth and did not remember putting it there. | 5 | 4 | 3 | 2 | 1 |

*Source:* From U.S. Department of Health and Human Services, *A Self-Test for Smokers* (Washington, DC: U.S. Government Printing Office, 1983).

## Scoring Your Test

Enter the numbers you have circled on the test questions in the spaces provided below, putting the number you have circled to question A on line A, to question B on line B, and so on. Add the three scores on each line to get a total for each factor. For example, the sum of your scores over lines A, G, and M gives you your score on "Stimulation," lines B, H, and N give the score on "Handling," and so on. Scores can vary from 3 to 15. Any score 11 and above is high; any score 7 and below is low.

A _____ + G _____ + M _____ = _____   Stimulation

B _____ + H _____ + N _____ = _____   Handling

C _____ + I _____ + O _____ = _____   Pleasure or relaxation

D _____ + J _____ + P _____ = _____   Crutch—tension reduction

E _____ + K _____ + Q _____ = _____   Craving—psychological addiction

F _____ + L _____ + R _____ = _____   Habit

A score of 11 or above on any factor indicates that smoking is an important source of satisfaction for you. The higher you score (15 is the highest), the more important a given factor is in your smoking.

| Why You Smoke | What to Do Instead |
|---|---|
| **Stimulation** | |
| You smoke to keep from slowing down, for a lift, to pep you up. | Find something else to pep you up—a hobby, brisk walks, simple exercises. |
| **Handling** | |
| You like the ritual of smoking, to have something in your hands and mouth. | Pick something else to handle: coins, pen or pencil, worry beads; try doodling, or chew on paper straws or minted toothpicks. |
| **Relaxation** | |
| You enjoy smoking; it is a reward, a time you feel good about yourself. | Consider the harm cigarettes cause you and the reward of quitting. Substitute social or physical activity; prove self-control and feel good about yourself. |
| **Crutch** | |
| You smoke to deal with problems and negative feelings. | Prove to yourself that smoking does not solve problems. Reduce tension other ways: Take deep breaths, call a friend, talk over feelings. Work on keeping your cool. |
| **Craving** | |
| You feel hooked and begin to think of the next cigarette before you put out the one you are smoking. You are aware of the need to smoke. | Recognize that quitting will be difficult and prepare to see it through. Plan to try to stop cold turkey, abstaining completely. The day before quitting, smoke to the point of distaste. |
| **Habit** | |
| You smoke automatically, often without realizing what you are doing. | Become aware of every cigarette you smoke. Ask yourself why you are smoking and if you really want it. Wrap up your cigarettes or put them in a place that is difficult to get to. |

Name _____     Date _____

Course _____     Section _____

AUDIT is a brief structured interview, developed by the World Health Organization, which can be incorporated into a medical history. It contains questions about recent alcohol consumption, dependence symptoms, and alcohol-related problems.

Begin the AUDIT by saying: "Now I am going to ask you some questions about your use of alcoholic beverages during the past year." Explain what is meant by alcoholic beverages (that is, beer, wine, liquor [vodka, brandy, and so on]).

**Record the score for each question in the box on the right side of the question [   ].**

1. How often do you have a drink containing alcohol?
   - [ ] Never (0)     [   ]
   - [ ] Monthly or less (1)
   - [ ] Two to four times a month (2)
   - [ ] Two to three times a week (3)
   - [ ] Four or more times a week (4)

2. How many drinks containing alcohol do you have on a typical day when you are drinking?
   - [ ] None (0)     [   ]
   - [ ] One or two (1)
   - [ ] Three or four (2)
   - [ ] Five or six (3)
   - [ ] Seven or nine (4)
   - [ ] 10 or more (5)

3. How often do you have six or more drinks on one occasion?
   - [ ] Never (0)     [   ]
   - [ ] Less than monthly (1)
   - [ ] Monthly (2)
   - [ ] Weekly (3)
   - [ ] Daily or almost daily (4)

4. How often during the last year have you found that you were unable to stop drinking once you had started?
   - [ ] Never (0)     [   ]
   - [ ] Less than monthly (1)
   - [ ] Monthly (2)
   - [ ] Weekly (3)
   - [ ] Daily or almost daily (4)

5. How often during the last year have you failed to do what was normally expected from you because of drinking?
   - [ ] Never (0)     [   ]
   - [ ] Less than monthly (1)
   - [ ] Monthly (2)
   - [ ] Weekly (3)
   - [ ] Daily or almost daily (4)

6. How often during the last year have you needed a first drink in the morning to get yourself going after a heavy drinking session?
   - [ ] Never (0)     [   ]
   - [ ] Less than monthly (1)
   - [ ] Monthly (2)
   - [ ] Weekly (3)
   - [ ] Daily or almost daily (4)

7. How often during the last year have you had a feeling of guilt or remorse after drinking?
   - [ ] Never (0)     [   ]
   - [ ] Less than monthly (1)
   - [ ] Monthly (2)
   - [ ] Weekly (3)
   - [ ] Daily or almost daily (4)

8. How often during the last year have you been unable to remember what happened the night before because you had been drinking?
   - [ ] Never (0)     [   ]
   - [ ] Less than monthly (1)

| ☐ Monthly | (2) |
| ☐ Weekly | (3) |
| ☐ Daily or almost daily | (4) |

**9.** Have you or someone else been injured
as the result of your drinking?

| ☐ Never | (0) | [  ] |
| ☐ Less than monthly | (1) | |

*Source:* Reprinted by permission of the World Health Organization.

| ☐ Monthly | (2) |
| ☐ Weekly | (3) |
| ☐ Daily or almost daily | (4) |

Record the total of the specific items [    ].

A score of 8 or greater may indicate the
need for a more in-depth assessment.

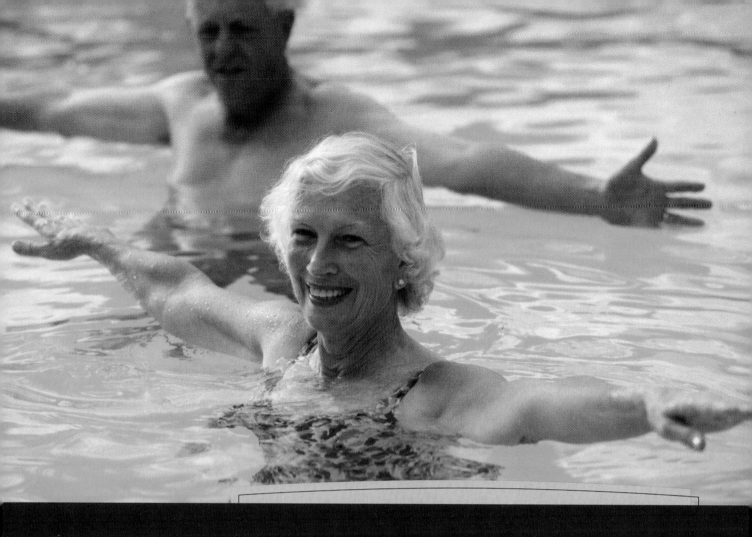

# Chapter Fourteen Aging, Dying, and Death

**OBJECTIVES** ■ Describe the profile of America's aging population.
■ Differentiate factors used to determine the three age categories.
■ Describe selected diseases and conditions that are common in the
elderly population. ■ **Describe factors that can enhance health during advanced years.** ■ Discuss the need for proper medical care and
appropriate use of medications by the elderly. ■ **Discuss the benefits
of having advance directives.** ■ Discuss the issues of health care cost
as it relates to the aging population. ■ **Identify safety issues involving
the elderly.** ■ Discuss the issues and options involved in caregiving.

ThomsonNOW™ Log on to ThomsonNOW at http://thomsonedu.com/
thomsonnow to access and explore self-assessments, interactive
tutorials, and practice quizzes.

"Come grow old with me, the best is yet to be." The U.S. population is graying. Life expectancy increased during the past century to 77 years for those born in 2001. Americans are living longer, and by 2030 the number of older Americans is expected to reach 71 million, or about 20% of the U.S. population.

Presently, Americans are particularly enamored with youth, beauty, and sexiness. Youth is portrayed as beautiful, vigorous, productive, efficient, and sexy. Older people are often viewed as being unattractive and "over-the-hill." The media uses older people to advertise medications, false-teeth cleaners, insurances, and various health-related products. When older people are portrayed positively, the aim is to make them feel and look younger. **Ageism** has a negative effect upon society. Although older adults have unique challenges and additional medical needs, it is imperative that this nation help them to thrive, increase research concerning their needs, intensify aging education, and improve support modalities.

**Senescence** (the process of aging) begins with conception and is a normal, positive, continuous physiological, emotional, social, and developmental process until death. Everyone living is aging. Our lives are in stages—infancy, toddler, childhood, adolescence, young adult, adult, middle age, old age, and death. Legally, adulthood begins at age 18 and old age begins at 65 years of age.

College students should be aware of and plan for aging by becoming familiar with physical and social issues facing their parents, grandparents, and other older individuals. This awareness can enhance living for the elderly through others' understanding of the aging process and empathy for the aging. In addition, it teaches young people how to enhance their own quality of life for its duration.

Aging is perhaps the least understood of all human processes. It differs from one person to another. Although most people start to show some signs of aging while in their thirties to sixties, some begin aging in their teens or twenties. Others live healthy lives relatively unmarred by health problems into their eighties, and beyond. The aging process can vary even within a single person. Some organs remain healthy and viable at the same time as other organs deteriorate.

As people get older, energy loss, muscle weakness, greater susceptibility to various diseases and illnesses, and problems with mobility are not entirely a result of aging itself but, instead, to poor nutrition and an inactive lifestyle. A healthy diet and regular exercise can slow and even reverse the deterioration in vitality; physical, emotional, and social fitness; and independence often associated with aging.

## A Profile of Aging

Although chronic diseases, communicable diseases, and various physical and neurological disorders are prevalent, people in the United States are living longer than ever, and living their lives in better health. The number of

Americans age 65 or older has increased to approximately 35 million—increasing 10-fold in the 20th century and accounting for about 13% of the population. Statisticians determine **life expectancy** by averaging the ages of death of all the people in a group for a certain period. **Life span** refers to the potential maximum number of years a person probably can live if everything goes well. Thanks to advanced technology, the potential life span now is approximately 110 years.

## LIFE EXPECTANCY

Among both people of color and whites, life expectancy from birth is greater for women than for men, with the greatest gaps (of nine years) reported between African-American women and men and between Puerto Rican women and men (see Figure 14.1). The life expectancy of white men exceeds that of all men of color, while the life expectancy of white women exceeds that of most women of color, except for Asian women living in Hawaii and for Puerto Rican women (living in Puerto Rico).

Based on current mortality data, the life expectancy for all Hispanics in the United States (both males and females) is 79 years. For the population living in Puerto Rico, female life expectancy from birth is close to 80 years, while for men it is nearly 71 years. Hispanic women have a longer life expectancy (more than 77 years) than either African-American or American Indian or Alaska Native women (more than 74 years). The predominantly black population of the U.S. Virgin Islands reports life expectancies at birth (for both women and men) that exceed these expectancies of other black Americans. Life expectancy for females in the Virgin Islands is 79 years, compared with slightly more than 74 years for African-American females elsewhere in the United States. Life expectancy at birth for all U.S. Asian populations (both males and females) is estimated at nearly 83 years.

Life expectancy in the United States ranks 48th (77.85) compared with other countries (Table 14.1). Andorra has the highest life expectancy. Macau, San Marino, Singapore, and Hong Kong round out the top five.

The drastic gain in life expectancy in this century is due to improved sanitation and disease prevention, improved medical care, progress in controlling pathogens that cause infectious diseases, improved nutrition, and increased use of preventive health services.

The graying of America has a challenging aspect, too. More and more elderly people will rely on government programs for food, housing, and medical care. Longevity can bring with it poverty, illness, inadequate health and medical care, and loneliness.

The need to plan for old age is perhaps most pressing for women. In 2001 women accounted for approximately 58% of the population age 60 and older and 70% of the population age 85 and older—currently the fastest growing segment of the older population. Older women often come face-to-face with the challenging issues of aging,

**FIGURE 14.1** ▶ Past and Projected Female and Male Life Expectancy at Birth, United States, 1900–2050

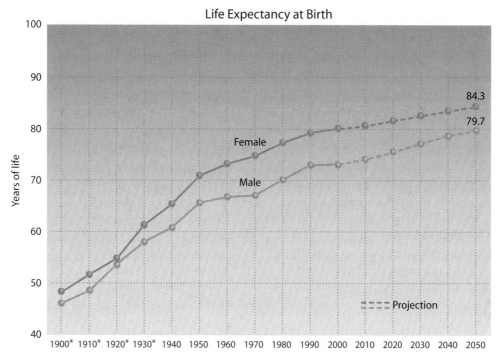

*Death registration area only. The death registration area increased from 10 states and the District of Columbia in 1900 to the entire United States in 1933.

*Source:* U.S. Department of Commerce, Bureau of the Census.

**TABLE 14.1** ▶ Countries with Highest and Lowest Life Expectancy, 2006

| COUNTRIES WITH HIGHEST LIFE EXPECTANCY, 2006 | | COUNTRIES WITH LOWEST LIFE EXPECTANCY, 2006 | |
|---|---|---|---|
| COUNTRY | LIFE EXPECTANCY (YEARS) | COUNTRY | LIFE EXPECTANCY (YEARS) |
| 1  Andorra | 83.51 | 226  Swaziland | 32.62 |
| 2  Macau | 82.19 | 225  Botswana | 33.74 |
| 3  San Marino | 81.71 | 224  Lesotho | 34.40 |
| 4  Singapore | 81.71 | 223  Angolo | 38.62 |
| 5  Hong Kong | 81.59 | 222  Zimbabwe | 39.29 |
| 6  Japan | 81.25 | 221  Liberia | 39.65 |
| 7  Sweden | 80.51 | 220  Mozambique | 39.82 |
| 8  Switzerland | 80.51 | 219  Zambia | 40.03 |
| 9  Australia | 80.50 | 218  Sierra Leone | 40.22 |
| 10  Guernsey | 80.42 | 217  Malawi | 41.70 |
| 48  United States | 77.85 | | |

*Note:* Life expectancy in the United States ranks 48 of 226 nations.

*Source:* The World Fact Book-Life Expectancy at Birth starting with births in 2006.

including economic security, access to community services, and health and long-term care. Older women are more likely to live alone, spend considerable years disabled, reside in a nursing home, and live in poverty.

# Age Determination

**Gerontologists** (professionals who study the aging process) have identified different ways of determining age. Only one involves the simple calculation of birth date. The others rely on more complex factors.

## KEY TERMS

**Ageism** discrimination that often denotes old age

**Senescence** the process of aging from birth to death

**Life expectancy** average length of time members of a population can expect to live

**Life span** potential maximum number of years members of a population could live

**Gerontologist** professional who studies the aging process

## Tips for Action Dare to Be 100

1. Aim for 100. Set your mind to living out your entire 100+ life span. Do not stop at 75. Dare to be 100.

2. Use it or lose it. Keep active physically and mentally.

3. Keep a positive attitude. Fill your life with hope, caring, and creativity.

4. Know your family medical history. Accept the good you have inherited, and commit to changing the not-so-good. Get regular checkups and enlist your doctor's help in your prevention program.

5. Let nature provide. The fewer processed foods in your diet, the better. Especially watch for foods processed with salt and sugar.

6. Trim the fat—especially saturated fat. It is a burden that weighs you down physically and emotionally.

7. Get your vitamins from foods whenever possible. Do not rely on pills.

8. Do not let 200 be your unlucky number. Have your cholesterol checked; then use diet to keep it in check.

9. Lighten up. Keep your sense of humor, and do not let temporary problems get you down. Laughter has healing properties.

10. Slow down aging by sticking to a strength and flexibility program.

11. Keep your brain sharp by using it. Read. Visit a planetarium. Take a class. You are never too old to learn.

12. Do not be put out to pasture. You, not your age, decide when to retire. Keep your job skills up-to-date. When you do retire, keep active. Return to life.

13. Stay fit. Take advantage of every opportunity to use your body and mind.

14. Get the sleep your body needs.

15. Walk every chance you get. Take the stairs. Park farther away. Take a brisk walk through the mall the next time you shop.

16. Take care of your heart with regular cardiovascular exercise, reduced salt intake, and a low-cholesterol diet.

17. Choose a doctor who shares your philosophy of prevention and health promotion. But remember, the best healer is you.

18. Do not end sexual activity until you want to. Staying in shape can help keep you looking and feeling sexy. See your doctor when you have problems.

19. Do not smoke. It not only shortens your life, but it also ages your skin.

20. It is your choice. You have the tools to lengthen and improve your life. Use them.

*Source:* Adapted from *Cooking Light*, October 1993, pp. 33–40.

### FYI AGES IN DECADES

Quadragenarian: 40–49 years of age
Quinquagenarian: 50–59 years of age
Sexagenarian: 60–69 years of age
Septuagenarian: 70–79 years of age
Octogenarian: 80–89 years of age
Nonagenarian: 90–99 years of age
Centenarian: 100–109 years of age
Supercentenarian: over 110 years of age

■ *Biological age* is a measure of the relative condition of the body. A 76-year-old man who has participated in cardiovascular conditioning for three decades may have a biological age of 40 years. A 32-year-old woman crippled with arthritis may have a biological age of 60 years.

■ *Functional age* is a measure of how a person compares with contemporaries—in seeing, hearing, walking, endurance, and reflexes.

■ *Psychological age* is a measure of how well a person adapts to changing circumstances. Even if impaired by physical illness or advanced years, a person may have a relatively young psychological age, determined by a sense of self-sufficiency and ability to meet life's challenges.

## Disorders Related to Aging

Among health concerns of people as they get older are sexual functioning, menopause, depression, osteoporosis, Alzheimer's, diabetes, Parkinson's disease, urinary incontinence, and influenza and pneumonia. These diseases and disorders can be managed with proper treatments and lifestyle changes.

### SEXUAL FUNCTIONING

Sexual enjoyment can last throughout old age if a couple acknowledges changes in sexual functioning and adjusts to those physical changes. The extent of physical change

Substantial differences are apparent in life expectancy among different population groups within the United States. For example, women outlive men by an average of six years. White women currently have the greatest life expectancy in the United States. The life expectancy for African-American women has risen higher than that of white men. People with an annual income of at least $25,000 live an average of three to seven years longer, depending on gender and race, than do people from households with annual incomes less than $10,000. Men have higher death rates for each of the 10 leading causes of death.

varies from one person to another. Women generally can anticipate the following changes.

1. The tissues of the vulva and vagina become thinner, making intercourse more painful.
2. The walls of the vagina lose their elasticity, which also makes intercourse more painful.
3. The amount of vaginal secretions diminishes, making penile penetration more difficult and painful.
4. The strength of vaginal orgasmic contractions is reduced.
5. The external genitals gradually get smaller.
6. The breasts lose firmness and fatty tissue.

In men, the following changes occur.

1. More time is required to achieve an erection.
2. An erection is more difficult to maintain.
3. The angle of the erection decreases.
4. Ejaculation is less forceful and contains less ejaculate fluid. Sperm production decreases. The orgasm is briefer than previously.
5. More time is required between orgasms.

Certain medications—such as tranquilizers, antidepressants, and some medications for high blood pressure—interfere with sexual function. A physician may be able to prescribe medication that has fewer side effects. Alcohol is known to delay orgasm in women and reduce potency in men.

Prostate surgery in men and hysterectomies in women affect the sexual performance of some. Diabetes, brain attack (stroke), arthritis, heart disease, and some other chronic debilitating diseases can interfere with sexual functioning. For example, the joint pain of rheumatoid arthritis responds to medication and surgery. Exercising, resting, taking warm baths, changing position, and changing the timing of sexual activity (avoiding the time of day when discomfort is worst) can help restore sexual enjoyment. Even the most serious conditions should not prevent couples from having a satisfying sex life.

## MENOPAUSE

**Menopause,** often called "change of life," is a natural part of the female life cycle, when ovaries cease functioning and the menstrual period stops, marking the end of the reproductive years. The range for onset of menopause varies widely—between ages 42 and 56. If the ovaries are removed surgically, menopause occurs at that time, regardless of the woman's age.

The lack of estrogen during menopause causes an increase in cholesterol levels, which places a woman more at risk for heart disease. In addition, most women have some symptoms. Indications of menopause include the following.

- Changes in the menstrual period—lighter bleeding, heavier bleeding, or irregularity in the time menstruation occurs each month; gradually the period stops completely
- Hot flashes or flushes (a sudden rush of heat that spreads over part or all of the upper body, sometimes accompanied by sweating)
- Vaginal dryness, itching, or burning and pain during intercourse
- Incontinence
- Increase in facial and body hair
- Headaches
- Fatigue
- Sleep disturbances
- Mild depression, irritability, anxiety, or mood swings
- Mild memory loss and inability to concentrate

For most women the symptoms associated with menopause are mild and require no medical treatment.

### KEY TERMS

**Menopause** stage in the life cycle when the ovaries stop functioning and hormone levels decrease

Men might expect to go bald as they get older. Roughly half of all men experience some balding as they age. Surprisingly, so do half of all women. A woman's baldness usually is distributed more evenly and is less extensive. To save as much hair as possible, a woman can do the following.

- Eat a well-balanced diet. Crash dieting causes hair loss.
- Wear hats or tight wigs only occasionally.
- Comb wet hair; do not brush it.

- Dry hair naturally. Curling irons, blow dryers, and hot curlers all damage hair.
- Avoid styles that pull hair, such as cornrows and braids.
- Protect hair from sunlight and harsh chemicals such as the chlorine in swimming pools.
- Use a mild shampoo and a gentle conditioner after every shampoo.

For those who have more severe problems, estrogen **hormone replacement therapy (HRT)** is available to relieve discomforts of hot flashes and night sweats on a short-term basis. However, there has been a decline in the use of HRT in which estrogen and progestin are combined, because this therapy increases the risk of heart disease, breast cancer, blood clots, and brain attacks.

Estrogen HRT is not for all women. Those with a personal or family history of breast or uterine cancer should not take estrogen. The decision to start HRT should be based on a woman's medical history and risk factors. Several newer drugs, including raloxifene, help increase bone mass and reduce blood cholesterol levels as estrogen does but, unlike estrogen, they do not affect uterine and breast tissue, stimulate uterine bleeding, or cause breast soreness. Raloxifene holds promise for the many postmenopausal women who do not take estrogen because of their aversion to the side effects of estrogen.

## DEPRESSION

Although depression strikes people of any age, it is more prevalent in older people. Approximately 20% of older persons living independently and 37% living in primary health facilities suffer from depression. This includes major depressive disorders, dysthymic disorders, or bipolar disorders. Depressive symptoms are not a normal part of aging. However, the elderly are particularly vulnerable to life events that lead to depression, such as loss of a mate, deteriorating health and medical problems, financial pressures, adjustments after retirement, and the challenge of living alone. Depression is a common side effect of some medications older people take for conditions such as arthritis, hypertension, and heart disease.

Depression can and should be diagnosed and treated. Many effective therapies are now available.

The newer antidepressants that enhance the activity of serotonin in the brain have few side effects and are not likely to interfere with medications for other conditions.

These include Prozac, Lexapro, Zoloft, and Paxil. Medications should be accompanied by psychological and social support. Psychotherapy can be as potent as medications. Three proven approaches are: 1) cognitive-behavioral therapy (CBT), which teaches the patient to counter negative thinking; 2) interpersonal therapy (IPT), which embraces better communication and conflict resolution skills; and 3) problem solving, in which the patient breaks down problems for manageability.

One outcome of untreated depression is suicide. Suicide rates increase with age and are highest among Americans age 65 years and older. The rates for both men and women are highest among those who are divorced or widowed.

## BRAIN HEALTH

At about 40 years of age, changes in the brain make it more difficult to filter out distractions and stay focused. Good brain health or cognitive health is achieved by maintaining and improving mental skills—memory, decision-making, learning, and planning. Many individuals believe that senility is a normal part of aging; it is not. Cognitive health changes normally with age to include slower pace when learning new information and the need to have new information repeated. However, some elderly go beyond change in cognition to cognition decline. Many with cognition decline have a higher risk of dementia and two-thirds with dementia have Alzheimer's disease.

Recent studies advocate being physically active, controlling hypertension, and participating in social activities as aids in maintaining and improving brain or cognitive health.

## Common Diseases and Conditions in Older People

Figure 14.2 shows the percentages of people over age 65 suffering from various chronic conditions. Conditions identified with older people include diabetes,

## Tips for Action When You Cannot Take Estrogen

If you and your doctor have decided against estrogen replacement therapy, do the following.

■ When a hot flash strikes, drink a glass of cold juice or icy water.

■ Try meditation, biofeedback, deep breathing, or yoga to beat hot flashes.

■ Dress in clothing made of natural fibers—cotton, linen, or wool.

■ Sleep in a cool room and use cotton sheets.

■ Open the windows and lower the thermostat.

■ Exercise. Women who exercise have half as many hot flashes as those who do not.

■ Steer clear of alcohol, caffeine, and spicy foods.

■ Eat tofu, tempeh, and other soybean products. They contain plant estrogen.

■ If intercourse is painful, use estrogen creams or vaginal lubricants that do not contain petroleum jelly.

■ Get plenty of calcium (ask your doctor about supplements).

**FIGURE 14.2 ▶** Common Chronic Conditions of Noninstitutionalized People over Age 65

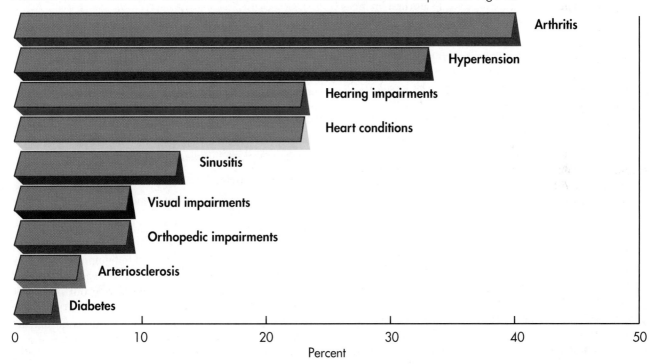

*Source:* U.S. National Center for Health Statistics.

osteoporosis, Alzheimer's disease, Parkinson's disease, urinary incontinence, influenza, and pneumonia.

### DIABETES

Diabetes is a serious disease in which the body is unable to process glucose properly and, as a result, the glucose accumulates in the blood (see Chapter 7). Approximately 7 million people aged 65 years or older have diabetes.

Early detection, improved health care, and better individual management are pivotal for preventing and controlling diabetes.

### KEY TERMS

**Hormone replacement therapy (HRT)** estrogen treatment after menopause or after the ovaries have been removed to offset the ill effects

## OSTEOPOROSIS

**Osteoporosis** is a disease that causes weak and fragile bones, which then may break with the least bit of trauma (see Figure 14.3). It is one of the leading causes of disability in the United States, affecting more than 25 million people. Some degree of bone loss is normal in both men and women of advancing age. However, the sharp decrease in estrogen following menopause accelerates the rate of bone loss in women. Osteoporosis is the major cause of bone fractures in women over age 50. It causes over 1.5 million fractures or breaks per year, mostly in the hip, spine, and wrist.

Experts estimate that half of all women over age 65 have osteoporosis. Of the approximately 25 million Americans who have osteoporosis, four out of five are women. A major risk factor for osteoporosis is early menopause (either naturally or from a hysterectomy). Additional factors include a small, thin frame, delicate bone structure, physical inactivity, low calcium intake, cigarette smoking, excessive use of alcohol, and a family history of osteoporosis (hence a genetic predisposition). Caucasians are at highest risk. Women who have never had a baby are at

increased risk. Certain drugs, such as cortisone, heparin, and several anticonvulsants, also weaken the bones and can aggravate osteoporosis.

Overweight women are less likely to develop osteoporosis because estrogen is stored in body fat. Even after the ovaries stop producing estrogen, it is produced in the body's fat layer.

Osteoporosis is sometimes called a silent disease because it has no symptoms during its early stages. For that reason, the condition usually is not recognized until it reaches an advanced stage. At that point fractures start occurring. In its later stages, osteoporosis causes debilitating pain, permanent disfigurement, and lasting disability.

Ordinary x-rays do not show bone loss until about 30% of the bone density has been lost, but three medical tests are available for diagnosing osteoporosis.

■ Single- and dual-photon absorptiometry
■ Dual-energy x-ray absorptiometry
■ Computerized tomography (CT scan)

The type of test chosen depends on the area of the body to be examined, the available equipment, and the patient's ability to pay (insurance coverage). Blood and urine tests usually are done first to rule out other diseases that can weaken the bones. A person at high risk for osteoporosis may want to ask about bone density measurement.

Various medical therapies are being used, including the drug calcitonin. It is prescribed for both men and women to slow bone breakdown and reduce the pain associated with osteoporosis. Other treatments include a calcium-rich diet (see Table 14.2) and a program of weight-bearing exercise.

## ALZHEIMER'S DISEASE

**Alzheimer's disease** is a form of dementia that causes deterioration of cognitive function due to loss of brain cells. It causes a loss of short-term memory and memory problems that interfere with daily life, job performance, and social functioning.

**FIGURE 14.3 ▶** Osteoporosis

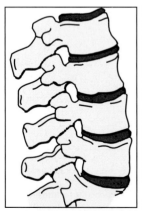
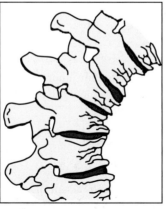

Healthy spine        Spine with osteoporosis

**TABLE 14.2 ▶** Sources of Calcium

| FOOD | AMOUNT | CALCIUM (MILLIGRAMS) | CALORIES |
|---|---|---|---|
| **Dairy products** | | | |
| Milk | | | |
| Whole, 3.5% | 1 cup | 288 | 159 |
| Nonfat (skim) | 1 cup | 296 | 88 |
| Cheese | | | |
| Cheddar | 1 inch cube | 129 | 68 |
| Cottage | 4 oz. | 107 | 180 |
| Swiss | 1-inch cube | 139 | 56 |
| American | 1-inch cube | 122 | 65 |
| Custard, baked | 1 cup | 297 | 305 |
| Ice cream | 1 cup | 194 | 257 |
| Ice milk | | | |
| Hardened | 1 cup | 204 | 199 |
| Soft serve | 1 cup | 273 | 266 |
| Pudding | | | |
| Chocolate | 1 cup | 250 | 385 |
| Vanilla | 1 cup | 298 | 283 |
| Yogurt | | | |
| From whole milk | 1 cup | 272 | 152 |
| From partially skimmed milk | 1 cup | 294 | 123 |
| **Meat, poultry, and seafood** | | | |
| Clams | 3 oz. | 53 | 65 |
| Salmon, pink | | | |
| Canned | 3 oz. | 167 | 120 |
| Sardines, canned | | | |
| In oil, drained | 3 oz. | 372 | 174 |
| Tuna, canned | | | |
| in water | 3 oz. | 17 | 135 |
| **Vegetables** | | | |
| Beans | | | |
| Lima | 1 cup | 80 | 189 |
| Red kidney | 1 cup | 74 | 218 |
| Snap (green or yellow) | 1 cup | 72 | 31 |
| Broccoli, cooked | 1 stalk | 158 | 47 |
| Collards, cooked | 1 cup | 289 | 51 |
| Mustard greens | 1 cup | 193 | 32 |
| Spinach | 1 cup | 200 | 41 |
| Turnip greens, cooked | 1 cup | 252 | 28 |
| **Fruit and fruit products** | | | |
| Oranges, fresh | 1 medium | 54 | 71 |
| **Grain products** | | | |
| Bread | 1 slice | 23 | 74 |
| Pancakes, plain or buttermilk | 1 cake | 58 | 61 |
| **Nuts and beans** | | | |
| Tofu, soybean curd | 3 oz. | 110 | 61 |

Over 4 million Americans over age 65 suffer from Alzheimer's disease. Alzheimer's is twice as common in women as in men, probably because women live longer. Alzheimer's affects one in 10 people over the age of 65 and almost half of those over 85. Researchers believe that the number of Alzheimer's victims will rise to 14 million by the middle of the 21st century, especially because technological advances are enabling people to live longer.

Former president Ronald Reagan's announcement that he had Alzheimer's disease drew much attention to this incurable disease. Although Alzheimer's disease is associated with the elderly, it has been diagnosed in individuals as young as the late forties. Alzheimer's is irreversible and cuts remaining life expectancy in half. It is now the fourth leading cause of death among older adults. The risk for developing Alzheimer's disease is greater if one or both parents develop the disease. Also, individuals with Down's syndrome are four times more likely than the general population to develop Alzheimer's disease.

Experts say that Alzheimer's disease is now the third costliest health problem affecting Americans, exceeded only by heart disease and cancer. Medical bills, nursing homes, home health care, and lost productivity from Alzheimer's cost an average of over $47,000 a year for each Alzheimer's patient, for a total of approximately $90 billion.

Two areas of the brain seem particularly affected by Alzheimer's disease:

1. The *cerebral cortex*, or outer layer, which is responsible for cognitive functions such as language

2. The *hippocampus*, located deep in the brain, believed to play an important role in memory

The death of neurons in areas of the brain has a severe impact on memory, thinking ability, and behavior. The disease progresses through three general stages.

—**Stage 1.** Forgetfulness and disorientation become noticeable. Victims also may be depressed, lack interest in their surroundings, and show poor judgment. During the first stage of Alzheimer's disease, victims become progressively unable to take care of routine tasks such as grocery shopping and doing the laundry.

—**Stage 2.** Existing symptoms worsen, and victims become restless and agitated. They often perform repetitive actions. Eyesight, hearing, taste, smell, and touch gradually diminish.

—**Stage 3.** The victims become completely dependent on caregivers. During this final stage they gradually lose all control of physical functions and become completely disoriented.

At present, no test is available to diagnose Alzheimer's disease in living patients. A diagnosis of probable Alzheimer's is based on medical history, physical examination, and tests of mental ability. When a person has symptoms of mental impairment, thorough medical, psychiatric, and

**KEY TERMS**

**Osteoporosis** condition in which the bones lose calcium and become brittle

**Alzheimer's disease** progressive, incurable disease in which nerve cells in the brain die; associated with elderly people

---

**Tips for Action** An Active Mind = A Healthy Mind

Research—one study involving a group of nuns in their nineties and older—has found that a lifetime of mind exercises can help delay the declining mental agility so common in old age. Start protecting your mind.

■ Strive for a broad range of experiences.

■ Be willing to try new things.

■ Stay flexible—mentally and physically.

■ Get to know a wide variety of people.

■ Surround yourself with people who are smarter than you are.

■ Seek out challenging activities.

The TV magazine *20/20* aired a segment featuring people who were not only living but were also living well after age 100. The interviewees had three commonalities.

1. They were engaged in living. They all had interests and meaningful activities.

2. They were physically active. One taught a dance class. Another raced automobiles.

3. They had the ability to face and bounce back from losses. One interviewee had just lost her 70-year-old daughter but insisted that the interview go on as scheduled. In it, she related fond memories of her daughter.

---

neurological evaluations should be done. This is especially important because many reversible conditions mimic Alzheimer's disease. Symptoms resembling those of Alzheimer's disease can be caused by poor nutrition, brain attack, adverse drug reactions, high fever, viral infection, minor head injuries, anxiety, boredom, loneliness, and depression. Physicians consider previous illnesses and use of medications, neurological tests that detect anatomical changes in the brain, and psychological tests that measure memory.

Unfortunately, the only certain diagnosis for Alzheimer's is during autopsy. Doctors examine the brain of a dead person for **plaques** and **tangles.** Scientists do not yet know whether the plaques and tangles are a cause or a result of the Alzheimer's disease. Scientists have identified mutations in several genes in Alzheimer's patients. They also have identified several enzymes and unique changes in the way the body processes proteins.

Although there is no cure for Alzheimer's, several drugs, vitamin E, and a group of plant extracts from India hold promise. Alzheimer's medications Aricept, Exelon, and Reminyl prevent an enzyme known as acetylcholinesterase from breaking down acetylcholine in the brain which Alzheimer's patients have too little of. Another drug protects brain cells by blocking Elixa, the release of excess glutamate. A "dream" drug, known only as compound 267, in tests with mice, reversed memory loss and reduced brain plaque and tangles linked to Alzheimer's disease. It is being tested in humans presently. The first human trial found compound 267 to be safe in young men. A second test, with healthy people ages 65 to 80, is aimed at determining correct dosages. Tests in patients on 267 started in 2006.

## PARKINSON'S DISEASE

Parkinson's disease is a debilitating central nervous system disorder that targets older people, affecting one out of every 100 persons over the age of 60. Actor Michael J. Fox was only 30 when he was stricken with the disease.

Parkinson's occurs when a depletion of dopamine, a neurotransmitter or a chemical that transmits nerve impulses from one cell to another, causes a gradual reduction in cells in specific parts of the brain. The signs of the disease are tremors, slowness of movement, stiffness in the arms and legs, and a decrease in facial expression, often called Parkinson's mask. Balance is affected, causing the patient to have an unusual posture. There is no cure for Parkinson's disease. However, a commonly used drug that alleviates the symptoms is Levodopa, usually known as L-dopa. Another option for advanced Parkinson's is injections of a drug called apomorphine which helps with episodes of decreased mobility. Other medicines are: COMT inhibitors, Dopamine agonists, and other medications.

## URINARY INCONTINENCE

**Urinary incontinence** affects more women than men. An estimated 40% of all women over age 60 have problems ranging from slight loss of urine to severe and frequent wetting. Most commonly, incontinence is caused by weakened pelvic muscles, especially in the elderly. This is a common aftereffect of pregnancy and childbirth, which is why the condition is more common among women. A common cause in men is obstruction or inflammation that can accompany prostatitis.

Urinary incontinence is not an inevitable consequence of aging. Instead, it is caused by specific changes in body function. Most often it stems from diseases or is a side effect of certain medications. The two general kinds of incontinence are:

1. **Urge incontinence.** The person has a sudden, strong urge to urinate and is unable to hold the urine long enough to reach a toilet.

2. **Stress incontinence.** Urine leakage occurs during physical exertion or when the person strains, laughs, coughs, or sneezes. Stress incontinence is the type caused by weakened pelvic muscles.

In most cases urinary incontinence responds to treatment. A wide variety of treatments are available.

- Surgery corrects structural problems (such as abnormalities in the position of the bladder) and severely weakened muscles; most cases of stress incontinence can be corrected surgically
- A set of specific exercises (Kegel) to strengthen pelvic muscles
- Medication to control urination or improve the bladder's capacity to hold urine
- Bladder training, which involves urinating at specific time intervals; a type of behavior modification often combined successfully with other techniques such as restricting liquids after a certain time of day

## INFLUENZA AND PNEUMONIA

Although influenza (the flu) and pneumonia strike people of every age, they are most serious in older people. According to the Centers for Disease Control and Prevention, of the approximately 60,000 adults who die every year from influenza and pneumonia, 95% are over age 65. Combined, influenza and pneumococcal pneumonia are the sixth leading cause of death in the United States.

The influenza virus attacks the respiratory tract and can lead to bronchitis or pneumonia. Pneumococcal pneumonia affects an estimated half-million Americans a year. Caused by a strep bacteria, it results in severe inflammation and infection in the lungs. Influenza initially exhibits the same symptoms as a cold, with a stuffy or runny nose and a cough. The flu is more severe, however, and lasts longer.

Prescribed drugs can reduce flu symptoms in nine out of 10 people if they are taken within 48 hours of the first symptoms. Pneumococcal pneumonia is treated with aggressive doses of antibiotics to kill the strep bacteria.

Vaccinations are available against both influenza and pneumococcal pneumonia, and they are recommended for people in high-risk groups, including those over age 65. People over age 60 who get a flu shot are only half as likely to develop the flu as those who do not get vaccinated. When adults have been vaccinated and are hospitalized for pneumonia, they are much more likely to survive than persons who were not vaccinated against a virulent bacterial form of pneumonia.

The pneumonia vaccine is required only once. Booster shots are given annually to those at highest risk for developing the disease (including those with chronic respiratory disease). Although the vaccination does not prevent pneumonia in all people who receive it, those who are vaccinated and develop pneumonia usually have milder symptoms and quicker recovery.

Because the viruses that cause the flu mutate constantly, becoming resistant to existing vaccines, an elderly person should get a flu shot every year. Most doctors recommend getting the vaccine in late October or November. Flu vaccines may become slightly less effective in preventing the flu as people age, but they still protect a high percentage of the elderly population from infection. Of those who do get infected, the flu vaccine makes symptoms less severe.

Influenza and pneumonia vaccinations do not cause the illness or symptoms of the illness, make any existing illnesses worse, interfere with other medications, or cause side effects other than temporary soreness or redness at the injection site.

## Healthy Aging

Developing good health habits should start early in life, but it is never too late. Adopting healthy habits, even later in life, offers many health benefits. Among them are improved general physical condition, enhanced mental well-being, and slowed physical decline.

## GOOD NUTRITION

Almost everyone can get all the needed nutrients by eating a variety of nutritious foods every day. Good nutrition, including a diet that is low in saturated fats, sodium, and

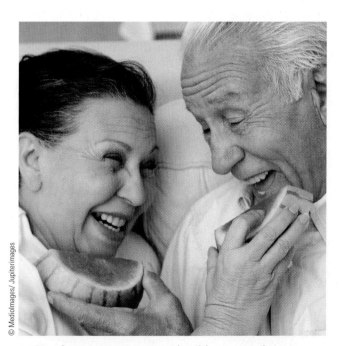

© Mediolmages/ Jupiterimages

▲ *Good nutrition promotes health as people age*

### KEY TERMS

**Plaques** dense deposits of protein found in the brains of Alzheimer's patients during autopsy

**Tangles** bunches of twisted nerve cell fibers found in the neurons of Alzheimer's patients during autopsy

sweets, and contains at least five servings of fresh fruits and vegetables each day, is vital for maintaining good health. For older people, the experts recommend the amounts presented in Table 14.3. Little research has been done to define how aging changes the body's use of various nutrients. Some studies show that aging may affect the need for certain vitamins and minerals. For example, the body's ability to absorb calcium and vitamin D decreases with age. Although Daily Values have been published for infants, children, and adults, guidelines for the specific nutritional needs of older people are scarce. Older people may need more protein because of weakened muscles and reduced ability to respond to physical stress.

## HEALTHY WEIGHT

Maintaining a healthy weight becomes more difficult for elderly people who tend to be less active and expend fewer calories. The U.S. Department of Agriculture Human Nutrition Research Center on Aging suggests that maintaining a healthy weight may be especially difficult for elderly men. When they gain weight, they retain the extra pounds, and when their weight drops below normal, they often are unable to regain it. Either way, the failure to adjust can increase the risk of serious illness. Poor weight control can worsen the effects of diseases common in the elderly population, including diabetes, hypertension, coronary artery disease, and arthritis.

The body's need for protein, carbohydrates, vitamins, and minerals stays the same as people age, but the need for calories decreases significantly. Therefore, elderly people have to make a special effort to eat foods that provide a good ratio of nutrients to calories. Fruits, vegetables, and natural grains are among the best. They should try to avoid empty calories, foods laden with calories but with few minimal nutrients. The most notorious culprits are processed foods high in fat, sodium, and refined sugar.

## REGULAR PHYSICAL ACTIVITY

Start walking. Good health depends on staying physically active in later years. Although older people may have to gradually modify the type and duration of exercise sessions, even those who have never exercised can improve their health by exercising regularly. Exercise also can prolong life.

People who exercise regularly, even when in their nineties, report more energy, improved oxygen in the lungs, endurance, and flexibility. They move more easily, sleep better, and are less anxious. Exercise even may help delay the physical effects of aging, which, according to some researchers, is not as much a function of passing years as it is of disuse. Some of the common signs of aging—stooped posture, shriveled muscles, memory loss—are effects of inactivity, not a function of advancing years.

Regular physical activity greatly reduces a person's risk of dying from heart disease, and decreases the risk for diabetes, colon cancer, and high blood pressure. Exercise also helps to control weight, keeps bones, muscles, and joints healthy, helps to relieve the pain of arthritis, reduces anxiety and depression, and can decrease the need for continuous medical care. Moderate exercise, such as walking or gardening, helps elderly people avoid stomach and intestinal bleeding. Exercise improves overall health and boosts resistance to disease.

## MIND POWER

The elderly should continue to keep the mind actively involved in creative and intelligent interests and hobbies. The key to maintaining sharp mental abilities is to stay involved in lifelong and satisfying activities. Reading, participation in book clubs, spiritual studies, word puzzles, word games, and physical activities are all useful in keeping the mind active.

## TOBACCO USE

Cigarette smoking—dubbed by former U.S. Surgeon General C. Edward Koop the No. 1 preventable cause of death in the United States—is a risk to good health for people of any age. The American Cancer Society reports that cigarette smoking is responsible for one of every five deaths in the United States, or more than 440,000 deaths each year. A person who smokes one pack of cigarettes a day deducts 12 years from his or her life.

Smoking is even more serious among older people. As people age, the blood flow to the lungs and oxygen exchange diminish. Cigarette smoking makes that already compromised situation even worse. In addition, smoking is the major cause of chronic obstructive lung diseases,

**TABLE 14.3 ▶** Recommended Amounts of Food for Elderly People

| RECOMMENDATIONS | EXAMPLES |
| --- | --- |
| At least two servings of dairy products | Low-fat or skim milk, reduced-fat cheese, low-fat cottage cheese, low-fat or nonfat yogurt |
| Two servings of proteins | Poultry, tuna, salmon, mackerel, lean meat, dried beans or peas, nuts |
| Four to five servings of fruits and vegetables | Apples, bananas, pears, plums, strawberries, oranges, grapefruit, broccoli, cauliflower, carrots, squash, beans, corn, tomatoes, spinach; include at least one citrus fruit or juice and at least one dark green leafy vegetable |
| Four servings of bread and cereal products | Whole-grain bread, whole-grain pasta, rice, oatmeal |

## FYI | MIXING MEDICATIONS AND ALCOHOL

The following reactions can occur when alcohol is mixed with:

- **Aspirin**—an increase in stomach irritation and bleeding
- **Pain relievers**—mental confusion, excessive drowsiness, impaired coordination, loss of consciousness, and impaired breathing
- **High blood pressure medication**—dizziness, fainting, lightheadedness, loss of consciousness
- **Diabetes medication**—weakness, headache, nausea, vomiting, rapid heartbeat, difficulty breathing

Mixed with sleeping pills, tranquilizers, antidepressants, some cough and cold products, and monoamine oxidase inhibitors, alcohol can be fatal.

*Source: Medication Education for Seniors and The Consumer's Guide to Drug Interactions (New York: Collier Books/Macmillan, 1993).*

which are much more common among the elderly. Smokers suffer more illnesses with longer durations, and smoking has been linked to pronounced wrinkling of the skin and premature baldness (see Chapter 13). Health begins to improve after the last cigarette has been smoked.

## ALCOHOL USE

As with smoking, alcohol can be detrimental to health for people of all ages. As people age, physical changes in the body affect the way alcohol is metabolized and eliminated. The body retains less body fluid, so alcohol is not readily diluted. With less body fluid, the blood alcohol concentration (BAC) increases much more rapidly. The elderly brain is affected more by lower levels of alcohol in the blood. Also, older people have a lower ratio of lean muscle mass and, thus, less mass in which the alcohol can be distributed (alcohol is not distributed in body fat). The liver, too, works more slowly to metabolize the alcohol, delaying the removal of alcohol from the body.

Alcohol consumption worsens many of the chronic disease conditions common among elderly people. Alcohol interferes with and diminishes the functioning of the most common medications taken by people over age 65. When alcohol is mixed with some medications, such as barbiturates, tranquilizers, and certain cough and cold products, the result can be fatal. The same drink that had few effects at 50 may have considerably more harmful effects at 75. Depending on existing health problems, regular medications, and physical condition, some elderly people may need to stop drinking. Others need to limit their intake of alcohol (see Chapter 13).

## Medical Care

Physical changes that take place during aging can result in chronic illnesses that demand frequent attention. Diseases that are common in the elderly population—glaucoma, diabetes, hypertension, and cancer—have few symptoms in the early stages and may go unnoticed by elderly individuals and their caregivers. Regular medical checkups, including eye examinations, allow early diagnosis and aggressive care, which can slow the deterioration these conditions cause.

Prior to age 65, healthy adults should have a complete physical exam every three years. The U.S. Preventive Services Task Force recommends a physical exam annually after age 65. Those at high risk for specific diseases, such as heart disease, cancer, and diabetes, may need more frequent checkups as advised by a physician.

In deciding which screening tests to recommend, experts take three factors into consideration: cost of the test, potential risks posed by the test, and whether knowing the test results will enable doctors to start treatment that will prolong life. Using those criteria, medical experts have identified several screening tests that should be done throughout adult life and more frequently in elderly people. After age 50, healthy adults should have the following medical tests annually.

- Rectal exam
- Test for occult (hidden) blood in the stool
- Proctosigmoidoscopy (an internal examination of the colon to detect abnormalities or cancerous growths)
- Blood pressure measurement
- Cholesterol test
- Tetanus-diphtheria booster (every 10 years)

Healthy women over age 50 should have mammograms, Pap smears, and breast exams annually. Every woman should perform a breast self-exam every month. Healthy men should have a prostate exam annually. All adults should be tested for glaucoma yearly starting at age 25.

The elderly take more medications than any other segment of the population. Of over-the-counter medications, aspirin and laxatives are the ones purchased most often. Because the older population has the highest rate of chronic or long-term illnesses (such as arthritis, diabetes, hypertension, and heart disease), this group tends to take more than one drug at the same time. Prolonged use of multiple drugs increases the risk of dangerous drug interactions. Damage to major organs, drug overdose, drug dependency, and death may result.

Because of the normal changes that occur with aging, drugs act differently in the body in later years than they do earlier in life. Those changes can affect the length of time a drug remains in the body and the amount of drug absorbed by body tissues.

---

**Tips for Action** Prescription Savvy

Before you accept a prescription from your doctor, make sure you can read it. And before you leave the pharmacy, make sure you have gotten the right prescription. Treatment errors from illegible prescriptions result in longer hospital stays and even death. The American Medical Association no longer tolerates poor handwriting by physicians. It wants prescriptions to be printed, typed, or computer-generated.

---

## Medical Cost

Under the Census Bureau's middle series projections the number of persons 65 years old and over would more than double by the middle of the next century to 80 million. About one in five would be elderly by the year 2030. The graying of America is causing a higher need for health care and social services. Currently about 80% of aging Americans have at least one chronic condition and 50% have at least two. Due to the increase in the number of older people, health care costs are projected to increase 25% by 2030. Medicare spending has increased from $33.9 billion in 1980 to over $260 billion and is projected to double again by 2012. Remaining healthy and preventing health problems/injuries is one way of cutting health care costs. Prevention of diseases and injuries helps the elderly to remain self-sufficient and independent as long as possible, thus delaying already high health care costs.

## Caregiving

Fifty-nine percent of adults in the United States are already family caregivers or expect to be one. The National Family Caregiver Association reports that the value of "free" service provided by family caregivers is estimated to be $257 billion a year. The medical technology that is enabling more and more people to reach old age is bringing with it a crisis in the caregiving arena. With the life span extending well into the eighties and nineties, people in their sixties and older are finding themselves caring for a parent, an aging mate, or a friend. **Caregivers** may be defined as people who help others who are unable to fulfill the tasks of daily living such as eating, bathing, dressing, or using the bathroom.

Caregiving has become a critical issue. The number of people over age 85—those in greatest need of daily help—is increasing rapidly and is expected to more than double in the next 15 years. As the baby boomers continue to age, more men and women will face the responsibility of caring for older relatives and friends.

Oftentime, family caregiving is more preferable and satisfying due to the level of care the older person receives. However, caregiving can be extremely detrimental. Of family members who provide at least 21 hours of care a week, 61% have suffered from depression. Older

**FYI | HOW TO SPOT PROBLEMS IN NURSING HOMES**

| Problem | Evidence |
|---|---|
| Not being taken to the bathroom when it is appropriate for the patient | Incontinence |
| Not receiving enough fluids | Dehydration |
| Not getting enough food | Malnutrition |
| Improper grooming | Poor hygiene conditions |
| Inattention to preventive skin care | Broken skin, sores |
| Insufficient exercise | Reduced mobility and range of motion |
| No encouragement to retain independence | Loss of interest in self-care |

*Sources:* Adapted from National Citizens' Coalition for Nursing Home Reform, *Nursing Homes: Getting Good Care There* (Washington, DC: NCCNHR).

caregivers with chronic health conditions themselves have a 63% higher death rate than their peers who are not caregivers. Researchers at Harvard Medical School and the University of Pennsylvania concluded that the risk of dying increased most among those with spouses who have mentally or physically disabling illnesses and that caregiving spouses need support as much as bereaved spouses.

American businesses lose up to $29 billion dollars each year as a result of employees having to be caregivers for an older family member.

## Injury Prevention and Safety in the Later Years

Falls are the most common cause of injuries to older adults. More than one-third of adults aged 65 or older fall each year, and of those who fall, 20%–30% suffer moderate

## Tips for Action 10 Warning Signs of Caregiver Stress

1. Denial about the disease and its effect on the person who has been diagnosed. ("I know mom's going to get better.")

2. Anger at the person with Alzheimer's, anger that no effective treatments or cures currently exist, and anger at others who do not understand what is going on. ("If he asks me that question one more time I'll scream!")

3. Social withdrawal from friends and activities that once brought pleasure. ("I don't care about getting together with the neighbors anymore.")

4. Anxiety about facing another day and what the future holds. ("What happens when he needs more care than I can provide?")

5. Depression begins to break your spirit and affects your ability to cope. ("I don't care anymore.")

6. Exhaustion makes it nearly impossible to complete necessary daily tasks. ("I'm too tired for this.")

7. Sleeplessness caused by a never-ending list of concerns. ("What if she wanders out of the house or falls and hurts herself?")

8. Irritability leads to moodiness and triggers negative responses and reactions. ("Leave me alone!")

9. Lack of concentration makes it difficult to perform familiar tasks. ("I was so busy, I forgot we had an appointment.")

10. Health problems begin to take their toll, both mentally and physically. ("I can't remember the last time I felt good.")

*Source:* Alzheimer's Disease and Related Disorders Association, Inc.

---

to severe injuries that reduce mobility and independence. More than 200,000 older people suffer serious fractures due to falls, and of those, 20% will die within the first year following the injury.

Additionally, older adults are involved in more automobile accidents. These occur more frequently because of less acute distance vision, reduced night vision, narrowed peripheral vision, and diminished ability to switch focus from objects in the distance to those that are close. Partly because of chronic illness and deteriorating health, automobile accidents not only are more frequent but also are more serious for older drivers. Data on car injuries released by General Motors show that if a car driven by a 20-year-old is involved in an accident with a car driven by a person over 65, the elderly person is five times more likely to be killed in the accident.

## Planning for the Later Years

The changes that occur as part of aging are not limited to physical and mental changes. Additionally, most elderly people have to adjust to changes in finances and possible changes in housing.

### FACING FINANCIAL CHALLENGES

Many older people are able to enjoy their retirement years with enough money to meet their basic needs and enjoy some leisure activities. Others face poverty for the first time in their lives. Retirement savings often must be used for expensive medical treatment not covered by insurance or Medicare. Many older people simply outlive their assets.

Even when benefits are available to elderly people who qualify for them, many do not take advantage. Many more either do not know about the benefits or do not know how to get them. Others, especially those for whom English is a second language, may not understand the complicated paperwork required.

Getting educated about benefits, and how to apply for them, is only part of what has to be done. Planning should start early, in the twenties and thirties, so adequate amounts of money can be put into interest-earning accounts for retirement income. Younger people would be wise to take advantage of tax-deferred savings plans such as the 401(k) plan and other tax shelter annuities to prepare for the financial challenges of retirement.

Older people often have to reconsider where they are able to live for the following reasons.

- Costly maintenance and utility bills
- Desire to live closer to children and other family members
- Desire to live in a smaller home
- Need to move from a home that has stairways and other structural barriers
- Desire to move from an unsafe neighborhood
- Need for regular nursing attention

Before making a move, issues of cost, independence, availability of medical care, and other aspects of personal

### KEY TERMS

**Caregiver** person who renders services to another person who is unable to take care of the activities of daily living

## Tips for Action Safety in the Home

Some easily implemented measures to promote safety of older people in the home are the following.

■ Get rid of throw rugs. Too many older people trip over or slip on them.

■ Place all extension cords and other wires or cords out of the walking area so people will not trip over them.

■ Leave sufficient space between furniture and other items in the home so older people who use canes, walkers, or wheelchairs, as well as those who get around independently, will have room to move about.

■ Have an emergency response system (ERS) installed.

■ Have railings installed on stairs and other places where needed to help the older person get around.

■ Wear low-heeled shoes, not slippers, socks, or stockings (the latter cause more slips).

■ Place rubber mats in the bathtub and have grab bars on the wall; a tub seat also may be helpful.

■ Keep an up-to-date list of emergency phone numbers within reach.

■ Have and maintain smoke detectors, checking the batteries regularly. Have an escape plan in mind in case of the need to leave immediately.

■ Maintain a constant and comfortable room temperature. Older people are not as sensitive to heat in particular and have died during heat waves simply because they did not feel the heat.

■ Get plenty of fluids. Dehydration can set in quickly in older people.

---

concern must be considered. Many types of housing offer support services such as nursing homes and continuing care communities. Some may arrange for in-home services that may include nursing care, home-delivered meals, transportation services, or escorts.

Options for older people encompass a broad range of possibilities. They include the following.

■ Staying in their own home and renting out part of it to a caregiver or helper

■ Moving to a smaller home

■ Moving in with family members

■ Moving to a group home where older people share a single residence

■ Moving to an apartment building where elderly residents share communal dining facilities and on-call nursing assistance

■ Moving to a community designed especially for older people

One of the most difficult decisions a person may have to make is how to care for an aging parent, other relative, or friend who needs assistance. The trend, for reasons of finance (the average yearly cost of living in a nursing home is more than $34,000) and personal preference, is toward staying in the familiar environment of the home. This often necessitates in-home services, which are increasing in number and range. Among the resources available are those listed below.

■ Area Agencies on Aging (AAAs), usually under the auspices of the county and listed that way in the phone book

■ Utility company financial breaks for those who qualify

■ Local churches, synagogues, and mosques (volunteer services)

■ Religious social services agencies such as Catholic Social Services and Jewish Family Services

■ Senior centers (provide transportation, volunteers, programs, and companions)

When dealing with any agency or agency representative, their qualifications, certification, experience, and reputation should be verified. Questions to ask include the following.

1. How long has the agency existed in your area?

2. Is the agency Medicaid- or Medicare-certified?

3. What type of training and certification are required for the employees?

4. What costs are involved?

5. Who pays, and how? Is insurance coverage accepted?

6. What is the duration of the contract? Can it be terminated before that time?

7. What are the days and times the services are delivered?

8. What are the exact services delivered?

9. How are disputes resolved? What recourse does a person have for unresolved issues?

10. Who is liable in case of theft, abuse, neglect, and other illegal activities?

One issue that has loomed larger than anyone had imagined is abuse of elders by those entrusted to care for them. The abuse can be physical, emotional, social, or psychological, and the abusers can be family members or contractual caregivers. In some cases caregivers are overwhelmed by the demands, spoken or unspoken, that the elderly person places on them, and they snap. These abusers can benefit from the support of others to relieve them of their heavy duties.

In other cases elderly people are exploited for the financial gain of those who sell them useless products or services, implore them to donate money for religious or other causes, and talk them into withdrawing money from bank accounts and entrusting it to strangers. In other cases the dynamics are similar to those of child abuse. Underlying the abuse is a pathological need for power, and that need is met by taking advantage of someone who is vulnerable.

Abuses of elderly people are not as difficult to detect and remedy as in children, because the former are typically eager to talk about anything that occurs in their life to those who are willing to listen and get involved. If the older person has memory loss or is otherwise mentally impaired, those entrusted with his or her care must be acutely sensitive to the person's needs and potential for abuse.

## Definitions of Death

Death occurs when the body can no longer adapt to the changes involved in disease or aging, and stops functioning. (The leading causes of death are presented in Table 14.4.) Traditionally, death was pronounced when a person stopped breathing and the heart stopped beating. Because of the ethics and issues surrounding organ transplants and other medical procedures, however, the medical and legal professions have had to devise more precise definitions of death.

Three general definitions of death are used to determine when death occurs: brain death, clinical death, and cellular death.

**Brain death** occurs when the brain stops functioning completely because there is no blood flow or oxygen. To measure whether the brain has stopped functioning, medical scientists use the following criteria.

- Whether the person has any reflexive movement
- Whether the person reacts to stimuli (such as being pinched), to light, or to pain
- Whether the person is breathing spontaneously (without the aid of a respirator) or showing any kind of spontaneous muscle movement
- Whether an electroencephalogram (EEG) shows any brain activity; a flat line indicates brain death

According to standards established by the Harvard University Medical School, two sets of readings must be taken 24 hours apart to establish brain death. A person can be brain dead while oxygenated blood is being circulated through the body with life-support equipment. In this way, vital organs can be kept alive for transplant after a person has been declared brain dead.

When a person stops breathing and the heart stops beating, **clinical death** has occurred. This determination is adequate in cases where medical procedures are not at issue.

The gradual breakdown of the body that occurs after the heart stops beating signals **cellular death.** Deprived of oxygen, body cells and tissues gradually stop functioning.

---

### KEY TERMS

**Brain death** complete loss of brain function

**Clinical death** cessation of heartbeat and breathing

**Cellular death** cessation of all metabolic processes

**TABLE 14.4 ▶** Leading Causes of Deaths for Persons 65 Years of Age and Older

| RANK | WHITE | BLACK | NATIVE AMERICAN | ASIAN OR PACIFIC ISLANDER | HISPANIC |
|---|---|---|---|---|---|
| 1 | Heart disease | Heart disease | Heart disease | Heart disease | Heart disease |
| 2 | Cancer | Cancer | Cancer | Cancer | Cancer |
| 3 | Stroke | Stroke | Diabetes | Stroke | Stroke |
| 4 | Chronic obstructive pulmonary disease (COPD) | Diabetes | Stroke | Pneumonia or influenza | COPD |
| 5 | Pneumonia or influenza | Pneumonia or influenza | COPD | COPD | Pneumonia or influenza |

*Source:* Centers for Disease Control and Prevention.

All metabolic processes cease. Eventually the muscles stiffen (**rigor mortis**) and blood pools in whatever body parts are resting against a surface.

# Dying

Dr. Elisabeth Kübler-Ross wrote her landmark work *On Death and Dying* after interviewing hundreds of people who were dying. In it she identified the five stages—denial, anger, bargaining, depression, and acceptance—encountered when coming to terms with death. Not everyone who is dying experiences all five stages. Among those who do, not everyone experiences them in the same order. Some go through two stages at the same time or bounce back and forth among the stages, repeating one or more. The stages are

1. **Denial.** ("No, not me.") This is a typical reaction when a person first learns that he or she is terminally ill. Kübler-Ross believes denial is important and necessary. It helps cushion the impact of the person's awareness that death is inevitable.

2. **Anger.** ("Why me?") The person resents the fact that others will remain healthy and alive while he or she must die. Kübler-Ross emphasizes the importance of allowing individuals to express their anger in natural, healthy ways.

3. **Bargaining.** ("Yes, me, but . . .") Individuals accept the fact of death but try to strike bargains, usually with God, for more time. They promise to be good or to do something in exchange for additional time.

4. **Depression.** ("Yes, it's me.") In this stage individuals now begin to consider their loss. First they mourn past losses, things left undone, wrongs committed. Then they enter a state of preparatory grief. They stop mourning all the small deaths and begin to conceive the final death. They mourn the things that never will be. This is a grief beyond words.

5. **Acceptance.** ("My time is very close now, and it's all right.") This stage is not one of resignation but, rather,

one of accepting what cannot be changed with a sense of peace and serenity. It is a time almost devoid of feeling—a letting go. Kübler-Ross notes that not everyone dies in a state of acceptance. The key is having another human being nearby who cares unconditionally.

Loved ones of the dying person experience a wide range of stressful emotions and denial of the impending death—anger and rage toward health caregivers, bargaining with God, despair, depression, and finally acceptance. Seeking the services of a thanatologist (a person knowledgeable of the psychological coping mechanisms for dealing with death) or support services can be helpful.

## THE RIGHT TO DIE

**Euthanasia** is derived from two Greek words—*eu*, meaning "good," and *thanatos*, meaning "death." There are two types of euthanasia.

1. *Active euthanasia* requires a direct action to bring about death. The two types of active euthanasia are suicide and mercy killing or physician-assisted suicide. Most often active euthanasia involves the use of strong chemical compounds that depress the central nervous system and induce death. Active euthanasia is illegal in the United States and most other countries. The best known public figure involved in assisted suicide is Dr. Jack Kevorkian, who has been called "Dr. Death" and the "suicide doctor." He has assisted with 45 physician-assisted suicides.

2. *Passive euthanasia* involves a protocol in which no action or medical intervention is taken to hasten death. It usually involves the removal of medical technology or refusal of medical intervention. Medical treatment or life-sustaining procedures (such as intravenous feeding or oxygen therapy) are withheld, or the decision is made not to initiate medical treatment (such as heart surgery) needed to save a person's life. In most states mentally competent adults have the legal right to refuse medical treatment. The most

impassioned controversies arise when patients are not responsive and family members or physicians have to make the decision on their behalf.

A landmark case involved Theresa Marie "Terri" Schiavo, who experienced cardiac arrest and collapsed early in 1990. She incurred massive brain damage and remained in a coma for 10 weeks. Three years after her collapse, she was diagnosed as being in a persistent vegetative state (PVS) with very little chance of recovery. Her husband and parents and others, including Governor Jeb Bush of Florida, differed over her right to live or die for seven years. Terri did not have a living will; therefore, a trial was held to determine her wishes regarding life-prolonging procedures. Arguments from both sides of the issue were heard. Her husband claimed that Terri would not want to be kept on a machine. Her parents claimed that Terri was a devout Roman Catholic who would not want to violate the Church's teachings on euthanasia by refusing nutrition and hydration. Despite 14 appeals, innumerable motions, petitions, hearings, five suits, and four denials of certiorari from the Supreme Court of the United States, her feeding tube was removed for a third and final time and she died on March 31, 2005, at age 41. What do you think would have happened if Terri had prepared an advance directive or a "Five Wishes" document before her illness occurred?

## ADVANCE PREPARATION FOR MEDICAL CRISES CAUSING DEATH

The Fives Wishes document and advance directive are the documents most commonly used to prepare for medical crises.

The Five Wishes document (www.agingwithdignity .org) allows the elderly and gravely ill to have their wishes carried out in case of medical crises or emergencies. It specifies the kind of medical treatment to be used, the person designated to make health care decisions, the patient's expected comfort level and treatment from persons around them, and the information that is to be given to loved ones.

The Five Wishes document is written with the aid of the American Bar Association's Commission on Legal Problems of the Elderly and is used in a majority of the states. A living will may also direct physicians to continue intervention, and different kinds of care.

## ADVANCE DIRECTIVE

An advance directive is a written document a person prepares indicating what medical decisions should be made if he or she loses the ability to make decisions due to some medical emergency or crisis. The two most commonly prepared documents are a living will and the power of attorney.

---

## FYI | THE DYING PERSON'S BILL OF RIGHTS

■ I have the right to be treated as a living human being until I die.

■ I have the right to maintain a sense of hopefulness, however changing its focus may be.

■ I have the right to be cared for by those who can maintain a sense of hopefulness, however changing this might be.

■ I have the right to express my feelings and emotions about my approaching death in my own way.

■ I have the right to participate in decisions concerning my care.

■ I have the right to expect continuing medical and nursing attention, even though "cure" goals must be changed to "comfort" goals.

■ I have the right not to die alone.

■ I have the right to be free from pain.

■ I have the right to have my questions answered honestly.

■ I have the right not to be deceived.

■ I have the right to have help from and for my family in accepting my death.

■ I have the right to die in peace and dignity.

■ I have the right to retain my individuality and not be judged for my decisions, which may be contrary to the beliefs of others.

■ I have the right to discuss and enlarge my religious or spiritual experiences, whatever these may mean to others.

■ I have the right to expect that the sanctity of the human body will be respected after death.

■ I have the right to be cared for by caring, sensitive, knowledgeable people who will attempt to understand my needs and will be able to gain some satisfaction in helping me face my death.

*Source:* "The Dying Person's Bill of Rights," *American Journal of Nursing*, vol. 75, January 1975, p. 99. Reprinted by permission of Lippincott Williams & Wilkins. From a workshop on "The Terminally Ill Patient and the Helping Person" in Lansing, Michigan, sponsored by the Southwestern Michigan Inservice Education Council and conducted by Amelia J. Barbus, associate professor of nursing at Wayne State University, Detroit Michigan, in 1975.

---

## KEY TERMS

**Rigor mortis** stiffening of the muscles after death

**Euthanasia** intentional and express termination of a life when quality is perceived to be such that it is not worth living

**FIGURE 14.4 ▶** A Sample of a Living Will

### SAMPLE LIVING WILL DECLARATION

Declaration made this _____ day of _____
     (month and year)

I, _____, being of sound mind willfully and voluntarily
     (Print full name)

make known my desires that my dying shall not be artificially prolonged under the circumstances set forth
below, do hereby declare:

If at any time I should have an incurable injury, disease, or illness certified to be a terminal condition
by two physicians who have personally examined me, one of whom shall be my attending physician, and
the physicians have determined that my death will occur whether or not life-sustaining procedures are utilized and where the application of life-sustaining procedures would serve only to artificially prolong the
dying process, I direct that such procedures be withheld or withdrawn, and that I be permitted to die naturally with only the administration of medication or the performance of any medical procedure deemed necessary to provide me with comfort care.

In the absence of my ability to give directions regarding the use of such life-sustaining procedures, it is
my intention that this declaration shall be honored by my family and the physician(s) as the final expression of my legal right to refuse medical or surgical treatment and accept the consequences from such
refusal.

I understand the full import of this declaration and I am emotionally and mentally competent to make
this decision.

Signed _____

City, County, and State of Residence _____

Date _____

The declarant has been personally known to me and I believe him or her to be of sound mind. I did not
sign the declarant's signature above for or at the direction of the declarant. I am not related to the declarant
by blood or marriage, entitled to any portion of the estate of the declarant according to the laws of intestate
succession or under any will of declarant or codicil thereto, or directly financially responsible for declarant's medical care.

Witness _____

Witness _____

Date _____

A **living will** can take the moral, legal, and ethical
pressure off survivors if a decision about treatment has to
be made in the event of a terminal illness or critical condition. In essence, the living will directs that life-sustaining
procedures be withheld if the patient is in a terminal

condition. Although the laws vary slightly from one state
to another, the will generally must be:

- drafted by a mentally competent adult
- drafted in the person's handwriting

- signed by the person making the will. If the person is physically unable to sign but is mentally competent, it may be signed by someone else in the person's presence
- dated
- witnessed by two adults. Neither can be the person who signed the will, and neither can stand to benefit financially from the person's death. (For example, a witness could not be named as a beneficiary on the person's life insurance policy.)
- delivered by the person or at the person's direction to his or her physician
- in accordance with the form prescribed by state law

Once drafted, a living will stands forever, unless the person who drafts it decides to revoke it. In that case, the person can destroy the will, issue a written revocation, or verbally revoke it in the presence of an adult witness. That witness must sign and date a notification of the revocation and deliver it to the person's physician. Figure 14.4 provides an example of a living will.

Some states also allow a person to give **power of attorney** to a trusted family member or friend. This proxy is entitled legally to speak on that person's behalf, make medical decisions for him or her, and see that the person's wishes are carried out.

## THE HOLOGRAPHIC WILL

A **holographic will** is a legal, completely handwritten document (in most states) in which the writer gives directives concerning his or her decisions and wishes in the event of the writer's death. The document usually contains

- a person named as executor
- a list of personal items or property and a list stating to whom the items and property are to be given
- a selectee or guardian if the writer has young children
- memorial, funeral, or burial arrangements
- the location of the holographic will

When a person dies without a will, he or she dies intestate. When no will exists, the state in which the dead person resides makes decisions concerning the welfare of any minor children and the dead person's property.

## HOSPICE CARE

In addition to choosing when to die, people may be able to choose where to die. Advances in technology have enabled most dying patients to choose to die either in the hospital or at home. Much of that choice is made possible by **hospice care,** a concept that originated in England.

Whether the patient is at home, in a hospital, or at a hospice center, hospice care provides comforting, kind, caring, humane services to people who are dying and to their families and caregivers. The hospice team focuses on the physical, social, emotional, and spiritual needs of the terminally ill person. The patient is made as comfortable as possible and is given personalized attention. Though hospice care can be offered in an institutionalized setting, most hospice patients are cared for in their own homes.

Additionally, the hospice team supports the family of the dying person by helping family members accept and prepare for the death. Family members are taught how to care for the dying person physically and emotionally. Hospice team members visit regularly to provide extra nursing care, emotional support, or other kinds of assistance and support.

## ORGAN DONATIONS

The **Uniform Anatomical Gift Act** provides for donation of the body or specific parts of the body when a donor dies. The act was approved in 1968 and is legal in all 50 states. Most commonly, the donor carries a **uniform donor card,** signed and witnessed, which specifies the donor's wishes. The uniform donor card allows donors to specify whether they want any needed organs or parts donated or whether the body can be used for anatomical study. Uniform donor cards are available from the National Kidney Foundation, and in some states they are available where driver's licenses are issued. Federal law requires that all families of brain-dead patients be offered the option of organ and tissue donation.

Although some people are disturbed by the thought of harvesting organs, the procedures used to remove organs are similar to those used in standard autopsies. Depending

### KEY TERMS

**Living will** legal written document stating what kind of treatment should or should not be given in the event of a terminal illness or critical condition

**Power of attorney** appointment of a friend or relative to make legal decisions for another

**Holographic will** legal handwritten document in which the writer leaves instructions to be carried out upon his or her death

**Hospice care** services for terminally ill patients and their families focusing on their comfort and social, emotional, and spiritual needs

**Uniform Anatomical Gift Act** legislation that provides for the donation of the body or organs upon a person's death

**Uniform donor card** document that specifies the wishes of a person to donate organs after death

on the organs being donated, the process may not vary significantly from what has to be done to prepare the body for burial. The body is treated with respect and dignity.

Many organs and parts can be transplanted successfully. Those used most often are the heart, lungs, liver, kidneys, bones, skin (used for grafting), corneas, pancreas, cartilage, and bone marrow. Organ donation offers life or a better quality of life to another person and gives the donor family the opportunity to help others at their time of tragedy and loss. The donor's family neither pays for nor receives payment for organ and tissue donation. All costs related to donation are paid for by the organ procurement center or transplant center. Most religions throughout the world support organ and tissue donation as a humanitarian act.

## DEATH

**Funeral** and memorial services are a rite of passage for people who have died. These services recognize the value of the dead person, comfort survivors, and play an important role in the grieving process by helping survivors say good-bye. Specific kinds of services are dictated by cultural beliefs. Some are somber occasions in which the dead person is paid tribute and eulogized. Wakes are joyous occasions in which survivors celebrate the person's life. In some cases terminally ill people plan their own funeral or memorial, choosing the type of ceremony and those who will participate.

Costs of services vary substantially (most are very expensive) and can include the casket, services of funeral home staff, use of facilities and equipment, the cemetery plot or crypt, the vault or liner, gravesite care, services of the clergy, and flowers. Costs also vary depending on how the body is disposed of; that is, whether it is embalmed or cremated.

**Embalming** preserves the body for an indefinite time after death, allowing funeral participants to view the corpse. In some states, embalming is not required by law. However, a body must be buried within a strict time frame if it is not embalmed or cremated.

**Cremation** reduces the body to ashes, called cremains. When a body is cremated, the survivors usually honor the deceased person with a memorial service. The cremains are kept in an urn or other containers, placed in a crypt, or buried in a cemetery. Some cemeteries have special vaults where the container of cremains can be stored.

## Summary

- Aging begins with conception and is an inevitable life-long process. As people age they may experience energy loss, muscle weakness, greater susceptibility to various diseases and illnesses, and problems with mobility. However, these changes are not entirely a result of aging itself but, instead, of poor nutrition and inactivity.

- Life expectancy increased drastically in the 1990s due to improved medical care, decreased infectious diseases, improved nutrition, and strides in sanitation and disease prevention.

- Life span and life expectancy are lengthening, giving rise to new issues surrounding the growing population of the elderly.

- Gerontologists have identified three ways of determining age: biological, functional, and psychological. Three particular concerns of aging are sexual functioning, menopause, and depression.

- Diseases and conditions common in the elderly population include osteoporosis, Alzheimer's disease, diabetes, urinary incontinence, influenza, and pneumonia.

- To counteract the ill effects of aging, people should eat healthy, remain or become physically fit, maintain a healthy weight, drink alcohol in moderation, and not smoke.

- Elderly people are more prone to accidents (in the home and on the road) because of poor eyesight, diminished hearing acuity, decreased coordination and balance, slower reactions, and the physical limitations posed by any disease.

- Caregiving for older people has become a major issue. The options range from remaining at home with possible in-home services to nursing home care.

- Death is classified according to the medical and legal communities as brain death, clinical death, and cellular death.

- When learning of impending death, the five stages a person experiences are denial, anger, bargaining, depression, and acceptance.

- Euthanasia has two forms: active (suicide or physician-assisted death) and passive.

- The living will allows a person to state the conditions for continuing his or her life. The holographic will is a legally binding, handwritten will giving various instructions to be followed upon the writer's death.

- Funeral options range widely in cost and require decisions regarding embalming, cremation, and burial.

## Personal Health Resources

ThomsonNOW Visit the ThomsonNOW website at http://thomsonedu.com/thomsonnow for valuable resources that will:

- Help you evaluate your knowledge of the material.

- Guide you through tutorials to help you understand and apply the material.

- Allow you to take an exam-prep quiz to better prepare for class tests.

AARP Global Aging Program. This site serves as an international clearinghouse of the most relevant and timely information on the aging population worldwide.

**www.aarp.org/globalageing**

Administration on Aging. This site provides information about varied issues surrounding the older population and programs that address the diverse needs of an aging society.

**www.aoa.gov**

Aging Research Center. This site provides statistical information concerning the older population.

**www.wrclab.org**

Centers for Disease Control and Prevention. This government agency provides statistical data for vital health concerns, diseases, and prevention.

**www.cdc.gov**

Gerontology Research Group. This site has the official tables of known supercentenarians.

**www.grg.org**

International Federation on Aging. This site promotes and improves the understanding of aging policies and practices globally.

**www.ifa-fiv.org**

Wikipedia. This site provides extensive information on aging, gerontology, and psychology.

**www.en.wikipedia.org/wiki/ageing**

## It's Your Turn for Study and Review

1. Aging does not begin on a certain birthday, but it begins at birth. It is a normal process of development throughout life that people experience at different rates. Fully discuss some life-enhancing factors that you may put into place now.

2. Research and write a short essay on the pros and cons of active euthanasia. Include your personal opinion of active euthanasia and explain your reasoning.

3. Interview several elderly persons. Collect data concerning their personal experiences of the aging process. Utilizing information from the interviews, develop a plan of action as to how you can start to confront the changes brought by aging.

4. Death is the final act, the completion of life. Because of death, many family members and friends are left bereaved. Coping with grief may evoke a wide range of emotions, including anger, anxiety, guilt, and depression. One way of coping is to express your feelings. List and discuss other ways of coping with grief.

## Selected Bibliography

*AARP Bulletin*—Discoveries. "Alzheimers: A Dream Drug." 47:4, April 2006, p. 28.

Administration on Aging. "The Many Faces of Aging: Facts and Figures," Fact Sheet. Washington, DC: U.S. Department of Health and Agency for Healthcare Research and Quality, Centers for Disease Control and Prevention. Physical Activity and Older Americans Benefits and Strategies. Accessed May 2004.

Bastian, D. "The Joy of Aging." *Christianity Today*, 50:1, January 2006, pp. 52–54.

Boyles, D. "Nostalgia." *AARP The Magazine*, January/February 2007, p. 84.

Bren, L. "Alzheimer's: Searching for a Cure." *FDA Consumer*, 37:4, July/August 2003, p. 18.

Birge, S. "The WHI and the Brain: What Have We Learned?" *Sexuality, Reproduction, and Menopause*, 2:2, June 2004, p. 71.

Cohen, E. and Kass, L. R. "Cast Me Not Off in Old Age." *Commentary*, 121:1, January 2006, pp. 32–39.

Cohen, G. "The Myth of Midlife Crisis." *Newsweek*, 147:3, January 16, 2006, pp. 82, 84–86.

Corbet, B. "Nursing Home Undercover." *AARP The Magazine*, January/February 2007, p. 70.

Curtis, P. "The Anti-Aging Pill." *Reader's Digest*, March 2007, p. 115.

Hawaleshka, D. "Can a Few Simple Moves Heal Her?" *Maclean's*, January 22, 2007, pp. 44–45.

Koerth-Baker, M. "Feats of Endurance." *AARP The Magazine*, January/February 2007, pp. 13–14.

Kübler-Ross, E. *On Death and Dying*. New York: Macmillan, 1969.

Matausek, M. "Dropping By." *AARP The Magazine*, January/February 2007, pp. 26–28.

Mather, M. and Carstensen, L. L. "Aging and Motivated Cognition: The Positivity Effect in Attention and Memory." *Trends in Cognitive Sciences*, 9, 2005, pp. 496–502.

Moran, J. and Simon, K. I. "Income and the Use of Prescription Drugs by the Elderly: Evidence from the Notch Cohorts." *The Journal of Human Resources*, XLI:2, Spring 2006.

## KEY TERMS

**Funeral** rites of passage for those who have died

**Embalming** procedure in which blood and body fluids are drained and formaldehyde and alcohol are injected

**Cremation** incineration of a body in a specialized furnace

Masoro, E. J. Austad, S. N. *Handbook of the Biology of Aging*, 6th ed. San Diego, CA: Academic Press, 2006.

Rando, T. *How to Go On Living When Someone You Love Dies.* New York: Bantam, 1988.

Research Notebook, "Disability Among Older Americans Continues to Decline." *FDA Consumer*, January/February 2007, p. 7.

Thoma, S. A. and Lincoln, N. B. "Factors Relating to Depression after Stroke." *British Journal of Clinical Psychology*, 45:1, March 2006, pp. 49–61.,

Updates "Expanded Use of Aricept." *FDA Consumer*, January/Febraury 2007, p. 3.

U.S. Census Bureau Population Division and Housing and Household Economic Statistics Division. January 18, 2001.

U.S. Department of Health and Human Services. *Healthy People 2010: Understanding and Improving Health.* Washington, DC: U.S. Government Printing Office, 2000.

Washburn, A. and Sands, L. "Social Cognition in Nursing Home Residents with and without Cognitive Impairment." *The Journal of Gerontology: Psychological Sciences*, 174: Vol. 61 B N 3 May 2006.

Weil, A. "Aging Naturally." *Time*, 166:16, October 17, 2005, pp. 60–66, 69–70.

Name _____    Course _____

Date _____    Section _____

The following are factors that will affect your life as you get older. Check each box that applies to you.

☐ I eat nutritional foods.

☐ My weight is within the recommended range.

☐ I exercise regularly and according to sound principles.

☐ I do not smoke cigarettes or misuse drugs.

☐ I get regular physical checkups and conduct self-exams.

☐ I get enough sleep.

☐ I stimulate my mind and stay mentally active.

☐ I have a good sense of self-worth and self-esteem.

☐ I have learned ways to deal with stress effectively.

☐ I maintain friendships and nurture interpersonal relationships.

☐ I help others and participate in volunteer activities.

☐ I buckle my seat belt, have an operational smoke detector in my home, and adhere to safety regulations and standards.

☐ I respect the environment and do what I can to preserve it by recycling and not being wasteful.

☐ I am planning financially for my retirement.

☐ I have a legal will covering disposition of my desires upon my death.

The more boxes you checked, the better off you will be as you get older. Reread the items you did not check, and make a commitment to work on them.

Name _____     Course _____

Date _____     Section _____

Complete the following questionnaire to determine your risk for developing osteoporosis.

| Question | Yes | No |
|---|:---:|:---:|
| **1.** Do you have a small, thin frame, or are you Caucasian or Asian? | ☐ | ☐ |
| **2.** Do you have a family history of osteoporosis? | ☐ | ☐ |
| **3.** Are you a postmenopausal woman? | ☐ | ☐ |
| **4.** Have you had early or surgically induced menopause? | ☐ | ☐ |
| **5.** Have you been taking excessive thyroid medication or high doses of cortisone-like drugs for asthma, arthritis, or cancer? | ☐ | ☐ |
| **6.** Is your diet low in dairy products and other sources of calcium? | ☐ | ☐ |
| **7.** Are you physically inactive? | ☐ | ☐ |
| **8.** Do you smoke cigarettes or drink alcohol in excess? | ☐ | ☐ |

The more times you answer "yes," the greater your risk for developing osteoporosis.
See your physician, and contact the National Osteoporosis Foundation for more information.

*Source:* Reprinted with permission from the National Osteoporosis Foundation, Washington, DC 2003.

Name _____     Course _____

Date _____     Section _____

The chart on the back of this sheet will give you a rough idea of how your life expectancy varies from the norm. To estimate how long you will live, begin by using the table below to find the median life expectancy for your age group. Then add or subtract years based on the risk factors listed on the chart on the following page (you should adjust your risk-factor score by the percentage at right if you are over 60).

| AGE | MALE | FEMALE | SCORING RISK FACTORS |
| --- | --- | --- | --- |
| 20–59 | 73 | 80 | Use table as shown |
| 60–69 | 76 | 81 | Reduce loss or gain by 20% |
| 70–79 | 78 | 82 | Reduce loss or gain by 50% |
| 80+ | Add five years to current age | | Reduce loss or gain by 75% |

| | Gain in life expectancy | | | No change | Loss in life expectancy | | | Start with your median life expectancy |
|---|---|---|---|---|---|---|---|---|
| **HEALTH** | **+3 YEARS** | **+2 YEARS** | **+1 YEAR** | | **–1 YEAR** | **–2 YEARS** | **–3 YEARS** | **TALLY** |
| Blood pressure | Between 90/65 and 120/81 | Less than 90/65 without heart disease | Between 121/82 and 129/85 | 130/86 | Between 131/87 and 140/90 | Between 141/91 and 150/95 | More than 151/96 | |
| Diabetes | — | — | — | None | Type II (adult onset) | — | Type I (juvenile onset) | |
| Total cholesterol | — | — | Less than 160 | 161–200 | 201–240 | 241–280 | More than 280 | |
| HDL cholesterol | — | — | More than 55 | 45–54 | 40–44 | Less than 40 | — | |
| Compared with that of others my age, my health is: | — | — | Excellent | Very good or fair | — | Poor | Extremely poor | |
| **LIFESTYLE** | **+3 YEARS** | **+2 YEARS** | **+1 YEAR** | | **–1 YEAR** | **–2 YEARS** | **–3 YEARS** | **TALLY** |
| Cigarette smoking | None | Ex-smoker, no cigarettes for more than five years | Ex-smoker, no cigarettes for three to five years | Ex-smoker, no cigarettes for one to three years | Ex-smoker, no cigarettes for five months to one year | Smoker, zero to 20 pack-years* | Smoker, more than 20 pack-years | |
| Secondhand-smoke exposure | — | — | — | None | Zero to one hour per day | One to three hours per day | More than three hours per day | |
| Exercise average (give yourself most positive category) | More than 90 minutes per day of exercise (for example, walking) for more than three years | More than 60 minutes per day for more than three years | More than 20 minutes per day for more than three years | More than 10 minutes per day for more than three years | More than five minutes per day for more than three years | Less than five minutes per day | None | |
| Saturated fat in diet | — | Less than 20% | 20%–30% | 31%–40% | — | More than 40% | — | |
| Fruits and vegetables | — | — | Five servings per day | — | None | — | — | |
| **FAMILY** | **+3 YEARS** | **+2 YEARS** | **+1 YEAR** | | **–1 YEAR** | **–2 YEARS** | **–3 YEARS** | **TALLY** |
| Marital status | — | Happily married man | Happily married woman | Single woman, widowed man | Divorced man, widowed woman | Divorced woman | Single man | |
| Disruptive events in the past year** | — | — | — | — | One | Two | Three | |
| Social groups, friends seen more than once per month*** | — | Three | Two | One | — | None | — | |
| Parents' age at death | — | — | Both lived past 75 | One lived past 75 | — | — | Neither lived past 75 | |

Your estimated life expectancy [        ]

*A pack-year is one pack per day for a year.
**Deaths of family members, job changes, moves, lawsuits, financial insecurity, and so on.
***People who offer support through disruptive events (applicable only in case of two or more such events).
*Source:* From Michael F. Roizen, M.D., using data abstracted from "The Real Age and Age-Reduction-Planning Programs of Medical Informatics." June 30, 1997, Newsweek, Inc., p. 65.

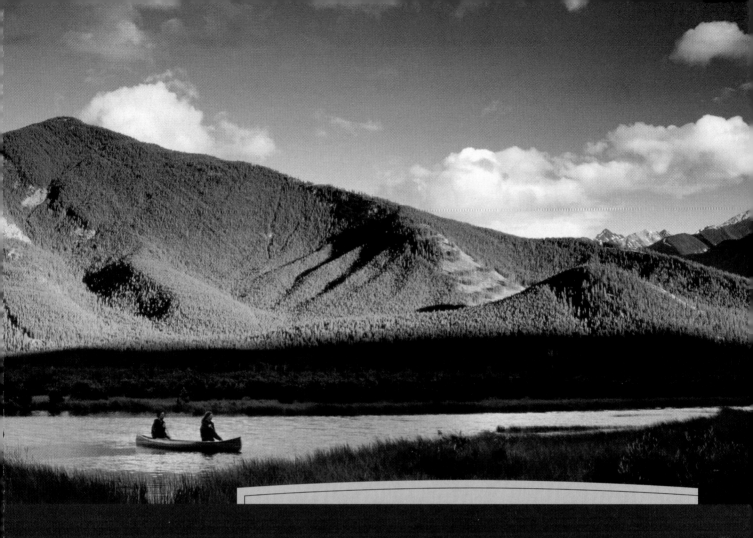

# Chapter Fifteen Consumerism and Environmental Health

**OBJECTIVES** ■ Outline issues surrounding self-care, including home health tests. ■ Identify and differentiate types of health care professionals. ■ Identify and differentiate types of health care facilities. ■ Identify responsible ways to use prescription drugs. ■ Differentiate brand-name and generic medications. ■ Identify different ways of paying for health care. ■ Recognize the techniques employed in health fraud. ■ List the various environmental threats to people. ■ Identify the sources and effects of various kinds of pollution.

ThomsonNOW™ Log on to ThomsonNOW at http://thomsonedu.com/ thomsonnow to access and explore self-assessments, interactive tutorials, and practice quizzes.

Taking responsibility for your health starts with wise self-care. This requires you to know when it is no longer smart to self-diagnose and self-treat. You need to familiarize yourself with the type of health care provider you need and how to find a good one. In addition, you need to know how to use medicines correctly, whether your doctor prescribes them or you buy them over-the-counter; what your options are for paying for health care; and how to avoid fraud.

When you take responsibility for yourself, you also take responsibility for the conditions in which you live, including those of the planet everyone shares. It means first being aware of what causes pollution and then doing your part to reduce pollution and the negative effects of other threats to the environment.

A number of government agencies can help in your quest to be responsible for yourself and your environment. You also can take many steps individually.

## Being a Smart Health Consumer

Your level of wellness is dynamic. Throughout your life many factors—some controllable, some not—influence your state of wellness: inherited conditions and your health at birth, your environment, your access to regular professional health care, and your behavior and lifestyle. You can do many things to influence your health, even to compensate for the factors you cannot control or modify, such as heredity.

Many resources for information about your health are available.

- Your health care professional (if your doctor does not volunteer the information, ask him or her)
- The library
- Information in newspapers, magazines, news programs, and health programs on radio and television
- Government agencies, such as the National Institutes of Health, the Centers for Disease Control and Prevention, the Environmental Protection Agency, and the Food and Drug Administration
- Nonprofit organizations, such as the American Heart Association and the American Cancer Society
- Labels on food and medications (by federal law, these labels, which provide certain health-related information, must be truthful and accurate)
- Consumer action groups, which provide information on health care fraud

### SELF-CARE

The growing trend toward **self-care** has stemmed from several factors.

- People want to be in control of their health, and more Americans than ever are learning the basics.

- The cost of health care has skyrocketed over the last decade, making self-care a necessity for many.
- *Prevention* has become a household term, and disease prevention entails many steps people can take on their own.

That does not mean you should stop going to the doctor. What it does mean is that you may be able to do some of the things you previously relied on health care professionals to do. It also means being wise enough to know the difference. Responsible self-care involves a number of elements.

- Knowing whether you are sick enough to need a physician
- Checking your own vital signs (such as your pulse and your temperature)
- Using home health tests (such as those that determine pregnancy and those that detect hidden blood in the stool) when appropriate
- Managing certain kinds of illnesses and injuries, such as common colds, indigestion, and minor abrasions
- Administering your own therapy, such as allergy shots, insulin for diabetes, and asthma treatments
- Preventing illness and injury
- Performing regular self-exams (such as monthly breast self-exam or testicle self-exam)
- Promoting your own health and wellness—starting an exercise program, losing weight, or reducing stress

Part of responsible self-care is knowing when self-care is no longer safe or smart. Knowing when you need to consult a health care provider is not always easy. Generally, you should seek medical help for any unusual symptoms that keep coming back, any serious injury or accident, unexplained changes in weight, or any unexplained bleeding. You also should consult a health professional if you develop any sudden, severe, or persistent symptoms, including the following.

- Chest pain
- Shortness of breath
- Bluish skin, lips, or fingernails
- Yellowing of skin or whites of the eyes
- High fever (102°F in adults, 103°F in children)
- Any significant and persistent change in bowel or bladder habits
- Diarrhea or vomiting that lasts more than two days or that comes back
- A sore that does not heal
- A lump, thickness, or swelling that gets bigger
- Numbness, paralysis, or slurred speech

## Tips for Action Safe Use of OTC Drugs

Over-the-counter (OTC) medications can be an effective weapon in one's self-care arsenal, if they are used safely. Always follow the manufacturer's directions exactly.

■ Do not take more than is recommended.

■ Do not take the medicine longer than is recommended.

■ Do not use medications that have expired.

■ Do not give medications to children under age 12 unless the label lists a recommended dose for children.

■ Do not continue taking the medication if the symptoms get worse or persist.

■ Allergic reactions to medication or an insect sting (severe swelling, dizziness, difficulty breathing, widespread hives, swelling of the throat or tongue)

■ Injury to the head followed by loss of consciousness, vomiting, or blurred vision

## HOME HEALTH TESTS

A number of consumer-controlled test kits or "home testing kits" on the market can be administered in the privacy of your own home. Many of them are available at local retail outlets; some are available by mail order or Internet-purchase only. It is particularly important to do a little research if you are purchasing online. For example, there are several brands of home testing kits for HIV being sold via the Internet. Keep in mind that the only home testing kit for HIV that is Food and Drug Administration (FDA) approved is the Access HIV-1 Test System®. Used properly, most home testing kits are accurate a high percentage of the time. To get the best results, follow these suggestions.

■ Ask your pharmacist or physician about the test before you buy it. These pros are qualified to give advice and answer questions.

■ Check the expiration date on the test before you buy it. Expired test kits may not yield accurate results.

■ Check the label before you leave the store. Some test kits should be protected from heat, cold, or light.

■ Read the instructions all the way through first; then follow directions carefully. If you are unsure about anything, talk to your pharmacist or doctor before using the test.

■ If the test has to be timed, use a watch with a second hand.

■ Write down your test results in case you need to compare them against a second test later.

Keep in mind that as useful as home health tests can be, they are not a substitute for professional testing or medical care.

## ACCESS TO HEALTH CARE

Health care in the United States is not available equally to all residents. One serious barrier is income. Many of the nation's poor cannot afford to go to the doctor, are too far from a health clinic, live in isolated areas, or cannot qualify for Medicaid or other subsidized programs. For some, the only health care that is available is the hospital emergency room, so they use this facility for nonemergency health care. This adds to the problem of health care delivery from an already overburdened hospital staff.

Poor people are at a disadvantage in getting health care. Many private doctors refuse to accept Medicaid patients or accept only a small quota. Some of the poorest areas of the United States traditionally are the least generous when qualifying people for Medicaid, so scores of the nation's poor have no medical help at all.

Studies have shown a direct relationship between health status and literacy skills. Half of those with the lowest literacy skills are Caucasians, according to the National Council on Patient Information and Education. Only a sixth-grade reading level is required to read a driver's license manual, but a 10th-grade reading level is necessary to understand the instructions on a bottle of aspirin. An informed consent form that must be signed before a test, treatment, or procedure requires college-level reading skills to understand.

Years of education also have been shown to relate directly to health status. Part of the reason is that educated people tend to practice better health behaviors, such as regular screening tests. When experts analyzed which women over age 40 were getting mammograms, the results told a grim story. More than 40% of those with more than 12 years of education had had a mammogram during the year preceding the study. For women of the same age who had less than a high school education, the figures indicate that only 20% (half the number of more educated women) had a mammogram.

## Health Care Practitioners

Medicine has become highly sophisticated during the last four decades. As a result, a seemingly endless variety of

### KEY TERMS

**Self-care** taking responsibility for one's own basic health care (to include self-diagnosis and self-treatment with OTC medications)

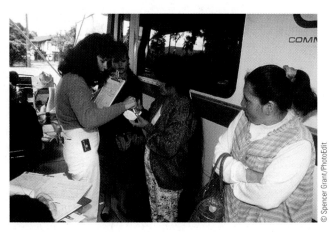

▲ *Access to professional medical care is a factor that influences health*

medical, dental, and other practitioners are present on the health care scene (less than 10% of all health care professionals are physicians). Some of these providers practice **orthodox medicine.** This traditional form of medical practice is based on scientifically validated procedures.

Nontraditional practitioners include chiropractors, acupuncturists, and other health care providers who rely on alternative methods of healing. The high costs of traditional health care are precipitating more interest in **integrative medicine**—a combination of conventional medical practices and natural, holistic, spiritual, lifestyle, and alternative approaches—according to Dr. Andrew Weil, a leading proponent. The American Holistic Medical Association has recommended that new patients ask 10 questions before making the final choice of a holistic physician. These questions would be appropriate to ask of an orthodox physician as well. One question of particular note is: "Does the practitioner appear to represent a healthy lifestyle, or does he or she show signs of overweight, overwork, smoking, or drinking?"

The most prevalent health care professionals are physicians, hospitalists, osteopathic physicians, dentists, podiatrists, optometrists, clinical psychologists, chiropractors, nurses, and allied health care practitioners.

## PHYSICIANS

Qualifying as a physician requires four years of undergraduate college work—with an emphasis on biology, anatomy, physiology, and chemistry—followed by at least four years of education at a school of medicine or osteopathy. To practice medicine, the person must graduate from an accredited school of medicine or osteopathy and pass a state licensing examination. The licensed physician's scope of practice covers medical problems of people of all ages.

Many physicians choose an area of specialty such as those listed in Table 15.1. They must complete a hospital-based residency program of an additional three to five years or more. After completing the residency, the

**TABLE 15.1** ▶ Selected Medical Specialties

| PHYSICIAN | SPECIALTY |
|---|---|
| Allergist | Allergies |
| Anesthesiologist | Sedating patients for surgery |
| Bariatrician | Prevention, control, and treatment of obesity |
| Cardiologist | Heart and blood vessel diseases |
| Dermatologist | Skin disorders and diseases |
| Endocrinologist | Gland disorders |
| Gastroenterologist | Diseases and disorders of the stomach and intestinal tract |
| Gerontologist | Diseases and disorders of elderly people |
| Gynecologist | Female reproductive health |
| Hematologist | Diseases and disorders of the blood and blood-forming tissues |
| Internist | Diagnosis and treatment of diseases of the internal organs by nonsurgical means |
| Neurologist | Diseases of the nervous system |
| Obstetrician | Prenatal care and childbirth |
| Oncologist | Cancer |
| Ophthalmalogist | Conditions of the eye |
| Orthopedic surgeon | Bone and joint disorders; bone fractures and injuries |
| Otolaryngologist | Ear, nose, and throat diseases |
| Pathologist | Study of the nature and cause of disease |
| Pediatrician | Diseases of children |
| Physiatrist | Physical disabilities |
| Psychiatrist | Mental and emotional disorders |
| Radiologist | Diagnosis and treatment using radiation |
| Surgeon | Manual and operative procedures to correct defects |
| Urologist | Diseases of the urinary tract and male reproductive tract |

physician is eligible to become board-certified in the selected specialty area (a diplomate).

## HOSPITALISTS

The nature of medical care evolves to meet the needs of the patient. In the mid-1990s, hospitals began hiring hospitalists or physicians who provide around-the-clock care for patients in hospital. A hospitalist is a primary-care physician who treats inpatients who do not have a primary-care physician or patients of primary-care physicians who do not provide inpatient services. There are more than 3,000 hospitalists practicing in the United States.

## FAMILY PRACTITIONERS

For their **primary-care physician,** most consumers choose a **family practitioner**—a physician (M.D.) or an **osteopathic physician** (D.O.) who treats all family members. Both professionals receive similar training. Osteopathic physicians, however, consider themselves to be more **holistic,** or oriented to treat the whole patient instead of a single disease or disorder. Within this overall orientation, osteopathy has specialty areas, too. If medical problems arise that cannot be handled by the primary-care physician, the patient generally is referred to a specialist for treatment.

> **VIEWPOINT** *The main professional organization for physicians is the American Medical Association (AMA). Should the AMA be able to endorse products and brands in the market? Proponents say this is the way to promote the best products. Opponents say medical organizations ruin their credibility when they accept money for endorsements. Which of these views do you support?*

## CHOOSING A PHYSICIAN

Choosing a primary care physician who is competent and empathetic requires some homework. It is much better to find your physician before a medical situation occurs. You will be able to make a more objective assessment, and the distractions will not mask your "gut feelings" about your selection. Remember, your doctor is your partner and your medical advocate, one whom you will appreciate if it becomes necessary for you to use more services of our complicated (and many times confusing) health care system. Family and friends are good sources for recommendations, as are other health care professionals (such as nurses) and the local hospital, university medical school, or medical association. The licensing board in your state has a list of physicians who have been disciplined either by state or by federal agencies. The offenses can be as minor as neglecting to take a continuing education course or as serious as harming a patient through negligence. Anyone can check with the board about a licensed physician.

## THE HEALTH EXAMINATION

After narrowing down your choices and choosing a physician based on answers to the questions you pose, the final step in choosing a physician is to make an appointment and visit the doctor. There are four components to a health examination (especially on your first visit) that are

vital. Your health history is so important that you will complete a questionnaire (usually 50 or more items). Based on your responses, the doctor will ask more questions about your health habits and family and social health. Be honest; this information is vital to your present and future health care plan. You are establishing a partnership with your medical advocate. Remember to take a copy of "My Portrait" (the family health history that you created in Chapter 1!) and share it with your doctor.

Many patients consider the physical examination the main event and become quite anxious. (Refer to FYI—What to Expect During An Examination.) Your health history is just as important during the physical examination. The doctor will ask follow-up questions and make notes. This is the time for you to ask questions, too. Do not be surprised about your anxiety. Remember, you will be sitting on a table dressed in an open-back, paper gown that covers very little. Laboratory tests will be performed on your blood and urine samples. The results of the exam and the lab tests will be reported to you.

If your visit to the doctor concerns a very serious health issue, it is wise to take someone you trust with you. Many times when patients are given the diagnosis of a serious medical condition, they become too emotional to hear and understand what the physician is telling them. This person (your second advocate) can calm you, take notes for you, and ask the doctor questions on your behalf.

Did you choose your physician wisely? Answers to the following questions will tell you.

- Were the waiting room and examination area clean and well organized?
- Was your wait reasonable?

### KEY TERMS

**Orthodox medicine** traditional or conventional form of medical practice using scientifically validated procedures

**Integrative medicine** a combination of orthodox, natural, holistic, spiritual, lifestyle, and alternative approaches to health care

**Primary-care physician** medical doctor seen initially for diagnosis, treatment, and management of health conditions of individuals or the family

**Family practitioner** physician who treats all family members

**Osteopathic physician** a doctor whose training is equivalent to a medical doctor's and includes emphasis on the musculoskeletal system and treatment of the whole person

**Holistic** treatment of patients that takes into account social and mental factors as well as physical condition

---

**Tips for Action** To Choose a Physician, Find out the Answers to These Questions

Ask the nurse or receptionist the following questions.

- How many years of training does the doctor have?
- How many years has the doctor practiced?
- Is the doctor licensed? If a specialist, is the physician board-certified?
- Where was the doctor trained?
- At which hospitals does the doctor have staff privileges?

- How many doctors are in the office? Will you always see the same one? Who takes over when the doctor is out of the office?
- Where is the office? Is it fast and easy to get to? Is parking convenient?
- What are the office hours? What will happen if help is needed after regular office hours?
- What method of payment or insurance does the doctor accept? What will happen if I cannot pay?

---

- Were you comfortable with the physician's gender, age, race, national origin, and his or her bedside manner?
- Did the physician seem comfortable with your gender, age, race, and national origin? Did the physician act patronizing, express negative racial stereotypes, or seem ignorant about cultural differences?
- Was the doctor easy to talk to? Did the doctor seem genuinely interested in you and take the time to answer all your questions, or did you feel rushed?
- Did the physician take a complete medical history as part of your initial visit? Did he or she take notes?
- Did the doctor explain what he or she was doing in terms you could understand? Did the doctor invite your questions?
- Did the doctor listen carefully to all your symptoms and complaints before making a diagnosis or recommending treatment? If the doctor was unsure of a diagnosis, was he or she willing to consult another doctor?
- Did the doctor ever talk about wellness, health promotion, or preventing disease, or was the emphasis on current symptoms and disorders?

If you do not like what you find, or if you feel uncomfortable, consult another physician.

## MULTICULTURAL CONCERNS

Health professionals naturally bring their own cultural background and beliefs to every patient encounter. This can influence their ability to communicate with and treat patients who are culturally different from themselves. Research has found, for example, that physicians spend more time communicating with younger patients than with older ones, more time with men than with women, and more time with people of higher socioeconomic status. In one classic study, authors P. L. Roter and J. A. Hall

reported that doctors tended to attribute the symptoms of Italian Americans to psychological causes—most likely because of their more verbal and descriptive style of talking about illness.

Although having the same cultural background or speaking the same language would clearly boost communication, it is not necessarily a prerequisite in a physician. As the National Council on Patient Information and Education stated, "Any health professional can develop better skills in dealing with the cultural factors surrounding medicine communication." The patient wants a physician who genuinely tries to communicate with everyone and who is not bogged down by common cultural myths.

You also need to be aware of your own cultural beliefs and habits and consider relating those to your physician. The National Council on Patient Information and Education points out, for example, that herbal treatments and other home remedies are popular among many cultures, including Asian, Hispanic, Brazilian, and American Indian. If you are using any alternative or herbal remedy, you should mention it to your doctor, as some of them may interfere with or counteract the effectiveness of medication the doctor prescribes for you. If the doctor is aware of such things, the treatment plan may be able to take advantage of both.

## OTHER PRACTITIONERS

The primary-care physician is only one of many professionals from whom you may seek medical help. Depending on your condition, you may need to consult one or more specialists.

**Dentists. Dentistry** involves diagnosis and treatment of the teeth, gums, and oral cavity. Dentists earn a bachelor's degree from a college or university and then complete an additional four-year program in a college of dentistry to earn a D.D.S. (Doctor of Dental Surgery) or a D.M.D. (Doctor of Medical Dentistry) degree. The dentist then must pass a state or regional licensing examination.

**Tips for Action** Making the Most of Your Doctor Visit

After making an appointment with the doctor, do the following.

■ **Put pen to paper.** Write down everything you can think of about your illness before you get to the doctor's office. If you do not write it down, you might forget to mention it.

■ **Play detective.** When did your symptoms start? What makes them worse? Better? Figure out all the clues so you can tell them to the doctor.

■ **Go over your list.** Talk to the doctor about all your concerns. Be specific. Do not leave out anything.

■ **Do not be afraid to ask questions.** If you do not understand something, ask. Do not give up until the doctor has explained it to you in terms you understand.

■ **Get it on paper.** Ask the doctor to write down any instructions. Ask if any pamphlets, brochures, or other written information is on hand that you can take home.

Some dentists choose to specialize, much like physicians do. Dental specialization requires additional coursework and clinical practice in the area of specialty. The specialties include:

■ *Endodontics*—treating the interior of the tooth, including the pulp and root (root canals)

■ *Orthodontics*—straightening irregularities of the teeth (installing braces)

■ *Periodontics*—treating diseases of the gum and bone, such as gingivitis and periodontitis

■ *Oral surgery*—operating to correct problems of the mouth, face, and jaw (such as removing impacted wisdom teeth)

The **dental hygienist** is the oral care specialist who takes x-rays of the teeth, cleans and polishes the teeth, and teaches patients how to take care of their mouth and teeth. A practicing dental hygienist must earn a bachelor's degree from an accredited school and pass a state licensing examination.

The **dental assistant** is the oral care professional who assists the dentist in the clinical setting. The duties include prepping the patient, preparing the instruments and handing them off to the dentist, clearing the patient's mouth during the procedure, and making impressions for dental prosthetics. Even though a degree is not required, the dental assistant may train at a community college/technical school or have on-the-job experience. Most states require passing a test.

Selecting a dentist requires just as much attention as selecting a physician, including recommendations from friends and family. You should make your choice before a dental emergency. The county dental society is another source for recommendations. If a dental school is established in your area, it can provide referrals. Again, the prospective patient should seek information concerning the office location, office hours, after-hours emergency care, billing procedures, and payment options. The dentist should examine your mouth thoroughly, explain all

treatment options, and answer questions carefully in understandable terms. The dentist's office should be clean, and anyone who touches the inside of the mouth—the dentist, any assistants, and the dental hygienist—should wear a mask and latex gloves to prevent the transmission of pathogens.

**Podiatrists.** **Podiatrists** diagnose and treat conditions of the feet, including corns, bunions, calluses, and malformations. Podiatrists complete an undergraduate degree, then a four-year academic and clinical program at an accredited school of podiatry. They earn either a D.P.M. (Doctor of Podiatric Medicine) or D.P. (Doctor of Podiatry) degree. Podiatrists can take x-rays, prescribe medication, prescribe therapies and therapeutic devices (such as corrective shoes), and perform surgery on the foot.

**Optometrists.** **Optometrists** complete an accredited academic and clinical program and receive an O.D. (Doctor of Optometry) degree. Then they must be licensed to practice. These practitioners examine the eyes, diagnose

### KEY TERMS

**Dentistry** practice involving diagnosis and treatment of teeth, gums, and oral cavity

**Dental hygienist** health care specialist, licensed to perform clinical tasks, who takes x-rays, cleans and polishes teeth, and teaches proper dental care

**Dental assistant** chairside assistant to the dentist who performs a variety of patient care, office, and sometimes laboratory duties

**Podiatrist** health care specialist who diagnoses and treats conditions of the feet

**Optometrist** licensed practitioner who examines the eyes, diagnoses problems, and prescribes eyeglasses or contact lenses

---

**Tips for Action** Boosting Your Oral Health

To maintain healthy teeth and gums:

■ Brush and floss the right way every day—after every meal, if possible.

■ Eat more whole-grain products, fresh fruits and vegetables, low-fat dairy products, lean meats, and dried peas and beans. Cut down on sugars, sweetened drinks, sweet snacks, and foods that stick to your teeth.

■ Watch for signs of trouble—chronic bad breath, a persistent bad taste in the mouth, aching teeth, loose teeth, or gums that are red, swollen, or bleeding.

■ Get regular dental checkups and attend to necessary dental work.

---

defects in eyesight, and prescribe eyeglasses or contact lenses to correct vision. An optometrist is not a physician, unlike an ophthalmologist, who can prescribe medication, treat diseases of the eye, and perform surgery.

**Clinical Psychologists. Clinical psychologists** complete both an undergraduate and a graduate program leading to the Ph.D. (Doctor of Philosophy) or Psy.D. (Doctor of Clinical Psychology). The scope of practice of the Ph.D. may be either clinical or counseling psychology. In most states psychologists also must be certified or licensed before they can practice. In many states they must meet further requirements. Many also earn credentials from professional societies and organizations. Clinical psychologists specialize in diagnosing and treating a variety of emotional and behavioral disorders without medication. They work with patients in individual or group settings. Some specialize in family or marriage counseling. Unlike psychiatrists, who hold the M.D. degree, clinical psychologists are not allowed to prescribe or dispense medication. However, legislation to allow prescribing authority within the scope of practice of psychology has been introduced in California, Connecticut, Georgia, Illinois, Tennessee, Texas, and New Mexico.

**Chiropractors. Chiropractors** employ a variety of techniques to manipulate the spine and relieve pain. As a type of alternative medicine (nontraditional medicine), **chiropractic medicine** is based on the belief that vital life forces flow from the spine to all parts of the body and that misalignment of the spine interrupts these life forces. Chiropractic methods often are successful in treating certain disorders, such as pain in the neck or lower back.

Chiropractors complete an intensive six-year academic program—emphasizing anatomy, physiology, biochemistry, and nutrition—combined with hands-on experience. They earn a D.C. (Doctor of Chiropractic) degree and are licensed and regulated by the states in which they practice. They are not allowed to prescribe or dispense medication or perform surgery. Chiropractors should adhere to standard chiropractic regimens, though specific techniques may differ. Chiropractors should not be used to take care of the medical needs of children.

**Nurses.** Nursing is concerned with providing information and clinical services that restore, maintain, or promote wellness and prevent illness. Nursing services are provided in a hospital, clinic, school, work site, or private physician's office. As with other disciplines, nursing has specialty areas that require additional classroom and clinical preparation. A nurse is the liaison between you and your physician.

The **registered nurse,** or R.N., completes an academic and clinical program at a college or school of nursing. The nurse then must pass a state licensing examination. The entry-level requirement for nursing is a college degree (B.S.N.) or associate degree in nursing.

Registered nurses who specialize in a clinical area and who diagnose and treat patients independent of a physician are called **nurse practitioners.** Examples are the family planning nurse practitioner and the certified nurse midwife. Nurse practitioners are required to complete advanced academic and clinical training. Many have master's or doctoral degrees in nursing. While they work under a physician's supervision, they perform many basic diagnostic and treatment procedures and prescribe medications, freeing physicians to handle more complex cases.

The **licensed practical nurse (LPN)** or licensed vocational nurse (LVN) have fewer educational requirements and a much shorter training period than the registered nurse—usually 12 to 18 months in a hospital-based program. Each must pass a state board examination before being able to work as a nurse. Their scope of practice is limited, and they must be supervised by a registered nurse or a physician.

**Allied Health Care Professionals.** Some of the allied health care professionals and paraprofessionals who help patients maintain and restore health are:

■ Nursing aides and physician assistants

■ Medical technologists

■ Emergency medical technicians

■ X-ray technicians

■ Occupational therapists

■ Physical therapists

■ Operating room technicians

## Tips for Action This Is Only a Test

Before you agree to any medical test, find out:

- Why the test is necessary.
- What the doctor expects to learn from the test.
- Whether the doctor could learn the same thing some other way.
- How long the test will take.

- What the test is going to feel like. (How much pain is involved? Will you be restricted afterward? How long before you can get back to your normal activities?)
- What risks are involved.
- How reliable the test is.

## FYI WHAT TO EXPECT DURING AN EXAMINATION

What should you expect from your next checkup? Your doctor should:

- Quiz you about major illnesses you have had, complaints you have now, drugs you are taking, any risky behaviors you engage in, and allergies you have.
- Check your skin for moistness, elasticity, and sores.
- Check your pulse and blood pressure.
- Check your eyes, ears, mouth, and nose with a flashlight, looking for signs of infection or disease.
- Check your neck for lumps in the thyroid gland or swollen lymph nodes.
- Listen to your heart and lungs with a stethoscope.
- Probe your abdomen for tenderness, rigidity, or hernia.
- Use a gloved finger to feel inside your rectum (a check for rectal cancer and an enlarged prostate gland in men).
- Check your joints for reflexes, swelling, or deformity.

If you are a woman, you also can expect a breast exam (the doctor will check for abnormal lumps) and a pelvic exam (the doctor will check the vagina and cervix for signs of disease).

years of specialized post-high school training. Many programs provide hospital-based training that leads to a college degree or associate degree. Most allied health care professionals must pass state or national licensing examinations before they are allowed to work in their field.

## Complementary and Alternative Medicine

As defined by the National Center for Complementary and Alternative Medicine (NCCAM), a component of the National Institutes of Health, **complementary and alternative medicine (CAM)** is a group of diverse medical and health care systems, practices, and products that are not presently considered to be part of conventional

### KEY TERMS

**Clinical psychologist** specialist in diagnosing and treating emotional and behavioral disorders without medication

**Chiropractor** health care practitioner who manipulates the spine to relieve pain

**Chiropractic medicine** a discipline founded on the belief that life forces flow from the spine to the rest of the body

**Registered nurse** health care practitioner who provides patient care and information that promote or restore health and wellness

**Nurse practitioner** registered nurse who is licensed to diagnose and treat patients independent of a physician

**Licensed practical nurse (LPN)** nurse with shortened training period and limited patient care responsibilities

**Complementary and alternative medicine (CAM)** a broad range of healing philosophies, approaches, and therapies not taught widely in medical schools, not generally used in hospitals, and not usually reimbursed by medical insurance companies; sometimes termed holistic therapy

- Phlebotomists
- Respiratory and inhalation therapists

Although not all of these areas of specialization require a college degree, all do require from one to five

medicine (medicine practiced by physicians with M.D. or D.O. degrees). The practices of complementary and alternative medicine change continually. Those therapies proven safe and effective become accepted as mainstream practices. Complementary medicine is used *together with* conventional medicine. Alternative medicine is used *in the place of* conventional medicine. The NCCAM classifies complementary and alternative medicine practices into five major categories or domains: alternative medical systems, mind-body interventions, biologically based treatments, manipulative and body-based methods, and energy therapies.

Alternative medical systems are built upon complete systems of theory and practice that may have evolved apart from or earlier than conventional systems used in the United States. Homeopathic medicine and naturopathic medicine are examples of alternative medical systems that developed in Western cultures.

Mind-body medicine uses various techniques designed to enhance the mind's capacity to affect bodily function and symptoms. Meditation, prayer, mental healing, and therapies that use creative expression are examples. Two alternative therapies that are popular and commercially successful are aromatherapy and music therapy.

Aromatherapy is a type of sensory therapy. In aromatherapy, essential oils extracted from flowers, leaves, barks, and other parts of plants are used to treat physiological or psychological health problems. These oils may be inhaled, applied to the skin, or added to bath water. The path to healing is through the olfactory nerves. Many are skeptical about the claims of aromatherapy in the treatment of physical ailments. However, smells do affect memory, and aromatherapy has been a component of treatment for some psychological disorders.

Music therapy is another type of sensory therapy. Its use has ancient roots, especially in China and India. Music may serve as an effective tool in therapy because it acts on the part of the brain that controls emotions and basic metabolic functions such as heart rate and blood pressure.

Biologically based therapies in CAM use substances found in nature for medical treatment and prevention. Examples include herbal products, foods, vitamins, and dietary supplements.

Manipulative and body-based methods use manipulation and/or movement of one or more parts of the body. Examples include chiropractic or osteopathic manipulation and various types of massage such as rolfing and shiatsu. Massage is a type of manipulative therapy that is associated with relaxation in the United States. However, massage is effective in treating back pain and relieving stress by lowering stress-related hormones such as norepinephrine.

Energy therapies such as biofield therapies (Reiki, pronounced "RAY-kee," and therapeutic touch or laying-on hands) involve manipulation of energy fields that purportedly surround a human body. Bioelectromagnetic-based therapies involve the unconventional use of electromagnetic fields (placing magnets on joints) to treat symptoms.

A savvy consumer of medical treatments must use a combination of factors to make appropriate choices, as individual needs are different. However, if you choose alternative medicine techniques to complement your orthodox or conventional health care, you should use the same precautions and ask the same questions of CAM practitioners as you would of orthodox practitioners. Remember that training and experience of CAM practitioners vary and that licensing and other regulations governing practice will vary by state or locality. Therefore, caveat emptor—research the practitioner's background.

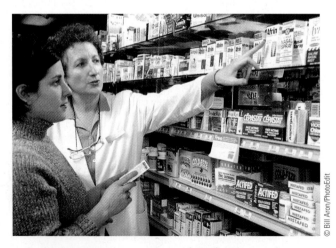

▲ *A pharmacist can provide useful information about prescription and over-the-counter medications*

## How to Choose Health Care Facilities

People who live in rural areas may have access to only a single health care facility. Those who live in urban areas may be able to choose from a private physician's office, a clinic, a nonprofit hospital, a for-profit hospital, a teaching hospital, a college health center, an outpatient surgery center, and a freestanding emergency center. Home health care may be available in some situations. The choice of a facility should be based on availability, convenience, the specific medical needs, ability to pay, and whether your physician has staff privileges at the facility. Hospitals are required to have a license. However, the Joint Commission on the Accreditation of Healthcare Organizations (JCAHO) is an independent organization that ensures the quality and safety of health care facilities. Even though it is not a requirement, for your protection, the hospital you use should be JCAHO accredited.

**TABLE 15.2 ▶** Health Care Facilities

| FACILITY | DESCRIPTION |
|---|---|
| Clinics | A group of practitioners work together in a single facility. They may cover only one specialty (such as internal medicine) or many specialties. Some include dental offices, x-ray facilities, and a pharmacy. |
| Not-for-profit hospitals | Typically administered by religious or other humanitarian groups, these hospitals provide care for patients regardless of whether the patient can pay for services. |
| For-profit hospitals | These hospitals are owned by a group of people or shareholders. They provide far less care for patients who are unable to pay. They generally stabilize these patients, then transfer them to nonprofit facilities. |
| Teaching hospitals | Affiliated with schools of medicine, these facilities provide a setting where students can study and practice alongside their professors. Experimental treatments and medications often are more available at teaching hospitals, used as part of studies and research programs. Teaching hospitals usually treat patients regardless of their ability to pay. |
| College health centers | These facilities are affiliated with colleges and universities. Some provide services only to students. Others extend services to staff, faculty, students, and family members. They range in size from small dispensaries to large multispecialty clinics. Patients generally receive treatment at a discount or for a co-pay. |
| Outpatient surgery centers | These facilities handle minor, low-risk surgical procedures that do not require the patient to stay overnight, such as vasectomies, breast biopsies, cataract removal, tonsillectomies, cosmetic surgery, hernia repair, dilation and curettage (D&C), and therapeutic abortions. Approximately 40% of all surgical procedures can be handled in these facilities. Those requiring prolonged anesthesia, complex skills, or extensive post-surgery care must be handled in a traditional hospital. |
| Freestanding emergency centers | These are emergency rooms that usually are not part of a hospital but do tend to be affiliated with one. Patients can get urgent care quickly and at less cost than the traditional emergency room, where they must become part of the hospital system. |
| Home health care | In some situations, physicians and other practitioners can arrange for patients to be cared for at home. Procedures such as dialysis and chemotherapy can be administered at home at a much lower cost than in the hospital. Approximately 80% of all insurance companies now pay for health aides, nurses, and other practitioners who give care in the home. |

Important distinctions between health care facilities are given in Table 15.2.

## Prescription Medication

**Prescription medications** are regulated by the Food and Drug Administration. Those regulated by both the Food and Drug Administration and the Drug Enforcement Agency have psychoactive properties and the potential to be abused. All prescription drugs bear the following warning on the label: *Caution: Federal law prohibits dispensing without prescription.* This does not apply only to practitioners. Sharing prescription medication with someone else is illegal, too. The only person who is legally permitted to take a prescription drug is the one for whom it was prescribed.

For a consumer to obtain a prescription medication legally, the practitioner writes an order that the patient takes to a pharmacist to be filled. The order is commonly called the **prescription**. Prescriptions are written in a type of shorthand of the profession that pharmacists are trained to translate. (Refer to FYI—Prescription Jargon.)

To get the intended benefits from prescription medications, they must be taken according to the directions on the prescription label. The doctor should explain how to take the medication. Upon obtaining the medication from the pharmacist, the patient should ask for any additional information that is important to know. Some medications, for example, must be taken with food or milk, and others on an empty stomach. The most important advice is to finish taking your prescription. Many antibiotics, for example, help a person feel better within a few days, but they must be continued for a full 10 days to completely kill the pathogen that caused the illness. Otherwise, the infection may recur.

To keep medications potent, store them away from direct sunlight, hot temperatures, and humidity. The prescription should be kept in its original container so the directions for use will be handy, and others (family members, roommates) will not take the medication by mistake.

---

### KEY TERMS

**Prescription medications** drugs that are used in patient care and are legal only when authorized by a physician or qualified health care practitioner

**Prescription** written order authorizing a pharmacist to dispense medication

## AVOIDING PROBLEMS WITH PRESCRIPTION DRUGS

When the doctor prescribes a drug, patients should mention any other medications they are taking. Serious problems can arise when some medications are taken at the same time. The same concept applies to food and drink. Serious (even life-threatening) interactions can take place if a person drinks or eats certain foods when taking certain medications. The doctor and the pharmacist can provide the needed information.

In general, you can avoid problems with prescription drugs if you:

■ Take any current medications along to a doctor's appointment. These drugs may have affected your current symptoms and may make a difference in what your doctor prescribes.

■ Take only the prescribed amount of medication at the prescribed times. If you have problems remembering when you take the medication, write it down.

■ Check with the doctor or pharmacist before opening capsules or crushing tablets. Some medications are not supposed to dissolve in the mouth.

■ Ask about possible food interactions. If you are supposed to take the medicine on an empty stomach, take it at least an hour before you eat or two hours after you eat.

■ Never drink alcohol or hot beverages when you take medication.

■ Watch for signs of an allergic reaction. Although reactions are not common, they can be serious. Call your doctor if you develop nausea, vomiting, weakness, a widespread rash or hives, or pale (ashy) skin after taking medication.

## BRAND-NAME VERSUS GENERIC MEDICATION

A **generic drug** is a medication that is chemically equivalent to the brand-name drug for which it is a substitute. It is also **bioequivalent.** Generic drugs must deliver the same amount of active ingredients into the patient's bloodstream in the same amount of time, have the same therapeutic action of the brand-name drug, and must be approved by the FDA.

Generic drugs in general are less expensive, mostly because manufacturers of generic drugs do not have to repeat the extensive clinical trials that were used in developing the brand-name drug. Though the active ingredients are the same, the fillers and binders used in generic drugs usually differ from those in brand-name drugs, which can affect how quickly they are absorbed or can make them less potent. Some people are allergic to the binders and fillers used in the generic substitute.

When a drug is first placed on the market, usually it is patented for 17 years. That means no one can manufacture another drug with the same chemical formulation during those years. Only when the patent has expired can other pharmaceutical companies manufacture generic versions of brand-name drugs. For that reason, some drugs currently on the market do not have generic versions.

Certain generic medications may not work as well as the brand-name originals. Doctors generally advise patients to stick with brand names for drugs to control epilepsy, other seizure conditions, heart problems, and psychiatric conditions.

## ONLINE PHARMACIES

For many consumers, shopping online for products and services has many advantages, convenience and saving

## FYI | PRESCRIPTION JARGON

Here is a quick translation of the abbreviations on prescriptions.

| | |
|---|---|
| **Rx** | Take |
| **c̄** | With |
| **a.c.** | Before meals |
| **p.c.** | After meals |
| **cap.** | Capsule |
| **tab.** | Tablet |
| **gtt.** | Drop |
| **h.s.** | At bedtime |
| **q.4.h.** | Every four hours |
| **q.d.** | Daily |
| **b.i.d.** | Twice a day |
| **t.i.d.** | Three times a day |
| **q.i.d.** | Four times a day |
| **p.r.n.** | As the circumstances may require |
| **p.o.** | By mouth |

## FYI | 9 PAIRS OF DRUGS THAT CAN HARM OR KILL YOU

Mevacor—Lopid
Coumadin—Tagamet
Calan—Duraquin
Theo-Dur—Tagamet
Lanoxin (Digoxin)—Calan
Prozac—Dilantin
Halcion—Erythromycin
Eldepryl—Norpramine
Tagamet—Dilantin

*Source: Worst Pills/Best Pills News, 1600 20th St., NW, Washington, DC 20009.*

time being just two. However, if you decide to purchase medications and health and cosmetic products via the Internet, be aware that you assume risks not faced by consumers who buy from traditional vendors. To increase consumer protection related to pharmacy practices on the Internet, the National Association of Boards of Pharmacy (NABP) developed the Verified Internet Pharmacy Practice Sites program, or VIPPS® (spring 1999). This is a voluntary program in which a VIPPS team reviews the applicant's policies and website, and performs an on-site inspection of the pharmacy's facilities. If a pharmacy qualifies, its website bears the VIPPS® seal. This certifies that the member pharmacy is in compliance with NABP standards for storing medications, quality control (to prevent the dispensing of diluted or counterfeit medications), and protecting the consumer's confidentiality.

VIPPS-approved online pharmacies are required to offer free telephone consultation with a pharmacist.

Regulation of pharmacies and pharmacy practice is primarily the jurisdiction of state board of pharmacy; the NABP does not regulate online pharmacies. Whether it is a traditional (brick-and-mortar) or online pharmacy, consumers should report problems or concerns regarding pharmacy pactices, medications, and medical devices to the state pharmacy board. To minimize the risk of buying counterfeit medications and other types of fraud, the FDA encourages consumers who purchase online medications to buy from pharmacies that participate in some type of certification program.

## Consumer Financing: Who Pays for Health Care?

More than 80 million people in the United States have chronic health problems that should be monitored and treated regularly. Everyone likely will need professional medical care at some time in their lives. Some people can afford to pay cash for the medical or dental services they need, but they are the exception.

Some people qualify for Medicaid, Medicare, or other government programs. Most people—about 75% of those age 65 and younger—have private health insurance and pay **premiums** to an insurance company, which then covers a percentage of the cost for surgery, hospitalization, or other medical care that may be needed. According to the U.S. Census Bureau, 39 million nonelderly Americans (14% of the population) lacked health insurance in 2000. Figure 15.1 shows the percentage of persons by age who did not have health insurance for an entire year (2000).

Enrollment in a health insurance plan does not guarantee quality health care. For one thing, the insurance plan restricts the kind of care the insured person can receive. Clients must have prior authorization for many procedures, and insurance plans place limits on what they will pay. In addition, few insurance plans will pay for preventive services, and almost none pay for what they consider experimental procedures (such as bone marrow transplants). Health insurance does help cover the cost of medical care if all the necessary requirements are met.

### KEY TERMS

**Generic drug** chemically equivalent medication substituted for a brand-name medication

**Bioequivalent** generic medication that the body can absorb and use at the same rate and level and has the same therapeutic action as a brand-name medication

**Premiums** payments to an insurance company for a percentage coverage of future medical expenses

**FIGURE 15.1 ►** Percentage of Uninsured Persons by Age

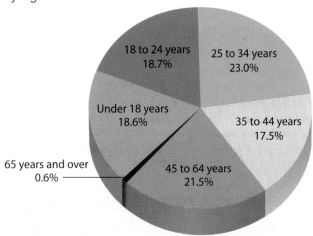

*Source:* U.S. Census Bureau, Statistical Abstract of the United States: 2006.

## AFFORDABLE HEALTH CARE

According to the Bureau of Labor Statistics, America's health care costs have have risen at twice the rate of inflation since 1970. We are in a health care crisis in this country. About half of the country cannot afford the health and medical services that are available in America. According to the U.S. Census Bureau, approximately 40 million (39,804,000) persons living in this country have no health insurance. As reported in a Reader's Digest poll of adults 21 and older, 66% reported that they could not afford to be sick. Of those polled who identified themselves as middle class and "underinsured," 50% have delayed medical treatment for a serious condition or having a prescription refilled, and 46% have postponed yearly health exams. About 25% reported that they had to withdraw money from a savings account to pay overdue medical bills.

## HEALTH INSURANCE

Health insurance policies are either **individual policies** (on your own) or **group policies** (combining the buying power of others, such as those at a place of employment). Health insurance does not automatically pay all the costs for a person's health care. All plans have certain restrictions. Depending on the health insurance, some or all of the following may apply.

- *Waiting period*—the amount of time that must pass after purchasing the policy before the insurance company will pay. For example, the waiting period may be three months. The newly insured would have to pay the full cost of any health care during that time.

- *Exclusion for preexisting conditions*—the circumstances under which the insurance company will pay

the cost of medical conditions the insured person had at the time the policy was bought. Some companies specify a waiting time. For example, they will begin to pay for preexisting conditions after six months. Others never will pay for preexisting conditions.

- *Deductible*—the part of the bill that has to be paid before the insurance starts to pay. For example, the insured might have to pay for the first $200 in medical care for each family member each year before the insurance will pay anything.

- *Co-payment*—a set dollar amount the insured is required to pay for each doctor's visit. For example, the insured may have to pay $10 or $20 for each visit to the doctor, and the insurance pays the rest of the bill.

- *Co-insurance*—shared cost of medical care between the insured and the insurance company on a set percentage determined by the insurance company. For example, the insured may be required to pay 20% of all medical costs, regardless of how high they are, and the insurance company will pay the other 80%.

- *Fixed indemnity*—a limit the insurance company will pay for certain procedures. For example, the company may have a limit of $1,200 for prenatal care. If the cost of prenatal care is $1,500, the insured will have to pay the $300 difference.

- *Exclusions*—procedures for which the insurance will not pay. For example, the insurance company may not pay for infertility testing and treatment.

- *Major medical coverage*—an amount the insurance will pay if the insured has a catastrophic condition and has exceeded the regular benefits.

- *Lifetime limit*—the total amount the insurance company will pay. For example, the policy may have a lifetime limit of $300,000. Once the company has paid $300,000 of the medical costs, it will pay no more.

The three general types of health insurance plans are: private fee-for-service plans (indemnity plans), managed care plans, and public or governmental plans.

## PRIVATE FEE-FOR-SERVICE PLANS OR INDEMNITY PLANS

With this kind of plan, the insured pays a premium to the insurance company. The insurance company may pay monetary benefits directly to the insured person or, at the direction of the insured person, pay the medical bills of the insured directly to the practitioners or facilities that provide the service. The practitioner or the facility sets

---

**Tips for Action** Making Health Insurance Work for You

To get the most out of your monthly premium to your health insurance company:

■ Obtain necessary approvals ahead of time. If you do not, you will end up paying the whole amount.

■ Follow the rules. If a particular claim form is provided, use it. If you are required to go to certain doctors, choose them.

■ Keep the company informed about changes in your life, such as marriage or birth of a child. Coverage of an additional person under your policy may involve a waiting period.

■ Plan ahead. Do not cancel one insurance policy before you've satisfied the waiting period for another one.

■ Keep good records. If your insurance company refuses to pay a claim that it should, you have the right to dispute it and will need the documentation.

■ Pay all your premiums on time. You cannot afford to be canceled.

■ Be absolutely truthful. If you lie or withhold important health information, your company can refuse to pay your claim or cancel your policy.

---

the fees. The insured is free to use any practitioner or facility that accepts that insurance.

## MANAGED-CARE PLANS

A managed-care plan provides and pays for health care services. A **preferred provider organization (PPO)** is a type of managed-care plan that many Americans have because it costs less than indemnity plans. It is a favorite of employers who provide health care coverage for their employees. With a PPO, the insurance company contracts with various physicians and hospitals; those physicians and hospitals in turn agree to charge a set fee for the services provided. The patient must receive any health care from a doctor or hospital that has contracted with the insurance company. Patients usually obtain services from the providers under contract to avoid paying a higher percentage of the cost of the care. If the managed-care plan is an exclusive provider organization (EPO), the plan will not pay for services provided by nonparticipating providers.

Another type of managed care is a **health maintenance organization (HMO)**. Five basic types or models of HMOs exist. Generally, in an HMO, the insured (or the employer) pays a monthly fee to a group practice. Once the insured has paid that monthly fee, he or she can use the services of practitioners in the HMO as many times as needed. The insured is not charged a fee for each service but is limited to the physicians who participate in the HMO. HMOs traditionally have been able to provide medical care at reduced cost because they emphasize preventive behaviors and they try various treatments before hospitalizing patients.

The trend is toward open HMOs, which allow their members to seek medical care from physicians outside the HMO. Patients who choose another doctor (one outside of the network) usually pay between 20% and 30% of the bill to that physician, and the insurance policy pays the remainder.

## HEALTH SAVINGS ACCOUNT

The health savings account (HSA) is not your typical health insurance. The HSA (available since 2004) is a savings account that works like an IRA. The idea of the HSA is that the majority of the money invested in it will be used to pay for the medical expenses that result from a catastrophic illness should one arise. With the HSA, a person establishes an account through a bank or credit union that is linked to a high deductible health plan. Each year the individual makes deposits to the HSA that are equal to the high deductible (example: $4,000). The money in the HSA belongs to the individual and can be withdrawn (tax-free) when used to pay for medical services, including

---

### KEY TERMS

**Individual policy** health insurance purchased by a person

**Group policy** health insurance purchased by a group of individuals, usually through a place of employment, at a reduced rate that is lower than an individual policy

**Preferred provider organization (PPO)** insurance plan in which the insured must obtain medical treatment from health care professionals with whom the insurance company has contracted services

**Health maintenance organization (HMO)** a system of managed care with emphasis on preventive medicine

routine health care. For a young, healthy person, the HSA may be advantageous. However, for people with low incomes, older individuals, or persons with chronic health problems, the HSA would be depleted paying for frequent visits to the doctor. A more serious concern is that an individual with chronic health problems might delay treatment or routine health care in order to preserve the money in the HSA account. Is this type of health plan right for you? Go to www.treasury.gov for more information on the HSA.

## PUBLIC AND GOVERNMENTAL PLANS

One example of a public insurance plan is **Medicare,** established in 1965 during President Lyndon B. Johnson's administration to help people over the age of 65 to pay their hospital bills. Part A of Medicare, which covers hospital room and board, is paid by Social Security taxes and is available to anyone over 65 who qualifies. Medicare Part B, which covers fees to doctors and other medical services during hospitalization, is voluntary. The consumer pays the premium for the Part B option.

After much controversy and debate, a Medicare prescription drug plan (Medicare Part D) was introduced in 2006. Like Part B, this program is voluntary and is available to anyone on Medicare. Part D provides insurance to help cover prescription medication expenses. The insurance is available from a variety of providers. Therefore, seniors are encouraged to weigh the benefits of each plan before choosing one. Senior advocacy groups such as AARP (American Association for Retired Persons) and for-profit pharmacy chains have established hotlines to answer questions and give advice about selecting a plan. Medicare Part D limits coverage of medications to those on the Medicare formulary (drug list) and requires prior authorization (which is obtained by your physician/health care provider) from your plan's administrators.

In an attempt to contain costs of Medicare, the federal government in 1983 instituted a system of paying hospital bills called **diagnosis-related groups (DRGs).** When a Medicare patient is admitted to the hospital, the price of the care is determined already by the DRG under which the patient is admitted. If the actual cost for treating the patient is less than the preset DRG, the hospital makes money. If the hospital stay is longer than expected or the bill exceeds the set amount, the hospital loses money. The Centers for Medicare and Medicaid Services (CMS) has created more than 500 DRGs.

A second public insurance plan is **Medicaid.** This plan provides limited coverage for people who cannot afford to pay for medical services—the medically indigent. It is financed through funds from the federal government combined with contributions from each state. Eligibility for Medicaid is based on income. CMS is responsible for the administration of both public programs.

## Medical Quackery and Health Care Fraud

Millions of dollars are lost each year to medical and health fraud—much of it to **quackery.** In some cases people are desperate and searching for a miracle when traditional medicine has failed them. In other cases patients (often elderly or less educated people) are taken advantage of intentionally by **quacks.** Regardless of the reason, the patients lose money. They also lose time—time that could mean the difference between successfully managing the health problem and death.

### CAVEAT EMPTOR (LET THE BUYER BEWARE)

Those engaging in health care fraud promote devices, treatments, medication, and services that are worthless. Most have little or no training in the medical field. Quacks have the ability to convince consumers that they are concerned about a patient's health status and that the product or service they offer will effect a cure.

According to the FDA, which is charged with protecting consumers against health fraud, the 10 most common health frauds in the United States are as follows.

1. Arthritis products
2. Cancer clinics
3. AIDS cures
4. Weight-loss schemes
5. Sexual aids
6. Baldness remedies
7. Nutritional cures
8. Chelation therapy (ridding the body of toxins)
9. Muscle stimulators
10. Candidiasis hypersensitivity

Contrary to popular belief, almost anyone can be the victim of a quack. Regardless of income, level of education, and experience, a person can be taken in. The best defense is sound knowledge about the products and services you are seeking—and the ability to spot the common signs of medical quackery. In general, a medical quack may

- Promise a quick cure or guarantee
- Diagnose a health problem by mail
- Change office locations or mailing addresses often
- Try to sell you one product to cure a wide variety of conditions
- Say a product will cure a condition for which no known cure exists (such as AIDS or certain kinds of cancer)

### Tips for Action Protect Yourself from Quacks

To avoid being a victim of medical fraud:

■ Do not abandon medical treatment even if you think it is not working. If you want to try something else, do it in addition to what your doctor has prescribed.

■ Do not agree to pay in advance for anything. Quacks want you to pay up front because they know your insurance policy will not pay—and neither will you when you catch on.

■ Do not agree to unorthodox tests to diagnose disease.

■ Ignore testimonials. Ask for published reports in legitimate journals that confirm the claim.

■ Ask your doctor or write to the appropriate professional organization, such as the American Cancer Society, if you have questions about a new treatment.

■ Claim to be persecuted or harassed by the government or the medical community

■ Say you must pay in advance

■ Use testimonials from previous patients or clients (a legitimate medical practitioner knows that what patients say is confidential)

■ Try to frighten you about legitimate products or services

■ Use titles such as "professor" or "specialist" that could be confused with legitimate credentials

## NUTRITIONAL FRAUD

Americans are bombarded with so much conflicting information about nutrition that knowing what to believe is difficult. The best sources of accurate, current information are registered dietitians; college faculty members who teach food science or nutrition; licensed dietitians in colleges, businesses, hospitals, and nursing homes; and cooperative extension agents in county extension offices.

In general, people should avoid anyone who is prescribing or selling vitamins out of an office or door-to-door; suggesting hair analysis as a basis for determining nutritional needs; using a computer-scored nutrition deficiency test as a basis for prescribing vitamins; or offering nutritional tests and products through the mail. Health-food stores often offer unsound nutritional advice, and some chiropractors, doctors, and dentists venture outside their practice, using unproven diagnostic tools and treatments.

## Agencies That Protect Consumers

Various official agencies and organizations have been created to protect consumers against health and medical fraud. Their scope varies. Governmental agencies are charged with enforcing regulations, making inspections, and suspending the services of violators. Voluntary and nongovernmental organizations monitor, advise, and provide consumer information and education.

## GOVERNMENTAL OR OFFICIAL AGENCIES

The governmental or official agencies that have the primary responsibility for consumer protection are the FDA, the Environmental Protection Agency (EPA), the Federal Trade Commission (FTC), and the U.S. Postal Service (USPS).

**Food and Drug Administration.** Part of the Department of Health and Human Services, the FDA ensures the safety of foods and food products and the safety and effectiveness of drugs, cosmetics, and medical devices and equipment. The FDA has jurisdiction over all products sold in interstate commerce. It has the authority to

■ Approve new drugs

■ Inspect plants where products are made

■ Set safety standards for diagnostic equipment

■ Set regulations for the proper labeling of foods, drugs, and cosmetics

■ Issue warnings to the public when a product is found to be unsafe

■ Request manufacturers to recall products

■ Take legal action against those in violation of the law

### KEY TERMS

**Medicare** public insurance plan, funded by federal taxes, for people age 65 and older

**Diagnosis-related groups (DRGs)** a system of predetermined payment made by Medicare based on the patient's diagnosis

**Medicaid** public insurance plan, funded by federal and state taxes, for people who cannot afford medical care

**Quackery** use of unproven methods of diagnosing and curing diseases

**Quacks** unqualified practitioners who take advantage of patients for their money

**Environmental Protection Agency.** The U.S. **Environmental Protection Agency,** created in 1970, has broad-based regulatory and enforcement powers over environmental matters. The mission of the EPA is to protect human health and safeguard the natural environment upon which life depends. Its jurisdiction covers indoor and outdoor air pollution, pollution of water supplies, chemical waste, pesticides, radiation, electromagnetic fields, nuclear waste, radon gas, and noise pollution. The EPA has jurisdiction over environmental issues that were under the direction of the Department of the Interior, the Department of Agriculture, and the Atomic Energy Commission.

**Federal Trade Commission.** The **Federal Trade Commission (FTC)** is an independent federal agency organized to protect consumers through the Bureaus of Consumer Protection, Competition, and Economics.

One of the most vital functions of the Bureau of Consumer Protection is to control advertising. If the FTC decides that a company's advertising methods are deceptive or false, the agency has the authority to investigate and then seek a court order to stop the advertising if the company will not do it voluntarily.

**U.S. Postal Service.** The Postal Service is responsible for protecting consumers from mail fraud and deception. It has the authority to file complaints and seek legal remedies to prevent unscrupulous vendors from using the U.S. mail to advertise or ship worthless products and services.

## NONGOVERNMENTAL AND VOLUNTARY AGENCIES

The **Better Business Bureau (BBB)** is a not-for-profit organization composed of member businesses that operate to ensure fair and reputable business practices in a locality. It has offices in the major cities and is listed in the White Pages of the telephone directory. One of its functions is to share with its members and consumers information about companies and their business practices.

Because the BBB is a voluntary agency, it has no legal powers. It is a clearinghouse for information and a place where consumers may register complaints. The BBB does not endorse or recommend products or services. If consumers have concerns or doubts about a business, a promoter, or a business practice, they can call the BBB for information before making a decision to purchase. In addition, the BBB offers a wide variety of pamphlets for consumer education and mediation services.

## Protecting Environmental Health

Environmental resources are abundant, but they are limited. They must be protected and preserved today so they will not be depleted for future generations. The common thread running through all the various threats to life on earth is pollution—the pollutants released into the environment by cars, products, and wastes.

## AIR POLLUTION

Exhaust from gasoline engines, black clouds belched out of industrial smokestacks, and chemicals released during manufacturing processes hang in the air over the earth, clogging it with **particulates** (tiny solid or liquid particles) that can contribute to respiratory disease, heart disease, cancer, and life-threatening changes in the immune system. Elderly people, people with chronic health problems, cigarette smokers, and people with existing respiratory diseases are at even greater risk.

The problem worsens when Mother Nature deals a blow known as **thermal inversion.** In thermal inversion a layer of warm air covers a layer of colder air, trapping pollutants and smog so they cannot rise from lower levels. Dangerous pollutants in the air remain close to the earth's surface, where they increase health risks. Figure 15.2 depicts this phenomenon.

The form of air pollution most familiar to Americans is probably **smog,** a brownish or grayish fog produced by chemical pollutants in the air. Smog develops when pollutants in the air react with sunlight, resulting in a dense, foggy cloud. Smog has been known to irritate the eyes and lungs and impair immunity. It can be hazardous to people with chronic respiratory diseases (such as emphysema, bronchitis, and lung cancer). Smog comes in two different colors.

**FIGURE 15.2 ▶** Thermal Inversion

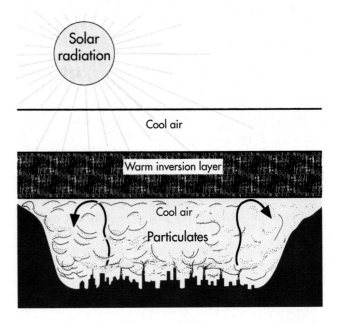

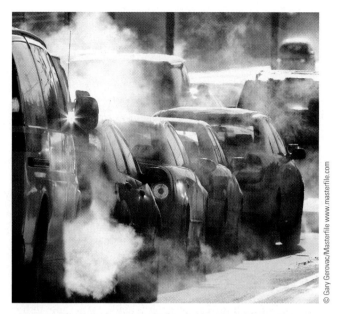

▲ *The number one air pollutant in urban areas is automobile exhaust*

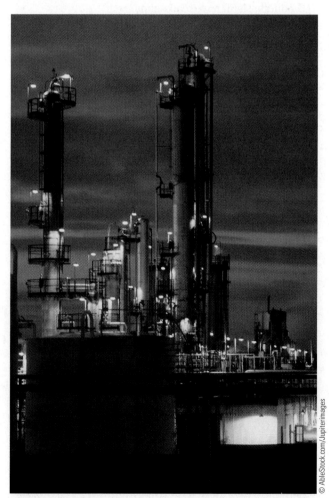

▲ *Industries follow guidelines of the Environmental Protection Agency (EPA) to prevent air and water pollution*

1. Gray smog (called **sulfur-dioxide smog**) results from burning oil that has high sulfur content. It is most common in the eastern United States and Europe.

2. Brown smog (called **photochemical smog**) results when the nitric oxide in automobile exhaust reacts with oxygen in the air. The end product is nitrogen dioxide, which becomes a brownish haze when exposed to sunlight. Exposure to sunlight also results in the formation of other pollutants, most notably ozone. (Among its other effects, ozone reduces plant yields in tomato, bean, soybean, snap bean, peanut, and corn crops; causes premature leaf dropping and lower growth rates in forests; and causes cracking of rubber products, weakening of textiles, changes in dyes, and premature cracking of paint.) Photochemical smog is most common in densely populated traffic centers of the world.

Amendments to the Clean Air Act enacted in 1977 mandated the reduction of pollutants in auto exhaust. This was done through the introduction of catalytic converters. As a result, emissions of carbon monoxide and hydrocarbons have dropped 96% since then. Nitric oxide emissions have fallen 88%. Another beneficial side effect has resulted from the unleaded gasoline that is now the norm, as leaded gasoline prevents catalytic converters from working.

Even though auto and industrial emissions are the major contributors to poor air quality, the activities of individuals also have adverse environmental effects. The smoke from barbeques is another source of air pollution.

### KEY TERMS

**Environmental Protection Agency (EPA)** federal office with regulatory and enforcement powers over environmental matters

**Federal Trade Commission (FTC)** U.S. agency organized to protect consumers

**Better Business Bureau (BBB)** not-for-profit organization composed of member businesses that promote fair and reputable business practices in a locality

**Particulates** tiny solid or liquid particles in the air that cause serious health problems

**Thermal inversion** atmospheric condition that occurs when a layer of warm air covers a layer of cold air and holds particulates at lower levels

**Smog** brown or gray fog caused by chemical pollutants

**Sulfur-dioxide smog** gray smog caused by burning oil with high sulfur content

**Photochemical smog** brown smog caused when automobile exhaust containing nitric oxide reacts with oxygen and forms nitrogen dioxide

The U.S. Department of Energy estimates that the 60 million barbeques used to celebrate July 4th release 225,000 metric tons of carbon dioxide into the air. According to the Pennsylvania Department of Environmental Protection, charcoal grills and lighter fluid contribute to ground-level ozone. Charcoal grilling produces health-harming carbon monoxide, particulate matter, soot, and carcinogenic hydrocarbons (formed when fat from the grilled meat hits the hot coals). As for conservation, the energy consumed (charcoal, lighter fluid, gas, electricity) while grilling on "The Fourth" is enough to power 20,000 households for one year and save the equivalent of 2,300 acres of forest.

## INDOOR AIR POLLUTION

Pollution that occurs indoors can impair health seriously. The tendency for people to conserve energy by insulating their homes well has increased the risk for indoor air pollution. The problem is worse during cold weather, when people take extra precautions to seal and insulate their homes. Indoor pollution is suspected as a cause of the increase in asthma cases in recent years.

**Carbon monoxide poisoning.** A colorless, tasteless, odorless, poisonous gas, **carbon monoxide** results from the incomplete combustion of fuel in furnaces, water heaters, space heaters, and engines. When inhaled, it reduces the oxygen level of the blood. If breathed in high enough concentrations, it is fatal. In its early stages carbon monoxide poisoning causes symptoms much like those of the flu: dizziness, weakness, fatigue, nausea, and vomiting. Carbon monoxide poisoning should be suspected if all members of a family are stricken.

**Asbestos.** A mineral that once was widely used as an insulating material and fire retardant in buildings, **asbestos** has been banned in new construction. In addition, materials containing asbestos have been removed from schools and other public buildings. Researchers discovered that microscopic asbestos particles and fibers were being released into the air, where unsuspecting victims inhaled them. The result sometimes was lung cancer and **asbestosis,** a progressive and fatal lung disease. Because this disease did not appear for 20 to 30 years, countless people were exposed to the hazard in the meantime.

Asbestos was used most commonly in attics and crawl spaces, around furnaces, and as insulation for pipes. People should never touch asbestos. If its presence is suspected, the house should be inspected professionally. A professional can recommend whether to seal the asbestos or to have it removed.

**Lead.** Once used in gasoline, paint, and food containers, lead has been shown to cause major health problems, especially in children. An estimated 98% of the lead in the

**FYI** | TO PREVENT CARBON MONOXIDE POISONING

- Have your furnace checked by a professional before you turn it on for the season.
- Have all natural gas appliances and wood-burning stoves professionally installed and maintained.
- Never use an oven to heat your home, cabin, or recreational vehicle.
- Never burn charcoal inside—not even in a small hibachi grill.
- Make sure you have proper fresh-air ventilation when using a wood-burning stove, fireplace, space heater, or gasoline-powered engine.

atmosphere comes from burning leaded gasoline. Other common sources of lead are

- Paint (an estimated 57 million houses and apartment buildings still have lead paint)
- Pipes (water that flows through lead pipes or pipes soldered with lead becomes contaminated with lead)
- Glazes on some ceramic cookware and dishes
- Imported metal cans (lead is used in the solder)

Once lead enters the body, it is absorbed by the bones. In high enough concentrations, it causes **lead poisoning.** The results are damage to the liver, kidneys, and major systems, including the nervous, cardiovascular, gastrointestinal, reproductive, and immune systems. In children, lead can retard intellectual development, resulting in impaired math and language skills, motor skills, and the ability to concentrate.

Lead is a natural metal, and it lasts forever in the environment. For most, lead in the body has come from past exposure to products such as leaded gasoline or leaded paint dust. Lead toxicity is associated with levels as low as 30 micrograms per deciliter of blood for adults and 10 micrograms per deciliter for children. The average American probably has 5 to 6 micrograms per deciliter in the blood.

The U.S. surgeon general says that even though lead poisoning poses one of the greatest environmental threats to American children, it can be prevented. Today many children remain at risk for lead poisoning from lead paint in older homes and from lead paint-contaminated house dust, drinking water, and soil. A comprehensive strategy that coordinates the activities of the Department of Health and Human Services, the Department of Housing and Urban Development, the Environmental Protection Agency, and the Department of Justice is aimed at preventing lead poisoning in children by eliminating and preventing residential

Most people associate unintentional carbon monoxide (CO) poisoning with motor vehicles or improperly vented space heaters with little relationship to race or gender. However, two physicians noticed that many of the patients being treated for unintentional CO poisoning in Washington State did not follow the typical pattern. After conducting a retrospective study using medical records of patients who were treated with hyperbaric oxygen (HBO$_2$) for acute unintentional carbon monoxide poisoning, these two physicians reported that the residents most at risk were Asians, Hispanic males, and black females. Drs. James Ralston and Neil

Hampton noted that Asians, Hispanics, and blacks are less than 12% of the population in Washington, but they were 26% of the patients treated for severe unintentional CO poisoning. Within each of the three racial and ethnic groups, charcoal briquettes were the most common source of CO poisoning (66.7% of Asian patients, 39.5% of black patients, and 65.8% of Hispanic patients). Ralston and Hampton noted that "cultural practices may explain the variation in typical sources of CO poisoning." Therefore, prevention messages and education strategies about the dangers of CO poisoning should be specific to the populations at risk.

lead paint hazards by funding hazard control; identifying and caring for children already poisoned through increased early intervention and expanded lead screening and follow-up services for at-risk children; refining lead poisoning prevention strategies; and conducting research.

Lead poisoning affects African Americans disproportionately. African-American male children have the highest lead exposure and blood lead levels of any measured group in the United States.

**Mercury.** Prior to 1990, when it was banned, mercury was added to latex paints to prevent the growth of mold and mildew. Researchers now have documented cases of **mercury poisoning** among those who use latex paint containing mercury. Health effects include peeling skin, aching limbs, hand tremors, profuse sweating, and racing pulse. Although some concern has been expressed over amalgam dental fillings, which contain mercury, long-term studies have not confirmed that these fillings pose a health threat.

**Formaldehyde.** **Formaldehyde** is an invisible gas used in home insulation, building materials (including plywood and particle board), carpet backing, and some furniture. The vapors and emissions from these materials have been shown to cause eye and lung irritation, headache, dizziness, and nausea. In tests on animals, formaldehyde has caused cancer. The vapors are worse when materials containing formaldehyde are exposed to heat and humidity.

Federal regulations have not yet been passed against materials containing formaldehyde. Many manufacturers, however, have stopped using it voluntarily in light of known health risks. State and county health departments offer formaldehyde testing to people who are concerned about exposure in their homes.

**Cigarette smoke.** The dangers of secondhand smoke are becoming well publicized, and much legislation against public smoking is being enacted. Chapter 13 includes a discussion of passive smoking and its effects on health. Following a report on environmental tobacco smoke by the U.S. surgeon general, most states have passed laws and ordinances that severely restrict or ban smoking in public buildings.

**Radon.** A naturally occurring radioactive gas, **radon** comes from the natural breakdown of uranium. High concentrations of radon are found in soil and rock containing uranium, granite, shale, phosphate, and pitchblende. It also is found in soils contaminated with certain kinds of industrial wastes, such as by-products from uranium or phosphate mining. In recent years well-insulated houses have tested positive for radon, most often in basements.

---

### KEY TERMS

**Carbon monoxide** colorless, tasteless, odorless, poisonous gas

**Asbestos** a mineral formerly used in construction as an insulator; now known to be a carcinogen

**Asbestosis** progressive and fatal lung disease caused by inhaling microscopic asbestos particles

**Lead poisoning** damage to liver, kidneys, and other body systems caused by absorption of lead into the body

**Mercury poisoning** deleterious effects on the body caused by overexposure to mercury

**Formaldehyde** chemical found in home construction materials that forms vapors that may cause eye and lung irritations

**Radon** naturally occurring radioactive gas; an air pollutant

Radon is attracted to dust particles, which may lodge in the lungs. Late in 1994 researchers backed off somewhat on earlier warnings regarding radon, saying the levels of radon in most homes do not warrant fear of illness. Exposure to very high levels of radon, however, have been known to cause cancer. Those who are concerned about the level of radon in their home should contact their state or local health department to measure the radon levels and receive information on how to bring down high levels.

## WATER POLLUTION

Nearly three-fourths of the earth's surface is covered by some kind of water: seas, oceans, lakes, rivers, streams, and groundwater. Of the more than 2,000 contaminants that have been found in these waters, almost 100 of them are known to cause cancer. Water pollution poses a significant threat to the water supply.

The most common sources of water pollution in the United States are

- Human and animal wastes, largely a result of poorly designed or structurally inadequate sewage treatment plants or improperly installed septic systems
- Improperly located landfills, which allow biological waste, industrial waste, household garbage, and other contaminants to leak into the water supply
- Corroded underground storage tanks for gasoline and petroleum products, many of them located near gas stations
- Oil resulting both from tanker accidents and from the seepage of crude oil into the soil and then the groundwater
- Excessive **fluoride** or **chlorine,** added to the water to prevent tooth decay and to kill microorganisms in the water
- The decay of vegetation and dead fish that fill ponds, lakes, and streams
- Mercury, lead, hydrocarbons, pesticides, arsenic, industrial by-products, and other toxic chemicals
- Natural sediments, such as sand and clay

Simply stated, anything that enters the air or soil can work its way eventually into the water and should be considered as a source of pollution. Any pollutant can contaminate drinking water—and can cause illnesses ranging in seriousness from indigestion to cancer.

Since 1977, federal law has required that suppliers of drinking water periodically sample and test the water supplied to household taps. Federal law also requires that the supplier correct any problems and that customers be notified. If a violation poses an acute risk to human health, notification must take place within 72 hours. Notification is made by a letter from your water supplier, a letter from the local health department, a notice in the newspaper, or an announcement on radio or television. Along with notification of the problem is notification of what the supplier is doing to correct the problem, as well as what the people notified can do to protect themselves. Finally, a person never should drink water directly from a lake, pond, river, or stream, no matter how clean it looks, without disinfecting it first.

## SAFETY OF WATER SUPPLY

Although problems with water contamination are increasing, tap water in the United States is still safe for the great majority in most communities. In the past decade, however, some major outbreaks of intestinal disease have been brought on by *Cryptosporidium* (crypto), a microscopic parasite that causes diarrhea, vomiting, and cramps. Complications may not appear until several days after drinking contaminated water. When healthy people become infected, the symptoms are usually mild and last about a week, or they have no symptoms at all. Federal officials recommend that people with a weakened immune system boil their water, as crypto can be life-threatening to them.

Crypto can get into the water system by excretion from cattle and other animals, which is washed by rainwater into rivers, lakes and reservoirs; overflow of sewage-treatment plants; swimming in contaminated lakes, ponds, or pools; eating contaminated food or water; handling feces from farm animals; and handling diapers of infected babies.

Not all water filters will protect against crypto, and bottled waters are not free of it. Proper filtration can remove 95% of crypto. The National Sanitation Foundation (NSF) operates a certification program for water-treatment devices, and the NSF label specifies which contaminants a device can remove. The filter should be labeled "absolute one micron" or "NSF-certified for Standard 53 cyst removal." "Nominal one micron" is not reliable to trap crypto.

Purifiers have to be maintained properly. The safest options are bottled waters that have been distilled or processed by reverse-osmosis. Reverse-osmosis filters and distillers are among the most expensive but also the most reliable.

## NOISE POLLUTION

If noise is loud enough or persistent enough, it is classified as pollution. Loud, prolonged noise can hurt a person. Taken to extremes, it can result in permanent hearing loss. Sounds so loud they hurt include a jet taking off from the runway and a jackhammer slamming through thick slabs of asphalt. Noises in the harmful range include loud arguing, a crying baby, the whir of a food blender, and the hum of a vacuum cleaner.

## FYI | I CAN'T HEAR YOU! ... TYPICAL NOISE LEVELS YOU'RE EXPOSED TO EVERY DAY

| | | |
|---|---|---|
| "Tricked-out" Car Stereo | 120 decibels | |
| Personal Stereo Player | 120–130+ decibels | Stock Car Race |
| Leaf Blower | 110 decibels | Car Horn |
| Lawn Mower | 90 decibels | Sound Effects (toys) |
| Typical Crowded Restaurant | 86 decibels | |
| Electric Razor | 85 decibels | Vacuum Cleaner |
| Someone Yelling | 75 decibels | |
| Dishwasher | 70 decibels | |
| Hair Dryer | 60–95 decibels | |

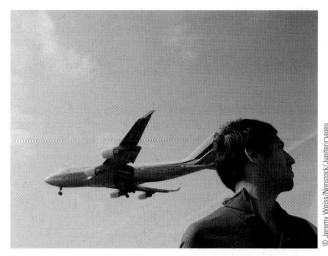

▲ *Even brief exposure to extremely loud sounds can cause hearing loss*

Sound is measured in decibels (see FYI—I Can't Hear You!). Every 10-point increase in decibels represents a 10-fold jump in intensity of the sound. Thus, traffic speeding along a highway (at 70 decibels) is 500 times more intense than someone whispering (at 20 decibels). The average sound level of a movie in the 1950s was 70 to 75 decibels; today, it's 85 to 135 decibels (depending on the scene). Even though a person begins to experience pain in the ears at a noise level of 125 decibels, researchers have concluded that repeated exposure to noise measuring 80 decibels or above causes temporary hearing loss. If prolonged, the hearing loss is permanent. Even brief exposure to extremely loud sounds (such as an explosion) can cause immediate, permanent hearing loss.

As many as 20 million Americans are exposed chronically to health-harming levels of noise. More than half of those people have partial hearing loss already. By the time they are 65, one-third of all Americans have hearing loss bad enough to interfere with communication. This is not strictly a function of age. In societies with less noise pollution, the incidence of hearing loss also is significantly lower in elderly people.

Hearing impairment caused by noise pollution can occur at any age, even during early infancy. It can range from a mild form such as **tinnitus** to permanent damage. Temporary hearing impairment usually disappears a few hours after the noise stops, but gradual damage to the delicate structures of the inner ear can result eventually in permanent hearing loss.

And the health consequences of noise are not limited to hearing impairment. Exposure to loud noise has been linked to stress-related health problems and certain chronic illnesses. According to Robert Fifer Ph.D., an audiologist at the University of Miami, the body's stress response increases when exposed to loud noise in the hazardous range. The physical reactions to loud noise include increased heart rate, breathing, and brain activity, elevated blood pressure, insomnia, and increased levels of stress hormones (epinephrine, norepinephrine, cortisol in the blood). More recent research is revealing that loud sounds "echo through our bodies." A study, reported in the *Journal of Occupational Health,* found that workers exposed to loud sounds during the day continued to be affected at nighttime. The workers experienced poor sleep quality, their nighttime heart rates did not drop as low as the workers in the control group, and their cortisol levels were still elevated the following morning.

## CHEMICALS AND PESTICIDES

**Pesticides** have become a significant source of pollution, partly because of overuse and partly because small amounts of pesticides are absorbed into food. Some pesticides known to be harmful to people, such as DDT (dichlorodiphenyltrichloroethane), have been banned from the market. Other pesticides are regulated fairly strictly by the Environmental Protection Agency. Pesticides work their way through the entire food chain by contaminating the soil, the groundwater, and eventually the food that is eaten.

### KEY TERMS

**Fluoride** chemical compound added to drinking water to prevent tooth decay

**Chlorine** chemical used to purify water

**Tinnitus** ringing in the ears

**Pesticides** chemicals used to kill insects, rodents, and other pests

Although the long-term effects of many pesticides are unknown, pesticides do accumulate in the human body. The effects are much more pronounced in children than adults. Some pesticides have been shown to cause birth defects and cancer. The chemicals in pesticides also may be related to nervous system disorders, liver damage, and kidney disease.

## RADIATION AND ELECTROMAGNETIC FIELDS

**Radiation** is not confined to nuclear power plants or atomic bombs. People are exposed to radiation every day. It is in video display terminals, microwave ovens, x-rays, and the ultraviolet (UV) rays of the sun. Food is bombarded with radiation to kill bacteria, prolong shelf life, destroy insects, inhibit sprouting, and delay ripening. Although the potential for a nuclear accident always exists, daily exposure to low levels of radiation from a variety of sources is a greater concern.

Another problem is radioactive waste. Most of the waste generated by nuclear plants, commercial industry, and military operations still is being stored temporarily in vats or barrels (many of them under water) at widespread sites. A permanent solution to the problem has not been found, yet more radioactive waste is generated every year. Some of the waste that is stored will not be considered safe for tens of thousands of years.

Some of the health effects of common sources of radiation remain unknown. For example, the jury is still out on video display terminals. Studies have shown that more harmful rays are emitted from the sides and back than from the front. You might suffer more harm from the computer next to you than from the one in front of you. Microwave ovens are relatively safe. The biggest potential danger comes from the chemicals in the plastic wrap used to cover food in the microwave. Damage from x-rays can be considerable.

Moderate exposure to radiation can damage the eyes and skin, affect egg and sperm production, and cause birth defects. Regular or prolonged exposure can cause cancer. Exposure to high levels of radiation can cause **radiation sickness,** characterized by nausea, vomiting, diarrhea, hemorrhage, and hair loss. In large enough doses, radiation can kill a person.

Of special concern are **electromagnetic fields (EMFs),** invisible fields (spaces that contain energy) caused by electrically charged conductors. Electromagnetic fields are generated by overhead power lines and a variety of common household products, including light fixtures, electrical wiring, telephone lines, computers, household appliances, refrigerators, radio and television signals, microwave ovens, hair dryers, electric blankets, and waterbed heaters.

Scientists think the fields that are emitted interfere with the electromagnetic fields created by the body's own cells. Early studies showed a statistical link between high-voltage power lines and cancer—especially in electrical workers and in children who live under overhead lines. More studies are needed. The Science Advisory Board of the Environmental Protection Agency says that current evidence is insufficient to prove that electromagnetic fields cause cancer.

Other possible health consequences of electromagnetic fields include infertility, spontaneous abortion, developmental problems, growth retardation, and mood disorders. The association between spontaneous abortion and slow fetal growth and use of electric blankets is so strong that federal officials urge pregnant women to use electric blankets with prudence.

## WASTE DISPOSAL

Possibly the greatest impact from pollution comes not from automobile exhaust or pesticides but, rather, from the wastes and garbage people generate daily. As the population increases, so does the amount of waste. In the United States alone, each person produces approximately a ton of garbage every year.

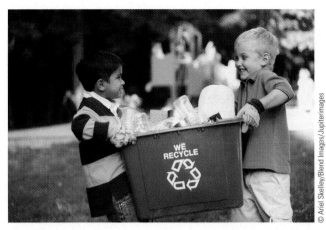

© Ariel Skelley/Blend Images/Jupiterimages

▲ *Only about 10% of the trash in the United States is recycled*

**FIGURE 15.3 ►** Total Solid Waste Generation in United States, 2003.

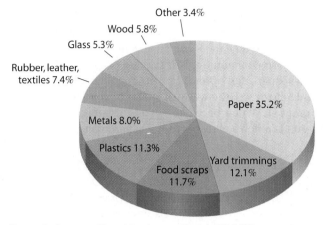

*Source:* Environmental Protection Agency, *Municipal Solid Waste Report,* 2006.

**Solid Wastes.  Municipal solid waste (MSW)** covers the spectrum of the American lifestyle: disposable diapers, newspapers, grass clippings, bottles, and food scraps. Figure 15.3 shows the proportional generation of solid wastes in the United States. In 2003 (latest figures available), 236 million tons (before recycling) of MSW were produced by residents, businesses, and institutions. According to the EPA, this equals about 4.5 pounds of waste per person per day. The EPA ranks the most environmentally sound strategies for handling MSW. Source reduction (altering the design, manufacture, or use of products to reduce what is thrown out) and reuse are the most preferred methods. These are followed by recycling and composting and disposal in combustion facilities and landfills.

Traditionally, people and governments have coped with solid wastes in four ways.

1. **Putting it in a sanitary landfill. A sanitary landfill** is a huge open pit where trash is compacted and buried. Landfills are supposed to be dug away from streams, ponds, and sources of groundwater to lessen the likelihood that water sources will be polluted by the garbage. Unfortunately, contaminants still filter into the soil and surrounding groundwater, creating a pollution source.

   Trash dumped in sanitary landfills is compacted. Each day a fresh layer of dirt is spread over any new trash. When the landfill is full, it is covered with a heavy layer of dirt, and trees and grass often are planted over it. The number of landfills has decreased from 8,000 in 1988 to 1,767 in 2002. Since new landfills are larger, the capacity has remained relatively constant. Landfills for MSW are regulated by the Resource Conservation and Recovery Act of 1976 (amended in 1984). About 80% of trash is buried in sanitary landfills.

2. **Burning it.** Various **incinerators** are used to burn solid waste. These include furnaces, cement kilns, and commercial incinerators designed for that purpose. Poorly designed incinerators contribute to air pollution by releasing particulates into the air. Approximately 10% of trash is incinerated.

3. **Dumping it in open pits.** In some areas solid waste is compacted and then dumped into open pits. The garbage in open pits rarely decomposes properly, smells putrid, and can be scattered by birds, animals, and the wind. Many urban areas have outlawed dumping garbage into open pits.

4. **Dumping it into the ocean.** Shoreline communities sometimes compact solid wastes and then ship it by barge to dump sites. Offshore sites have the potential for polluting the oceans, and their capacity is limited.

### KEY TERMS

**Radiation**  energy from waves and particles such as ultraviolet rays and x-rays

**Radiation sickness**  illness caused by overexposure to radioactive substances, possibly causing death

**Electromagnetic fields (EMFs)**  invisible spaces of energy caused by electrically charged conductors

**Municipal solid waste (MSW)**  trash or garbage generated by residences, businesses, or institutions that consists of everyday items such as product packaging, newspapers, bottles, food scraps, appliances, and furniture.

**Sanitary landfill**  large, open pit where trash is buried

**Incinerator**  container used to burn solid waste

Because the resources for disposal are being depleted, trash is being transported to sites in rural and unpopulated areas of the country and to developing countries. Only about 10% of trash is **recycled**—collected, reprocessed, and marketed—though officials estimate that eight to nine times that much could be recycled.

More communities are starting programs to recycle newspapers and other paper products, aluminum, glass, and plastics. Others are encouraging homeowners to **compost.** When bacteria eat the organic material, the result is a rich soil that is useful in gardening.

**Recycling—"Closing the Loop."** Recycling as a method of waste reduction is a win for the consumer, the manufacturer, the government, and the environment. Recycling, including composting, diverts more than 72 million tons of material away from disposal. The typical recycled materials include batteries (rate of 93%), paper and cardboard (rate of 48%), and yard trimmings (rate of 56%). There are more than 4,500 recycled-content products on the market. These everyday products include aluminum cans, cereal boxes, newspaper, carpeting, car bumpers, and anything made from steel.

**Hazardous Wastes.** Some waste products generated by industry, laboratories, and medical facilities are classified as **hazardous wastes** because they are contaminated with pathogens or toxic chemicals. By law, hazardous wastes cannot be dumped in a sanitary landfill.

Before federal laws were enacted to regulate the disposal of hazardous wastes, these toxic materials were dumped in canals, open pits, and other areas that now are called **hazardous waste sites.** The worst of these sites has been scheduled for clean-up by the federal government under the Superfund law. The government has identified 1,219 sites as hazardous and an additional 32,000 as potentially hazardous.

As many as 40 million Americans live within four miles of the nation's worst hazardous waste sites. As a result they have birth defects, nervous system disorders, cancer, cardiovascular problems, respiratory irritation, and skin irritation. Poor people and minorities are affected more profoundly by the placement of landfills and the disposal of toxic waste in proximity to where they live. A 1987 study published by the United Church of Christ's Commission for Racial Justice found that three to five African Americans and Hispanics live in communities with uncontrolled toxic waste sites, including abandoned production operations and unregulated dumps.

**Liquid Wastes.** Liquid wastes—generally, what is flushed down the toilet—are handled in most cities and municipalities by sewage treatment plants. At these treatment facilities, sewage is processed, removing bacterial

**FYI** *HOW MUCH GASOLINE DOES IT TAKE...? SAVE ENERGY—BUY LOCALLY GROWN WHEN YOU CAN

| Produce | Gasoline |
| --- | --- |
| **Pineapple** | |
| Costa Rica | 0.3 gallons |
| Hawaii | 2.8 gallons |
| | |
| **Apple** | |
| Iowa | 1.7 teaspoons |
| Washington | 1 cup |
| | |
| **Potato** | |
| North Dakota | 0.6 cup |
| Idaho | 1.3 cups |
| | |
| **Grapes** | |
| California | 1.9 cups |
| Chile | 2.2 cups |

*Energy it takes to transport from point of orgin to Des Moines, Iowa (Richard Pirog and others, Leopold Center for Sustainable Agriculture, Iowa State University)

contaminants and **polychlorinated biphenyls (PCBs).** Once treated, the water is returned to the river or lake from whence it came.

## Food Safety

A number of food hazards have been identified by **food toxicologists.** Food is often adulterated with

- Pesticides, used to kill the pests that destroy crops
- Antibiotics, used to prevent infections in animals intended for slaughter
- Hormones, used to increase milk production in cows
- Radiation, used to prolong the shelf life of canned food, inhibit the sprouting of vegetables, and delay the ripening of some fruits

Every time you sit down to a delicious meal, you may be getting more than you bargained for. In a single year the average person eats 160 pounds of food additives and 140 pounds of sweeteners.

**Additives** (sometimes called **preservatives**) are put into food to lengthen storage life, prevent the growth of microorganisms, prevent nutrients from breaking down, alter taste, enhance color, and make foods more appealing to consumers. Processed foods purchased at the grocery store may contain

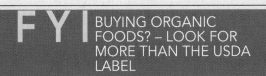

## FYI BUYING ORGANIC FOODS? – LOOK FOR MORE THAN THE USDA LABEL

**Milk**

"rBGH free"—made without using bovine growth hormone

"USDA organic"—milk is hormone and antibiotic free

**Seafood**

"Country-of-origin labeling" (COOL)—indicates where product came from and if farm raised or wild caught

**Meat**

"Grass fed"—meat comes from animals that graze in open pastures vs. animals raised in feedlots

"Certified humane raised & handled"—meat poultry, eggs, dairy products comes from animals raised using ASPCA animal-care standards to include no antibiotics or growth hormones

**Produce**

"Certified naturally grown"—produce comes from USDA-independent, small-scale farmers who use organic practices

**Coffee**

"Fair Trade certified"—the coffee (tea or chocolate) is organic and shade-grown, and the farmer receives a fair price for the product

- Sodium and calcium propionate, sodium benzoate, sodium nitrate, potassium sorbet, and sulfur dioxide, to prevent the growth of bacteria, yeast, and mold in baked goods
- Sulfites, to prevent browning
- Nitrites and nitrates, to prevent botulism and improve the color and flavor of meats
- Antioxidants, such as BHA (butylated hydroxyanisole), BHT (butylated hydroxytoluene), citric acid, and vitamin E, to prevent fats and oils from turning rancid and fruits and vegetables from turning brown
- Emulsifiers (such as lecithin, diglycerides, monoglycerides, and polysorbates), to keep oil and water suspended in foods such as mayonnaise, ice cream, and salad dressings
- Monosodium glutamate (MSG) and disodium guanylate (GMP), to improve the natural flavors of food

- Acetone peroxide (a bleaching agent) and azodicarbonamide (a maturing agent), to bleach flour white and improve its baking qualities
- Agar, gelatin, pectin, carrageenan, locust bean gum, sodium alginate, and carboxymethylcellulose, to thicken foods and improve their texture
- Wax coatings (made of fats, mineral oil, vegetable oil, shellac, beeswax, paraffin, or synthetic resin), to preserve the moisture in fresh fruits and vegetables

Although many food additives are safe, some are under scrutiny by the Food and Drug Administration because of their potential health risks. The FDA has banned the use of sulfites on fresh fruits and vegetables, including those in salad bars, because of fatal allergic reactions in sensitive individuals. The FDA also requires labeling foods containing sulfites. Nitrites and nitrates, which can be converted into a cancer-causing agent called nitrosamine in the digestive tract or during the cooking process, have been reduced by law in products including bacon, luncheon meats, and sausage.

The federal government also discourages the use of **fungicides** (agents that kill fungi) in wax coatings used on fruits and vegetables. According to the National Academy of Sciences, 90% of all fungicides can cause cancer.

## OTHER FOOD SAFETY ISSUES

Mad cow disease—To strengthen the 1997 animal feed regulations, in October 2005, the FDA amended its regulations on animal feed, including pet food, to further protect

### KEY TERMS

**Recycling** collecting, reprocessing, and reusing trash

**Compost** rich soil resulting from the decomposition of leftover food mixed with lawn clippings and leaves

**Hazardous waste** trash contaminated with toxic substances that can cause diseases

**Hazardous waste site** any area where toxic waste was dumped before laws were enacted to regulate proper disposal of toxic substances

**Polychlorinated biphenyls (PCBs)** industrial chemicals found in sewage that cause cancer and central nervous system damage

**Food toxicologist** specialist who detects dangerous substances in food

**Additives (preservatives)** chemical substances added to foods to make them safer and more appealing to consumers

**Fungicides** agents that kill fungi

consumers against mad cow disease or bovine spongiform encephalitis (BSE). Though the risk for BSE in humans is low in the United States, three of the "high-risk cattle materials" banned are:

- the brains and spinal cords from cattle ages 30 months and older
- the brains and spinal cords from cattle of any age not inspected and passed for human consumption
- the entire carcass of cattle not inspected and passed for human consumption if the brains and spinal cords have not been removed

Food-borne illnesses—Because of improper handling, preparation, and storage, food becomes contaminated with pathogens and many cases of food-borne illness (often called "food poisoning") occur annually. Those persons especially vulnerable to food-borne illnesses include young children, seniors, and persons with compromised immune systems. Food-borne illness is largely preventable. The following recommendations will help.

- **Sponges.** Researchers have found that about half of the sponges used for wipe-ups and cleaning surfaces contain fecal bacteria and 20% harbored the *Salmonella* bacteria. Use paper towels to clean up spills; wash between uses and let dry thoroughly; sanitize weekly by placing them through a dishwasher or washing-machine cycle or soaking them in a mild bleach solution; change sponges each month.

- **Fingers.** According to the National Restaurant Association, fingers are common transmitters of food-borne bacteria. Wash the hands for 20 seconds with hot, soapy water both before and after preparing foods (especially when handling raw poultry, meat, or seafood), using the bathroom or changing a diaper, and after sneezing or coughing.

- **Leftovers.** Never allow them to sit at room temperature for more than two hours. Cooking kills bacteria, but it is a myth that reheating food that has been left unrefrigerated for too long will render it safe. When reheating leftovers, get them steaming hot.

- **Marinating.** Keep meat in the refrigerator while marinating so harmful bacteria cannot multiply. Discard the marinade.

- **Cross-contamination.** Handling raw meat, poultry, fish, and eggs and then touching other foods and surfaces can spread hazardous bacteria including *Salmonella*, *Listeria*, and *E. coli*. A trace of bacteria can survive for hours (days if it is wet). Plain soap and hot water can adequately clean contaminated surfaces. For added protection, use an antibacterial cleaner or chlorine bleach.

## FYI | COMMON FOOD STORAGE TIMES

| Food | Cupboard | Refrigerator | Freezer |
|---|---|---|---|
| Jam | Read label | Six months | Not advised |
| Fruit (dried) | One month | Six months | Not advised |
| Steak (cooked) | Never | Three to four days | Six to 12 months |
| Tuna fish (canned) | Unopened Two to five years | Opened Three to four days | Opened One to three months |
| Vinegar | Opened (one year) | Not advised | Not advised |

*Source:* U.S. Department of Agriculture.

- **Eggs.** After cracking an egg, wash your hands and spills with soap and hot water. Remove eggs from the refrigerator only when you are ready to begin baking or cooking. If an egg contains *Salmonella*, the bacteria levels could still be dangerously high after two hours. Especially if you are at high risk for food-borne illness, avoid eating anything containing raw eggs. If recipes call for raw eggs, use substitutes with powdered egg whites or pasteurized eggs, both of which are *Salmonella*-free.

- **Squash and melons.** Foods grown on the ground, such as melons and squash, can have dangerous bacteria on their skins. Rinse them under cold water and scrub clean to remove any clinging soil before cutting.

- **Thawing.** If frozen food sits at room temperature or warmer, bacteria multiplies to dangerous levels. Thaw foods in the refrigerator or in a basin of cold water that you refill frequently. Thaw in the microwave if you are ready to cook. You can safely refreeze defrosted food that was thawed in the refrigerator.

- **Cutting boards (wooden or plastic).** The U.S. Department of Agriculture recommends that nonporous plastic boards be cleaned in the dishwasher. Wooden boards are fine, too, as long as you sanitize them. Pour on a bleach solution (two tablespoons bleach mixed in one quart of water), and let it sit for several minutes.

- **Canned foods.** Do not use foods from bulging or dented cans, even if the food looks fine. These foods may contain *Clostridium botulinum*, which causes deadly botulism.

- **Refrigerator.** Research shows that one in five households keeps the refrigerator above 50°F. Your refrigerator should be set at or below 40°F. The freezer should be 0°F.

## Summary

- One's state of wellness is controlled by inheritance, environment, access to regular health care, and lifestyle.
- Traditional or orthodox medicine is based on scientifically validated procedures developed over time.
- Health care facilities may be clinics, not-for-profit hospitals, for-profit hospitals, teaching hospitals, college health centers, outpatient surgery centers, and freestanding emergency centers, as well as home health care.
- Health insurance may be private fee-for-service, preferred provider, private prepaid group plans, or public or governmental plans.
- People should guard against quackery, particularly promised cures for progressive diseases such as arthritis, cancer, and AIDS.
- Governmental agencies that protect consumers are the Food and Drug Administration, Environmental Protection Agency, Federal Trade Commission, and U.S. Postal Service. The Better Business Bureau is a nongovernmental consumer protection organization without legal powers of enforcement.
- Air pollution and smog cause respiratory irritation and damage, in addition to other ill health effects.
- Indoor air pollution can be caused by carbon monoxide, asbestos, lead, mercury, formaldehyde, and radon.
- The most common sources of water pollution are human and animal wastes, improperly located landfills, corroded storage tanks, oil, excessive fluoride or chlorine added to the water, decaying vegetation and dead fish, natural sediments, and toxic chemicals.
- Continuing elevated noise pollution levels can cause permanent hearing loss.
- Food additives, some of which may be harmful, are regulated by the Food and Drug Administration.
- Taking food safety precautions can prevent many bacterial infections, including food poisoning.

## Personal Health Resources

ThomsonNOW Visit the ThomsonNOW website at http://thomsonedu.com/thomsonnow for valuable resources that will:

- Help you evaluate your knowledge of the material.
- Guide you through tutorials to help you understand and apply the material.
- Allow you to take an exam-prep quiz to better prepare for class tests.

Healthfinder. This site links to federal government publications about health topics and consumer sites on the Internet that have been evaluated for quality by the U.S. Department of Health and Human Services.

**www.healthfinder.gov**

Internet FDA. This site provides information about the Food and Drug Administration (FDA) and its regulatory activities. It includes the weekly *FDA Enforcement Report*, *FDA Consumer*, other FDA publications, summaries of laws that the FDA enforces, information about how to report problems with food and products that the FDA regulates, telephone numbers to FDA offices, and links to other FDA Internet sites.

**www.fda.gov**

Mayo Health O@sis. Operated by the Mayo Clinic and providing hundreds of articles on virtually every health and medical topic, this site provides information on selected prescription and over-the-counter medications, allows users to submit questions to Mayo practitioners, and has a glossary of medical terms.

**mayohealth.org**

National Association of Boards of Pharmacy (NABP). This association developed the Verified Internet Pharmacy Practices Sites™ (VIPPS®) program to assist consumers in the identification of Internet pharmacies whose practices comply with state dispensing regulations, respect patient privacy rights, and provide meaningful consultation between patients and pharmacists. Consumers can use this site to search for a VIPPS® Internet pharmacy that matches their needs. The pharmacy is identified by the VIPPS® hyperlink seal display on its website. The NABP was established in 1904 to assist state licensing boards in developing, implementing, and enforcing standards to protect public health.

**www.nabp.net**

National Center for Complementary and Alternative Medicine (NCCAM). This center is part of the National Institutes of Health. It conducts and supports basic and applied research and training and disseminates information about complementary and alternative medicine (CAM) to practitioners and the public. The NCCAM Clearinghouse provides information on various CAMs in the form of fact sheets, frequently asked questions (FAQs), searches of federal databases of scientific and medical

literature, and selected federal links. The Clearinghouse does not provide medical advice, treatment recommendations, or referrals to practitioners.
1-888-644-6226
TTY 1- 866-464-3615 (toll free)

**www.nccam.nih.gov/**

National Coalition on Health Care. This is a not-for-profit, nonpartisan alliance of 96 groups working to improve America's health care. "Did You Know?" health care facts, press releases, information on careers, and policy studies are available.

**www.americashealth.org/**

National Institute of Environmental Health Sciences (NIEHS). This site provides information on environmental disease and research related to pesticides, gene links to breast, ovarian, and prostate cancers, and other basic research on health and the environment. NIEHS is part of the National Institutes of Health.

**www.niehs.nih.gov/**

National Lead Poisoning Information Center. The center gathers and provides information on environmental lead poisoning and prevention for consumers and professionals. Information includes a quarterly newsletter, fact sheets, and lead poisoning alerts from the Lead Program, which is a project of the National Safety Council's Environmental Health Center. This site has direct links to other sites with environmental information.

**www.nsc.org/ehc/lead.htm**

National Poison Control Center Hotline
1-800-222-1222

Quackwatch. This site provides information on health fraud, including signs of quackery, questionable products, services, advertisements, and organizations, and information on consumer protection.

**www.quackwatch.com**

TOXNET. Information is presented on environmental hazards and environmental problems in communities.

**www.toxnet.nlm.nih.gov/**

U.S. Department of Agriculture (USDA). Information is available about the agency's offices, programs, and services; current consumer news; and issues ranging from biotechnology and trade to food safety and nutrition to "USDA for Kids."

**www.usda.gov/**

USDA Meat and Poultry Hotline 1-800-535-4555
Agriculture and Agri-Food Canada 613-225-2342

**www.arg.ca/**

## It's Your Turn for Study and Review

1. Describe two differences between orthodox medicine or health care and complementary and alternative medicine and therapies.

2. Identify the specialty of the following practices, give the educational degree required, and indicate if the practitioner is a physician: chiropractic, endocrinology, gynecology, internal medicine, nurse midwifery, periodontics, physiatry, psychiatry, and optometry.

3. You and your grandmother are having a discussion about generic and brand-name medications. She said that her pharmacist gave her a generic substitute for the medication that she takes and told her that the generic and the brand-name medication are essentially the same or "bio-e something." She knows that you are enrolled in a personal health class this semester and will be able to "break it down" so she will understand what the pharmacist meant. Identify the term and identify the attributes of a generic medication that are essential before it can be substituted for a brand-name medication. Name the agency responsible for making this determination.

4. You have just transferred to a university in another state and need to find a physician to provide your medical care. Despite the advice given to you by your physician at home, you find a physician by choosing one in the telephone directory. While asking questions about your health history, the doctor shows you a notebook of cards and letters from satisfied patients. Describe briefly your concerns about what happened in the office and the process that you used to find the health practitioner.

5. Caveat emptor—consumer protection begins with you. However, there are agencies that fight health fraud. Identify by name and function four official consumer protection agencies and one voluntary consumer protection agency.

6. You use the Internet to pay bills and shop online and are thinking of using the Internet to purchase your prescription asthma medication. Identify one resource (and three reasons to use it) sponsored by the NABP that you should access before making a decision to purchase prescriptions from an Internet pharmacy.

7. Identify a source and at least two health effects of each of the following pollutants: asbestos, carbon monoxide (CO), formaldehyde, lead, noise at 80 decibels, and radon. What measures can you take to reduce your risk of exposure?

8. List three benefits of recycling.

9. List safety measures that should be observed related to the following: leftovers, thawing, cutting boards,

handling raw meat or eggs, temperature of refrigerator and freezer.

## Thinking about Health Issues

Is the FDA's iPLEDGE registry consumer protection or an invasion of privacy?

Helen Fields, "The New Cost of Taking Accutane." *U.S. News & World Report*, March 31, 2006.

The prescription medication Accutane, which is "practically a miracle cure for severe acne," can cause two serious side effects—birth defects and spontaneous abortions (miscarriages). Beginning spring 2006, the physician prescribing Accutane is required to add the patient's name to the iPLEDGE registry (ipledgeprogram.com) and the pharmacist is required to verify registration before filling the prescription. For the Accutane users:

1. Should sexually active females be required to use two contraceptives and all females be required to take monthly pregnancy tests?

2. Should males have to promise never to share the medication with anyone?

3. Are these "pledges" and the FDA's registration requirements for Accutane users measures to protect public health or an infringement on the rights of the patient?

4. Name at least one medical procedure with a "patient pledge" requirement.

## Selected Bibliography

Adler, J., et al. "Going Green." *Newsweek*, 147:3, July 17, 2006, pp. 43–52.

Bren, L. "Agencies Team Up in War against Internet Health Fraud." *FDA Consumer*, 35:5, September/October 2001, pp. 9–10.

Chillot, R. "Clean Home, Health Hazard?" *Health*, 15, October 2001, pp. 84–92.

"FDA Proposes Additional Mad Cow Safeguards." *FDA Consumer*, 39:6, November–December 2005, p. 6.

Fields, H. "The New Cost of Taking Accutane." *U.S. News & World Report*, 140:9, March 13, 2006, p. 63.

Geiger, D. "TLC for Your Ear." *Health*, 20:3, April 2006, pp. 79–82.

Gleick, P. "Global Water: Threats and Challenges Facing the United States—Issues for the New U.S. Administration." *Environment*, 43:2, March 2001, pp. 18–26.

Henkel, J. "Buying Drugs Online." *FDA Consumer*, 34:1, January/February 2000, pp. 24–29.

Howley, K. "'I Can't Afford to Get Sick'." *Reader's Digest*, April 2006, pp. 91–99.

Krimsky, S. "Hormone Disruptors: A Clue to Understanding the Environmental Causes of Disease." *Environment*, 43:5, June 2001, pp. 22–31.

Kyle, A. D., et al. "Evaluating the Health Significance of Hazardous Air Pollutants Using Monitoring Data." *Public Health Reports*, 116:1, January/February 2001, pp. 32–43.

Johansen, B. "The Paul Revere of Global Warming." *The Progressive*, 70:8, August 2006, pp. 26–28.

Johnson, K. A. "The Color of Health Care." *Heart and Soul Magazine*, Spring 1994.

Lewis, C. "Home Diagnostic Tests: The Ultimate House Call?" *FDA Consumer*, 35:6, November/December 2001, pp. 18–22.

McGrath, T. "Is Life Too Loud?" *Men's Health*, 21:2, March 2006, pp. 106–109, 146.

Mushak, B. "Environmental Equity: A New Coalition for Justice." *Environmental Health Perspectives*, 101:6, November 1993, pp. 478–483.

National Association of Pharmacy Boards. *VIPPS®* (Verified Internet Pharmacy Practice Sites). Available at www.nabp.net/vipps/intro.asp. Accessed August 12, 2006.

National Center for Complementary and Alternative Medicine. "What Is Complementary and Alternative Medicine?" 2006. Available at www.nccam.nih.gov/health/whatiscam. Accessed August 12, 2006.

Porter, M. and Teisberg, E. O. "Information Is the Best Medicine—Doctor Know." *The New Republic*, 235:4773, 4774, July 10–17, 2006, pp. 13–14.

Quinn, J. B. "What We Need Is Policy." *Newsweek*, 147:3, July 17, 2006, p. 53.

Ralston, J. D. and Hampson, N. B. "Incidence of Severe Unintentional Carbon Monoxide Poisoning Differs across Racial/Ethnic Categories." *Public Health Reports*, 115:1, January/February 2000, pp. 46–51.

Rauber, P. "Miles to Go Before You Eat." *Sierra*, 91:3, May–June 2006, pp. 34–35.

Roizen, M. and Oz, M. "Secrets of Great Doctors." *Reader's Digest*, March 2006, pp. 110–115.

Satcher, D. S. "The Surgeon General on the Continuing Tragedy of Childhood Lead Poisoning." *Public Health Reports*, 115:6, November/December, 2001, pp. 579–580.

Schulte, B. "Rising Temperature." *U.S. News & World Report*, 140:21, June 5, 2006, pp. 35-43.

Smith, K. "Environment and Health: Issues for the New U.S. Administration." *Environment*, 43, May 2001, pp. 34–42.

Spake, A. "Natural Hazards." *U.S. News and World Report*, February 12, 2001, pp. 42–49.

Solomon, B. and Lee, R. "Emissions Trading Systems and Environmental Justice." *Environment*, 42:8, October 2000, pp. 32–45.

Stevens, S. "P's and Q's of BBQ—A Guide to Guilt-free Grilling." *Sierra*, 90:4, July–August 2005, pp. 20–21.

Tanner, M. "The Slippery Slope to National Health Care." *USA Today*, 135:2734, July 2006, pp. 10–14.

U.S. Department of Health and Human Services. *Healthy People 2010: Understanding and Improving Health.* Washington, DC: U.S. Government Printing Office, 2000.

U.S. Census Bureau, *Statistical Abstract of the United States: 2006*, 125th ed. Washington, DC, 2005, p. 110.

U.S. Environmental Protection Agency. Municipal Solid Waste. February 22, 2006. Available at www.epa.gov/. Accessed July 30, 2006.

# Self Assessment 15.1 Are You a Savvy Health Consumer?

Name _____  Course _____

Date _____  Section _____

Answer each of the questions below. For each "yes" give yourself 1 point. For each "no" give yourself 2 points. If a question does not apply to your situation, leave it blank and score 0 points.

|  |  | Yes | No |
|---|---|---|---|
| 1. | Do you know which signs and symptoms indicate that you are sick enough to see a physician? | ☐ | ☐ |
| 2 | Do you know how to check your own vital signs, such as temperature and pulse? | ☐ | ☐ |
| 3. | When appropriate, do you purchase and use home health tests? | ☐ | ☐ |
| 4. | Do you know how to manage most minor illnesses and injuries, such as a common cold, temporary indigestion, or a minor abrasion? | ☐ | ☐ |
| 5. | If appropriate, do you administer your own therapy, such as allergy shots? | ☐ | ☐ |
| 6. | Do you regularly perform monthly self-exams, such as breast self-exams or testicular self-exams? | ☐ | ☐ |
| 7. | Do you participate in a regular exercise program? | ☐ | ☐ |
| 8. | Is your weight within 10% of the range considered ideal for your age, gender, and height? | ☐ | ☐ |
| 9. | If you need to lose or gain weight, are you actively involved in an appropriate nutrition and exercise program? | ☐ | ☐ |
| 10. | Before you take any over-the-counter medications, do you read the label and carefully check and follow instructions for use? | ☐ | ☐ |
| 11. | Do you have a primary care physician? | ☐ | ☐ |
| 12. | Before you take any prescription medication, do you check the label carefully and follow the physician's instructions? | ☐ | ☐ |
| 13. | Do you follow instructions on medications strictly, taking only the recommended dose and using the medication only as long as recommended? | ☐ | ☐ |
| 14. | Do you check for expiration dates on over-the-counter and prescription medication, and do you discard medications when they expire? | ☐ | ☐ |
| 15. | If your symptoms persist or get worse while you are taking medication, do you check with your physician? | ☐ | ☐ |
| 16. | Have you checked your physician's credentials, such as years of training, years of practice, and licensing compliance? | ☐ | ☐ |
| 17. | Before visiting your physician, do you write a list of your symptoms or your questions ahead of time? | ☐ | ☐ |
| 18. | If your physician recommends medical tests, do you question the need for tests and explore alternatives with your physician? | ☐ | ☐ |
| 19. | Do you have regular physical and dental checkups? | ☐ | ☐ |
| 20. | Do you have some type of health insurance, either private, group, or government-funded? | ☐ | ☐ |
| 21. | If a practitioner offers you an unorthodox diagnosis or treatment, do you insist on seeing published reports in legitimate sources first? | ☐ | ☐ |
| 22. | If you live in an area of heavy traffic, do you try to avoid outdoor exercise and exposure between the hours of noon and 4 p.m.? | ☐ | ☐ |

23. If you live near a smelter, refinery, industrial plant, or coal-powered furnace, do you take measures to protect yourself from possible air pollution? ☐ ☐

24. Do you resist smoking yourself, and do you avoid exposure to the cigarette smoke of others? ☐ ☐

25. Do you take regular measures to protect yourself from loud noise, including turning down the volume on your stereo? ☐ ☐

26. Do you read labels and avoid food additives whenever you can? ☐ ☐

27. Do you wash your hands before and after eating? ☐ ☐

28. Do you store food according to accepted methods? ☐ ☐

29. Do you wash your hands after using the bathroom? ☐ ☐

30. Do you keep your kitchen or eating area clean? ☐ ☐

Add up your scores. If you scored:

**20–30** Congratulations. You are a savvy health consumer. Continue to do what you can to protect yourself against threats from the environment and to practice good preventive health practices.

**32–46** Some of the areas in your life could use improvement. Go back over the assessment and review the questions to which you answered "no." Those questions will give you a blueprint for improving your consumer health.

**48–60** You are not doing everything you can to protect your health and wellness. Review the suggestions in this chapter, and then work to design a plan that will help you be a better health consumer.

# Appendix A National Health Information Center 2007 National Health Observances

## The YEAR 2007 AT A GLANCE

### January

Cervical Health Awareness Month

National Blood Donor Month

Thyroid Awareness Month

National Birth Defects Prevention Month

National Glaucoma Awareness Month

8–14  National Folic Acid Awareness Week

### February

AMD/Low vision Awareness Month

International Prenatal Infection
Prevention Month

National Wise Health Consumer Month

2  National Wear Red Day 2007

7–14  Congenital Heart Awareness Week

12–17  National Condom Week

16  National Women's Heart Day

American Heart Month

National Children's Dental Health
Month

2  Give Kids A Smile Day

4–10  National Burn Awareness Week

11–17  Children of Alcoholics Week

14  National Donor Day

25–March 3  National Eating Disorders
Awareness Week

### March

National Brain Injury Awareness Month

National Endometriosis Awareness Month

National Multiple Sclerosis Education
and Awareness Month

Save Your Vision Month

4–10  National Patient Safety Awareness Week

5–11  National Problem Gambling Awareness Week

5–9  National School Breakfast Week

12–18  Brain Awareness Week

24  World Tuberculosis Day 2007

National Colorectal Cancer Awareness Month

National Kidney Month

National Nutrition Month®

Workplace Eye Health and Safety Month

5–11  Multiple Sclerosis Awareness Week

5–11  National Sleep Awareness Week®

8  World Kidney Day

18–24  National Inhalants and Poisons
Awareness Week

27  American Diabetes Alert Day

# April

Alcohol Awareness Month

Counseling Awareness Month

Irritable Bowel Syndrome Awareness Month

National Child Abuse Prevention Month

National Facial Protection Month

Occupational Therapy Month

Women's Eye Health and Safety Month

2–8  National Public Health Week

5  National Alcohol Screening Day

21–28  National Infant Immunization Week

28–May 6  National SAFE KIDS Week

28  World Tai Chi & Qigong Day

Cesarean Awareness Month

Foot Health Awareness Month

National Autism Awareness Month

National Donate Life Month

National Youth Sports Safety Month

Sports Eye Safety Month

1–7  Root Canal Awareness Week

5  A Day To End Sexual Violence

7  World Health Day

23–29  Cover the Uninsured Week

28–29  2007WalkAmerica

# May

American Stroke Month

Better Sleep Month

Hepatitis Awareness Month

Melanoma/Skin Cancer Detection and
Prevention Month

Multiple Chemical Sensitivity Awareness Month

National Celiac Disease Awareness Month

National Neurofibromatosis Month

National Physical Fitness and Sports Month

Sturge-Weber Awareness Month

Ultraviolet Awareness Month

2  National Anxiety Disorders Screening Day

6–12  National Mental Health Counseling Week

6  High Blood Pressure Sunday

12  Cornelia de Lange Syndrome

13–19  Food Allergy Awareness Week

13–19  National Women's Health Week

14–18  Bike to Work Week

14  National Women's Check-up Day

Asthma and Allergy Awareness Month

Clean Air Month

Lyme Disease Awareness Month

Mental Health Month

National Bike Month

National High Blood Pressure Education Month

National Osteoporosis Awareness and
Prevention Month

National Teen Pregnancy Prevention Month

Tuberous Sclerosis Awareness Month

1–7  National Physical Education and Sport Week

2  National Teen Pregnancy Prevention Day

6–12  North American Occupational Safety and
Health Week

7  Melanoma Monday

12  Fibromyalgia Awareness Day

13–19  National Alcohol- and Other
Drug-Related Birth Defects Week

14–20  National Stuttering Awareness Week

14–18  National Neuropathy Week

15  Sex Differences in Health Awareness Day

16 National Employee Health and Fitness Day

18 HIV Vaccine Awareness Day

20–26 National Emergency Medical Services Week

20–26 Schizophrenia Awareness Week

20–26 Tinnitus Awareness Week–Take Action Today!

21–27 Recreational Water Illness Prevention Week

31 World No Tobacco Day

## June

1–July 4 Fireworks Safety Month

Home Safety Month

Myasthenia Gravis Awareness Month

National Aphasia Awareness Month

National Scleroderma Awareness Month

Vision Research Month

3–9 National Headache Awareness Week

3–9 Sun Safety Week

3 National Cancer Survivors Day

11–17 National Men's Health Week

21 National ASK Day

24–30 Helen Keller Deaf–Blind Awareness Week

27–July 5 Eye Safety Awareness Week

27 National HIV Testing Day

## July

Hemochromatosis Awareness Month

International Group B Strep Awareness Month

National Group B Strep Awareness Month

UV Safety Month

10–14 National Youth Sports Week

## August

Cataract Awareness Month

Children's Eye Health and Safety Month

National Immunization Awareness Month

Psoriasis Awareness Month

Spinal Muscular Atrophy Awareness Month

1–7 World Breastfeeding Week

1 National Minority Donor Awareness Day

## September

America On the Move's September Campaign

Childhood Cancer Month

Fruit and Vegetable Month

Healthy Aging® Month

Leukemia & Lymphoma Awareness Month

National Acceptance Month

National Alcohol and Drug Addiction Recovery Month

National Cholesterol Education Month

National Pediculosis Prevention Month/Head Lice Prevention Month

National Sickle Cell Month

Ovarian Cancer Awareness Month

Prostate Cancer Awareness Month

Reye's Syndrome Awareness Month

Sports and Home Eye Safety, Month

9–15 National Suicide Prevention Week

10 STOP A Suicide Today Day

16–22  National Farm Safety & Health Week

16–22  Reye's Syndrome Awareness Week

21  World Alzheimer's Day

30–October 6  Hearing Aid Awareness Week

16–22  National Rehabilitation Awareness Celebration

18  Take a Loved One for a Check-up Day

26  National Mesothelioma Awareness Day

30  World Heart Day

# October

"Talk About Prescriptions" Month

Halloween Safety Month

Let's Talk Month

National Breast Cancer Awareness Month

National Chiropractic Month

National Disability Employment Awareness Month

National Family Sexuality Education Month/ Let's Talk

National Physical Therapy Month

Sudden Infant Death syndrome Awareness Month

1  National Child Health Day

10  Stop America's Violence Everywhere Today

11  NDSD Mental Health Screening™

15–19  National Health Education Week

16  World Food Day

21–27  Respiratory Care Week

24  Lung Health Day

Eye Injury Prevention Month

Healthy Lung Month

Lupus Awareness Month

National Celiac Disease Awareness Month

National Dental Hygiene Month

National Down Syndrome Awareness Month

National Medical Librarians Month

National Spina Bifida Awareness Month

1–5  Drive Safely Work Week

7–13  Fire Prevention Week

10  World Mental Health Day

12–20  Bone and Joint Decade National Action Week

15–19  National School Lunch Week

19  National Mammography Day

22  International Stuttering Awareness Day

# November

American Diabetes Month

Foot Health Issues Related to Diabetes Awareness Month

Lung Cancer Awareness Month

National Alzheimer's Disease Awareness Month

National Healthy Skin Month

Pancreatic Cancer Awareness Month

Pulmonary Hypertension Awareness Month

15  Great American Smokeout

Diabetic Eye Disease Month

Jaw Joints—TMJ Awareness Month

National Adoption Month

National Family Caregivers Month

National Hospice Palliative Care Month

Prematurity Awareness Month

13  Prematurity Awareness Day

18–24  Gastroesophageal Reflux Disease Awareness Week

# December

1–7  National Aplastic Anemia and MDS
Awareness Week

2–8  National Handwashing Awareness Week

1  World AIDS Day

# Appendix B Eat a Variety of Fruits and Veggies Every Day

## How Many Fruits & Vegetables Do You Need?

Everybody is different. Find the amount that's right for you. Go to *www.fruitsandveggiesmatter.gov* to calculate how many fruits and vegetables you need according to your age, gender, and physical activity level. Individual results will be provided.

## Fruits and Vegetable Benefits: Nutrient Information

Fruits and vegetables are sources of many vitamins, minerals, and other natural substances that may help protect you from chronic diseases. Some of these nutrients may also be found in other foods. Eating a balanced diet and making other lifestyle changes are key to maintaining your body's good health.

### FIBER

Diets rich in dietary fiber have been shown to have a number of beneficial effects including decreased risk of coronary artery disease.

Excellent vegetable sources: navy beans, kidney beans, black beans, pinto beans, lima beans, white beans, soybeans, split peas, chick peas, black eyed peas, lentils, artichokes

### FOLATE*

Healthful diets with adequate folate may reduce a woman's risk of having a child with brain or spinal cord defect.

Excellent vegetable sources: black eyed peas, cooked spinach, great northern beans, asparagus

### POTASSIUM

Diets rich in potassium help to maintain a healthy blood pressure.

Good fruit and vegetable sources: sweet potatoes, tomato paste, tomato puree, beet greens, white potatoes, white beans, lima beans, cooked greens, carrot juice, prune juice

### VITAMIN A

Vitamin A keeps eyes and skin healthy and helps to protect against infections.

Excellent vegetable sources: sweet potatoes, pumpkins, carrots, spinach, turnip greens, mustard greens, kale, collard greens, winter squash, cantaloupe, red peppers, Chinese cabbage

## VITAMIN C

Vitamin C helps heal cuts and wounds and keep teeth and gums healthy.

Excellent fruit and vegetable sources: red and green peppers, kiwi, strawberries, sweet potatoes, kale, cantaloupe, broccoli, pineapple, Brussels sprouts, oranges, mangoes, tomato juice, cauliflower

Good sources: These foods contain 10 to 19 percent of the Daily Value per reference amount.

Excellent sources: These foods contain 20 percent or more of the Daily Value per reference amount.

*The Institute of Medicine recommends that women of childbearing age who may become pregnant consume 400 micrograms of synthetic folic acid per day to supplement the folate they receive from a varied diet. Synthetic folic acid can be obtained from eating fortified foods or taking a supplement.

# Glossary

**Acquired immune deficiency syndrome (AIDS)** an incurable, sexually transmitted viral disease caused by the human immunodeficiency virus (HIV)

**Acquired immunity** protection from reacquiring an infectious disease because the first occurrence triggered specific antibodies against it

**Acute myocardial infarction** a condition that occurs when blood supply to heart muscle is cut off and the tissue dies; heart attack

**Addiction** a state of biochemical or psychological dependence produced by habitual drug taking

**Additives (preservatives)** chemical substances added to foods to make them safer and more appealing to consumers

**Adequate Intake (AI)** the recommended average daily nutrient intake level of a nutrient by healthy people when there is not enough research to determine the full RDA

**Adrenocorticotropic hormone (ACTH)** hormone released by the pituitary gland that stimulates the adrenal glands to release other hormones in the initial stage of stress

**Aerobic exercise** activity that requires oxygen to produce the necessary energy to carry out the activity

**Ageism** discrimination that often denotes old age

**AIDS dementia** deteriorated mental and motor capacity caused by HIV-inflicted damage to the central nervous system

**Air displacement** a relatively new technique to assess body composition by calculating the body volume from the air displaced by an individual sitting inside a small chamber

**Alcohol poisoning** death attributed to BAC at 0.50% and above

**Alcoholic cirrhosis** scarring, shriveling, and hardening of liver tissue resulting from chronic alcohol consumption

**Alcoholic hallucinosis** mental disorder characterized by mental disorientation and mood disturbance

**Alcoholic hepatitis** chronic inflammation of the liver tissue caused by alcohol drinking

**Alcoholic pellagra** condition caused by deficiency of protein and niacin due to prolonged alcohol consumption

**Alcoholism** chronic, progressive condition of dependence on alcohol characterized by consumption above social and controllable limits

**Alpha-fetoprotein (AFP) screening** a fetal testing procedure that analyzes AFP levels in a blood sample taken from the mother

**Alveoli** air sacs in the lungs where the exchange of gases takes place

**Alzheimer's disease** progressive, incurable disease in which nerve cells in the brain die; associated with elderly people

**Amino acids** chemical compounds that contain carbon, oxygen, hydrogen, and nitrogen

**Amniocentesis** a fetal test in which fluid is removed from uterus through a long, thin needle inserted into abdominal wall and uterus into amniotic sac

**Amniotic sac (amnion)** tough, transparent fluid-filled membrane that surrounds the fetus like a balloon

**Amphetamines** a group of synthetic amines affecting portions of the brain that control breathing, heart rhythm, blood pressure, and metabolic rate

**Anabolic steroids** synthetic derivatives of the male hormone testosterone

**Anabolic-androgenic steroid** a synthesized version of the male hormone testosterone

**Anaerobic exercise** high-intensity activity that does not require oxygen to produce the desired energy to carry out the activity

**Androgynous** showing behaviors that are not gender-specific; they are identified with males and females alike

**Anemia** a deficiency in the oxygen-carrying material in the red blood cells

**Aneurysm** sac formed by distention or dilation of an artery wall

**Anger** temporary emotion that combines physiological and emotional arousal; can range from mild irritation to intense rage

**Angina pectoris** chest pain that occurs when the heart muscle does not get enough blood

**Anorexia nervosa** an eating disorder involving extreme weight loss at least 15% below recommended body weight

**Antibodies** protein substances that interact with antigens and form the basis of immunity

**Antigen** a substance that triggers the immune response

**Antihypertensives** medications used to lower blood pressure

**Antioxidants** disease-fighting vitamins that protect the body from the harmful effects of free radicals

**Anxiety disorders** psychological conditions characterized by exaggerated fear

**Aorta** artery through which oxygen-rich blood is transported from the heart to arteries that nourish the body systems

**Apgar score** an evaluation of baby's health at birth based on heart rate, respiration, color, reflexes, and muscle tone; maximum score is 10

**Aphrodisiac** a substance that stimulates sexual desire

**Aplastic crisis** interruption in the body's production of RBCs; may occur in persons with sickle cell disease

**Aromatherapy** relaxation from scents of oils, plant extracts, and candles

**Arrhythmia** irregular heartbeat

**Arteries** blood vessels leaving the heart with blood full of oxygen

**Arterioles** very small arteries

**Arthritis** general classification of numerous diseases that cause swelling and pain in the joints, muscles, and bones

**Asbestos** a mineral formerly used in construction as an insulator; now known to be a carcinogen

**Asbestosis** progressive and fatal lung disease caused by inhaling microscopic asbestos particles

**Asthma** chronic respiratory disease characterized by attacks of wheezing and difficulty breathing caused by narrowing of the bronchi that may be triggered by allergens

**Asymptomatic** without signs of illness

**Atherosclerosis** condition that results when the blood vessel walls become coated with plaque, obstructing blood flow

**Atria** the two upper chambers of the heart, which receive the blood (atrium is singular)

**Atrophy** to decrease in strength or size of tissue from disuse

**Attitude adjustment** changing the way a person thinks about things

**Aura** sensory warning signals that may precede migraine headache

**Autoerotic** sexual behaviors aimed at self-stimulation

**Autoimmunity** a disorder of the immune system in which the immune system attacks the body's own cells and tissues

**Autoinoculation** spreading a pathogen from one part of one's body to another part

**Autonomic nervous system** the portion of the nervous system that controls involuntary bodily functions, especially the glands, smooth muscle tissue, and the heart

**Axon** a long cable connected to the neuron, receiving information from the cell body, relaying it to another neuron

**Bacteria** a type of disease-causing microorganism

**Bacterial endocarditis** infectious disease involving the heart valves or tissues

**Barbiturates** sedative-hypnotic substances that depress the central nervous system

**Basal body temperature (BBT) method** NFP method that uses a woman's temperature fluctuations to indicate when coitus is safe or unsafe

**Basal cell carcinoma** common type of skin cancer that usually does not metastasize

**Basal metabolic rate (BMR)** amount of energy (calories) a person uses when totally inactive

**B-cells** a type of lymphocyte that produces antibodies capable of deactivating invading pathogens

**Behavioral psychology** theory holding that all behavior is learned

**Benign prostatic hypertrophy (BPH)** or **enlargement** noncancerous enlargement of prostate gland

**Benign tumor** tumor that remains self-contained; noncancerous

**Bereavement** intense grief associated with the process of disbonding from a significant person who has died

**Beta-blockers** medications prescribed to control high blood pressure and heart conditions

**Beta-carotene** plant source of vitamin A; helps guard against free radicals

**Better Business Bureau (BBB)** not-for-profit organization composed of member businesses that promote fair and reputable business practices in a locality

**Bidis** skinny, sweet-flavored clove look-alikes sold in various flavors, prepared with unprocessed tobacco, and more potent than regular cigarettes

**Binge drinking** consuming five or more drinks consecutively for men and four consecutively for women

**Binge eating disorder (BED)** an eating disorder characterized by consuming large quantities of food in a short time

**Bingeing** consuming a large amount of food in a short time; gorging

**Bioelectrical impedance analysis (BIA)** method of determining body composition by analyzing electrical conduction through the body

**Bioequivalent** generic medication that the body can absorb and use at the same rate and level and has the same therapeutic action as a brand-name medication

**Biofeedback training** method of measuring physiological functions controlled by the autonomic nervous system

**Biopsy** microscopic examination of a small piece of tissue that has been removed with a special needle; one of the cancer diagnostic tests

**Bipolar disorder** a mood disorder characterized by sudden, dramatic, and alternating shifts in emotion; manic-depressive disorder

**Bisexual** having a physical attraction both to the same sex and to the opposite sex

**Blackout** inability to remember recent events when drinking

**Blood alcohol concentration (BAC)** or **blood alcohol level (BAL)** ratio of alcohol measured in the blood to total blood volume; expressed as a decimal

**Blood lipids** or **lipoproteins** fatty substances carried through the blood

**Bod Pod** commercial name of the equipment used to assess body composition through the air displacement technique

**Body composition** proportionate amounts of fat tissue and nonfat tissue in the body

**Body language** nonverbal communication; body positions, gestures, postures, and movements that send various messages to others

**Body mass index (BMI)** technique incorporating height and weight to estimate critical fat values

**Bradycardia** heart rate of fewer than 60 beats per minute

**Brain death** complete loss of brain function

**Braxton-Hicks** contractions normal uterine contractions that occur periodically throughout pregnancy

**Breathalyzer** device used to measure blood alcohol

**Breech** positioning of fetus so buttocks are seen first at birth

**Bronchi** two main passageways that connect to each lung from the trachea

**Bronchitis** inflammation of the bronchial tubes in the lungs

**Bulimia nervosa** an eating disorder in which a person consumes large quantities of food in a short time, followed by self-induced vomiting or taking laxatives or diuretics

**Burnout** physical and mental exhaustion caused by chronic stress

**Bursae** fluid-filled sacs that keep muscles, bones, ligaments, and tendons moving smoothly against each other

**Caffeine** mild stimulant found in coffee, tea, chocolate, and medications

**Calcium** an essential mineral needed for growth and maintenance of strong bones and teeth

**Calendar method** form of NFP that requires refraining from coitus during ovulation

**Caliper** instrument used to measure the thickness of fat under the skin

**Calorie** a term meaning the same as kilocalorie; measurement of energy

**Cancer** group of diseases characterized by uncontrolled growth and spread of abnormal cells that kill normal cells

**Candida** common STD caused by the fungus Candida albicans

**Capillaries** extremely small blood vessels with thin walls that allow nutrients and oxygen to pass through

**Carbohydrates** compounds composed of carbon, hydrogen, and oxygen used by the body to create 90% of its energy

**Carbon monoxide** colorless, tasteless, odorless, poisonous gas in tobacco smoke

**Carcinogen** cancer-causing agent or substance

**Carcinoma in situ** an early cancer that does not extend beyond the surface layer

**Cardiologist** physician trained in the diagnosis and treatment of heart conditions

**Cardiopulmonary resuscitation (CPR)** manual method of providing oxygen to the brain, heart, and other vital organs, reversing sudden cardiac death

**Cardiorespiratory endurance** the ability of the heart, lungs, and blood vessels to deliver blood and nutrients to the cells efficiently to meet the demands of prolonged, aerobic physical activity

**Caregiver** person who renders services to another person who is unable to take care of the activities of daily living

**Carotenoids** a nutrient occurring in plants, which lowers the risks for heart disease, cancer, and other chronic diseases

**Carotid endarterectomy** removal of fatty deposits from one of the two main arteries in the neck that supply blood to the brain

**Carotid pulse** pulse taken by locating the carotid artery in the neck

**Cartilage** elastic tissue at ends of bones that acts as a shock absorber and buffer between bones

**Caudal anesthesia** anesthetic injected through a tiny tube into the tip of the spine to dull sensation

**Cellular death** cessation of all metabolic processes

**Cellulite** fat that appears lumpy

**Central nervous system (CNS)** the portion of the nervous system composed of the brain and the spinal cord

**Cerebral embolism** moving blood clot that partially blocks a blood vessel in the brain

**Cerebral hemorrhage** bleeding from a ruptured blood vessel in the brain

**Cerebral thrombus** blood clot that gets caught on plaque in a blood vessel in the brain, causing complete blockage of the blood vessel

**Certified nurse-midwife** registered nurse who is certified to care for women during pregnancy and delivery

**Cervical cap** small rubber cap that fits firmly over the cervix and is used with a spermicide to prevent fertilization

**Cervical mucus method** NFP that requires judging the thickness of cervical mucus to determine ovulation

**Cervicitis** inflammation of the cervix

**Cervix** lower portion of the uterus that connects with the vagina

**Cesarean section (C-section)** delivery of fetus through opening in abdomen and uterus created by a surgical incision

**Challenge** the capacity to see change as an opportunity for excitement and growth

**Chancre** a painless ulcer that develops at the site where the bacteria enters the body and is the primary symptom of syphilis

**Chancroid** STD named for the genital lesions it produces; caused by bacterium Haemophilus ducreyi

**Chemotherapy** drugs taken intravenously to kill cancer cells

**China white** a designer drug with more potent effects than heroin

**Chiropractic medicine** a discipline founded on the belief that life forces flow from the spine to the rest of the body

**Chiropractor** health care practitioner who manipulates the spine to relieve pain

**Chlamydia** a common STD caused by the bacteria *Chlamydia trachomatis*

**Chlorine** chemical used to purify water

**Cholesterol** yellow, waxy substance produced by the liver and found in animal products; used by the body for metabolism and production of certain hormones

**Chorionic villus sampling (CVS)** a fetal test of a tiny piece of chorionic villi containing fetal cells, removed from the cervix through a catheter

**Chronic fatigue syndrome (CFS)** a viral illness that produces extreme fatigue and other symptoms similar to mononucleosis

**Chronic obstructive lung disease (COLD)** lung diseases characterized by decreased breathing functions; includes chronic bronchitis, emphysema, and chronic asthma; COPD or COBD

**Cilia** hairlike projections inside of the fallopian tubes

**Circumcision** surgical removal of foreskin of penis

**Client-centered therapy** a focus on clients and their beliefs and needs as more important than the counselor's (Rogers)

**Clinical death** cessation of heartbeat and breathing

**Clinical depression** extreme emotional low stemming from a physical problem such as a chemical imbalance in the body

**Clinical psychologist** specialist in diagnosing and treating emotional and behavioral disorders without medication

**Clitoridectomy** excision of the clitoris

**Clitoris** sensitive female sex organ, which becomes erect when sexually excited

**Closed adoption** adoption in which exchange of parental information is not allowed

**Clove cigarettes** cigarettes containing about 40% cloves, with a numbing ingredient, eugenol

**Cluster headaches** headaches that occur in groups and cycles, characterized by intense pain

**Cocaine** powerful stimulant derived from the coca plant

**Codeine** a natural derivative of opium used as a cough suppressant or mild painkiller

**Cohabitation** living together as spouses without being married

**Coitus interruptus** withdrawal of the penis from the vagina before ejaculation

**Coitus** sexual intercourse by insertion of a penis into a vagina

**Colitis** recurring inflammation of the large intestine

**Collagen** fibrous protein found in connective tissue

**Colon** large intestine where wastes are processed

**Colostrum** yellowish liquid secreted from the breasts preceding lactation; contains antibodies and protein

**Colposcopy** an internal medical examination performed to detect the presence of genital warts in women who are asymptomatic

**Colpotomy** incision of the vagina with entry into the cul-de-sac

**Commitment** a deep and abiding interest and dedication to something

**Common cold** inflammation of the upper respiratory tract (nose and throat) caused by any of 200 or more viruses

**Communal marriage** a marriage of three or more individuals who share all family functions; also known as group marriage

**Complementary and alternative medicine (CAM)** a broad range of healing philosophies, approaches, and therapies not taught widely in medical schools, not generally used in hospitals, and not usually reimbursed by medical insurance companies; sometimes term

**Complex carbohydrates** important source of energy for the body found in fruits, vegetables, legumes, and grains

**Compost** rich soil resulting from the decomposition of leftover food mixed with lawn clippings and leaves

**Computerized axial tomography (CAT scan)** use of radiation to view internal organs that do not show up on an x-ray

**Conception** the start of pregnancy, when a sperm cell fertilizes an egg cell

**Condom** thin sheath placed over the penis that prevents semen from entering the vagina

**Conflict** the stress that results from two opposing and incompatible goals, demands, or needs

**Congenital anomalies** defects that are present in a baby at birth

**Congenital heart defects** heart malformations present at birth

**Congenital syphilis** a condition that is present at birth when the bacteria are transmitted by the mother during pregnancy

**Congestive heart failure** condition caused when blood flow from the heart slows and blood returning to the heart backs up in the veins, causing blood to collect in the tissues

**Contraceptives** any device, drug, or practice that prevents ovulation, fertilization, or implantation

**Control** the belief that one can influence the effects of life experiences on oneself

**Cool-down** the ending phase of a workout that helps the body begin to return to its resting state

**Coronary arteries** blood vessels that surround the exterior of the heart and supply heart muscle with blood

**Corpus luteum** enlarged follicle that continues to secrete progesterone

**Cortisol** hormone released by the adrenal glands in the first stage of stress

**Cowper's glands** two pea-sized organs that produce preejaculatory fluid

**Crack** small pieces or rocks formed from a dried mix of cocaine hydrochloride, baking soda, and water

**Cremation** incineration of a body in a specialized furnace

**Cross-training** combining more than one activity to attain cardiorespiratory fitness and allow some muscles to rest

**Crowning** the top of the fetus's head appearing at the vaginal opening during labor

**Cue (to action)** a construct of the health belief model that addresses a circumstance or event that motivates a person to act

**Cyanotic defect** heart defect characterized by too little oxygen in the blood

**Daily Reference Values (DRVs)** Recommended amounts of macronutrients such as total fat, saturated fat, and cholesterol

**Daily Values (DVs)** the RDIs and DRVs together make the Daily Values seen on food and supplement labels

**Date rape** sex without the consent of both of the dating partners

**Defibrillator** a device that delivers electrical shocks to the heart in an attempt to restore normal rhythm

**Dehydration** abnormal depletion of body fluids

**Demerol** short-acting synthetic narcotic used as an analgesic or a painkiller; usually injected

**Dendrites** branches of neurons that convey impulses to the cell body

**Dental assistant** chairside assistant to the dentist who performs a variety of patient care, office, and sometimes laboratory duties

**Dental hygienist** health care specialist, licensed to perform clinical tasks, who takes x-rays, cleans and polishes teeth, and teaches proper dental care

**Dentistry** practice involving diagnosis and treatment of teeth, gums, and oral cavity

**Depo-Provera®** progestin contraceptive that is injected and lasts three months

**Depressants** a classification of drugs that inhibit neural activity and slow physical and mental functions; downers

**Designer drugs** manufactured drugs that mimic the effects of other drugs

**Detoxification** ridding the body of poisons or the effects of poisons

**Developmental tasks** work to be done at various stages in a person's life (Erikson)

**Diabetes mellitus** chronic condition characterized by excessive amounts of glucose in the blood due to abnormal metabolism of glucose

**Diabetic coma** unconsciousness induced by ketoacidosis

**Diagnosis-related groups (DRGs)** a system of predetermined payment made by Medicare based on the patient's diagnosis

**Diaphragm** rubber or plastic cup that fits over the cervix and prevents semen from entering the uterus and fallopian tubes

**Diastole** relaxation of the heart between beats

**Diastolic blood pressure** force in the blood vessel during the heart's relaxation phase

**Dietary Reference Intake (DRI)** a set of nutritional values, new combined listing, including more than 26 essential vitamins and minerals, which apply to healthy people

**Digestion** process of breaking down food and drink into substances the body can absorb

**Dilation and curettage (D&C)** surgical procedure that removes the embryo and placenta from the uterus by scraping

**Dilation and evacuation (D&E)** abortion procedure in which the cervix is dilated and the fetus removed by suction

**Dilation** or **dilatation** opening of the cervix to 10 centimeters; occurs during first stage of labor

**Dilaudid** derived from morphine, legitimately used as cough suppressant and as analgesic for treating severe pain

**Disease-prone personality** personality that tends toward illness

**Distress** negative stress

**Diuretic** any drug that speeds up elimination of salts and water from kidneys and other body organs

**Diverticulosis** a painful condition caused by weakened places on the large intestine that bulge, fill with fecal matter, and become irritated

**Dopamine** brain chemical that controls pleasure sensations; the key to cocaine's addiction

**Drug abuse** the use of a chemical substance that results in physical, mental, emotional, or social impairment

**Drug misuse** the occasionally inappropriate or unintentional use of a medication

**Dynamic** or **ballistic stretching** technique using rapid, bouncy, or bobbing movements to stretch muscle fibers

**Dyspareunia** painful intercourse

**Dysplastic nevi** flat, irregularly shaped moles, mottled in color with indistinct borders; a warning sign of malignant melanoma

**Eating disorder** severe disturbance in eating behavior; three forms are anorexia nervosa, bulimia nervosa, and binge eating

**Eclampsia** coma and seizures that may occur beginning about the 20th week of pregnancy associated with high blood pressure during pregnancy

**Ecstasy** or **MDMA** a hallucinogen with amphetamine-like properties

**Ectopic pregnancy** implantation outside of the uterus

**Effacement** thinning of cervix during the first stage of labor

**Ego** the part of the psyche that controls and regulates basic drives

**Ejaculation** sudden discharge of semen from the penis as a culmination of the sexual response

**Electrocardiogram (ECG)** measurement of electrical activity in the heart

**Electromagnetic fields (EMFs)** invisible spaces of energy caused by electrically charged conductors

**Embalming** procedure in which blood and body fluids are drained and formaldehyde and alcohol are injected

**Embryo** product of conception from weeks two through seven

**Emphysema** progressive lung disease that eventually destroys the alveoli and greatly reduces lung functioning

**Endocrine system** body system composed of glands that manufacture and secrete hormones directly into the blood; ductless glands

**Endometriosis** a condition in which pieces of the endometrium migrate to fallopian tubes, ovaries, or abdominal cavity

**Endometrium** interior lining of the uterus

**Endorphins and enkephalins** naturally occurring narcotics in the body, produced by the immune system

**Endorphins** natural painkillers released by the brain

**Energy value** the result of multiplying the number of grams of each energy nutrient in a serving of food by the caloric values per gram of carbohydrate, protein, and fat

**Energy-balancing equation** formula stating that when caloric input equals caloric output, an individual does not gain or lose weight

**Environmental Protection Agency (EPA)** federal office with regulatory and enforcement powers over environmental matters

**Enzyme-linked immunosorbent assay (ELISA or EIA)** a blood test that diagnoses HIV by exposing the presence of HIV antibodies

**Epidermis** top layer of skin

**Epididymis** storage structure along the top of each testicle where sperm cells mature

**Epidural anesthesia** spinal anesthesia administered over a period of hours to desensitize lower back

**Epilepsy** a seizure disorder caused by abnormal electrical activity in the brain

**Epinephrine** hormone released by the adrenal glands during the first stage of stress, affecting metabolism, the muscles, and circulation

**Episiotomy** procedure in which an incision is made from the bottom of the vaginal opening toward the anus to prevent tearing of vagina during birth

**Erectile dysfunction (ED)** inability to obtain or maintain an erection for coitus; impotence

**Erection** the engorged, rigid state of the penis during sexual arousal

**Essential fat** body fat needed for normal physiological functioning

**Essure** permanent sterilization of the female

**Estrogen** hormone produced by the ovaries that controls female sexual development

**Ethyl alcohol** colorless liquid and central nervous system depressant made by the process of fermentation and found in alcoholic beverages

**Eugenol** (oral anesthetic), has a numbing effect in the back of the throat that enables users to inhale the smoke more deeply

**Euphoria** a heightened sense of well-being associated with drug use

**Eustress** positive stress

**Euthanasia** intentional and express termination of a life when quality is perceived to be such that it is not worth living

**Explanatory style** the way people perceive the events in their lives optimistic or pessimistic

**Extrovert** an outgoing personality

**Fallopian tubes** four-inch tubular passage leading from upper portion of the uterus to each of the two ovaries

**Family practitioner** physician who treats all family members

**Fat cell theory (hypertrophy and hyperplasia)** theory stating that the quantity of fat in the body is the result of the size and number of fat cells a person has

**Fat substitutes** substances that taste like fat and contain fewer calories, fat, and cholesterol

**Federal Trade Commission (FTC)** U.S. agency organized to protect consumers from fraud

**Female condom** sheath inserted into vagina to prevent fertilization and sexually transmitted diseases

**Female genital mutilation (FGM)** or "**female circumcision**" the practice of cutting away the entirity or parts of the female external genitalia (clitoris, labia)

**Fertility Awareness-Based Methods (FAMs)** any method of preventing pregnancy based on avoiding coitus during ovulation

**Fertilization** union of egg and sperm cells; conception

**Fetal alcohol effects (FAE)** aberrant behavior patterns in newborns resulting from the mother's alcohol consumption during pregnancy

**Fetal alcohol syndrome (FAS)** group of physical and behavioral defects in a newborn caused by the mother's alcohol use during pregnancy

**Fiber** or **roughage** nondigestible complex carbohydrate needed to keep the digestive system in good working order

**Fibromyalgia** arthritis-related disease marked by widespread pain, fatigue, stiffness, but no evidence of inflammation, or joint or muscle degeneration

**Fight** or **flight** series of physiological changes that stress evokes: alarm, resistance, and exhaustion

**Fimbriae** fingerlike projections at the end of fallopian tubes

**First degee relative** a family member that is a person's biological parent, sibling, or offspring

**FITT formula** frequency, intensity, time, and type of workout applied to each of the physical fitness components

**Flashback** recurrence of a drug trip (experience)

**Flavonoids** phytochemicals that have anticlotting properties

**Flexibility** the ability of a joint to move freely through its full range of motion

**Fluoride** chemical compound added to drinking water to prevent tooth decay

**Follicle** egg sac in ovary

**Follicle-stimulating hormone (FSH)** a hormone that stimulates growth of the follicle in the ovary and spermatogenesis in the testes

**Fomite** an object contaminated with a pathogen

**Food and Drug Administration (FDA)** the regulatory agency charged with establishing criteria for all drugs and reviewing active ingredients in all over-the-counter drugs

**Food intoxication** a kind of food poisoning in which a food is contaminated by natural toxins or by microbes that produce toxins

**Food irradiation** process that exposes food to gamma rays to destroy contaminants

**Food toxicologist** specialist who detects dangerous substances in food

**Forcible rape** unlawful sexual activity with a person without consent by force (to include substantial impairment of the victim with drugs) or threat of injury

**Formaldehyde** chemical found in home construction materials that forms vapors that may cause eye and lung irritations

**Fraternal twins** two babies conceived about the same time as the result of fertilization of two separate egg cells

**Free radicals** unstable molecules produced when the body burns fuel for energy; can damage body cells and lead to heart disease, a weakened immune system, and other serious illnesses

**Frostbite** a skin condition caused by overexposure to cold temperatures

**Functional foods** foods that may help prevent disease, usually because health-promoting ingredients have been added to them.

**Funeral rites** of passage for those who have died

**Fungi** plantlike organisms that lack chlorophyll; some are pathogens

**Fungicides** agents that kill fungi

**Gallstones** structures composed of mineral salts and cholesterol that form in the gallbladder

**Gamete intrafallopian transfer (GIFT)** eggs and sperm are collected, mixed, and inserted into fallopian tube

**Gametes** sex cells

**Gastric ulcers** chronic inflammation of the lower end of the esophagus and the stomach

**Gastritis** chronic inflammation of the stomach lining that is common in alcoholics

**Gastroesophageal reflux disease (GERD)** a condition of the digestive tract characterized by persistent heartburn, esophagitis, and other serious symptoms due to back flow of acid from the stomach up into the esophagus

**Gender identity** a person's sense of being female or being male

**Gender roles** the different behaviors and attitudes that society expects of females and males

**General adaptation syndrome (GAS)** the body's attempt to react and adapt to stressors

**Generic drug** chemically equivalent medication substituted for a brand-name medication

**Genetic code** chemicals in genes designated in combinations of the letters A, T, C, and G

**Genetic predisposition** theory stating that inherited genes influence a person's propensities, including weight

**Genetically modified (GM) organisms** organisms whose genetic makeup has been changed to produce desirable traits.

**Genital** or **venereal warts** an STD caused by the human papillomavirus (HPV)

**German measles** or **rubella** viral infection that can damage eyes, ears, brain, or heart of the fetus during pregnancy if the mother contracts the disease

**Gerontologist** professional who studies the aging process

**Gestation** period from conception to birth (259–287 days)

**Gestational diabetes** form of diabetes (a metabolic disorder) that occurs only during pregnancy

**Glans** sensitive tip of the penis

**Glucose** a simple sugar; body's basic fuel

**GnRH analogs** gonadotropin-releasing hormone analogs; a drug treatment for endometriosis

**Gonads** sex glands, the primary reproduction organs

**Gonorrhea** STD caused by the bacteria *Neisseria gonorrhoeae*

**Granuloma inguinale** STD caused by bacterium *Calymmatobacterium granulomatis*

**Grief** emotional reaction to a significant loss

**Group policy** health insurance purchased by a group of individuals, usually through a place of employment, at a reduced rate that is lower than an individual policy

**Hallucinogens** a group of mind-altering drugs that affect the brain and nervous system

**Hangover** effects associated with consuming excessive amounts of alcohol

**Hardiness** a set of personality traits characteristic of people who are resistant to stress

**Hassles** various minor annoyances that occur daily

**Hay fever** mild respiratory ailment caused by environmental agents that provoke the body to produce histamines

**Hazardous waste site** any area where toxic waste was dumped before laws were enacted to regulate proper disposal of toxic substances

**Hazardous waste** trash contaminated with toxic substances that can cause diseases

**Health belief model (HBM)** an intrapersonal theory that analyzes the relationship between a person's perception of a threat to health and the willingness of the person to reduce the perceived threat by changing behavior

**Health maintenance organization (HMO)** a system of managed care with emphasis on preventive medicine

**Health** the condition of being fit in body, mind, and spirit, free from pain or disease, with the ability to adapt to the environment

**Health-related fitness** the five components are body composition, cardiovascular

endurance, muscular flexibility, muscular strength, and muscular endurance

**Heart rate reserve (HRR)** the difference between resting heart rate and maximal heart rate

**Heat cramps** muscle spasms in the arms, legs, or abdomen as a result of overexercise in warm weather

**Heat exhaustion** fatigued condition resulting from depletion and inadequate fluid replacement during heavy exercise

**Heat stroke** an emergency condition resulting from overexercise in hot weather

**Height and weight table** assessment tool used to determine ideal or healthy weight

**Hemochromatosis** iron toxicity due to ingesting too many iron-containing supplements

**Hemoglobin** a chemical in red blood cells that carries oxygen and is responsible for the RBCs' color

**Hemoglobin** the protein that makes the blood red and transports oxygen from the lungs to the rest of the body

**Hemoglobinopathy** abnormal hemoglobin in the blood

**Hemorrhage** excessive blood loss

**Hepatitis** inflammation of the liver caused by a virus; several types have been identified

**Hepatotoxic trauma** disease of the liver caused by alcoholism; commonly called fatty liver

**Heroin** narcotic drug derived from morphine that is 35 times stronger than morphine

**Herpes** an STD caused by the herpes simplex virus (HSV)

**Heterosexual** having a physical attraction to the opposite sex

**High density lipoprotein (HDL)** fatty substance that picks up cholesterol in the bloodstream and returns it to the liver; "good" cholesterol

**High-Density Lipoprotein (HDL)** "good cholesterol" molecule containing high concentration of protein

**High-impact aerobics** aerobic exercise that has a running or jumping component

**HIV-positive** determined to have HIV infection by testing

**Hobbies** chosen activities that one enjoys doing for relaxation

**Holistic treatment** total treatment of patients that takes into account social and mental factors as well as physical condition

**Holographic will** legal handwritten document in which the writer leaves instructions to be carried out upon his or her death

**Home Access HIV-1 Test System** the only Food and Drug Administration approved HIV test for home use

**Homeostasis** the body's internal sense of balance

**Homocysteine** an amino acid not produced in the body and not present in foods; plays a role in methionine metabolism

**Homophobic** exaggerated fear of homosexuals

**Homosexual** having a physical attraction to the same sex

**Hormone replacement therapy (HRT)** estrogen treatment after menopause or after the ovaries have been removed to offset the ill effects

**Hospice** care services for terminally ill patients and their families focusing on their comfort and social, emotional, and spiritual needs

**Hostility** chronic form of anger characterized by lack of trust in others

**Human chorionic gonadotrophin (HCG)** a hormone produced by the placenta that signals the pituitary gland not to release FSH and LH

**Human immunodeficiency virus (HIV)** a fragile virus spread through the exchange of blood and semen that circulates freely in the bloodstream and always precedes the onset of AIDS

**Humanistic psychology** theory that behavior is motivated by a desire for personal growth and achievement

**Humor therapy** treatment using laughter to increases endorphins, which decreases stress

**Hydrogenated trans-fatty acids (TFAs)** fats or oils that have been treated by a process that adds hydrogen to some of the unfilled bonds in the fat molecule, thereby hardening the fat or oil

**Hydrostatic weighing** method of determining body composition by measuring the amount of water displaced when a person exhales and sits under water

**Hymen** membrane partially covering the vaginal opening

**Hyperglycemia** high blood sugar caused by the body's inability to process glucose in the blood

**Hypertension** also known as high blood pressure; a chronic increase in blood pressure above the normal range

**Hyperthermia** abnormally high body temperature

**Hypertrophy** an increase in size and strength of muscles that are used regularly and vigorously

**Hypervitaminosis** a toxic condition caused by overuse of vitamin supplements

**Hypoglycemia** low blood sugar

**Hypokinetic** underactive

**Hypothermia** a condition in which body temperature drops below 95°F and loses its ability to produce heat because heat is lost faster than it can be produced

**Hysterectomy** total or partial surgical removal of the uterus

**Hysterotomy** surgical procedure in which the fetus and placenta are removed surgically through an abdominal incision

**Iatrogenic illness** medically induced sickness caused by adverse reactions to drugs

**Id** the part of the psyche that seeks pleasure and satisfaction of basic drives

**Identical twins** two babies conceived at the same time as the result of a single fertilized egg that divides into two cells that develop separately

**Immune response** body's reaction to first exposure to a pathogen

**Immune-competent personality** personality that enables a person to handle pressure without becoming ill

**Immunity** resistance to disease; may be natural or acquired

**Immunodeficiency** failure of the immune system to react to pathogens

**Immunotherapy** use of the body's own immune system to fight cancer; desensitization to allergens through periodic injections of weakened allergens

**Implantation** attachment of embryo to lining of the uterus

**Implants** pieces of endometrium that have migrated to other areas

**In vitro fertilization** procedure in which a woman's eggs are placed in a glass dish and incubated with donor sperm

**Incest** sexual activity between close relatives father-daughter, stepfather-stepdaughter, mother-son, brother-sister

**Incinerator** container used to burn solid waste

**Incontinence** inability to control urination voluntarily

**Individual policy** health insurance purchased by a person

**Infarct** area of tissue deprived of oxygen that dies

**Infectious diseases** conditions in which a pathogen can be spread from person to person; also called communicable or contagious diseases

**Infertility** inability to achieve pregnancy after trying for 12 months or six months for a woman 35 years old or older

**Infibulation** the practice of fastening the prepuce or labia minora together with clasps, stitches, or other devices to prevent coitus

**Inflammation** body's reaction to pathogens or trauma characterized by redness, pain, and swelling

**Influenza (flu)** a viral infection of the nose, throat, bronchial tubes, and lungs

**Inhalants** drugs that produce vapors that cause psychoactive effects when inhaled or sniffed

**Insoluble** not dissolvable in water

**Insomnia** prolonged and usually abnormal inability to obtain adequate sleep

**Insulin** hormone essential for processing glucose in the body

**Insulin reaction** low blood sugar caused by too much insulin; insulin shock

**Integrative medicine** a combination of orthodox, natural, holistic, spiritual, lifestyle, and alternative approaches to health care

**Interpersonal needs** a theory proposing that all humans have three basic psychologial needs inclusion, control, and affection

**Intimacy** a close association, contact, or familiarity with someone

**Intoxication** temporary state of mental confusion when alcohol content is consumed more rapidly than the body can metabolize it

**Intracytoplasmic sperm injection (ICSI)** a procedure to induce conception by injecting a single sperm directly into an egg cell

**Intrauterine device (IUD)** small plastic contraceptive device placed in the uterus by a health care practitioner to prevent implantation

**Intrauterine insemination (IUI)** a procedure in which sperm from a donor is placed in contact with one or more female ova; better known as artificial insemination

**Introitus** vaginal opening

**Introvert** a reflective, inner-centered personality

**Invasive tumor** tumor that continues to grow and encroaches upon surrounding tissues and organs

**Iron-deficiency anemia** anemia caused by an iron deficiency. It can be cured with an iron supplement

**Ischemia** lack of oxygen to body tissue

**Islets of Langerhans** cells in the pancreas that produce insulin

**Isokinetic (constant speed contraction) exercises** isotonic concentric activities utilizing constant resistance machines that regulate movement and resistance to overload muscles

**Isometric (static) muscle contraction** muscle remains the same length and no movement occurs while a force is exerted against an immovable object

**Isotonic (dynamic) muscle contraction** muscle changes in length, either shortening or lengthening

**Journaling** recording personal occurrences, experiences, situations, and observations

**Karvonen formula** a method for determining if exercise is demanding enough to condition the heart and lungs by ascertaining the optimal target zone

**Karyotype** photograph of a cell during cell division; shows chromosomes in order of size from largest to smallest; used to detect chromosome defects

**Kawasaki disease** childhood disease most common to Asian children; affects the heart in about 20% of the cases

**Keloid** raised scar that results from overgrowth of fibrous tissue following a cut, piercing, or burn to the skin

**Ketoacidosis** or **ketosis** accumulation of acid substances (ketones) caused by incomplete burning of fat for energy

**Kilocalorie (kcal)** the amount of energy required to raise the temperature of 1 gram of water 1°C

**Korsakoff's syndrome** psychosis caused by deficiency of B vitamins resulting from alcoholism

**Labia majora** two outer folds of tissue covering vaginal opening

**Labia minora** two folds of skin within labia majora

**Labor** regular contraction of the uterus and dilation of cervix to expel the fetus

**Lactation** milk secretion from the breasts

**Lacto-ovo-vegetarian** a vegetarian who eats no meat, poultry, or fish but does eat eggs and milk products

**Lactose** intolerance a digestive disorder caused by a deficiency of the enzyme lactase that is characterized by stomach pains and gas when a person consumes dairy products

**Lacto-vegetarian** a vegetarian who includes milk and cheese products in the diet

**Laminaria** wand made from dried seaweed used to expand the cervical opening as part of an abortion procedure

**Laparoscope** a fiber-optic instrument inserted through the abdominal wall to give an examining doctor a view of the abdominal organs

**Laparoscopy** a procedure that uses an optical device (laparoscope) to view the abdominal cavity

**Laparotomy** female sterilization; a surgical procedure in which the fallopian tubes are cut or blocked

**Lead poisoning** damage to liver, kidneys, and other body systems caused by absorption of lead into the body

**Lean body mass** nonfat body tissue made up of muscle, bone, and organs (heart, brain, liver, kidneys)

**Lecithin** fatlike substance occurring in foods such as liver, eggs, peanuts, and soybeans

**Legumes** vegetables such as peas and beans that are high in fiber and are also important sources of protein

**Leukoplakia** condition in which tissue in the oral cavity turns white, thickens, and hardens; a common effect of smokeless tobacco

**Libido** sex drive

**Licensed practical nurse (LPN)** nurse with shortened training period and limited patient care responsibilities

**Life expectancy** average length of time members of a population can expect to live

**Life expectancy** the average number of years of life remaining to a person at a particular age; the average number of years at a given year of birth that a person is expected to live

**Life span** potential maximum number of years members of a population could live

**Ligaments** structures that attach muscles to bones

**Likelihood of taking action** a construct of the health belief model that addresses the chances a person will behave or take certain actions

**Lipids** blood fats

**Lipoprotein** form of cholesterol combined with protein when traveling through the body

**Living will** legal written document stating what kind of treatment should or should not be given in the event of a terminal illness or critical condition

**Local infection** an inflammation that remains in the area of the body where the invasion of the pathogen occurred

**Lochia** discharge of blood and mucus after childbirth

**Locus of control** a concept in personality theory based on a person's perception of control, whether internal or external factors are more controlling

**Loneliness** feeling of emptiness when a person's social network is significantly lacking in quality or quantity

**Low density lipoprotein (LDL)** fatty substances produced by the liver that carry cholesterol to arterial walls; "bad" cholesterol

**Low-impact aerobics** activities that place minimal stress on the joints and are recommended for people with low fitness levels

**LSD** lysergic acid diethylamide-24; a psychedelic drug that produces distorted reality

**Lupus** an arthritic, chronic disorder of the immune system accompanied by inflammation of various parts of the body

**Luteinizing hormone (LH)** a hormone that stimulates ovulation in females and testosterone in males

**Lyme disease** a bacterial infection transmitted by a tick bite

**Lymph** nodes larger glands of the lymph system found in the head, neck, armpits, small of the back, and groin

**Lymphatic system** specialized groups of vessels that network throughout the body and cleanse body tissues

**Lymphocytes** specialized white blood cells produced in the bone marrow that identify pathogens and help macrophages fight pathogens

**Lymphogranuloma venereum (LGV)** an STD that affects the lymph nodes and is caused by a type of chlamydia

**Macrominerals** the seven major minerals the body needs in relatively large quantities daily (100 mg or more per day)

**Macrophages** specialized white blood cells (phagocytes) that destroy pathogens

**Macrosomia** literally, "large body"; refers to a condition in which fetus converts extra glucose from mother to fat

**Magnetic resonance imagery (MRI)** use of radio waves and magnetic fields that produce a computer image of the body to locate abnormalities

**Major depressive disorder** or **depression** a serious medical condition that is characterized by depressed mood or loss of interest or pleasure in nearly all activities, including the ability to function on a day-to-day basis

**Malignant melanoma** a more serious type of cancer in the form of a pigmented mole or tumor

**Malignant tumor** a tumor that is cancerous

**Malnutrition** effects on body due to prolonged deficiency of necessary nutrients

**Mammography** an x-ray used to detect breast cancer

**Mantra** a word or phrase repeated silently during meditation

**Marijuana** the drug derived from the cannabis plant, Cannabis sativa, that contains THC, an ingredient that causes mild euphoria when inhaled or eaten

**Marriage** a legally and socially sanctioned union between a man and a woman

**Massage therapy** increases serotonin and dopamine that aid in reducing stress

**Masturbation** self-stimulation of genitals or other erogenous areas

**Maximum heart rate (MHR)** the fastest heart rate obtained during all-out exercise

**Medicaid** public insurance plan, funded by federal and state taxes, for people who cannot afford medical care

**Medicare** public insurance plan, funded by federal taxes, for people age 65 and older

**Meditation and relaxation** relaxation of the mind and body

**Melanocytes** pigment-producing cells of the skin

**Menarche** the initial menstrual period

**Menopause** stage in the life cycle when the ovaries stop functioning and hormone levels decrease

**Menstruation** monthly discharge of blood from the uterus through the vagina

**Mercury poisoning** deleterious effects on the body caused by overexposure to mercury

**Mescaline** hallucinogen derived from peyote cactus

**Metabolic rate (MR)** total amount of energy the body expends in a given amount of time

**Metabolism** process of converting nutrients into body tissue and functions

**Metastasis** the process of new cancers forming when cells from a malignant tumor break off and travel to other parts of the body

**Metazoa** multicellular animals that live as parasites in and on humans and animals

**Methadone** a synthetic narcotic used as a heroin substitute

**Methamphetamines** powerful stimulants that induce intense euphoria; one form is ice

**Methionine** an essential amino acid

**METs** measurement of body's expenditure of energy

**Microminerals** or **trace minerals** those the body requires daily in minute quantities (100 mg or less per day)

**Migraine headache** a vascular form of headache characterized by severe pain

**Minerals** inorganic substances that make up 4% of body weight and are vital to mental and physical functioning

**Minilaparotomy** female sterilization; a procedure in which the fallopian tubes are cut or sealed

**Monogamy** marriage of a man and a woman

**Mononucleosis** a contagious viral illness that attacks the lymph nodes in the neck and throat; commonly called mono

**Monounsaturated** fats fats with only one double bond of unsaturated carbons in carbon atom chain

**Mons pubis** mound of fatty tissue covering the pubic bone

**Mood disorder** a condition characterized by emotional extremes without apparent reason

**Morphine** main alkaloid found in opium; used medically to kill pain and sedate

**Mucous membranes** moist tissues that help protect the interior surfaces of the body from invasion by pathogens

**Multiple birth** birth of twins, triplets, or more babies

**Municipal solid waste (MSW)** trash or garbage generated by residences, businesses, or institutions that consists of everyday items such as product packaging, newspapers, bottles, food scraps, appliances, and furniture

**Muscular endurance** the ability of muscles to exert force or sustain a muscle contraction repeatedly for an extended period

**Music therapy** instrumental and vocal sounds for listening and relaxing pleasure

**Mutation** a disruption in the order of chemicals in the genetic code that produces an anomaly or, in the case of cancer, growth and spread of tumors

**Myocardium** heart muscle

**Myoma** a mass of muscle and connective tissue growing in the uterus; surgically removed by myomectomy

**MyPyramid Plan** grouping of foods into five groups plus oils indicating serving sizes for each

**Narcotic** a drug that induces stupor and insensibility; in legal terms, any addictive drug subject to illegal use

**Neonatal abstinence syndrome (NAS)** set of withdrawal symptoms occurring shortly after birth in newborns who have been exposed to heroin in utero

**Neuron** a nerve cell that is the foundation for the electrochemical communication system in the brain

**Neurons** nerve cells

**Neurotransmitters** chemicals that send messages across a synapse from the axon of a nerve cell to another nerve cell

**Nicotine** addictive chemical component found in tobacco

**Nicotine patch** pad worn on the arm that delivers a steady amount of nicotine through the skin as an aid to quitting

**Nitrosamines** cancer-causing substances that are found in tobacco

**Nonaerobic exercise** activity that has frequent rest intervals between outlays of energy

**Nongonococcal urethritis (NGU)** infection in the urethra of men, usually caused by the Chlamydia bacteria

**Norepinephrine** hormone released by the adrenal glands during the first stage of stress that affects circulation

**Norplant®** long-lasting hormonal contraceptive implanted under the skin of upper arm by a health care practitioner to prevent ovulation

**Nurse practitioner** registered nurse who is licensed to diagnose and treat patients independent of a physician

**Nutrients** chemical substances or nourishing elements found in food

**Nutrition** the study of nutrients in foods and in the body

**Obesity** a condition in which a person has an excessive amount of body fat, usually about 30% accumulation above recommended body weight according to body size

**Obsessive compulsive disorder** an anxiety disorder in which a person has constant unpleasant and unacceptable thoughts and performs repetitive acts that are unnecessary

**Obstetrician** physician who specializes in the care of women during pregnancy, delivery, and the period immediately following birth

**Omega-3** oils oils found in fish

**Oncologist** physician who specializes in treating cancer (tumors)

**Open adoption** adoption in which some parental information is exchanged and some contact is allowed between the birth parents and the adoptive parents

**Opiates** drugs obtained from the juice of the opium poppy

**Opioids** synthetic narcotics

**Opium** base compound for all natural narcotics

**Opportunistic infections** illnesses that normally would not be serious but attack a person's body because of a weakened immune system caused by HIV

**Optometrist** licensed practitioner who examines the eyes, diagnoses problems, and prescribes eyeglasses or contact lenses

**Oral contraceptives** hormonal tablets taken by women to prevent ovulation

**Orthodox medicine** traditional or conventional form of medical practice using scientifically validated procedures

**Osteoarthritis** most common form of arthritis (affects primarily the hands and weight-bearing joints), caused by erosion of cartilage resulting in joint deformation, stiffness, and pain

**Osteopathic physician** a doctor whose training is equivalent to a medical doctor's and includes emphasis on the musculoskeletal system and treatment of the whole person

**Osteoporosis** condition in which the bones lose calcium and become brittle

**Ova** female gametes; eggs

**Ovaries** almond-shaped female sex glands that produce eggs, or ova, and the hormones estrogen and progesterone

**Overload** principle gradually subjecting the body to more stress than it is accustomed to

**Ovulation** release of a mature egg from the ovary in the middle of the menstrual cycle

**Pacemaker** device implanted near the heart to regulate heartbeat

**Panic attack** a condition in which a person is overwhelmed by feelings of anxiety and loss of control

**Pap test** diagnostic test for cancers of the cervix, uterus, and vagina, performed by taking a sample of cells from the cervix for examination under a microscope

**Paracervical block** local anesthetic injected around opening of the uterus to eliminate pain and feeling from lower vagina

**Partial vegetarian, semivegetarian, or pesco-vegetarian** a vegetarian who includes eggs, dairy products, and small amounts of poultry and seafood in the diet

**Particulates** tiny solid or liquid particles in the air that cause serious health problems

**Parturition** live birth at end of pregnancy

**Patent ductus arteriosus** heart defect caused by a duct remaining open between the pulmonary artery and the aorta allowing the blood to mix

**Pathogen** disease-causing organism

**PCP** an anesthetic that blocks nerve receptors from pain and temperature without producing numbness; angel dust

**Pediculosis** infestation with lice

**Pelvic inflammatory disease (PID)** inflammation of the uterus, fallopian tubes, and ovaries

**Penis** male organ of sexual activity

**Peptic ulcers** irritations in the lining of the stomach or the small intestine caused by an infection and the corrosive effect of digestive juices

**Percent body fat** adipose (fat) tissue as a percent of total body tissue

**Percodan** a cough-suppressing and analgesic medication

**Perineum** the area between the back of the vaginal opening and the anus

**Pernicious anemia** or **vitamin B$_{12}$ deficiency anemia** a condition in which the stomach does not produce intrinsic factor to combine with and transport vitamin B$_{12}$ to the bloodstream

**Personality** the total of all individual characteristics that make each person unique

**Pesticides** chemicals used to kill insects, rodents, and other pests

**Peyote** a type of cactus that yields mescaline

**Phagocytosis** the destruction of pathogens by macrophages

**Photochemical** smog brown smog caused when automobile exhaust containing nitric oxide reacts with oxygen and forms nitrogen dioxide

**Physical abuse** an act of physical harm intentionally inflicted on another

**Physical activity** bodily movement produced by skeletal muscles that requires an expenditure of energy and has health benefits

**Physical fitness** the general capacity to adapt and respond favorably to physical effort

**Physiological dependence** a biochemical need to repeat administration of a substance; addiction

**Phytochemicals** compounds found in vegetables and fruits; have antioxidant properties

**Pituitary gland** a pea-sized body in the brain, which releases hormones including follicle-stimulating hormone and luteinizing hormone

**Placenta** organ through which fetus receives nourishment and empties waste via mother's circulatory system; the afterbirth

**Plaque** material composed of fat and cholesterol that adheres to the walls of the blood vessels

**Plaques** dense deposits of protein found in the brains of Alzheimer's patients during autopsy

**Pleurae** membranes that line the chest cavity and reduce friction during respiration

**Pneumonia** an inflammation of the bronchial tubes and air sacs of the lungs

**Podiatrist** health care specialist who diagnoses and treats conditions of the feet

**Polyandry** a marriage in which one woman has more than one husband simultaneously

**Polychlorinated biphenyls (PCBs)** industrial chemicals found in sewage that cause cancer and central nervous system damage

**Polycystic ovarian syndrome (PCOS)** a female endocrine disorder characterized by irregular menstrual periods, infertility, and excessive body and facial hair

**Polygamy** a marriage simultaneously to more than two people

**Polygyny** a marriage in which one man has more than one wife simultaneously

**Polyneuritis** inflammation of several peripheral and central nerves caused by thiamine deficiency attributable to alcoholism

**Polyps** small growths on the wall of the colon or rectum

**Polyunsaturated fats** fats that contain two or more double bonds between unsaturated fats along the carbon atom chain

**Portion** amount one chooses to eat at any one time and may be more or less than a serving on food labels.

**Postpartum depression (PPD)** a psychiatric disorder consisting of severe depression that can affect a woman soon after giving birth

**Postpartum** the first three months after childbirth

**Post-traumatic stress disorder** a condition in which a person mentally reexperiences a violent event

**Power of attorney** appointment of a friend or relative to make legal decisions for another

**Preferred provider organization (PPO)** insurance plan in which the insured must obtain medical treatment from health care professionals with whom the insurance company has contracted services

**Pregnant** having a developing embryo or fetus in the uterus

**Premature ejaculation** emission of semen and loss of erection within 30 seconds to two minutes of beginning coitus

**Prematurity/low birthweight (LBW)** weighing less than five and one-half pounds at birth

**Premenstrual syndrome (PMS)** a hormone-induced condition of physical discomfort occurring about 10 days before menstruation

**Premiums** payments to an insurance company for a percentage coverage of future medical expenses

**Prepuce** single fold of skin that covers the clitoris and the glans of uncircumcised penis

**Prescription medications** drugs that are used in patient care and are legal only when authorized by a physician or qualified health care practitioner

**Prescription** written order authorizing a pharmacist to dispense medication

**PRICE** recommended treatment for acute injuries: protect, rest, ice application, compression, and elevation

**Primary prevention** taking steps to prevent health problems from developing

**Primary-care physician** medical doctor seen initially for diagnosis, treatment, and management of health conditions of individuals or the family

**Progesterone** hormone that prepares uterus for pregnancy

**Progression** principle placing additional stress on the body once it has adapted to its current stress factor

**Progressive relaxation** exercise to relieve stress, involving tensing and relaxing muscle groups

**Proof** amount of alcohol in a beverage, expressed as twice the percent of alcohol

**Proper training intensity** the intensity that gives the best cardiorespiratory development results as determined by heart rate

**Prophylactic penicillin therapy** use of penicillin to prevent infections from occurring in infants and young children with sickle cell anemia

**Proprioceptive neuromuscular facilitation (PNF)** technique based on the contraction and relaxation of muscles

**Prostaglandins** hormones that cause the uterus to contract; used to induce abortion

**Prostate** gland organ that produces seminal fluid

**Protease inhibitors** class of anti-AIDS drugs that target a later point in the viral life cycle and block action of the HIV protease enzyme

**Proteins** chains of amino acids

**Protozoa** one-celled animals that can live as parasites in humans

**Pseudofolliculitis barbae** a skin condition of black males in which the sharp points of shaved hair penetrate points of the face causing a painful rash (razor bumps)

**Psilocybin** primary psychoactive agent in psychedelic mushrooms

**Psyche** all conscious and unconscious mental functions (Freud)

**Psychedelic** literally, "revealing to the mind"

**Psychoactive substance** any agent that has the ability to alter mood, perception, or behavior

**Psychoanalysis** literally, "analyzing the psyche"

**Psychological dependence** a state in which individuals crave drugs to satisfy some personality or emotional need

**Psychological/emotional abuse** negative and hostile verbal or nonverbal treatment of another

**Psychology** the study of the human psyche

**Psychoneuroimmunology (PNI)** a science focusing on how the mind affects the immune system and physical condition

**Puberty** the stage in life ushering in adolescence, marked by major physiological changes dominated by increased production of sex hormones

**Pubic lice** small insects (metazoa) that infest the host's pubic hair; Phthirius pubis

**Pudendal block** a local anesthetic that eliminates feeling from the lower vagina

**Puerperium** 42-day period following childbirth when the uterus and vagina usually return to normal

**Purging** self-induced vomiting

**Quaaludes** a depressant often used interchangeably with barbiturates; high potential for physical and psychological dependence

**Quackery** use of unproven methods of diagnosing and curing diseases

**Quacks** unqualified practitioners who take advantage of patients for their money

**Radial pulse** pulse taken by locating the radial artery in the wrist

**Radiation** emission of rays of energy from a common center that can destroy cancerous cells

**Radiation energy** from waves and particles such as ultraviolet rays and x-rays

**Radiation sickness** illness caused by overexposure to radioactive substances, possibly causing death

**Radiologist** a physician who specializes in the use of radiation to diagnose and treat disease

**Radon** naturally occurring radioactive gas; an air pollutant

**Rate of perceived exertion (RPE)** an alternative method of determining the intensity of exercise, associated with Gunnar Borg

**Rebound headache** a headache induced by pain medication that is not used according to the manufacturer's dosing instructions

**Receptors** components of a neuron that combine with the neurotransmitter to receive messages from another neuron

**Recovery heart rate** heartbeats per minute after exercising

**Recycling** collecting, reprocessing, and reusing trash

**Reference Daily Intake (RDI)** Recommended amounts of 19 vitamins and minerals, also known as micronutrients.

**Refractory period** the time immediately following orgasm when a male cannot be sexually stimulated

**Registered nurse** health care practitioner who provides patient care and information that promote or restore health and wellness

**Relaxation response** an inborn bodily reaction that counteracts the harmful effects of stress

**Resting heart rate** heartbeats per minute while at rest

**Resusceptibility** vulnerability to reinfection with a disease after having recovered from it

**Retrogression** principle leveling of performance for a period of time before performance improves again

**Reversibility** the physical effects of exercise are lost due to inactivity or disuse

**Reye's syndrome** a disease that affects the brain of children ages two to 16 years following a viral infection; associated with aspirin

**Rh factor** chemical in bloodstream of most people that can cause complications during pregnancy when a mother who is Rh- (no Rh chemical) carries an Rh+ fetus

**Rheumatic diseases** disorders that involve inflammation and swelling of the joints and that restrict range of motion

**Rheumatic heart disease** damage to the heart caused by strep throat

**Rheumatoid arthritis** more severe form of arthritis that causes inflammation and swelling

of tissues lining the joints; affects all joints of the body

**RhoGAM** vaccine administered to counteract complications of Rh incompatibility

**Rickettsiae** microorganisms similar to bacteria that are transmitted to humans through insect bites

**Rigor mortis** stiffening of the muscles after death

**Risk factor** a familial or environmental situation or a behavior that increases the likelihood that a person will develop a health problem

**Ritalin** a central nervous system stimulant prescribed for attention deficit/hyperactivity disorder (ADHD)

**Rohypnol** a benzodiazepine that sedates a person and makes him or her vulnerable to assault; "rape drug"

**RU 486** known as the abortion pill; (mifepristone), a drug used to induce menstruation by preventing uterine lining from supporting embryo

**Sanitary landfill** large, open pit where trash is buried

**Saturated fats** fats mainly found in animal products; increase levels of blood fat cholesterol

**Scabies** condition caused by the Sarcoptes scabiei parasite, which burrows under the skin and lays eggs

**Schizophrenia** a psychological disorder characterized by severe disturbances in perceptions, thoughts, moods, and behaviors

**Scrotum** loose pouch of skin containing the testes

**Seasonal affective disorder (SAD)** form of depression caused by lack of exposure to sunlight during the winter

**Secondary prevention** early detection and intervention to reduce the consequences of a health problem

**Self-actualization** fulfillment of one's potential

**Self-care** taking responsibility for one's own basic health care (to include self-diagnosis and self-treatment with OTC medications)

**Self-esteem** a way of looking at oneself; may be high or low

**Self-help groups** addicts participating with others who have similar experiences and can offer personal support

**Semen** thick, milky fluid containing sperm that is expelled through the urethra

**Seminal vesicle** glands that produce a fluid suitable for sperm motility

**Seminiferous tubules** hollow, cylindrical structures that make up most of the testes and produce sperm

**Senescence** the process of aging from birth to death

**Septal defect** heart defect characterized by abnormal blood flow between the left and right heart chambers

**Septum** wall that bisects the heart lengthwise

**Serving** recommended amount you should consume

**Setpoint theory** theory stating that individuals have a weight-regulating mechanism in the hypothalamus of the brain that controls how much one weighs

**Sex** the quality of being male or female

**Sexual abuse** unwanted and inappropriate sexually motivated acts toward another person

**Sexual harassment** unwanted sexual pressuring of someone in a subordinate, vulnerable, or dependent position by another in a position of power

**Sexual orientation** one of the components of sexuality that is characterized by emotional, romantic, or sexual attraction to a person of a particular biological sex

**Sexuality** the total biological, psychological, emotional, social, environmental, and cultural aspects of sexual behavior

**Sexually transmitted diseases (STDs)** illnesses caused by pathogens that are transmitted during sexual acts

**Sickle cell disease** an inherited form of anemia that produces sickle-shaped cells that clump together and clog tiny blood vessels

**Simple carbohydrates** sugars found naturally or added in the processing of foods

**Skinfold measurement** method of determining body composition by measuring the thickness of fat under the skin

**Smog** brown or gray fog caused by chemical pollutants

**Soluble** dissolvable in water

**Sonogram** visual image of developing fetus in uterus

**Special K or ketamine hydrochloride**; an opiate-like drug that impairs motor movements and respiration when smoked or snorted.

**Specificity of training** aiming overload specifically at the desired outcome of the fitness component

**Specificity principle** holds that exercise must target the muscles identified for development

**Sperm** male gametes

**Spermatogenesis** sperm cell production

**Spermicides** chemicals in the form of creams, foams, or jellies that are placed in the vagina and kill live sperm

**Sphygmomanometer** instrument used to measure blood pressure

**Spinal anesthesia** anesthetic to block pain, injected between fourth and fifth vertebrae of lower back

**Spirituality** a belief in a power higher than oneself and a faith that affirms one's life

**Spontaneous abortion** or miscarriage termination of pregnancy prior to 20th week

**Spot-reducing** exercising to reduce fat in a specific location of the body

**Squamous cell carcinoma** common type of skin cancer that affects the squamous layer of the epidermis

**Stalking** repeated communications or actions with the intent of harassing, annoying, or alarming another person

**Static or slow-sustained stretching technique** in which muscles are relaxed and lengthened gradually through a joint's complete range of motion and held for a short time (10–60 seconds)

**Statutory rape** unlawful sexual intercourse with an individual who has not reached the legal age of consent, regardless of whether it is against that person's will

**Stenoses** heart defects characterized by obstructions to a valve, artery, or vein

**Sterilization** surgical procedure that leaves a person infertile

**Stimuli** external agents that incite responses

**Storage fat** fat found beneath the skin and around major organs that acts as an insulator, as padding, and as a source of energy for metabolism

**Strep throat** an extremely contagious infection caused by a bacteria and treated with antibiotics

**Stress** demands that place physical and emotional strain on an individual

**Stroke (cerebrovascular accident or CVA)** disruption of blood flow to the brain, causing destruction of brain cells; also known as brain attack

**Structural analog** a designer drug that mimics the effects of another drug

**Sudden cardiac death (SCD)** result of an electrical malfunction that throws the heart off rhythm and ends with the abrupt loss of heart function

**Sudden infant death syndrome (SIDS)** death of a baby by an undetermined cause, usually while sleeping at night

**Sulfur-dioxide** smog gray smog caused by burning oil with high sulfur content

**Sun protection factor (SPF)** the numerical rating given to a product that informs the consumer how effectively the product protects from the sun's ultraviolet rays

**Superego** internal voice or conscience; determines acceptable and unacceptable behavior

**Superovulation** production and release of multiple ova as a result of taking fertility drugs

**Surgery** removal of a tumor and surrounding tissue

**Synapse** a gap between each neuron that requires a special chemical to send messages across

**Synergism** the combined action of two or more drugs that is greater than the effects of any drug taken alone

**Synovial membranes** lining of joints that releases a lubricating fluid

**Syphilis** a sexually transmitted disease caused by the spirochete bacterium *Treponema pallidum*

**Systemic infection** an infection that spreads throughout the body via the blood or lymphatic system

**Systemic** pertaining to the whole body

**Systole** contraction segment of heartbeat

**Systolic blood pressure** force in the blood vessel during the heart's contraction

**Tachycardia** heart rate of more than 100 beats per minute

**Tangles** bunches of twisted nerve cell fibers found in the neurons of Alzheimer's patients during autopsy

**Tar** yellowish-brown sticky residue in tobacco that causes cancer

**Target heart rate** the number of heartbeats desired during exercise for maximum benefit

**Tay-Sachs disease** an enzyme deficiency occurring almost exclusively in children of Eastern European Jewish ancestry

**T-cells** lymphocytes that activate additional B-cells, stop B-cell activity when the pathogen is destroyed, kill normal cells that have become cancerous, and attack pathogens

**Telomerase** enzyme that allows the cells to reproduce indefinitely, forming a tumor

**Tendons** cordlike structures that connect bones to each other

**Tertiary prevention** taking care of a health problem that has already caused illness

**Testes** almond-shaped male sex glands that produce sperm and testosterone

**Testosterone** hormone produced by the testes that regulates male sexual development

**Therapeutic communities** self-help group homes programmed to assist addicts in remaining drug-free

**Thermal inversion** atmospheric condition that occurs when a layer of warm air covers a layer of cold air and holds particulates at lower levels

**Tinnitus** ringing in the ears

**Tobacco** plant (*Nicotiana tobacun* or *Nicotiana rustica*) with leaves that are dried and processed for smoking

**Tolerable Upper Intake Level (UL)** the highest amount of a nutrient an individual can consume daily without the risk of adverse health effects

**Tolerance** condition in which an individual must increase drug dosage to experience the same effects over time

**Toxic** core group of personality traits most detrimental to physical health: cynicism, frequent anger, and aggression

**Toxoplasmosis** parasitic disease resulting from exposure to uncooked meat or cat litter; can produce blindness or mental retardation in fetus

**Trachea** tube that connects the larynx to the lungs; windpipe

**Tranquilizers** psychoactive drugs that depress the central nervous system but have milder effects than the other depressants

**Transient hemispheral attack** form of TIA in which difficulty in thinking and communicating occurs along with numbness in one arm, leg, or the face because of less blood flow to one side of the brain

**Transient ischemic attack (TIA)** brief or temporary interference with blood supply to the brain; a mini stroke

**Transient monocular blindness** form of TIA characterized by blurred vision in one eye

**Trichomoniasis (trich or TV)** STD caused by the protozoan *Trichomonas vaginalis*

**Triglycerides** fatty substances used for energy or stored by muscle or fat cells

**Trimester** a three-month period of pregnancy

**Tubal ligation** female sterilization procedure in which the fallopian tubes are cut, sealed, or blocked to prevent sperm from reaching the ovary

**Tubal occlusion** a closing or shutting off of the fallopian tubes

**Tuberculin test** a skin test used to diagnose tuberculosis

**Tuberculosis (TB)** a bacterial infection in the lungs characterized by coughing blood, pain in the chest, fever, and fatigue

**Tumor** an abnormal mass of tissue that grows independently of surrounding tissue and serves no useful function; neoplasm

**Two-drug induced abortion method** injection of methotrexate followed in several days by insertion of misoprostol into vagina to expel embryo

**Type 1 diabetes** or **insulin-dependent diabetes (IDDM)** form of diabetes in which the pancreas does not produce insulin

**Type 2 diabetes** or **noninsulin-dependent diabetes (NIDDM)** form of diabetes in which the pancreas produces some insulin but the body's cells are insensitive to it

**Type A personality** characterized by being impatient, aggressive, ambitious, hot-tempered, and hard-driving; has higher risk for heart disease

**Type B personality** characterized by being calm, casual, and relaxed

**Type C personality** characterized by those who are easily distressed but do not express their hostility

**Ultrasound** a technology using high-frequency soundwaves to produce visual image of developing fetus

**Ultraviolet (UV) rays** beams of radiation from the sun that contribute to the development of skin cancer when a person is exposed to them

**Umbilical cord** attachment of tissue containing blood vessels connecting the fetus to the placenta, through which fetus receives nourishment

**Uniform Anatomical Gift Act** legislation that provides for the donation of the body or organs upon a person's death

**Uniform donor card** document that specifies the wishes of a person to donate organs after death

**United States Recommended Daily Allowances (USRDAs)** dietary guidelines developed by the FDA and USDA

**Urethra** duct through which urine from the bladder is released from the body; long duct running through center of penis, which carries and releases urine as well as semen

**Urethritis** inflammation of the urethra

**Uterus** pear-shaped, muscular organ within the pelvic cavity where the fetus develops; also called the womb

**Vacuum curettage** or **aspiration induced abortion** procedure in which uterine contents are removed by suction

**Vagina** three- to five-inch tubular passage leading to internal reproductive areas that connects with the uterus

**Vaginal sponge** foam sponge containing a spermicide, inserted in the vagina to prevent fertilization

**Vaginismus** strong, involuntary contractions in the muscles of the lower part of the vagina

**Vaginitis** inflammation of the vagina

**Valsalva effect** an increase in pressure in the abdomen and chest that results from holding one's breath during exercise (as in straining to lift a heavy object)

**Vas deferens** tubes that carry the sperm from the epididymis up the ejaculatory duct

**Vasectomy** male sterilization procedure in which vas deferens are cut and tied to block the transport of sperm

**Vector** insect carrier of pathogen

**Vegan** a vegetarian who eats no animal products at all

**Vegetarian** person who eats foods of plant origin and not meat

**Veins** blood vessels that return the blood with carbon dioxide to the heart

**Vena cava** either of the two largest veins in the body that return blood to the right atrium inferior vena cava brings blood from the lower limbs and abdomen; superior vena cava brings blood from the head, neck, and upper limbs

**Ventricles** the two lower chambers of the heart, which pump the blood

**Venules** very small veins

**Vernix** waxy, protective substance covering the fetus in the uterus

**Very low density lipoproteins (VLDL)** largest of the lipoproteins; allows cholesterol to circulate in bloodstream

**Viruses** microorganisms without their own metabolism that reproduce within the living cells of the person they invade

**Visualization** focusing in on a mental image that one is comfortable with

**Vitamins** organic substances essential for normal growth

**Vitiligo** an autoimmune skin disorder characterized by gradual destruction of the pigment-producing cells

**Vulva** outer female genitalia

**Waist-to-hip ratio** waist circumference measurement divided by measurement of the widest circumference around the hips

**Warm-up** the beginning phase of each workout session that helps the body progress gradually from rest to exercise

**Wellness** adoption of healthy lifestyle habits that enhance well-being and reduce the risk of disease

**Wernicke's disease** syndrome caused by thiamine deficiency resulting from excessive alcohol

**Western blot** a blood test done to confirm results of the ELISA tests

**Wind chill** real temperature as affected by wind so as to feel colder and increase the effects on the body

**Withdrawal** physical and psychological symptoms that occur when an individual who is addicted to a drug discontinues its use

**Yoga** exercise done to calm and stimulate the mind

**Yo-yo dieting** losing and regaining weight again and again

**Zidovudine (AZT)** drug used to treat AIDS and HIV infection

**Zygote** fertilized egg

# PHOTO CREDITS

# Index